Manual of Neonatology

Manual of Neonatology

Edited By:

Vineet Bhandari *MD, DM*
New Haven
CT, USA

PEEPEE
PUBLISHERS AND DISTRIBUTORS (P) LTD.

Manual of Neonatology
Published by
Pawaninder P. Vij

Peepee Publishers and Distributors (P) Ltd.
Head Office: 160, Shakti Vihar, Pitam Pura
Delhi-110 034 (India)

***Corporate Office:* 7/31, First Floor, Ansari Road, Daryaganj**
Post Box-7243, New Delhi-110002 (India)

Ph: 65195868, 23246245, 9811156083

e-mail: peepee160@yahoo.co.in

e-mail: peepee160@rediffmail.com

e-mail: peepee160@gmail.com

www.peepeepub.com

First Edition: 2008

ISBN: 81-8445-048-6
978-81-8445-0484

Printed at: Lordson, C-5/19, Rana Pratap Bagh, Delhi-110007

With Respect To

My Parents, Rajni and Jagdish Bhandari

and All My Teachers

Contributors

Ramesh Agarwal
MD, DM
Assistant Professor
Division of Neonatology
Department of Pediatrics
All India Institute of Medical Sciences
New Delhi, India
Email: aranag@rediffmail.com

Pankaj B Agrawal
MD
Instructor of Pediatrics
Harvard Medical School
Attending Neonatologist
Division of Neonatology
Children's Hospital Boston
300 Longwood Avenue
Boston, MA, USA
Email: pagrawal@enders.tch.harvard.edu

Zubair H Aghai
MD
Associate Professor of Pediatrics
Division of Neonatalogy
Department of Pediatrics
Cooper University Hospital
Robert Wood Johnson Medical School
Camden, NJ 08043, USA
E-mail: aghai-zubair@cooperhealth.edu

Namasivayam Ambalavanan
MD
Associate Professor
Division of Neonatology
Department of Pediatrics
University of Alabama at Birmingham
Birmingham, AL, USA
Email: ambal@uab.edu

Muhammad Aslam
MD
Instructor of Pediatrics
Harvard Medical School
Chief Clinical Fellow
Division of Neonatology
Children's Hospital Boston
300 Longwood Avenue
Boston, MA, USA
Email:
Muhammad.Aslam@childrens.harvard.edu

Praveen Ballabh
MD
Associate Professor of Pediatrics
(Neonatology)
Regional Neonatal Intensive Care Unit
Maria Fareri Children's Hospital at
Westchester Medical Center
Valhalla, NY
Email: pballabh@msn.com

Vineet Bhandari
MD, DM
Associate Professor
Division of Neonatal-Perinatal Medicine
Department of Pediatrics
Yale School of Medicine
P.O. Box 208064
New Haven, Connecticut 06520-8064
Email: vineet.bhandari@yale.edu

Manoj Biniwale
MD, MRCP (UK)
Assistant Professor
Division of Neonatology
Department of Pediatrics
State University of New York
Stony Brook, NY
Email: mbiniwale@notes.cc.sunysb.edu

Deepak Chawla
MD, DM
Senior Lecturer
Department of Pediatrics
Government Medical College
Chandigarh, India
Email: drdeepak.chawla@gmail.com

Dinesh Kumar Chirla
MD, DM
Clinical Director
Division of Neonatal-Perinatal Medicine
Rainbow Children's Hospital
Hyderabad, Andhra Pradesh, India
Email: dchirla@gmail.com

Heather Christianson
BA
Research Coordinator
Perinatal Follow Up Program
Alberta Children's Hospital
2888, Shaganappi Trail NW
Calgary, AB, Canada T3B6A8
Email: christia@ucalgary.ca

Girish Gupta
MD, DM
Professor and Head
Department of Pediatrics
INHS Asvini
Colaba, Mumbai, Maharashtra, India
Email: dscnnf@rediffmail.com

Shruti Gupta
MD
Fellow
Division of Neonatology
Department of Pediatrics
State University of New York
Stony Brook, NY
Email: shgupta@notes.cc.sunysb.edu

Anantha Harijith
MD, MRCP (UK)
Fellow in Neonatology
Children's Hospital of New York
Presbyterian
Columbia University Medical Center
New York, NY 10032
Email: harijitha@yahoo.com

Shaik Ashfaq Hussain
MBBS, DCH
Registrar
Genesis Hospital
Hyderabad, Andhra Pradesh

Vasanth H Kumar
MD
Assistant Professor of Pediatrics
(Neonatology)
State University of New York
The Women and Children's Hospital at
Buffalo
Buffalo, NY
Email: vkumar@upa.chob.edu

Satyan Lakshminrusimha
MD
Assistant Professor of Pediatrics
Associate Program Director
Neonatal-Perinatal Medicine Fellow
Program
State University of New York at Buffalo
Buffalo, NY
Email: slakshmi@buffalo.edu

Abhay Lodha
MBBS, MD, DM, MSc.
Assistant Professor
Department of Pediatrics
Staff Neonatologist
Calgary Health Region
Foothills Medical Centre
Rm C211, 1403-29th St NW
Calgary, AB, Canada T2N2T9
Email:
abhay.lodha@calgaryhealthregion.ca

Wendy McKenney
MS, ARNP
Instructor in Pediatrics
Division of Neonatology
Children's Hospital at Dartmouth
Lebanon, NH, USA
Email: mck@hitchcock.org

Akhil Maheshwari
MD
Assistant Professor
Divisions of Neonatal-Perinatal Medicine and Pediatric Gastroenterology
Departments of Pediatrics and Cell Biology
University of Alabama at Birmingham
NHB 525, 619 19th St South
Birmingham, AL 35233
Email: akhil@uab.edu

Srinivas Murki
MD, DM
Consultant in Neonatology
Fernandez Hospital, Boggulakunta
Hyderabad, Andhra Pradesh
Email: srinivas_murki@yahoo.com

Raghavendra Rao
MD, DCH, DM, Dip NB
Assistant Professor of Pediatrics (Neonatology)
University of Minnesota
Minneapolis, MN
Email: raoxx017@umn.edu

M. Jeeva Sankar
MD, DM
Senior Research Associate
Division of Neonatology
Department of Pediatrics
All India Institute of Medical Sciences
New Delhi
Email: jeevasankar@gmail.com

Subrata Sarkar
MD
Clinical Assistant Professor of Pediatrics
Neonatal-Perinatal Medicine
University of Michigan Health System
Ann Arbor, MI 48109-0254
E-mail: subratas@med.umich.edu

Reg Sauvé
MD, FRCPC, MPH
Professor, Departments of Pediatrics and Community Health Science
University of Calgary
Director, Perinatal-Neonatal Follow-up Program
Heritage Medical Research Building
3330, Hospital Drive NW
Calgary, AB, Canada T2N4N1
Email: rsauve@vcalgary.ca

Prem Shekhawat
MD
Associate Professor of Pediatrics, Biochemistry and Molecular Biology
Medical College of Georgia
1120 15th Street, Augusta, GA 30912
E-mail: pshekhawat@mail.mcg.edu

Vishal Sondhi
MD
Department of Pediatrics
INHS Asvini
Colaba, Mumbai, Maharashtra, India
Email: vishalsondhi@gmail.com

Amuchou Singh Soraisham
MD, DNB, DM
Assistant Professor
Division of Neonatology
Department of Pediatrics
Alberta Children's Hospital
University of Calgary
Calgary, Canada
E-mail:
Amuchou.soraisham@calgaryhealthregion.ca

Hari B Srinivasan
MD
Assistant Professor
Division of Neonatology
Department of Pediatrics
Sinai Children's Hospital
15th and California
Chicago, IL 60606, USA
E-mail: srih@sinai.org

Gautham Suresh
MD, DM, MS
Associate Professor
Division of Neonatology
Children's Hospital at Dartmouth
Lebanon, NH, USA
Email: gautham.suresh@hitchcock.org

Rhishikesh Thakre
MD, DM
Consultant in Neonatology
Neo Clinic
27, Samarth Nagar
Aurangabad, Maharashtra
Email: rhishikeshthakre@hotmail.com

PREFACE

This **Manual of Neonatology** has been the fulfillment of a long-awaited dream. It is meant to provide practical and useful information of various aspects of the care of the newborn for medical students, pediatric residents, neonatology fellows, pediatricians and neonatologists. It has been my attempt to cover all topics in this **Manual** using my "rule of 9", i.e., under the following 9 headings: definition, incidence, etiopathogenesis, clinical features, diagnosis (including differential diagnoses), investigations, management, complications and prognosis. To accomplish this goal, I have been very fortunate to acquire the participation of extremely accomplished neonatologists. These neonatologists are currently practising in India, Canada and USA. An important commonality is their experience in taking care of sick newborns in India. It is my hope that the collective wisdom of this remarkable group of physicians, researchers and teachers will help guide the coming generation the art and science of neonatal medicine. I hope the profusion of tables and figures in the chapters will ensure easy readability and understanding of the topics. I am extremely grateful to all the contributing authors for the selfless contribution of their time and effort to the **Manual**.

Mr. Pawaninder P Vij, the director of Peepee Publishers and Distributors (P) Ltd., New Delhi has been outstanding in his efforts and support to ensure that the **Manual** was completed on schedule.

Finally, I am most grateful for the constant support and continual encouragement of **Anita Bhandari,** MD which has been instrumental in the successful compilation of the **Manual**.

Vineet Bhandari

Contents

1

EXAMINATION AND CARE OF THE NORMAL NEWBORN (Including Small for Gestational Age and Infant of Diabetic Mother)

Anantha Harijith

HISTORY

A detailed history is very important in the care of newborn. Neonatal history should include history of current pregnancy as well as previous ones. In the details of current pregnancy enquire about last menstrual period (LMP), probable gestational age, presence of fetal movements and problems, if any, during pregnancy. The problems that one should usually look into are vaginal bleeding, maternal infection, early onset of labor, rupture of membranes, pre-eclampsia; maternal details such as age, chronic maternal illness (e.g. kidney disease, anemia, hepatitis B infection, HIV infection), gestational diabetes and past history of sexually transmitted diseases.

Problems with previous pregnancies such as prematurity, abortion and fetal demise should also be looked into. Illness in the previous newborn babies such as jaundice or sudden neonatal death might point towards inherited disorders. In addition, enquire about family history of inherited disorders. If the pregnant woman is presenting in labor ask about regular follow-up and history of previous sonogram.

Risk of infection in the newborn increases with prematurity, prolonged rupture of membranes (>18 hours), maternal chorioamnionitis, and colonization of the birth tract with pathogenic organisms such as Group B Streptococci, Gonococci and Herpes simplex virus. Maternal chorioamnionitis is indicated by maternal fever, foul smelling amniotic fluid and abdominal tenderness.

Polyhydramnios (amniotic fluid volume more than 2 liters) could be due to upper gastrointestinal tract (GIT) obstruction, abdominal wall defects, neural tube anomalies or inability of the fetus to concentrate urine. Oligohydramnios is usually associated with intrauterine growth retardation. This may indicate amniotic fluid leak or renal dysgenesis. Oligohydramnios contributes to pulmonary hypoplasia.

Meconium stained amniotic fluid suggests fetal distress. Thick meconium staining necessitates preparation for prevention of meconium aspiration. This includes visualization of vocal cords using a laryngoscope and aspirating meconium from the pharynx or larynx if indicated.

Postnatal history must include mode of delivery, history of maternal anesthesia or sedation, need for resuscitation after delivery and Apgar scores. History of administration of Vitamin K at birth reduces the risk of hemorrhagic disease of newborn. Application of erythromycin ointment to the eye at birth protects against chlamydial conjunctivitis but only delays the onset of gonococcal conjunctivitis to the second postnatal week. Level of alertness, activity and feeding since birth gives an idea of the general well-being of the newborn. A newborn baby is expected to pass meconium within 24 hours and pass urine within 48 hours of birth (Table 1.1).

Table 1.1: Clinical relevance of history-taking

History	*Clinical relevance*
Family	Increased risk of specific congenital anomalies or inherited disorders
Pregnancy induced hypertension (PIH; pre-eclampsia)	Increased risk of small for gestational age (SGA)
Diabetes	Increased risk for large for gestational age (LGA), congenital anomalies
Vaginal bleeding	Placenta previa
Maternal infections (STDs, UTI)	Increased risk of preterm labor/birth
Premature rupture of membranes	Increased risk of preterm labor/birth
Polyhydramnios	Increased risk of GIT obstruction, neural tube and urinary tract anomalies
Oligohydramnios	Increased risk of renal agenesis, pulmonary hypoplasia
Meconium-stained liquor	Post dates, fetal distress
No Vitamin K given at birth	Hemorrhagic disease of the newborn
Eye discharge	Gonococcal or chlamydial conjunctivitis

CLINICAL EXAMINATION

Initial physical examination of the newborn must be a detailed one and preferably be performed within 24 hours of birth. The aim of this initial exam, apart from assessing the general well-being of the neonate, should include detection of congenital anomalies, problem in the neonate arising from maternal illness and initiation of health promotion advice.

Weight and head circumference of the infant should be measured and plotted to the appropriate centile. A head to foot examination with the neonate completely naked is preferred. General activity and alertness should be recorded. Watch for movement of all four limbs. A normal newborn maintains tone and holds the limbs in normal flexed position. Floppiness may be indicative of very sick infant or significant neuromuscular disorder. In general appearance, one should also look for abnormal color changes such as plethora, pallor, jaundice or cyanosis.

Abnormal facial appearance or facies may be suggestive of a syndrome. Palpate the head over the sutures and fontanelle. Overriding of coronal sutures as a result of molding is common. A bulging tense fontanelle is abnormal. Eyes should be examined both by inspection and with an ophthalmoscope. Leukocoria (white pupil) or absent red reflex must get urgent attention from an ophthalmologist. Position of ears is important. Low set ears may be suggestive of an underlying syndrome. Low set ears are positioned such that the top of the pinna falls below a horizontal line connecting the two outer canthi of the eyes. Palpate the palate anteriorly and posteriorly, look for submucous cleft in the posterior palate. Neonatal teeth can be rarely seen. This is usually an isolated finding. Neonatal tooth usually lacks the root and is at risk for separation followed by aspiration. Neonatal tooth is also seen in Ellis Van Creweld syndrome. Examine the neck for swelling or webbing.

Examine the chest for breathing. Normal respiratory rate should be 40-60 per minute with no chest retraction, grunting or nasal flaring. Respiratory distress needs immediate further evaluation. Listen for the heart sounds and presence of any murmur. Normal heart rate is 110-150 per minute. Heart sounds must be normally heard loudest on the left side of the chest. Femoral pulses should always be felt on both sides. Bounding peripheral pulses are felt in patent ductus arteriosus (PDA).

Abdomen appears full in a normal newborn. **Scaphoid abdomen** is seen in congenital diaphragmatic hernia. Liver is normally palpable 1-2 cm below coastal margin. The spleen and the left kidney may also be normally palpated. Examine the umbilical cord for the presence of 3 vessels.

Examination of the perineum: Inspect the position and appearance of the anus. In boys check the penis for length and position of urethral orifice. Presence of testes in the scrotum must be confirmed. In a full term newborn girl labia majora covers clitoris and labia minora.

Examine the extremities for extra digits and normal proportion of length. Hips are checked for developmental dysplasia. In order to examine the hip properly the infant must be placed supine on a flat firm surface. The examiner should stabilize the pelvis with one hand; place the middle finger of the other hand over greater trochanter with thumb along the middle thigh. Flex the hip to 90 degrees, adduct and push the femoral head gently downward. Movement of the femoral head posteriorly with a 'clunk' is suggestive of dislocatable hip. This is **Barlow's test**. The opposite movement of the femoral head will result in a dislocated femoral head returning to the acetabulum with a 'click'. This is the **Ortolani test**.

Examine the spine for any defect, sinuses or abnormal tuft of hair. A symmetric complete **Moro reflex** is indicative of a healthy infant (Table 1.2).

Table 1.2: Common clinical presentations

Clinical feature	*Clinical relevance*
Abnormal facies	Suggestive of specific syndromes
Scalp swelling	Caput, cephalhematoma
Low set ears	Specific syndromes, renal disorders
Absent "red reflex"	Corneal opacity, cataract
Plethora	Polycythemia
Pallor	Anemia, shock
Jaundice	Hyperbilirubinemia
Cyanosis (central)	Congenital heart disease, severe pulmonary disease
Scaphoid abdomen	Congenital diaphragmatic hernia

ABNORMAL PHYSICAL SIGNS THAT RESOLVE SPONTANEOUSLY

Swelling of the scalp is commonly noted in neonates following delivery.

The most common swelling is caput succedaneum, a collection of subcutaneous, extra periosteal fluid at the presenting part. The borders are diffuse and not confined to the borders of skull bones. Caput resolves spontaneously in the first week of life.

Cephalhematoma is sub-periosteal collection of blood. This is usually fluctuant and is confined to the borders of skull bone. This condition resolves spontaneously though there is risk of hyperbilirubinemia from the broken down hemoglobin.

Subgaleal hematoma is a rare condition associated with vacuum extraction. The loss of circulating blood volume due to collection of blood in the extensive space below the aponeurosis could result in pallor and life threatening shock. Hyperbilirubinemia must be looked for upon follow up of this condition.

Subconjunctival hemorrhages are common in normal delivery and resolve by 1-2 weeks. Capillary hemangiomas are normally seen over the eyes and resolve spontaneously in a year whereas portwine stain, a capillary malformation, darkens with advancing age.

Pin head sized white cysts in the nose and cheeks are called milia and represent retention of keratin and sebaceous material in the pilaceous follicles.

Small white pearlish lesions seen in the midline of palate are the benign Epstein pearls. Harlequin color change is referred to a condition where one side of the body becomes red with the other side blanching. This is attributed to vasomotor instability.

Breast enlargement can occur in newborn boys and girls under the influence of maternal hormones. A small amount of milk called "witch's milk" may be produced. It is important to observe and not to manipulate breast tissue.

Soft systolic heart murmur (grade 1-2/6), with no audible clicks, a normal second heart sound and normal pulses, point towards an innocent murmur.

Vaginal discharge and small amount of bleeding from maternal

Table 1.3: Gestational age assessment

External characteristic	*28 weeks*	*32 weeks*	*36 weeks*	*40 weeks*
Skin	Smooth, red-pink, veins visible	Smooth, pink, few veins visible	Smooth, pink	Cracking, pale pink
Breast tissue	Flat areola, no bud	Stripped areola, scant bud	3-4 mm bud palpable	5-10 mm bud palpable, areola raised
Ear cartilage	Pinna flat, remains folded	Pinna soft, remains folded	Pinna firm, springs back into place when folded	Pinna firm, instant recoil
Lanugo	Abundant	Thinning	On shoulders, upper back	Little on shoulders
Male genitalia	Testes high in canal, scrotal surface smooth	Testes descending, a few scrotal rugae	Testes high in scrotum, more scrotal rugae	Testes descended, scrotum pendulous, covered in rugae
Female genitalia	Prominent clitoris with small labia minora	Prominent clitoris, enlarging labia minora	Labia majora more prominent, labia minora small	Clitoris and labia minora covered by labia majora
Plantar surface of foot	Scant anterior creases	1/3 anterior creases	Sole has creases	Creases over the entire sole

hormone withdrawal may be noted in the newborn girls in the first week of life.

Mongolian bluish black spots are normally seen in Asian infants and fade slowly over the first few years of life.

GESTATIONAL AGE ASSESSMENT

The best way to assess gestational age is using the Ballard scoring system based on neuromuscular and physical maturity.[1] In addition examination of the eyes for blood vessel pattern in the anterior lens has been used as quick methods to assess gestational age. Complete disappearance of blood vessels from the anterior lens capsule takes place at 34 weeks gestation. Table 1.3 is a simplified method to assess gestational age in newborns of 28 weeks gestation and above.

HIGH-RISK NEWBORNS

High-risk newborns should preferably be delivered in a tertiary level neonatal intensive care unit (NICU) (Table 1.4).

Table 1.4: High-risk newborns

Risk factor	*Associated risk for the newborn*
Maternal history	
Advanced maternal age (>40 years)	Chromosomal abnormalities, SGA
Low maternal age (<16 years)	Preeclampsia, prematurity, child abuse
Substance abuse	SGA, drug withdrawal syndrome, fetal alcohol syndrome, sudden infant death syndrome, child abuse
Trauma	Prematurity, Fetal death
Medical conditions	
Diabetes mellitus	Congenital anomalies, stillbirth, respiratory distress syndrome (RDS), hypoglycemia
Urinary tract infection	Prematurity, sepsis
Renal disease, heart, lung disease	Prematurity, IUGR, stillbirth
Hypertension (chronic, preeclampsia)	Prematurity, IUGR, stillbirth, asphyxia

Contd.

Contd.

Anemia	Prematurity, IUGR, stillbirth, asphyxia, hydrops fetalis
RBC Isoimmunization	Stillbirth, anemia, jaundice, hydrops
Platelet Isoimmunization/ Thrombocytopenia	Stillbirth, bleeding
Thyroid disease	Goiter, hypothyroidism, hyperthyroidism
Systemic lupus erythematosus	Fetal demise, permanent congenital heart block
Obstetric history	
Heavy bleeding during pregnancy	Stillbirth, anemia, premature labor
Premature rupture of membranes, fever, Infection, Chorioamnionitis	Infection
Past history of premature labor	Recurrent prematurity
Complications of labor and delivery	
Premature labor	Respiratory distress, asphyxia, infection
Postmaturity	Stillbirth, asphyxia, meconium aspiration
Maternal fever	Infection
Precipitous (Rapid) labor	Birth trauma, intracranial hemorrhage (ICH)
Prolonged labor	Stillbirth, asphyxia, birth trauma
Meconium-stained amniotic fluid	Meconium-aspiration syndrome, persistent pulmonary hypertension, stillbirth, asphyxia
Prolapsed cord	Asphyxia, ICH , anemia due to blood loss
Small placenta	SGA
Large placenta	Hydrops, maternal diabetes
Abruptio placentae, Vasa praevia	Blood loss
Fetal conditions	
Multiple gestation	Prematurity, twin-transfusion syndrome, asphyxia, birth trauma

Contd.

Contd.

Intrauterine growth restriction (IUGR)	Stillbirth, congenital anomalies, asphyxia, hypoglycemia, polycythemia
Abnormal fetal position	Congenital anomalies, birth trauma, bleeding
Large for gestational age	Congenital anomalies, birth trauma, hypoglycemia
Abnormality of fetal heart rate/rhythm	
Hydrops, asphyxia, congestive heart failure, heart block	
Acidosis	Asphyxia, RDS
Decreased fetal activity	Fetal distress, stillbirth, asphyxia
Polyhydramnios	Anencephaly, neuromuscular disorders, problems with swallowing (e.g., esophageal atresia), chylothorax, omphalocele, gastroschisis, hydrops, intrauterine infection, polyuria–poor renal urine concentration inability
Oligohydramnios	Postmaturity, IUGR, placental insufficiency, fetal demise, renal agenesis, pulmonary hypoplasia, deformation sequence

SKIN CARE

Mature skin protects against heat loss and infections. Skin of term newborn is covered with vernix caseosa. Vernix is a combination of sebaceous gland secretions and exfoliated epidermis, serving as protective barrier. Once the infant is stable after delivery, blood and meconium should be wiped from the body. Vernix is cleaned using water and sterile cotton sponge.

Place the baby under a warmer until the skin is dried. Term babies may be transferred to crib/cot. Preterm babies may need to be placed in an incubator if temperature control is not achieved in a crib/cot.

Term infants are bathed with warm water and a low alkaline or neutral soap. Preterm infants weighing >2 kg may be bathed in the first week of life in warm water only. Do not use soap in preterm infants in the first two weeks of life.

Immature skin of the premature infant contributes to increased insensible water loss, especially in the first 72 hours of life. This is due to poorly developed stratum corneum of the epidermis. Epidermis matures by two weeks of life. Covering the extreme premature infant with transparent plastic sheet reduces water loss. Alcohol (70% ethanol or isopropanol), chlorhexidine and iodine are used to clean the skin before performing procedures. These agents cause chemical burns, and hence, the contact time should be kept to a minimum. Iodine could be absorbed resulting in deranged thyroid function tests. Chlorhexidine should not be used in newborns weighing <1 kg.

FEEDING

Well infants of gestational age >34 weeks are usually able to establish breast or bottle feeding. This is because they coordinate sucking, swallowing, and breathing well. Oral feeding may not be possible in less mature infants, because of neurological immaturity or respiratory compromise. In such cases milk can be given as an intermittent bolus or a continuous infusion through a fine feeding tube passed orally or nasally to the stomach. Expressed breast milk (EBM) is preferred over formula. Term babies may be breast fed adlib. Term intrauterine growth restricted (IUGR) babies with very low birth weight (<1.5 kg) may be fed EBM orally or through a nasogastric (NG) tube. Human milk fortifier may be added.

In preterm infants below 30 weeks gestation, IV fluids may be started after birth. Feeding may be delayed for 24 hours after birth. In babies weighing more than 1 kg start EBM through NG tube. Preferably start bolus feeds every 2-3 hours or continuous at the rate of 1ml per kg per hour, initially increasing by 1 ml every 12 hours, gradually increasing to full feeds, aiming for 165 ml/kg/day. [2,3]

In babies weighing <1 kg start EBM through NG tube. Preferably start bolus feeds every 2 hours or continuous at the rate of 1ml per kg per hour, initially increasing by 0.5 ml every 12 hours, gradually increasing to full feeds aiming for 165 ml/kg/day.

CORD CARE

Umbilical cord care involves exposing the cord to room air and allowing the cord to dry. Cord may be cleaned with sterile alcohol twice a day. Do not apply antibiotic ointment to the cord as it promotes development of resistant bacteria.

Summary of the recommendations of World Health Organization on umbilical care is given below:[4] (Table 1.5)

Table 1.5: Recommendations on cord care

Intervention	*Home delivery*	*Institutional delivery*
Cord Care at Birth		
Cleanliness	Wash hands with clean water and soap before delivery and before cutting/tying cord. Clean surface to receive baby. Wear gloves (institutions)	
When to cut/clamp the cord	Wait until cord stops pulsating or placenta is delivered	Same for normal deliveries; if active management is used, clamp cord early
What kind of ties	Clean string ties, threads or narrow tapes, at least 15 cm in length, tied tightly in 2 places (infant end and maternal end)	Sterile ties (at least 15 cm in length), clamps or rubber bands applied/tied tightly in 2 places
Length of stump left	2-3 cm or longer, according to local custom	
Cutting instrument	Sterile blade (razor blade in original packing is considered sterile); if unavailable, knife or scissors that have been boiled for 10 minutes	Sterile scissors or blade
Topical antimicrobial on stump after cutting cord	None unless necessary, as a temporary measure, according to local situation (e.g. in neonatal tetanus endemic areas, or to replace a harmful traditional substance)	24-hour rooming-in: none unless necessary, according to local situation Nurseries/intensive care units: chlorhexidine, tincture of iodine, povidone-iodine, triple dye or silver sulphadiazine

Contd.

Contd.

Postnatal Care of Cord Stump		
Cleanliness and protection from contamination	Wash hands with clean water and soap before and after care. Keep the stump exposed to air or loosely covered with clean clothes. Fold napkin below stump Avoid applying unclean substances, touching the cord and covering it with bandages	
Beneficial practices that may decrease the risk of cord infection	Keep the baby with the mother (in institutions: 24-hour rooming-in, no nurseries), skin-to-skin contact, early and frequent breastfeeding	
How to clean the cord when soiled	Wash with clean water and soap, dry thoroughly	
Topical antimicrobials on cord stump	None unless necessary, according to local situation (e.g. in neonatal tetanus endemic areas, or to replace a harmful traditional substance) as a temporary measure	Rooming-in: none unless necessary, according to local situation Nurseries/intensive care units: chlorhexidine, tincture of iodine, povidone-iodine, triple dye, silver sulphadiazine (once daily for 3 days)

SGA INFANT

SGA is defined as two standard deviations below the mean for gestational age. A small for gestational age baby may be small because of genetic factors and hence need not reflect pathological intrauterine growth retardation. This may be due to maternal, placental or fetal factors.

Maternal Factors

- Genetic factors including race.
- Maternal malnutrition.
- Chronic diseases.
- Pre-eclampsia.
- Complicated diabetes mellitus.
- Multiple gestation.
- Uterine anomaly.
- Exposure to teratogen – alcohol, radiation.

Placental Factors

- Placental insufficiency due to maternal vascular disease.
- Malformation.

Fetal Factors

- Constitutional small infant.
- Chromosomal abnormality.
- Congenital malformation – example, skeletal system.
- Congenital infection – rubella and cytomegalovirus.

MANAGEMENT OF SGA

It is important to identify the cause of small for gestational age during pregnancy itself. If IUGR is suspected further investigation is necessary. Detailed ultrasonography must be done *in utero* to look for fetal anomaly. Doppler evaluation of placental flow helps to identify *in utero* placental insufficiency. Poor placental blood flow is an indication to plan for early delivery. With maternal hypertension, accelerate fetal lung maturity with IM betamethasone 12 mg—two doses separated by 24 hours. Deliver the baby weighing the risk of complications of prematurity against the risk of continuing pregnancy. Premature delivery must be attempted only where tertiary neonatal intensive care services are available.

If fetal distress is noted before delivery, the resuscitation team must be present at delivery. IUGR is 'symmetric' when the retarded growth begins early in pregnancy, decreasing the length, weight and head circumference proportionately. These babies have significant problems. Growth retardation beginning in late stages spare the brain growth and hence head circumference is usually normal.

Complications Associated with IUGR

- Congenital anomalies.
- Fetal distress.
- Neonatal depression with low Apgar scores.
- Meconium aspiration.
- Hypothermia.
- Hypoglycemia.

- Hypocalcemia.
- Hyponatremia.
- Pulmonary hypoplasia.
- Pulmonary hemorrhage.
- Persistent pulmonary hypertension.
- Polycythemia.

Once the infant is stabilized start feeding in the first hour of life. Give IV fluids if feeds are not tolerated. Monitor for complications. SGA babies with IUGR need long-term follow-up for growth and development.

INFANT OF DIABETIC MOTHER

Diabetes mellitus in pregnant women increases the risk to the fetus. The problems in the fetus could range from hypoglycemia to major congenital malformations. Better control of glucose during pregnancy reduces the complications in the newborn infant.[5] Sudden fetal death in pregnancy complicated by diabetes mellitus is associated with ketoacidosis, pre-eclampsia and maternal vascular disease of placenta.

Complications in Infants of Diabetic Mothers (IDM)

- Large for gestational age (LGA).
- Hypoglycemia.
- Respiratory distress syndrome.
- Hypocalcemia.
- Polycythemia.
- Neonatal jaundice.
- Transient hypertrophic obstructive cardiomyopathy.
- Renal vein thrombosis.
- Caudal regression syndrome.
- Neural tube defects.
- Small left colon syndrome.
- "IUGR"– associated with maternal vascular disease.

PATHOPHYSIOLOGY

Maternal hyperglycemia with accompanying fetal hyperglycemia results in hypertrophy of fetal pancreatic islet cells (Pedersen's Hypothesis). This results in hyperinsulinemia in the fetus. Hyperinsulinemia blocks cortisol induction of lung maturation. Insulin also causes increased erythropoietin. Hypocalcemia in these infants may be due to vitamin D antagonism at the intestinal level from elevated cortisol and hyperphosphatemia due to tissue breakdown.

MANAGEMENT DURING PREGNANCY

Control of blood sugar is very important right from the first trimester of pregnancy. Monitor HbA1C at least once every trimester. If hyperglycemia is not controlled by dietary therapy, insulin must be used. Oral hypoglycemic agents should not be used as they cross placenta. Maternal serum alphafetoprotein is measured at 16-18 weeks of gestation. Detailed ultrasonography at 18 weeks must be done to rule out congenital anomalies and assess fetal growth. Mother should be monitored for pre-eclampsia, polyhydramnios and reduced renal function. A large for gestational age fetus may necessitate delivery by cesarean section.

MANAGEMENT OF IDM

A detailed physical examination for congenital anomalies must be done after delivery. Blood glucose levels are checked hourly for the first three hours of life followed by every six hours in the first 24 hours. If hypoglycemia is noted and the infant is asymptomatic (blood sugar under 40 mg/dL) feed the infant immediately and recheck the blood sugar. Management of persistent hypoglycemia is discussed below. Check hematocrit levels at one and 24 hours of life. If the infant is jittery, check calcium levels. Watch for jaundice.

MANAGEMENT OF HYPOGLYCEMIA

Infants weighing less than 2 kg with hypoglycemia should be started on intravenous dextrose in the first hour of life even if they are asymptomatic. Persistent hypoglycemia by 3 hours of life in a larger infant necessitates intravenous dextrose. Symptoms of hypoglycemia are lethargy, apnea, respiratory distress, shock and seizures. Initial specific treatment of symptomatic hypoglycemia is administration of IV 10% dextrose at 2 ml/kg over 2 minutes. This is followed by IV 10% dextrose at 80-120 ml/kg per day. Start oral feeds and gradually wean the IV dextrose. In cases where the blood sugar does not get corrected with IV 10% dextrose, increase the concentration of dextrose. Dextrose solution of concentration 15% or more should be administered only through central venous catheter (umbilical venous catheter). In intractable hypoglycemia not responding to IV dextrose, start hydrocortisone at 5 mg/kg per day IM in two divided doses. In the absence of intravenous access subcutaneous or intramuscular glucagon (300 microgm/kg to a maximum of 1mg) may be given. However, glucagon may not be effective in small for gestational age infants with poor glycogen stores.

REFERENCES

1. Ballard JL, Khoury JC, Wedig K, Wang L, Eiler-Walsman BL, Lipp R: New Ballard Score, expanded to include extremely premature infants, J Pediatrics 1991;119:417-423.
2. Williams AF: Early enteral feeding of the preterm infant, Arch Dis Child Fetal Neonatal Ed 2000;83:F219-F220.
3. Cooke RJ, Embleton ND: Feeding issues in preterm infants, Arch Dis Child Fetal Neonatal Ed 2000;83:F215-F218.
4. World Health Organization, Division of Reproductive Health (Technical Support). Care of the umbilical cord: A review of the evidence WHO/RHT/MSM/98.4.
5. American College of Obstetricians and Gynecologists, ACOG Practice Bulletin No.30, Obstet Gynecol 2001;89:525.

2 DELIVERY ROOM RESUSCITATION

Vasanth H. Kumar

Approximately 10% of newborns require some form of **resuscitation** soon after birth. Approximately 1% requires extensive resuscitative measures. Although vast majority of newborn infants do not require intervention to make the transition from intrauterine to extrauterine life, because of the large number of births, a sizable number will require some degree of resuscitation.

Effective and successful resuscitation requires a team approach to resuscitation. The personnel involved in resuscitation should have basic understanding of the principles of resuscitation and perinatal physiology and practice in the skill set required in resuscitating these infants. Certification of the each caregiver by the **Neonatal Resuscitation Program (NRP)** of the American Academy of Pediatrics ensures a consistent approach to resuscitation.

PREPARATION FOR DELIVERY

Anticipation of high risk deliveries that might need resuscitation soon after birth is the first step in successful resuscitation. Table 2.1 summarizes the conditions associated with delivery of **high risk newborns**. Even though this list is by no means exhaustive, clinical and maternal history should dictate attending a particular delivery.

Table 2.1: Conditions associated with risk to newborns

Antepartum risk factors
- Maternal diabetes
- Pregnancy-induced hypertension
- Chronic hypertension
- Chronic maternal illness
  - Thyroid, neurological, renal, pulmonary
- Anemia or isoimmunization
- Previous fetal or neonatal death
- Bleeding in second or third trimester
- Maternal infection
- Polyhydramnios/Oligohydramnios
- Premature rupture of membranes
- Post-term gestation/multiple gestation
- Size-date discrepancy
- Drug therapy
  - Lithium carbonate, magnesium, adrenergic blocking drugs
- Maternal substance abuse
- Fetal malformation
- Diminished fetal activity
- No prenatal care
- Age < 16 years or > 35 years

Intrapartum risk factors
- Emergency cesarean section
- Forceps or vacuum-assisted delivery
- Breech or other abnormal presentation
- Premature labor/precipitous labor
- Prolonged rupture of membranes (> 18 hours before delivery)
- Chorioamnionitis
- Prolonged labor (>24 hours)/Prolonged second stage of labor (>2 hours)
- Fetal bradycardia/Non-reassuring fetal heart rate patterns
- Use of general anesthesia/Narcotics within 4 hours of delivery
- Meconium-stained amniotic fluid
- Prolapsed cord/Abruptio placenta/placenta previa

Personnel capable of initiating resuscitation should attend every delivery. More than one experienced person should attend an anticipated high risk delivery. Resuscitation of severely depressed newborn infants requires at least 2 persons, one to ventilate and intubate if necessary and another to monitor heart rate and perform chest compression if required. A third person may be required during extensive resuscitation that includes administration of medications. A clean and warm environment with a complete inventory of resuscitation equipment and drugs should be maintained at hand and in fully operation condition whenever delivery occurs. Table 2.2 presents a list of suggested neonatal supplies, medications, and equipment. Make sure that all equipment is in working order. Radiant warmer should be on and dry, warm blankets available for receiving the infant upon delivery.

Table 2.2: Neonatal resuscitation supplies and equipment[1]

Suction equipment
- Bulb syringe
- Mechanical suction and tubing
- Suction catheters, 5F or 6F, 8F, and 10F or 12F
- 8F feeding tube and 20-mL syringe
- Meconium aspiration device

Bag-and-mask equipment
- Neonatal resuscitation bag with a pressure-release valve or pressure manometer (the bag must be capable of delivering 90% to 100% oxygen)
- Face masks, newborn and premature sizes (masks with cushioned rim preferred)
- Oxygen with flowmeter (flow rate upto 10 L/min) and tubing (including portable oxygen cylinders).

Intubation equipment
- Laryngoscope with straight blades, No. 0 (preterm) and No. 1 (term)
- Extra bulbs and batteries for laryngoscope
- Tracheal tubes, 2.5, 3.0, 3.5, and 4.0 mm ID
- Stylet (optional) / Scissors / Tape or securing device for tracheal tube
- Alcohol sponges
- CO_2 detector (optional) / Laryngeal mask airway (optional).

Medications
- Epinephrine 1:10 000 (0.1 mg/mL) - 3-mL or 10-mL ampules
- Isotonic crystalloid (normal saline or Ringer's lactate) for volume expansion—100 or 250 mL
- Sodium bicarbonate 4.2% (5 mEq/10 mL)—10-mL ampules
- Naloxone hydrochloride 0.4 mg/mL—1-mL ampules; or 1.0 mg/mL—2-mL ampules.

Contd.

Contd.

- Normal saline, 30 mL / Dextrose 10%, 250 mL
- Feeding tube, 5F (optional)
- Umbilical vessel catheterization supplies
  - Sterile gloves; Scalpel or scissors; Povidone-iodine solution; Umbilical tape
  - Umbilical catheters, 3.5F, 5F; Three-way stopcock
- Syringes, 1, 3, 5, 10, 20, and 50 mL
- Needles, 25-, 21-, and 18-gauge or puncture device for needleless system.

Miscellaneous

- Gloves and appropriate personal protection
- Radiant warmer or other heat source
- Firm, padded resuscitation surface
- Clock (timer optional) / Warmed linens / Stethoscope / Tape, 1/2 or 3/4 inch
- Cardiac monitor and electrodes and/or pulse oximeter with probe (optional for delivery room)
- Oropharyngeal airways.

Newborn infants who do not require resuscitation can generally be identified by a rapid assessment of the infant. Infants born at term gestation, clear amniotic fluid, breathing and/or crying and with good muscle tone need routine care which includes providing warmth, clearing of the airway (if needed) and keeping them dry. Preterm delivery, meconium stained amniotic fluid, infant who is not crying or breathing, infant who is cyanotic or floppy, infant with weak or absent responses need further assessment under a radiant warmer and likely intervention. Management of such infants is based on the rapid assessment of infant's respiration, heart rate and color. Figure 2.1 depicts the flow algorithm of the management of such infants.[2]

The initial steps of resuscitation are to provide warmth by placing the infant under a radiant warmer, position the head in a "sniffing" position to open the airway, clearing the airway with a bulb syringe or suction catheter, drying the infant and to stimulate breathing. Some points that should be noted on initial resuscitation steps include the following:

Temperature Control

Very low birth weight preterm infants are likely to become

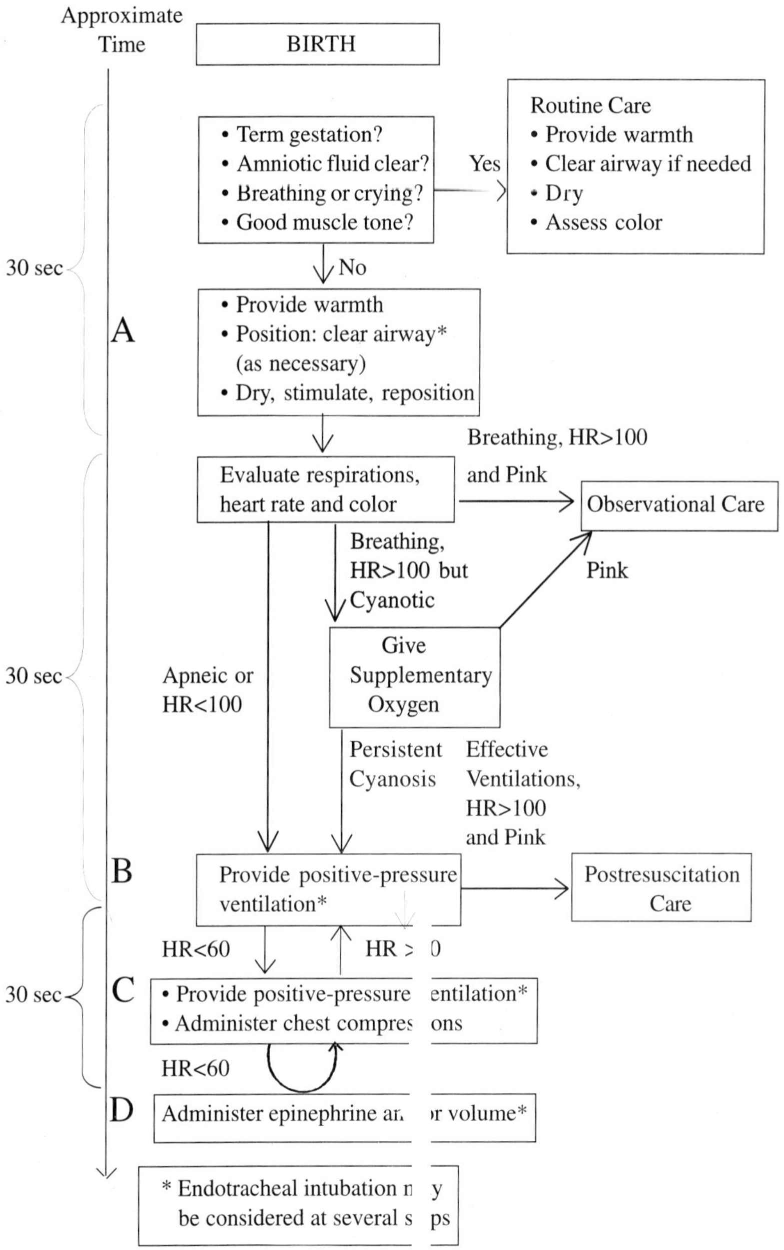

Fig. 2.1: Neonatal flow alg rithm of resuscitation

hypothermic despite the use of traditional techniques for decreasing heat loss. For this reason it is recommended that additional warming techniques be used, such as covering the infant in plastic wrapping or polyethylene bags or placing under radiant warmer. *The goal is to achieve normothermia, but at the same time hyperthermia should be avoided.*

Clearing the Airway of Meconium

Aspiration of meconium before delivery, during birth or during resuscitation can cause severe aspiration pneumonia. Current NRP guidelines no longer recommend routine intrapartum oropharyngeal and nasopharyngeal suctioning for infants born to mothers with meconium staining of amniotic fluid. Similarly suctioning of meconium using an endotracheal tube after birth is not recommended if the infant is vigorous. A vigorous infant is defined as the one who has strong respiratory efforts, good muscle tone and a heart rate of > 100 beats per minute (bpm). *Endotracheal suctioning for infants who are not vigorous should be performed immediately after birth.*

Periodic Evaluation at 30-second Intervals

After initial assessment soon after birth and administration of initial steps of resuscitation, further resuscitative efforts should be guided by simultaneous assessment of respirations, heart rate and color periodically every 30 seconds. While Apgar scores (Table 2.3) are assigned at 1 and 5 minutes of postnatal life, resuscitative efforts should begin soon after initial stabilization and assessment. A newborn infant who is uncompromised will achieve and maintain pink mucous membranes without administration of supplemental oxygen. Evidence obtained from continuous oximetry, however, has shown that neonatal transition is a gradual process. Healthy term infants may take > 10 minutes to achieve a preductal oxygen saturation of > 95% and may need even longer time to achieve a postductal saturation of > 95%.

Administration of Oxygen

There are concerns about the potential adverse effects of 100% oxygen on respiratory physiology and cerebral circulation and the potential tissue damage from oxygen free radicals. Conversely there are also concerns about tissue damage from oxygen deprivation during and after asphyxia. Meta-analysis of 4 human studies showed a reduction in mortality rate and no evidence of harm in infants resuscitated with room air versus those resuscitated with 100% oxygen, although these results should be viewed with caution because of significant methodological concerns. Current evidenced is insufficient to resolve all questions regarding supplemental oxygen use during neonatal resuscitation. Following are the guidelines for babies born at term:

1. Use 100% oxygen when infant is cyanotic or when **positive pressure ventilation** (PPV) is required during neonatal resuscitation.
2. However, research suggests that resuscitation with something less than 100% oxygen may be just as successful.
3. If resuscitation is started with less than 100% oxygen, supplemental oxygen up to 100% oxygen should be administered if there is no appreciable improvement within 90 seconds following birth.
4. If supplemental oxygen is not available, use room air to deliver positive pressure ventilation.

To reduce excessive tissue oxygenation in a preterm infant (< 32 weeks gestation) 2005 AHA guidelines[3, 4] recommend the following in these infants:

1. Use an oxygen blender and pulse oximeter during resuscitation.
2. Begin PPV with oxygen concentration between room air and 100% oxygen. No studies justify starting at any particular concentration.
3. Adjust oxygen concentration up or down to achieve an oxyhemoglobin concentration that gradually increases towards 90%. Decrease the oxygen concentration as saturations rise over 95%.
4. If the heart rate does not respond by increasing rapidly to > 100 bpm, correct any ventilation problem and use 100% oxygen.
5. If your facility does not have an oxygen blender or pulse oximeter in the delivery room (DR), it is OK to use 100% oxygen. There is no convincing evidence that a brief period of 100% oxygen during resuscitation will be detrimental to the preterm infant.

Table 2.3: Apgar scoring system [5, 6]

Sign	*Score*		
	0	*1*	*2*
Heart Rate	Absent	< 100 bpm	> 100 bpm
Respiratory Effort	Absent	Slow (irregular)	Good, crying
Muscle Tone	Limp	Some flexion of extremities	Active motion
Reflex Irritability	No response	Grimace	Cough or sneeze
Color	Blue, pale	Pink body, blue extremities	All pink

If the infant is breathing spontaneously, heart rate is > 100 bpm and the color is becoming pink, the infant should be wrapped and returned to parents. Some newborns do not immediately establish respirations but will rapidly respond to gentle tactile stimulation including flicking the soles of the feet or rubbing the back. If breathing does not start after two attempts at tactile stimulation, then secondary apnea probably exists and respiratory support should be initiated.

Infant who is spontaneously breathing, heart rate is > 100 bpm and is cyanotic needs supplemental oxygen. Oxygen can be administered at a rate of 5L/minute either by mask or by tubing held about 1 cm from the nose. Oxygen should be withdrawn as color improves.

Infant who is apneic despite ***tactile stimulation*** *or has a HR < 100 bpm and infants who are persistently cyanotic despite supplemental oxygen need positive pressure ventilation.*

1. PPV is administered initially with bag and mask ventilation.
2. Bag volume – 750 mL; flow – 5 – 8L/min; mask of appropriate size.
3. The mask should cover the chin and nose but leave eyes uncovered. The primary measure of adequate ventilation is prompt improvement in heart rate. Chest wall movement should be assessed if heart rate does not improve.
4. The initial peak pressures needed are variable and unpredictable and should be individualized to achieve an increase in heart rate and/or movement of the chest with each breath. If inflation pressure is monitored, an initial inflation pressure of 20 cm H_2O may be effective. But some term infants

may need higher initial inflating pressures of 30-40 cm H_2O. Assisted ventilation should be delivered at a rate of 40 to 60 breaths per minute.

Endotracheal intubation is initiated if the infant remains apneic or heart rate < 100 bpm despite 30 seconds of bag and mask ventilation. *Endotracheal intubation is indicated at several points of neonatal resuscitation that includes ineffective or prolonged bag and mask ventilation, while performing chest compressions or when endotracheal administration of medication is desired.* Suggested endotracheal tube size and depth of insertion at various birth weight and gestational age is shown in Table 2.4.

Table 2.4: Suggested tracheal tube size and depth of insertion according to weight and gestational age [1]

Weight (gms)	*Gestational age (wks)*	*Tube size mm (ID)*	*Depth of insertion from upper lip, cms*
< 1000	< 28	2.5	6.5 - 7
1000 - 2000	28 - 34	3.0	7 - 8
2000 - 3000	34 - 38	3.5	8 - 9
> 3000	> 38	3.5 – 4.0	> 9

ID indicates internal diameter.

***Chest compressions** are indicated for a heart rate of < 60 bpm despite adequate ventilation with supplemental oxygen for 30 seconds.*

1. Ventilation is the most effective action in neonatal resuscitation and because chest compressions are likely to compete with effective ventilation, personnel should ensure that assisted ventilation is being delivered optimally before starting chest compression.
2. Compression should be delivered on the lower third of the sternum, to a depth of approximately 1/3rd of anterior posterior diameter of the chest. Chest compression can be delivered either by a 2 thumb-encircling hand technique or by compression with 2 fingers with a second hand supporting the back.
3. Compression and ventilation should be coordinated to avoid simultaneous delivery. There should be a 3:1 ratio of compression to ventilations with 90 compression and 30 breaths to achieve around 120 events per minute to maximize ventilation.

4. The chest should be permitted to fully reexpand during relaxation phase of chest compressions for adequate ventilation, but the rescuers thumb should be in contact with the chest.

Devices/Effectiveness of Assisted Ventilation

1. Flow controlled pressure limited mechanical devices (e.g., T-piece resuscitators) are recognized as an acceptable method of administering positive pressure ventilation during resuscitation of the newborn and in particular the premature infant.
2. Self inflating and flow inflating bag and mask equipment and technique remains the cornerstone of achieving effective ventilation in most resuscitations.
3. Laryngeal mask airway has been shown to be an effective alternative for assisting ventilation of some newborns who have failed bag and mask ventilation or endotracheal intubation.
4. Increasing heart rate is the primary sign of effective ventilation during resuscitation. Other signs are improving color, spontaneous breathing and improving muscle tone. Check these signs of improvement after 30 seconds of PPV. This requires the assistance of another person.
5. An increasing heart rate and CO_2 detection (using end tidal CO_2 detector) are the primary methods for confirming endotracheal tube placement. Poor or absent pulmonary blood flow may give false negative results on the CO_2 detector (i.e., no CO_2 detected despite tube placement in trachea), but endotracheal tube placement is correctly identified in nearly all patients who are not in cardiac arrest. Other clinical indicators such as condensed humidified gas in endotracheal tube and the presence or absence of chest movement may also help in correctly identifying endotracheal tube placement.

Medications[6]

Drugs are rarely indicated in resuscitation of the newborn infant. Bradycardia in the newborn infant is usually the result of inadequate lung inflation or profound hypoxemia and establishing adequate ventilation is the most important step to correct it. But if the HR is <60 bpm despite adequate ventilation with 100%

oxygen and chest compression, administration of epinephrine or volume expansion or both may be indicated.

EPINEPHRINE

1. Doses of 0.01 to 0.03mg/kg (0.1-0.3 mL/kg of 1:10,000 epinephrine) will likely be ineffective via the endotracheal tube.
2. Therefore, IV administration of 0.01 to 0.03 mg/kg per dose (0.1-0.3 mL/kg of 1:10,000 epinephrine drawn in 1 mL syringe) is the preferred route.
3. While access is obtained, administration of higher dose (upto 0.1mg/kg or 1mL/kg of 1: 10,000 epinephrine, drawn in 3 mL or 5 mL syringe) through the endotracheal tube may be considered, but the safety and efficacy of this practice has not been evaluated.

VOLUME EXPANSION

1. Consider volume expansion when blood loss is suspected or the infant appears to be in shock (pale skin, poor perfusion, weak pulse) and has not responded adequately to other resuscitative measures.
2. Isotonic saline is the solution of choice at a dose of 10 mL/kg which may be repeated if necessary.
3. In premature infants care should be taken to avoid giving volume expanders too rapidly.

NALOXONE

1. Naloxone is not recommended during the primary steps of resuscitation.
2. Two criteria need to be fulfilled prior to administering naloxone. They include *continued respiratory depression after PPV has restored a normal heart rate and color, and a history of maternal narcotic administration within the past 4 hours.*
3. There are no studies reporting the efficacy of endotracheal naloxone. This route is not recommended. Intravenous route is preferred. Intramuscular route is acceptable but has delayed onset of action.
4. The recommended dose is 0.1 mg/kg.

BICARBONATE

1. It is discouraged during brief cardiopulmonary resuscitation.
2. Used in *prolonged arrests unresponsive to other therapy and should be given only after establishing ventilation and circulation.*
3. Uses—Persistent metabolic acidosis or hyperkalemia after documenting them on arterial blood gas or serum chemistries.
4. Dose 1–2 mEq/kg of 0.5 mEq/mL (4.2% sodium bicarbonate) by a slow intravenous push.

Table 2.5 gives an overview of special conditions that need appropriate and immediate management during resuscitation.

Table 2.5: Special circumstances in resuscitation of the newborn infant [1]

Condition	*History/Clinical signs*	*Actions*
Mechanical blockage of the airway		
Meconium or mucus blockage	Meconium stained amniotic fluid Poor chest wall movement	Intubation for suctioning /ventilation
Choanal atresia	Pink when crying Cyanotic when quiet	Oral airway Endotracheal intubation
Pharyngeal airway malformation	Persistent retractions Poor air entry	Prone positioning Posterior nasopharyngeal tube
Impaired lung function		
Pneumothorax	Asymmetrical breath sounds. Persistent cyanosis/bradycardia	Needle thoracocentesis
Pleural effusion / ascites	Diminished air movement Persistent cyanosis/ bradycardia	Immediate intubation Needle thoracocentesis Abdominal paracentesis Possible volume expansion
Congenital diaphragmatic hernia	Asymmetrical breath sounds Persistent cyanosis/ bradycardia Scaphoid abdomen	Endotracheal intubation Placement of orogastric catheter

Contd.

Contd.

Pneumonia/sepsis	Diminished air movement Persistent cyanosis/ bradycardia	Endotracheal intubation Possible volume expansion
Impaired cardiac function		
Congenital heart disease	Persistent cyanosis/ bradycardia	Diagnostic evaluation
Fetal/maternal hemorrhage	Pallor, poor response to resuscitation	Volume expansion, possibly including red blood cells

INDUCED HYPOTHERMIA

Hypothermia may reduce the extent of brain injury following hypoxia-ischemia. There is insufficient data to recommend routine use of selective and/or systemic hypothermia after resuscitation of infants with suspected asphyxia. Further clinical trials are needed to determine which infants benefit most and which method of cooling is most effective.

Hyperthermia may worsen the extent of brain injury following hypoxia-ischemia. The goal should be to achieve normothermia and to avoid iatrogenic hyperthermia in resuscitated newborns.

WITHHOLDING OR WITHDRAWING RESUSCITATION

1. Noninitiation of resuscitation and discontinuation of life-sustaining treatment during or after resuscitation are ethically equivalent, and clinicians should not hesitate to withdraw support when functional survival is highly unlikely.
2. In conditions associated with high rate of survival and acceptable morbidity, resuscitation is nearly always indicated. This generally includes babies > 25 weeks (unless there is evidence of fetal compromise such as intrauterine infection or hypoxia ischemia) and those with most congenital malformations.
3. In conditions with uncertain prognosis in which survival is borderline, the morbidity rate is relatively high, and the anticipated burden to the child is high, parental desires concerning initiation of resuscitation should be supported.

DISCONTINUING RESUSCITATIVE EFFORTS

After 10 minutes of continuous and adequate resuscitative efforts, discontinuation of resuscitation may be justified if there are no signs of life (no heart rate and no respiratory effort).

REFERENCES

1. International guidelines for neonatal resuscitation: An excerpt from the guidelines 2000 for cardiopulmonary resuscitation and emergency cardiovascular care: International consensus on science, *Pediatrics* 2000;106;e29.
2. 2005 American Heart Association (AHA) guidelines for cardiopulmonary resuscitation (CPR) and Emergency cardiovascular care (ECC) of pediatric and neonatal patients: Neonatal resuscitation guidelines, *Pediatrics* 2006;117:e1029-e1038.
3. The 2005 AAP/AHA guidelines for neonatal resuscitation: www.americanheart.org/eccguidelines.
4. Evidence based worksheets: www.C2005.org.
5. Apgar, V: A proposal for a new method of evaluation of the newborn infant, Anesth Analg 1953;32:260.
6. 'Resuscitation in the delivery room' by Ringer SA in *Manual of Neonatal Care*, Editors: Cloherty JP & Stark AR; 4th edition; Lippincott Williams & Wilkins, Pp-53-64.

3 HYPOGLYCEMIA AND HYPERGLYCEMIA IN THE NEONATE

Prem Shekhawat

INTRODUCTION

Glucose, like oxygen is of fundamental importance for any living being and it is the major energy source for the fetus and neonate. While the fetus receives adequate amount of maternal glucose via the placenta, in sharp contrast, the neonate becomes independent immediately after birth and has to balance between glucose deficiency and excess states. Preterm and term neonates differ substantially in their ability to maintain **euglycemia** since in the preterm infant various enzymes required for endogenous glucose production and utilization are in a state of development. The maintenance of euglycemia in the sick neonate with associated metabolic derangements is even more challenging; thus, neonates are prone to glucose disequilibrium. In this chapter we will briefly discuss the processes by which a neonate maintains euglycemia and elaborate on a practical approach to diagnosing and managing hypo- and hyperglycemia. The long-term outcome of any sick neonate depends on several factors but maintenance of euglycemia constitutes a significant role.

HYPOGLYCEMIA

Definition

Hypoglycemia is one of the most commonly encountered metabolic problems in the neonatal period but, to date, there are no uniformly accepted standards defining the range of euglycemia. Blood glucose levels are frequently lower in the neonate, more so in the preterm neonate, thus defining a lower limit of euglycemia is critical when intervention becomes necessary to avoid long-term injury. The situation is complicated further in the preterm neonate who lacks the neural capacity to demonstrate any overt symptomatology. The current definition of hypoglycemia is derived from statistical measures of blood glucose levels in healthy term neonates.[1] Whole blood glucose values are 10-15% lower than plasma/serum values.

Normally, in the healthy term neonate, mean serum glucose values reach a nadir of 55 to 60 mg/dl at 1-2 hours after birth and then rise to 70 to 80 mg/dl after 48-72 hours (Figure 3.1).[1] No such data exists for preterm, very low birth weight (VLBW) neonates, since some form of intervention is usually started to provide exogenous glucose by the intravenous (IV) route. The fall in serum glucose in extremely low birth weight (ELBW) neonates is even more pronounced. Hence, it is virtually impossible

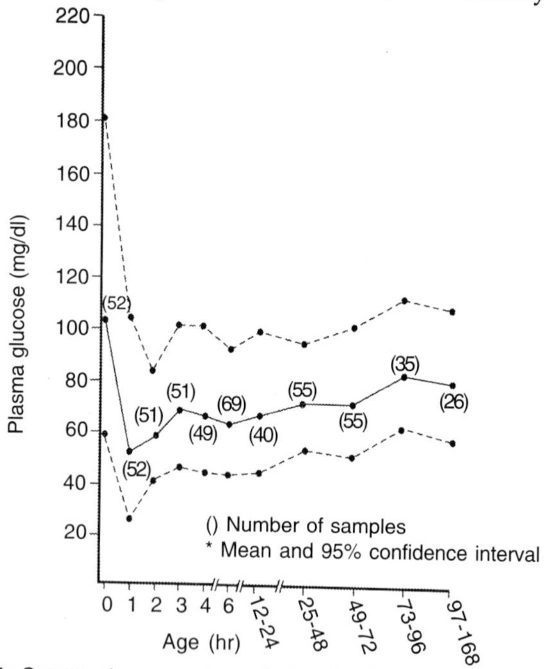

Fig. 3.1: Serum glucose values during the first week of life in healthy newborn appropriate gestational age infants (Adapted from: Srinivasan G, Pildes RS, Cattamanchi G *et al.* J Pediatrics 109:114;1986)

to define a normal range of euglycemia in this population. Recent investigations have shown that at serum glucose levels below 40 mg/dl a prolongation in latencies in brain stem auditory evoked response (BAER) are seen. The current consensus is that in the first few days after birth, hypoglycemia is defined as any **blood glucose level of <45 mg/dl** in both the term and preterm neonate.[2]

Epidemiology

Hypoglycemia is an extremely common condition in the neonates, seen in 5-30% of term neonates and upto 25-75% of preterm neonates.[2]

Pathology

Hypoglycemia occurs in a neonate born with low glycogen and fat stores who has limited capacity to generate glucose via the gluconeogenesis pathway or has excessive peripheral tissue utilization of glucose like in the **infant of a diabetic mother (IDM)**.[3]

Pathogenesis

Euglycemia after birth is maintained by a combination of finely controlled metabolic adjustments. Neonates, especially the ELBW preterm neonates are born with low stores of glycogen and adipose tissues which play a critical role in providing glucose and ATP. This situation is further complicated by the fact that several enzymes involved in gluconeogenesis viz. Phosphoenolpyruvate carboxykinase (PEPCK), Glucose-6-phosphatase, Fructose-1,6-diphosphatase, and Pyruvate caroboxylase are expressed at very low levels thus limiting gluconeogenesis. Thus preterm ELBW and intrauterine growth restricted (IUGR) infants are highly likely to become hypoglycemic in the immediate neonatal period.[4]

Neonates have poorly developed counterregulatory mechanisms to react to hypoglycemia which makes them highly vulnerable. The hypoglycemic neonate defends itself by decreasing insulin secretion and increasing glucagon, epinephrine, growth hormone and cortisol secretion which leads to glucose production and mobilization of fatty acids from adipose tissues. The increase in glucose production comes initially from the breakdown of glycogen (upto 1-2 hours) and later there is protein breakdown with increasing levels of cortisol. This process is evident by increased plasma levels of gluconeogenic amino acids, alanine and glutamine. Hypoglycemia occurs when there is excessive production of insulin (overutilization), poor gluconeogenesis (underproduction) or failure of counterregulatory mechanisms (pituitary or adrenal failure).[4] Figure 3.2 illustrates how insulin secretion is tightly controlled by serum glucose.

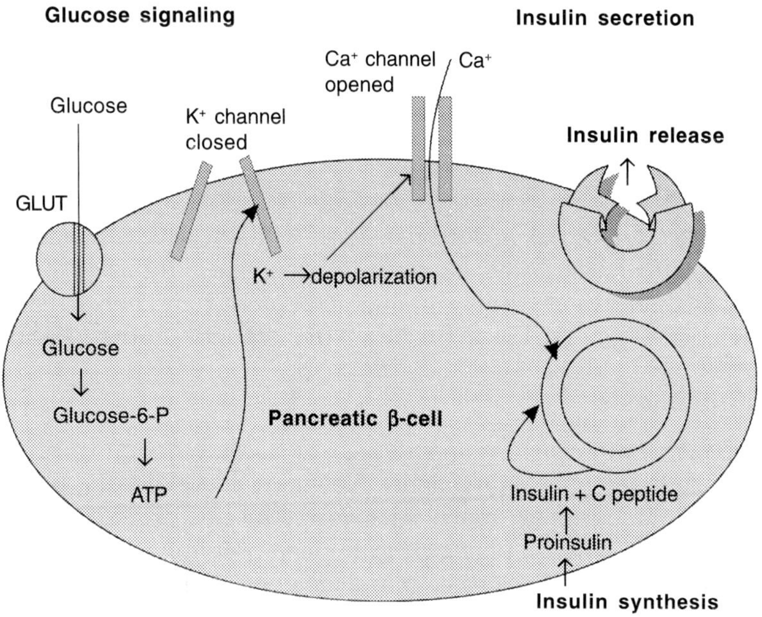

Fig. 3.2: Insulin secretion by pancreatic β-cells and its control by serum glucose

Clinical Features

Preterm, IUGR, small-for-gestation (SGA) and large-for-gestation (LGA) neonates are much more likely to experience hypoglycemia. Some infants may have macroglossia, macrosomia, ear pits/ creases, hemihypertrophy, abdominal wall defects, cardiac defects, clitoromegaly, Wilm's tumors and visceromegaly (**Beckwith-Wiedemann syndrome**). Infants with pituitary developmental defects may have micropenis, colobomas of iris, midline defects, a central incisor and eye ball defects.

Signs and symptoms of hypoglycemia are **nonspecific**, they are either autonomic nervous system mediated or secondary to neuroglycopenia. Some of the commonly seen signs are jitteriness, irritability, lethargy, tachycardia, hypothermia, flushing, seizures, apnea, grunting and sweating especially on the forehead. **Remember hypoglycemic infants are not always symptomatic.** Therefore, **routine glucose monitoring for at-risk infants is mandatory.**[5] Lack of symptoms in a neonate also **does not** guarantee absence of long-term sequelae.

Etiology of neonatal hypoglycemia may also be divided into the following categories:

A. *Inadequate production of glucose*
   1. Pre-term infants—born before late pregnancy storage of glycogen.
   2. IUGR—low glycogen and fat stores, impaired gluconeogenesis. The incidence of symptomatic hypoglycemia is highest in SGA infants.
   3. Post-term infants—glycogen depletion from placental insufficiency.
   4. Delayed feedings or conditions causing vomiting or malabsorption.
   5. Sepsis.

B. *Increased utilization of glucose*
   1. Very immature or severely ill infants. Perinatal asphyxia/anoxia; respiratory distress—increased energy needs.
   2. Cold stress—rapid depletion of glycogen.
   3. Polycythemia—increased utilization of glucose by red blood cells.
   4. Heart failure.
   5. Erythroblastosis fetalis, SGA infants.

C. *Increased uptake of glucose related to hyperinsulinism*
   1. IDM.
   2. Erythroblastosis fetalis.
   3. Beckwith-Wiedemann syndrome.
   4. Pancreatic islet cell adenoma/nesidioblastosis.
   5. High glucose infusion or tocolytics used prior to delivery.
   6. **Panhypopituitarism**.
   7. Maternal chlorpropamide therapy.
   8. Maternal benzothiazide therapy.

Chapter 3

D. *Other etiologies*

1. Inborn errors of metabolism (e.g., fatty acid oxidation disorders, galactosemia, glycogen storage disease, tyrosinemia, maple syrup disease).
2. Endocrine disorders (e.g., panhypopituitarism, adrenal failure, glucagon deficiency, epinephrine production defects).

Diagnosis

Hypoglycemia needs to be suspected in neonates. Routine measurement of glucose using glucose strip test like the accucheck (Roche Diagnostics India Pvt. Ltd.) of all neonates in first few days of life is recommended.

Caution

An accucheck is just a screening tool since the correlation between serum glucose and accucheck is very poor when the serum glucose is below 45 mg/dl. **A serum glucose level must be obtained for an accucheck of < 45 mg/dl for confirmation.** Clinical signs could help the clinician suspect hypoglycemia but the rule of thumb is that **every sick neonate deserves to have an accucheck.**

If hypoglycemia persists after the initial steps in management (see next section), then further testing is warranted. These tests include plasma insulin level, insulin-like growth factor-1 (IGF-1), plasma and urine ketones, urine organic acids, free fatty acids. Estimation of carnitine, ammonia, lactate and pyruvate levels, growth hormone, cortisol, epinephrine, and glucagon can be diagnostic in some cases. In rare cases a urine drug screen may be helpful. **The plasma insulin levels should be close to zero in any hypoglycemic infant.** Some infants with persistent hypoglycemia due to hyperinsulinemia may require further sophisticated tests which are available only at tertiary care centers, thus **appropriate and timely referral of these infants with persistent hypoglycemia is critical**.

Management

Initial management of hypoglycemia should by done using a protocol in each nursery or neonatal intensive care unit (NICU) as suggested below. **Remember it is important to draw a blood**

sample before initiation of therapy to diagnose the cause of persistent hypoglycemia.

A. *Symptomatic:* Do not feed but give an IV bolus of 2 mL/kg of D10W over 2-3 minutes and begin peripheral plain D10W infusion at 100mL/kg/d (Figure 3.3) to deliver glucose of 5-7 mg/kg/min.*

B. If accucheck is < 45 mg % and patient is asymptomatic, obtain serum glucose and begin enteral feeds. If infant is to breast-feed, take infant to mother for feeding; if this is not possible supplement with formula.
   1. If serum glucose is ≤ 30, start IV therapy.
   2. If serum glucose is ≥ 45, continue with normal newborn care.
   3. If serum glucose is 31-44, repeat accucheck and serum glucose in 30 minutes after feed.
      a. If serum glucose <45, start IV therapy.
      b. If serum glucose ≥45, obtain accuchecks q 30 min × 2, q hour × 2 then prefeed. Once there have been 3 accuchecks in a row ≥45, stop measuring accuchecks.

C. *Once IV therapy has been started*
   1. Monitor accuchecks q 30 min × 2, q hour × 2, then, prefeed.
   2. Wean by 3-5 cc/hr for each good feed if prefeed accucheck is ≥45 mg %.
   3. If unable to maintain accuchecks at ≥45 mg %, determine glucose delivery and increase delivery (mg/kg/min) either by increasing volume or glucose concentration.
   4. Infants requiring > D12.5W glucose should be transferred to the NICU.

D. *Criteria to transfer to the NICU*
   1. If low glucose has not been controlled and stabilized in first 4 hours.
   2. If IV access is not dependable.
   3. Symptomatic baby.

E. *In an emergency situation where an IV cannot be obtained one may give:*
   1. Glucagon intramuscular (IM), subcutaneous (SC) or IV 0.2 mg/kg/dose (max 1 mg) q 30 min prn.
   2. Nasogastric (NG) feed D5W.

3. Place an umbilical venous catheter (UVC) in order to get blood return and bolus D10W.
4. Hydrocortisone 2 mg/kg IV q 6 hours.

All of these should be done while preparing to transfer to the NICU.

*__Appendix:__ Glucose delivery calculation: (cc/kg/day) × (%CHO)/ 144.

Rule of thumb: 100cc/kg/day of D10W = 7 mg/kg/day.

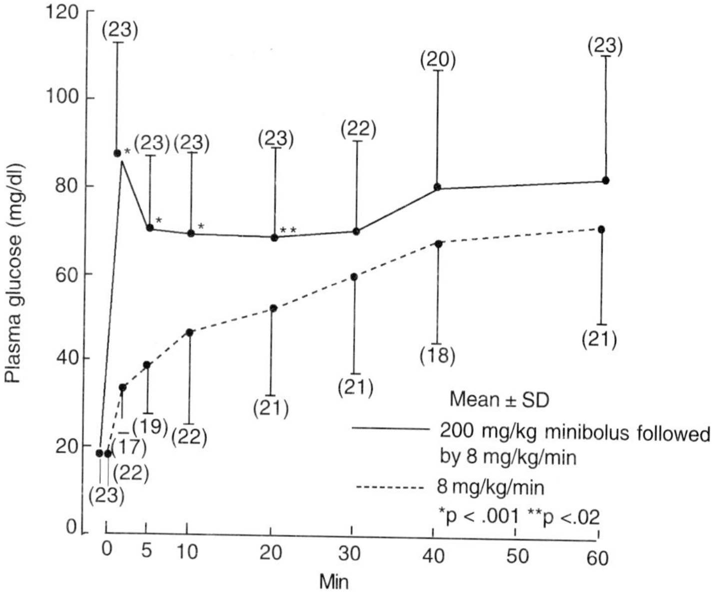

Fig. 3.3: Effect of IV bolus glucose followed by a constant infusion on serum glucose versus IV infusion alone (Adapted from: Lilien LD, Pildes RS, Srinivasan G *et al.* J Pediatrics 97:295;1980)

Complications

Hypoglycemia is a potentially life-threatening condition and requires prompt and appropriate management. Any delay in treatment may lead to serious long-term consequences. In the short-term, infants may experience apnea, respiratory failure and seizures. Hypoglycemia leads to diffuse neuronal injury especially in the parietal and occipital lobes. The extent of injury is dependent on the degree and duration of hypoglycemia.[5] Follow-up examinations of hypoglycemic infants have demonstrated a steep fall in motor and sensory development (Figure 3.4). Brain imaging studies in infants who suffered severe and prolonged hypoglycemia initially show abnormal hyperintensity of the parietal and occipital cerebral cortex (Figure 3.5) followed by marked neural tissue loss.[6]

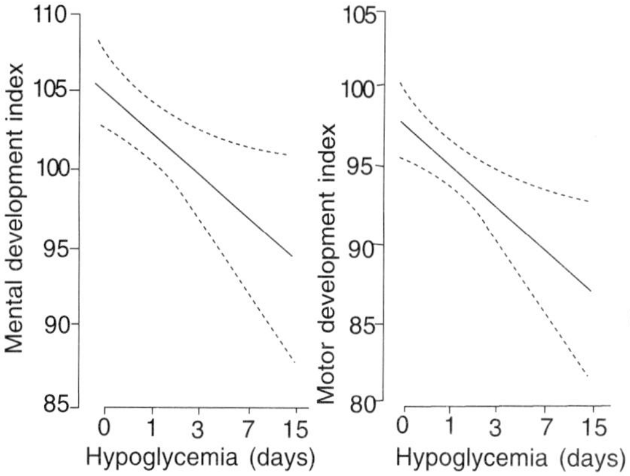

Fig. 3.4: Duration of hypoglycemia and Bayley Mental Development Index and Bayley Psychomotor Development Index at 18 months in 433 premature infants (Adapted from: Lucas A, Morley R, Cole TJ: BMJ 1988;287:1304)

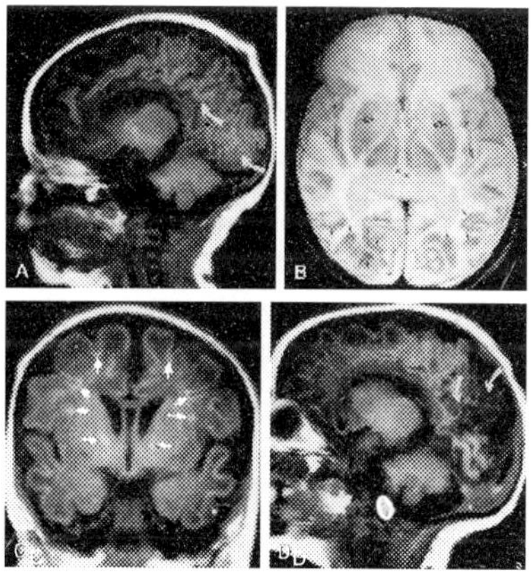

Fig. 3.5: Hypoglycemia leads to permanent neuronal injury: Figure A to C, MRI images at age 13 days and Figure D at 27 days. A: There is abnormal hyperintensity (arrows) of the parietal and occipital cerebral cortex. B: Abnormal hyperintensity (open arrows) in the globi palladi and mixed hypointensity and hyperintensity (solid arrows) in the occipital cortex and white matter. C: Hyperintensity of the globi palladi (open arrows). D: Marked tissue loss, most prominently in the parietal and occipital lobes (arrows) (Adapted from: Barkovich JA, Ali FA, Rowley HA *et al.* AJNR Am J Neuroradiol 19;523:1998)

Prognosis and Follow-up

Several neonates develop partial epilepsy after prolonged hypoglycemia. Other neurologic problems include developmental delays, learning and behavior problems, hyperactivity and attention difficulties, autistic features, microcephaly and cortical blindness.

HYPERGLYCEMIA

Definition

Hyperglycemia constitutes a significant risk factor for morbidity and mortality in sick VLBW infants. It is generally defined as blood glucose level of >150 mg/dl regardless of the neonates gestational age, weight or postnatal age.[7]

Epidemiology

40-80% of VLBW infants less than 1000 grams experience hyperglycemia during the course of their hospital stay.[7] Hyperglycemia occurs 15 times more frequently in infants less than 1000 grams at birth than those weighing more than 2000 grams. Some term neonates present with transient diabetes which improves with time; permanent diabetes mellitus is relatively rare in the neonatal period.

Pathology

Glucose homeostasis is poor in VLBW infants. Insulin secretion is tightly controlled by plasma glucose levels and availability of ATP in pancreatic beta cells (Figure 3.2). This control mechanism does not function well in preterm neonates and growth restricted neonates also exhibit a state of insulin resistance. High exogenous glucose infusion in a stressed neonate is a common cause of hyperglycemia. Insulin resistance may be mediated through insulin receptors, glucose transporters (GLUT 4), or enzymes regulating glycolysis, glycogenolysis or gluconeogenic pathways.[8]

Pathogenesis

Conditions that cause stress to the infant, such as asphyxia, respiratory distress, intraventricular hemorrhage, sepsis, or a surgical procedure, can increase the risk of hyperglycemia. Continuous infusion of glucose, or lipids and the administration of some drugs, such as corticosteroids, aminophylline, and caffeine, may also induce hyperglycemic reactions in neonates.[8] In these VLBW infants there may be a state of deficient insulin secretion, production of biologically inactive insulin, or altered conversion of proinsulin to insulin. Transient neonatal diabetes mellitus may present in first 10 days of life and in rare cases it may become permanent. Concentration of C-peptide and plasma insulin is low and there is family history of diabetes in a third of these patients. The exact cause of **neonatal diabetes** is not known.[9]

Clinical Features

Hyperglycemic infants are typically preterm, SGA or IUGR and undergoing stressful clinical situations like surgery or painful procedures. Hyperglycemia is commonly seen in infants receiving dexamethasone or hydrocortisone. Positive correlation of hyperglycemia with low Apgar scores, high fractional concentration of inspired oxygen, and respiratory distress score has been described.[9]

Diagnosis

Hyperglycemia, in most cases is a chance finding on routine laboratory screening unless accuchecks are monitored in critically ill neonates. All abnormal accucheck readings should be confirmed with a laboratory blood sugar estimation.

Management

The treatment of neonatal hyperglycemia must be based on the diagnosis and suspected etiology in each case. The exogenous glucose infusion rate and medications must be reviewed.[10] Urine output, urine glucose and serum glucose and serum electrolytes must be measured. When the blood glucose reaches 150-350 mg/dl, start by reducing the exogenous glucose intake. It is recommended to continue enteral feeding if possible in the meantime. If hyperglycemia persists, use of continuous insulin infusion with glucose restriction is necessary[10]. Caloric restriction may cause caloric deprivation and may lead to growth restriction and neurodevelopmental delay in the VLBW infant. On the other hand continuous insulin infusion may cause hypoglycemia and hypokalemia, thus cause neuronal injury and long-term disabilities.[11] The long-term clinical significance of large doses of exogenous insulin in association with early high caloric intake in the preterm neonate is not well studied. A recent review of six controlled studies in VLBW infants using insulin infusion to improve caloric intake reported hypoglycemia ranging from 0.2% to 11% of subjects. Insulin therapy led to improved glycemic control with higher caloric intake but no major difference in weight gain was noted in the short term.[12] Thus, currently, insulin infusion is not recommended for improving caloric intake or weight gain.

Exogenous insulin can be administered by three methods: intramuscularly (IM); intravenous bolus; or, continuous intravenous infusion. Insulin given IM is generally precluded for infants <1000 grams as the available tissue sites are limited and the absorption is variable. Intravenous bolus generally will cause a reduction in the glucose level but may cause transient hypoglycemia. Continuous intravenous infusion of insulin administered concurrently with glucose and titrated according to the blood glucose levels will minimize adverse effects of both hyperglycemia and hypoglycemia while allowing for increased glucose loads to meet maintenance and growth requirements.[13]

Continuous insulin intravenous infusion has been used to optimize parenteral nutrition. Exogenous insulin is infused constantly at a prescribed rate with the continuous glucose infusion and is titrated according to the blood glucose levels. Depending on the estimated fluid requirements of the infant, the dextrose concentration can reach as high as 25%, as long as the insulin infusion rate is less than <0.5 unit/kg/hr to keep blood glucose levels stable between 100 and 200 mg%, and glucose induced diuresis has not occurred.[13]

The decision to begin insulin for any of these conditions is never made lightly. Take into consideration, the gestational age, day of life, and current condition of the infant, estimated fluid requirements based on the hydration status of the infant, current urine output, and recent trending of laboratory tests, such as sodium, potassium, glucose, creatinine, and BUN levels. Based on this information, it may be decided that temporarily decreasing the glucose load would be of greater benefit than would be immediately initiating insulin to control hyperglycemia. Glucose loads may be decreased gradually to a minimum 5 to 6 mg/kg/min, equaling basal glucose production. After the infant's condition has stabilized or hyperkalemia has developed, insulin should be initiated and the glucose load increased.[14] A concerted effort to identify the cause of hyperglycemia should be made while treating the problem adequately.

After the decision has been made to initiate insulin, the rate of the infusion is determined. For glucose levels of <400 mg %, the infusion rate is 0.01 unit/kg/hr; for ≥400 mg %, the rate is 0.1 unit/kg/hr is used. The insulin concentration is calculated so that 0.1 cc/hour will give the desired units/kg/hr, either 0.01 unit/kg/hr or 0.1 unit/kg/hr. The same dextrose concentration is ordered for both the maintenance and the insulin fluids to allow for a constant glucose load while titrating the insulin. Titration of the insulin rate is accomplished according to the desired glucose levels of 100 to 200 mg/dl. The total hourly fluid volume calculated for the infant is maintained constant by inversely changing the maintenance fluid rate to equal the change in the insulin rate[14]. For instance, if the insulin rate is increased by 0.1 cc/hr, the maintenance fluid rate is decreased by 0.1 cc/hr. Maintenance and insulin fluids are infused through the same line, ideally via the umbilical venous catheter, leaving the umbilical arterial catheter as a non-glucose line for blood glucose measurements. The hourly intravenous rate at which insulin is infusing should not exceed 0.5 cc/hr for a prolonged period. The insulin concentration may need to be doubled or quadrupled when the infusion rate is ≥ 0.5 cc/hr to allow maximal infusion of parenteral nutrition or maintenance fluids.

Onset of action for insulin is approximately one half to 1 hour after insulin reaches the infant. Insulin is unstable in extremes of pH so if the infant is acidotic or alkalotic, the efficacy of insulin is affected and may result in persistent hyperglycemia. Corticosteroid therapy, such as dexamethasone, may result in hyperglycemia either through a direct effect or by enhancing the release of catecholamines.[9] The rise in blood glucose levels within the first 2 to 4 hours following the administration of corticosteroids should be responded to with great caution because hypoglycemia may result after the transient effect of heightened catecholamine release eases. Continuous insulin therapy is required until the infant's ability to adequately manage glucose loads with endogenously produced insulin matures, generally during the first 7 to 10 days of life. After enteral feedings are initiated, further stimulation of endogenous insulin production and reactivity apparently occurs, enabling the infant to wean off from exogenous insulin. Continued careful monitoring of blood glucose levels is **extremely important** to **prevent hypoglycemia** during this time.[14]

Complications

Hyperglycemia in premature neonates can cause osmotic diuresis with resultant loss of water and electrolytes, leading to dehydration. The increased serum osmolarity with dehydration causes intracellular fluid to move to the extracellular space. The resultant fluctuations in cerebral blood flow may lead to intracranial hemorrhage.[15] Use of insulin inappropriately with poor monitoring can cause hypoglycemia and brain injury. SGA infants who are noted to be hyperglycemic have been shown to suffer from a metabolic syndrome which includes insulin resistance as adults.

Prognosis and Follow-up

Prognosis is excellant in most cases if appropriate therapy is instituted in time and these infants do not require any long-term follow-up.

REFERENCES

1. Srinivasan G, Pildes RS, Cattamanchi G *et al.*: Plasma glucose values in normal neonates: A new look, J Pediatrics 1986;109:114-117.
2. Cornblath M, Hawdon J, Williams A, *et al.*: Controversies regarding definition of neonatal hypoglycemia: Suggested operational thresholds, *Pediatrics* 2000;105:1141-1145.
3. Ogata ES: Glucose metabolism during pregnancy, In: Polin RA, Fox WW, Abman SH, eds, *Fetal and Neonatal Physiology*, 3rd ed, Philadelphia: W. B. Saunders; 2004.
4. Tyrala E, Chen X, Broden G: Glucose metabolism in the infant weighing less than 1100 grams, *J Pediatrics* 1994;125:283-287.
5. Lucas A, Morley R, Cole TJ: Adverse neurodevelopmental outcome of moderate neonatal hypoglycaemia, BMJ 1988;287:1304-1308.
6. Dekelbab BH, Sperling MA: Hypoglycemia in newborns and infants, *Advances in Pediatrics* 2006;53:5-22.
7. Pildes RS: Neonatal hyperglycemia, *J Pediatrics* 1986;109:905-07.

8. Pollak A, Cowett R, Oh W: Glucose disposal in low-birth-weight infants during steady state hyperglycemia: Effects of exogenous insulin administration, *Pediatrics* 1978;61:546-549.
9. Meetze W, Bowsher R, Compton J, Morehead H: Hyperglycemia in extremely low-birth weight infants, *Biology of the Neonate* 1998;74:214-21.
10. Binder N, Raschlo P, Benda G, Reynolds J: Insulin infusion with parenteral nutrition in extremely low-birth weight infants with hyperglycemia, *J Pediatrics* 1989;114:273-280.
11. Simeon P, Geffner M, Levin S, Lindsey A: Continuous insulin infusions in neonates: Pharmacologic availability of insulin in intravenous solutions, *J Pediatrics*1994;124; 818-820.
12. Kairamkonda V: Does continuous insulin infusion improve glycaemic control and nutrition in hyperglycaemic very low birth weight infants? *Arch Dis Child* 2006;91:76-9.
13. Shannon L: Insulin usage in the neonate: *Neonatal Network* 1988;6:31-39.
14. Farrago H, Nawrath L, Healey J, *et al.*: Persistent glucose production and greater peripheral sensitivity to insulin in the neonate vs. the adult, *American J Physiology* 1997;272:E86–E93.
15. Efron D, South M, Volpe JJ, Inder T: Cerebral injury in association with profound iatrogenic hyperglycemia in a neonate, *Eur J Paediatr Neurology* 2003;7:167-71.

4 DISORDERS OF CALCIUM, PHOSPHORUS AND MAGNESIUM METABOLISM IN THE NEONATE

Prem Shekhawat

INTRODUCTION [1-3]

Calcium, the most abundant mineral in the human body plays several critical roles in cellular physiology besides providing structural integrity to the skeleton. Serum calcium concentration represents a minute fraction of total body calcium and its cytosolic and extracellular fluid (ECF) concentration is very tightly regulated. Serum concentration of calcium is inversely proportional to serum phosphorus concentration and it is intimately regulated by **parathormone** (PTH), vitamin D, calcitonin and serum magnesium concentration. Approximately 50-55% of total plasma calcium is diffusible (ionic) and the rest is bound to protein (mainly albumin). Ionic calcium is the only biologically available fraction and is intimately involved in cell-cell signaling, coagulation, cell division, neuromuscular excitability, enzyme activation, and membrane integrity and membrane permeability. Measurements of calcium levels are affected by pH and heparin content of the sample. Heparin can bind ionized calcium and decrease its concentration; for every change in pH by 0.1 unit, ionized calcium changes inversely by 0.16 mg/dL (0.04 mmol/L).

Blood inorganic phosphate concentration is highest in the neonatal period (4.5 to 9.0 mg/dL) and it declines with increasing age (3.0 to 4.5 mg/dL in adults). In contrast to serum calcium, only 10-12% of phosphorus is protein bound. The majority of body phosphorus (80-85%) is complexed with hydroxyapatite in the skeleton. Cytosolic and ECF concentrations of phosphorus are less rigorously regulated than calcium and magnesium. Dietary phosphorus is absorbed throughout the small intestine. The proximal renal tubule regulates plasma phosphorus levels by varying its reabsorption. This reabsorption process is facilitated by PTH.

PTH, an 84 amino acid hormone secreted by the four parathyroid glands is the principal regulator of serum calcium concentration. PTH acts on various PTH-responsive tissues through its receptor (PTH-R), a G-protein coupled receptor. PTH mobilizes skeletal calcium and phosphorus, stimulates calcium reabsorption in renal tubules and stimulates synthesis of activated vitamin D ($1,25[OH]_2D_3$). This leads to an increase in serum calcium level with a decline in serum phosphorus level (Figure 4.1). Several fragments of PTH are found circulating in blood but the two-site "intact PTH" assay measures the bioactive hormone. The normal circulating levels of PTH varies from 10 to 60 pg/mL. Parathyroid cells respond to changes in ambient ionized calcium (Ca^{++}) through calcium-sensing receptor (CaSR). Loss-of-function mutations in

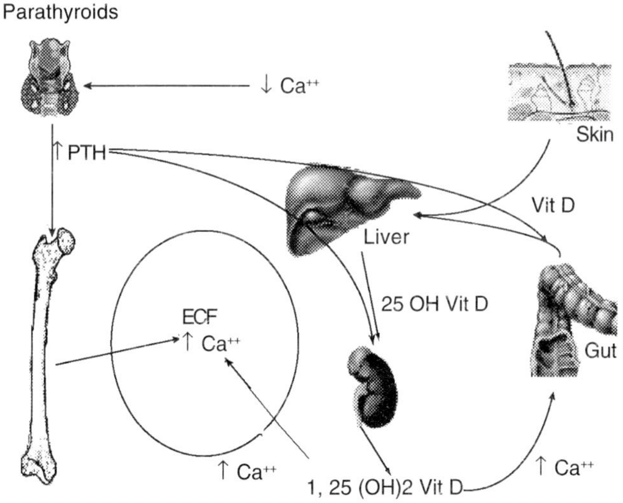

Fig. 4.1: Hormonal regulation of serum calcium by PTH and Vitamin D

the CaSR are seen in neonatal hyperparathyroidism and hypercalciuric hypercalcemia and likewise a gain-of-function mutations in CaSR is responsible for autosomal dominant neonatal hypocalcemia (Figure 4.2). The extracellular domain of CaSR is sensitive to the pH and Mg^{++} concentration in the ECF and in the face of hypomagnesemia, PTH release is impaired. PTH-related protein (PTH-rP), a homologue of PTH, plays a significant role in fetal and neonatal calcium metabolism. PTH-rP is secreted by fetal parathyroid glands and placenta. It was initially identified as the cause of hypercalcemia in some malignancies; PTH-rP acts through PTH-R and knockout of PTH-rP gene leads to embryonic lethality underpinning its crucial role during fetal development. Human milk contains high levels of PTH-rP and it has been postulated to help calcium absorption.

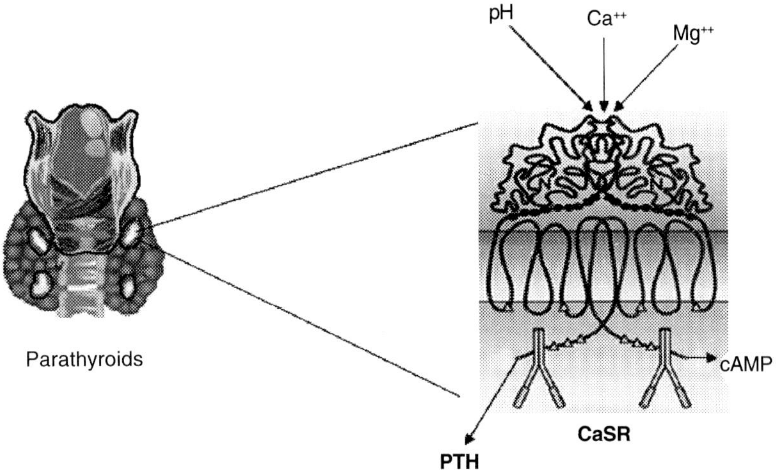

Fig. 4.2: Control of PTH release from parathyroid glands by calcium sensing receptor (CaSR) and effect of ambient concentration of calcium, magnesium and pH

Vitamin D, a steroid hormone synthesized in the skin from 7-dehydrocholesterol and absorbed from the diet, plays a crucial role in calcium and phosphorus homeostasis. Vitamin D undergoes 25-hydroxylation in the liver to form 25-hydroxyvitamin D (25(OH)D); subsequent hydroxylation in the proximal tubules of kidney forms the biologically active 1,25 $(OH)_2D_3$. Measurement of 25(OH)D level reflects Vitamin D status of the neonate. The normal circulating level of 25(OH)D is 15-55 ng/mL, whereas the concentration of 1,25 $(OH)_2D_3$ ranges from 25-80 pg/mL. 1,25 $(OH)_2D$ leads to increase in intestinal absorption of calcium and phosphorus. PTH helps convert 25(OH)D into 1,25 $(OH)_2D_3$ in the proximal tubules of kidney, thereby increasing the intestinal absorption of calcium and phosphorus. 1,25 $(OH)_2D_3$ enters the cell and binds to cytosolic Vitamin D receptors (VDR). VDR with its ligand 1,25 $(OH)_2D_3$ then enters the nucleus to bind to specific response elements (VDRE) of several genes to modulate their transcription. PTH secreted in response to hypocalcemia is the main regulator of 1,25 $(OH)_2D_3$ production, which in turn suppresses PTH gene expression.

Calcitonin, a 32-amino acid peptide secreted by thyroid parafollicular C cells, has anti-PTH action, and it plays a significant calcitropic function in pregnant and lactating women as well as in the fetus and neonate. Neonatal calcitonin levels are much higher than adult levels. During pregnancy approximately 30 g of calcium and 16 g of phosphorus is transferred across the placenta, mainly during the third trimester. Thus, preterm neonates are especially vulnerable to metabolic bone disease since they are deprived of this maternal mineral transfer (Figure 4.3).

Chapter 4

HYPOCALCEMIA [4-6]

Definition

Hypocalcemia is frequently observed in neonates, especially the sick preterm infant. Hypocalcemia is often asymptomatic, and its treatment in neonates currently is controversial. Hypocalcemia is defined as a total serum calcium concentration of <8.0 mg/dL in term neonates, and less than 7 mg/dL in preterm neonates.

Epidemiology

Incidence of neonatal hypocalcemia varies in different populations. Hypocalcemia occurs in up to 30% of infants with very low birth weight (<1500 g). High incidence is also reported in infants of diabetic mothers (IDM) and in infants with birth asphyxia. Late-onset hypocalcemia is common in infants in developing countries

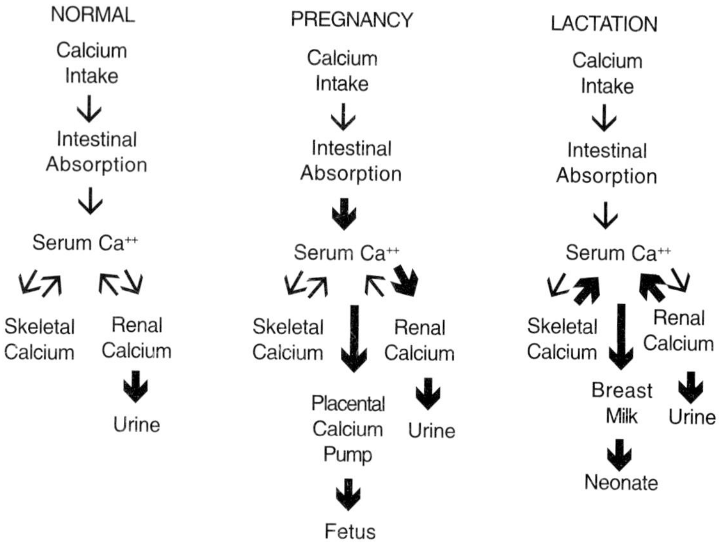

Fig. 4.3: Adaptive mechanisms involved in calcium homeostasis during pregnancy and lactation. The *thickness of arrows* indicates a relative increase or decrease with respect to the normal, non-pregnant state (Adapted from: Kovacs CS, Kronenberg HM, Endocrine Reviews 1997;18:832-872)

where babies are fed cow's milk or formulas containing high amounts of phosphate.

Pathology

Infants who develop hypocalcemia are typically preterm or large for gestational age (LGA) infants who are IDM. Majority of infants who experience perinatal birth asphyxia develop hypocalcemia. It is also commonly seen in infants with aortic arch anomalies like coarctation of aorta, bicuspid aortic valve and ventricular septal defect (**DiGeorge syndrome**).

Pathophysiology

Over 99% of the body's total calcium is in bone, and serum levels constitute less than 1%. Several factors regulate this homeostasis of calcium and maintain serum calcium within a narrow defined range. These include parathormone (PTH), vitamin D, hepatic and renal function (to convert vitamin D to active metabolites), and serum phosphate and magnesium levels. Hypocalcemia in the neonate is broadly divided into two categories (Table 4.1):

Table 4.1: Common causes of neonatal hypocalcemia

Early onset hypocalcemia (<48 h of age)	Maternal hyperparathyroidism
Prematurity	Kenny-Caffey syndrome
Intrauterine growth restriction (IUGR)	Osteogenesis imperfects type II
Perinatal depression/asphyxia	PTH resistance
Infant of diabetic mother (IDM)	Vitamin D deficiency
Late onset hypocalcemia (>48 h of age)	Resistance to Vitamin D action
High phosphate load in formulas	Metabolic or respiratory alkalosis
Neonatal hypoparathyroidism	Sepsis, septic shock
Vitamin D deficiency	"Hungry bone syndrome"
Hypomagnesemia	Rhabdomyolysis-induced renal failure
Phototherapy	Pseudohypocalcemia (hypoalbuminemia)
Infantile osteopetrosis	Medications: Bicarbonate, Furosemide, Lipid infusions, rapid blood transfusions, plasmapheresis with citrated blood.
DiGeorge syndrome	

- **Early neonatal hypocalcemia** (within 48 hours of birth)
  1. *Prematurity:* Possible mechanisms include poor intake, decreased responsiveness to vitamin D, increased calcitonin, and hypoalbuminemia leading to decreased total but normal ionized calcium.
  2. *Birth asphyxia:* Delayed introduction of feeds, increased calcitonin production, increased endogenous phosphate load, and alkali therapy all may contribute to hypocalcemia.
  3. *Diabetes mellitus in the mother:* Functional hypoparathyroidism induced by magnesium deficiency plays a predominant role, increases the risk of prematurity and asphyxia.
  4. *Intrauterine growth restriction (IUGR):* Infants with IUGR may have hypocalcemia if they also are preterm or have had perinatal asphyxia.

- **Late neonatal hypocalcemia** (3-7 days after birth)
  1. Increased exogenous phosphate load: Most commonly seen after feeding with phosphate-rich formula or cow's milk.
  2. Magnesium deficiency.
  3. Transient hypoparathyroidism of the newborn.
  4. **Hypoparathyroidism** due to other causes.
  5. Aplasia or hypoplasia of the parathyroid glands - DiGeorge syndrome; velocardiofacial syndrome; gestational diabetes mellitus, fetal exposure to retinoic acid; complex of vertebral defects, anal atresia, tracheoesophageal fistula with esophageal atresia, and radial and renal abnormalities (VATER), association of coloboma, heart defects, choanal atresia, renal abnormalities, growth retardation, male genital anomalies, and ear abnormalities (CHARGE).
  6. PTH receptor defects – **Pseudohypoparathyroidism**.
  7. Activating mutations of the calcium-sensing receptor leading to inappropriately suppressed PTH secretion.
  8. Abnormal vitamin D production or action: Vitamin D deficiency-dietary insufficiency, maternal use of anticonvulsants, acquired or inherited disorders of vitamin D metabolism and rarely resistance to actions of vitamin D.
  9. **Hyperphosphatemia:** This could be due to excessive phosphate intake in cow milk based formulas, total parenteral nutrition (TPN), increased endogenous loading caused by anoxia, chemotherapy, or rhabdomyolysis and renal failure.
  10. Others causes include: malabsorption syndromes, alkalosis - respiratory alkalosis caused by hyperventilation; metabolic alkalosis with the administration of bicarbonate, diuretics, or chelating agents, such as the high doses of citrates taken in during massive blood transfusions. One should be aware of pseudohypocalcemia secondary to hypoalbuminemia. Some infants may show "**Hungry bones syndrome**" related to rapid skeletal mineral deposition seen in infants with rickets or hypoparathyroidism after starting vitamin D therapy.

Clinical Features

Hypocalcemia is asymptomatic in many cases. Symptoms of hypocalcemia include jitteriness, tetany, and hyperactivity with muscle jerking and twitching. Some infants will develop frank clonic seizures. Laryngospasm, inspiratory stridor, and wheezing have been attributed to hypocalcemia. Some infants may develop vomiting and feeding intolerance due to pylorospasm; frank intestinal obstruction has been described in rare cases. Extensor hypertonia, tachycardia, carpopedal spasm with positive Chvostek sign are rarely seen in neonates.

Diagnosis

1. Serum calcium, total and ionized levels: Measuring ionized calcium level is essential to differentiate true hypocalcemia from a mere decrease in total calcium concentration. A decrease in total calcium is commonly associated with low serum albumin concentration and abnormal pH.
2. Serum magnesium: Serum magnesium may be low in patients with hypocalcemia and hypocalcemia may not respond to calcium therapy if hypomagnesemia is not corrected.
3. Serum electrolytes and glucose: Seizures or jitteriness in newborns can be associated with hypoglycemia and sodium abnormalities.
4. Serum phosphorus: Determining the phosphate level is essential to establish the etiology of hypocalcemia. Phosphate levels are higher in cases of exogenous and endogenous phosphate loading, renal failure and hypoparathyroidism.
5. PTH levels are indicated if hypocalcemia persists in the presence of normal magnesium and normal or elevated phosphate levels. **Always order an "intact PTH" level since there are several circulating isoforms of PTH.** Low PTH levels suggest hypoparathyroidism and serum calcium will rise in response to a PTH challenge. PTH levels could be elevated in patients with vitamin D metabolism abnormalities and pseudohypoparathyroidism (resistance to action of PTH), and calcium levels will not rise in response to a PTH challenge.
6. Serum levels of Vitamin D metabolites ($25[OH]D_2$) and

Chapter 4

(1,25[OH]$_2$D$_3$): 25-hydroxyvitamin D levels are commonly used clinically and reflect the true vitamin D status of infant, **1,25 hydroxyvitamin D** levels remain near normal even in the face of severe vitamin D deficiency. These assays can help eliminate uncommon causes of hypocalcemia such as malabsorption or disorders of vitamin D metabolism.

7. Urine calcium, magnesium, phosphorus, and creatinine levels are helpful in neonates with suspected renal tubular defects and renal failure.
8. Serum alkaline phosphatase is generally elevated in patients with rickets.
9. Chest radiography to evaluate thymic shadow, which may be absent in patients with DiGeorge syndrome.
10. Ankle and wrist radiography for evidence of rickets. Changes appear at an early stage in the radius and ulna; distal ends are widened, concave, and frayed.
11. Electrocardiography: A prolonged QTc (>0.4 s), a prolonged ST segment, and T wave abnormalities may be observed.
12. Total lymphocyte and T-cell subset analyses by flow cytometry are helpful in patients with DiGeorge syndrome.
13. Maternal and family screening may be required in cases of familial forms of hypocalcemia, such as those caused by activating mutations of the calcium-sensing receptor.

Management

Treatment of an asymptomatic neonate with hypocalcemia remains controversial. In contrast, symptomatic hypocalcemia should be treated promptly because of its serious implications for neuronal and cardiac function. Infants with seizure activity need stabilization with management of their airway and breathing and anticonvulsants are commonly given before confirmation of hypocalcemia in any patient. Seizures usually may not respond to the usual anticonvulsant therapy until calcium is administered intravenously. Intravenous treatment is usually indicated in patients having seizures. Oral calcium therapy is commonly used in asymptomatic patients and as follow-up to intravenous calcium therapy. A diet high in calcium and low in phosphate is recommended in most instances. Patients with renal failure should be prescribed a low-phosphate formula, such as Similac PM 60/40.

Calcium therapy is the mainstay of treatment for hypocalcemia. Therapy with intravenous calcium is the most effective and rapid means of elevating serum calcium concentration. Once hypocalcemia is controlled, follow-up treatment with oral therapy can be given. However, in patients with asymptomatic hypocalcemia, therapy with oral calcium alone may be sufficient. Vitamin D, in one of its various forms, is also indicated depending on the metabolic abnormality present. However, the use of vitamin D formulations in newborns to prevent hypocalcemia has not been effective. The most important aspect of management is resolution of the primary cause (e.g., hyperphosphatemia, hypomagnesemia).

Calcium, intravenous and oral preparations:

- Calcium gluconate 10% (i.e., 100 mg/mL) IV solution contains 9.8 mg/mL (0.45 mEq/mL) elemental calcium. 10-20 mg/kg elemental calcium (1-2 mL calcium gluconate/kg) IV slowly is given over 5-10 min to control seizures; may be continued by 50-75 mg/kg/d IV infusion over 24 hours. Use extreme care in peripheral infusion because extravasation can cause severe tissue necrosis. Rapid IV infusion may cause bradycardia and hypotension; may cause liver necrosis, if administered in an umbilical venous catheter lodged in a branch of portal vein.
- Calcium chloride 10% (i.e., 100 mg/mL) contains 27 mg/mL (1.4 mEq/mL) elemental calcium. Calcium chloride is more irritating to the veins and may affect pH; therefore, it is typically avoided in pediatric patients. Prolonged use of calcium chloride may lead to hyperchloremic acidosis.
- Calcium Glubionate (Neo-Calglucon)—Calcium supplement for PO use. The glubionate salt (Neo-Calglucon) (1800 mg/5 mL) contains 115 mg elemental calcium/5 mL.
- Oral Calcium carbonate salt (Oystercal, Caltrate, Tums, Os-Cal)—Supplement for PO use. In many ways, the carbonate salt is the calcium supplement of choice because it provides 40% elemental calcium. Thus, 1 g of calcium carbonate provides 400 mg of elemental calcium. Well absorbed orally and unlikely to cause diarrhea. Available in tab and liquid forms and its dosage in neonates is: 30-150 mg/kg/d PO divided qid; may be added to formula (e.g., Similac PM

60/40 to make a calcium-phosphorous ratio of 4:1). For older children: 20-65 mg/kg/d PO divided bid/qid.

Magnesium administration is necessary to correct any hypomagnesemia because hypocalcemia does not respond until the low magnesium level is corrected. A sick neonate with severe hypocalcemic-hypomagnesemic tetany or if suspected of having hypomagnesemic-hypokalemic ventricular arrhythmias should receive IV Magnesium sulphate (10%) containing 0.8 mEq/ml to give 0.2 mEq/Kg/dose slowly over 20-30 minutes and repeated until a plasma magnesium levels of >1.0 mg/dL (0.4 mmol/L or 0.8 mEq/L) is achieved. This should be followed by a maintenance dose of 0.25-0.5 mEq/day added to IV infusion.

Vitamin D

Calcitriol (Rocaltrol)—Active metabolic form of vitamin D (i.e., 1,25-dihydroxycholecalciferol). Especially useful in impaired liver or renal function causing inability to hydroxylate vitamin D to its active forms. It is generally rapid-acting; however, may act more slowly in neonates (over 36-48 hours). Preterm infants may be resistant to its actions. It is also used to treat acute hypocalcemia. It is used in a dose of 0.01-0.05 mcg/kg/d IV qd/bid; adjust dosage until normocalcemia is attained. The other alternative is Dihydrotachysterol (DHT, Hytakerol) – it is a synthetic analog of vitamin D, which does not require activation by renal 1-hydroxylase for activity. It is also available in liquid form facilitating administration of variable doses in infants and young children. 1 mg equivalent to 120,000 U (i.e., 3 mg) vitamin D-2. The neonatal dose is 0.05-0.1 mg/d PO.

Regular follow-up monitoring of serum calcium concentration and appropriate monitoring of the underlying disease (e.g., PTH concentration in hypoparathyroidism) is necessary. This monitoring is important because no definitive measures exist to determine whether an infant has transient hypoparathyroidism that may last for several years or is at risk for recurrence of hypoparathyroidism and hypocalcemia; recurrence has been reported as late as adolescence.

Prevention

Late-onset hypocalcemia in neonates, which is typically caused by hyperphosphatemia, can be prevented by avoiding high-phosphate containing diets like regular cow's milk. Ensuring adequate vitamin D stores in mothers during pregnancy will prevent neonatal hypocalcemia. Feeding a low-phosphate diet such as human milk or Similac PM 60/40 formula will prevent hypocalcemia in hyperphosphatemic states, such as renal failure, hypoparathyroidism, or endogenous phosphate loading. Enhancing the calcium-phosphorus ratio to 4:1 in the diet (by adding calcium supplements to a low-phosphate diet) also reduces intestinal absorption of phosphate.

Prognosis

Most cases of early neonatal hypocalcemia resolve within 2-3 days without any significant complications. Late neonatal hypocalcemia secondary to exogenous phosphate load and magnesium deficiency responds to phosphate restriction and magnesium repletion. Hypocalcemia due to hypoparathyroidism requires continued therapy with vitamin D metabolites and calcium supplements. The period of therapy depends on the nature of the hypoparathyroidism; transient hypoparathyroidism lasting several weeks to months. Rapid infusion of calcium-containing solutions through peripheral or central lines could lead to chemical burns with disfigurement and sterile calcified abscess in the liver.

HYPERCALCEMIA

Definition

Hypercalcemia is rare, it is defined as total serum calcium of >10.3 mg/dL or ionized calcium of >5.0 mg/dL. Common causes of hypercalcemia are listed in Table 4.2.

Pathogenesis

An increase in net calcium mobilization from the skeleton and renal handling of calcium are the two most common causes of hypercalcemia. Skeletal calcium mobilization occurs due to hyperparathyroidism due to inactivating mutations of CaSR. Hypophosphatemia due to inadequate provision of dietary phosphorus, especially in very low birth weight (VLBW) infants, stimulates renal calcitriol synthesis which in turn activates intestinal calcium absorption and skeletal resorption. Subcutaneous fat necrosis is a common cause of hypercalcemia. It is commonly seen after forceps application or vacuum extraction. Hypercalcemia occurs due to excessive and uncontrolled production of calcitriol from macrophages at sites of necrotic fat.

Table 4.2: Common causes of neonatal hypercalcemia

Iatrogenic hypercalcaemia	Subcutaneous fat necrosis
Hypophosphatemia	Williams syndrome
Vitamin D excess	Idiopathic infantile hypercalcaemia
Excessive calcium supplementation	Inborn errors of metabolism
Thiazide diuretics	Lactase deficiency
Functional hyperparathyroidism	Disaccharidase deficiency
Maternal hypocalcaemia	Hypophosphatasia
Congenital parathyroid hyperplasia	Adrenal insufficiency
Inactivating mutations in the CaSR	Severe congenital hypothyroidism
Familial hypocalciuric hypercalcaemia	Thyrotoxicosis
Neonatal severe hyperparathyroidism	Down syndrome (unknown cause)
Jansen's metaphyseal chondrodysplasia	IMAGe syndrome (Intrauterine growth retardation, Metaphyseal dysplasia, Adrenal hypoplasia congenita, Genital abnormalities)
Persistent PTH-rP	
Non-parathyroid hypercalcaemia	
Disorders of vitamin D metabolism	Hypervitaminosis A
Phosphate depletion	Prolonged ECMO

Clinical Features

Hypercalcemia may be asymptomatic in mild cases or it could be an incidental finding on routine screening. Severe hypercalcemia (>14 mg/dL) may present dramatically and could be life threatening. The common clinical features include vomiting, poor feeding, tachypnea, hypotonia, lethargy, constipation, drowsiness or irritability and hypertension. Some chronic cases present with failure-to-thrive, marked dehydration due to polyuria, which is secondary to renal resistance to vasopressin. Hypertension is due to direct vasoconstrictor effect of calcium, and there may be shortening of ST segment with various degrees of heart blocks. Later these patients will develop nephrocalcinosis, hematuria, hypertensive encephalopathy, extraskeletal calcification and nephrolithiasis.

The clinical examination of these infants is normal, except in infants with subcutaneous fat necrosis or **Williams-Beuren syndrome**. Williams-Beuren syndrome is characterized by hypercalcemia in about 15% cases; these infants have an "elfin" facies with supravalvular aortic stenosis, developmental delays and dental malformations. Patients with Williams-Beuren syndrome have IQ in the 50-80 range and later develop kyphoscoliosis, pectus excavatum, renal defects and an abnormal gait.

Diagnosis

Laboratory evaluation of hypercalcemia must include a serum phosphorus level and alkaline phosphatase levels. A family history of hypercalcemia indicates mutations in the CaSR of parathyroid glands. Other useful diagnostic tests include:

1. Simultaneous urine and serum calcium and phosphorurs levels.
2. Intact PTH.
3. Vitamin D_2 and D_3 levels.
4. An exaggerated response to vitamin D_2 and elevated calcitriol levels.
5. Plain abdominal X-ray, a skeletal survey and renal ultrasound.
6. Magnetic resonance imaging (MRI) of the area of subcutaneous fat necrosis is indicated as it may show pathognomonic needle-shaped clefts in fat.
7. Echocardiographic studies are indicated if Williams-Beuren syndrome is suspected.
8. Investigations for congenital lactase and sucrose-isomaltase deficiency.
9. Genetic studies are indicated in familial cases of hypercalcemia, looking for common microdeletions at chromosome 7q11.13, 6(q22.2q23) and 4[46,XX, del(4)(q33)]. A fluorescent in situ hybridization (FISH) probe for elastin gene (ELN) is diagnostic for Williams-Beuren syndrome.

Management

Treatment of neonatal hypercalcemia depends on the severity of disorder. Mild cases are managed conservatively with avoidance of excessive calcium and vitamin D intake and adequate hydration. Intravenous saline boluses with loop diuretics like frusemide are indicated for management of severe hypercalcemia. When hypercalcemia is associated with hypophosphatemia, 30-50 mg/kg/day of oral or IV Na/K phosphate may be used. **Glucocorticoids** (prednisolone 2 mg/kg/day) can suppress intestinal calcium absorption and increase renal excretion and help reduce serum calcium. Recently IV bisphosphonates (pamindronate 0.5-2.0 mg/kg) has also been used. Familial cases of hypercalcemia with persistent problems may require subtotal parathyroidectomy. A low-calcium containing formula like Calcilo XD (Ross Laboratories, North Chicago, IL) can be beneficial for long-term management. Treatment monitoring should be done by checking serum and urine calcium and phosphorus levels.

Prognosis

Prognosis for transient hypercalcemia is excellent but infants with familial disease due to mutations in CaSR will develop skeletal defects and infants with Williams-Beuren syndrome have developmental delays.

HYPERMAGNESEMIA[7]

Definition

Hypermagnesemia is defined as serum magnesium level of > 2.8 mg/dL.

Etiology

Maternal treatment with magnesium sulphate therapy for preterm onset of labor or severe preeclampsia is the most common cause of neonatal hypermagnesemia. Sometimes excessive magnesium could be added to parenteral nutrition solution. Rarely, use of magnesium-containing antacids has led to neonatal hypermagnesemia.

Clinical Features

Most term neonates are asymptomatic. Preterm neonates may

present in the immediate neonatal period with hypotonia, flaccidity, apnea, respiratory failure, lethargy, poor feeding, abdominal distension with poor gut motility. Some neonates present with delayed passages of meconium when their mothers were chronically treated with magnesium. Most clinical effects of hypermagnesemia disappear within hours to 1-2 days since magnesium is excreted in the urine. Preterm neonates with limited excretory capacity may continue to have higher levels for upto 3-4 days after birth. Hypermagnesemia rarely may suppress PTH secretion.

Diagnosis

Serum magnesium level should be obtained in all neonates whose mothers are treated with magnesium during pregnancy before any enteral feeds are started. It is helpful to obtain a serum calcium level at the same time. Normal neonatal serum magnesium levels range from 1.5 to 2.8 mg/dL.

Management

Most often the only treatment necessary is to provide IV fluids and avoid feeding these infants. Rarely, some neonates may require intubation and ventilation due to severe apnea for a few days. Intravenous calcium is effective in antagonizing clinical effects of hypermagnesemia. Begin feeding only after serum levels have fallen in the normal range.

Prognosis

Excellent with no long-term or residual effects.

REFERENCES

1. Guise TA, Mundy GR: Evaluation of hypocalcemia in children and adults, J Clin Endocrinol Metab 1995;80:1473-1478.
2. Gertner JM: Disorders of Calcium and Phosphorus Homeostasis. Pediatr Clin N Amer 1990;37:1441-1465.
3. Reichel H, Koeffler Hp, Norman AW: The role of Vitamin D endocrine system in health and disease, N Engl J of Med 1989;320:980-991.
4. Mimouni F, Tsang RC: Neonatal Hypocalcemia: To Treat or Not To Treat, J Amer Coll Nutr 1994;13: 408-415.
5. Sanchez GJ, Venkataraman PS, Pryor RW, et al.: Hypercalcitoninemia

and hypocalcemia in acutely ill children: Studies in serum calcium, blood ionized calcium, and calcium-regulating hormones, J Pediatr 1989; 114: 952-956.

6. Hsu SC, Levine MA: Perinatal calcium metabolism: Physiology and pathophysiology, Sem Neonatol 2004;9:23-36.
7. Broner CW, Stidham GL, Westenkirchner DF, Tolley EA: Hypermagnesemia and hypocalcemia as predictors of high mortality in critically ill pediatric patients, Crit Care Med 1990;18:921-928.

5 FLUIDS AND ELECTROLYTES IN THE NEWBORN

Namasivayam Ambalavanan

PRINCIPLES OF WATER AND ELECTROLYTE BALANCE

Fluid and electrolytes management is particularly important in the neonatal intensive care unit (NICU) as sick neonates require IV fluids and are prone to develop fluid and electrolyte imbalance. Inappropriate management may result in serious short-term or long-term complications. It is important to understand normal postnatal changes in fluid and electrolyte balance and the factors that alter these changes before proceeding to evaluation and management.

NORMAL BODY WATER ALTERATIONS IN THE POSTNATAL PERIOD

Neonates are born with an excess of **total body water** (TBW), primarily in the extracellular fluid compartment [TBW = extracellular fluid (ECF) + intracellular fluid (ICF)]. This excess of TBW is normally lost over the first postnatal week. TBW in adults is approximately 60% of body weight, of which two-thirds (40%) is intracellular and one-third (20%) is extracellular. Total body water in normal term neonates has about 75%, of which 40% is extracellular and 35% is intracellular. Preterm infants have more TBW, which may be as high as 90% at 23 weeks' gestation, and a larger proportion is extracellular (upto 60%). Therefore, while a term infant loses 5-10% of body weight over the first week, a preterm infant may lose upto 10-15% over the same period. Small for gestational age (SGA) infants have higher proportional body water content as they have lower body fat content.

Water may be lost in both easily measured ways (urine, stool, orogastric drainage), or as **insensible water loss** (IWL). IWL is water loss that is not readily measured, and is mostly that is lost by evaporation from the skin (2/3rd) or from the respiratory tract (1/3rd). It is necessary to have a rough estimate of IWL in order to calculate fluid losses, and therefore, the fluid required for the neonate.

FACTORS IMPACTING UPON THE NORMAL FLUID AND ELECTROLYTE STATUS IN THE IMMEDIATE POSTNATAL PERIOD (Table 5.1)

Table 5.1: Factors affecting fluid and electrolyte status

Factors	*Comments*
Gestational age	The lower the gestational age, the greater is the IWL
Postnatal age	IWL also decreases over the first postnatal week as the skin thickens over time
Immature renal function	Compared to older infants, neonates have a reduced ability to concentrate or dilute urine and hence, are more prone to become dehydrated or fluid overloaded with inadequate or excessive fluid intake, respectively
Ambient and body temperature	Higher temperatures increase IWL
Ambient humidity	Higher ambient humidity reduces IWL
Activity level	Increased activity will slightly increase IWL
Radiant warmer	Increases IWL of upto 50%
Phototherapy	Increases IWL of upto 50%
Surgical conditions	Gastroschisis, omphalocele, neural tube defects etc. will increase IWL, depending upon the surface area of the defect
Other sources of fluid/electrolyte losses	Stool (e.g. diarrhea or ostomy output) and gastric drainage (via orogastric or nasogastric tubes)

IWL: Insensible Water Loss.

Clinical and Laboratory Assessment of Water and Electrolyte Balance

Clinical Evaluation

Body weight is often regarded as an important indicator of changes in fluid status. However, an infant's weight does not always correlate with changes in intravascular volume. Body weight may increase significantly despite a reduction in intravascular volume, as in disorders such as peritonitis or use of muscle relaxants due to "third-spacing" in which interstitial fluid increases at the expense of intravascular volume. Growth charts are useful for following nutritional status over time, but they are of little use in daily management.

Manifestations of **dehydration** such as poor skin turgor, dry mucosa, sunken fontanelle are late indicators of dehydration in neonates. Tachycardia may be seen early in hypovolemia, but may also be noted with fluid overload (leading to congestive heart failure). Poor capillary refill is often seen with dehydration, but may also be noted with cold stress. Hepatomegaly is often noted in infants with excessive extracellular fluid, especially in congestive heart failure. Blood pressure changes are late, and usually indicate severe hypovolemia or cardiogenic shock.

Laboratory Evaluation

Laboratory tests need to be evaluated in light of the clinical setting. It is necessary to remember that in the first or second postnatal day, many serum levels (e.g. creatinine) may reflect maternal values. Common lab evaluations include blood glucose, serum electrolytes, urea, creatinine, and plasma osmolarity. It is important to use non-hemolyzed samples, and analyze samples quickly. Especially when taking care of premature infants, a laboratory that can handle microsamples is essential. Many modern blood gas analyzers can measure blood glucose and electrolytes, in addition to **blood gas** values. An arterial (or arterialized capillary) blood gas demonstrating metabolic acidosis may help in the recognition of poor tissue perfusion.

Urine output and total fluid intake are critical items of information in the intensive care unit. Infants in diapers (napkins) need to have their diapers weighed soon after voiding to avoid errors due to evaporation from the diaper.[1] Urinary electrolytes, specific gravity, and calculation of the **fractional urinary excretion of sodium** in relation to creatinine (FENa) give additional information useful in infants with disturbances of fluid and electrolyte balance. However, these data may be difficult to interpret in infants on diuretics.

The normal range of values is shown in Table 5.2.

Table 5.2: Normal range of laboratory values to guide fluid/electrolyte balance in the neonate

Measurements	*Normal range*	*Comments*
Blood Glucose	50-100 mg/dL	Avoid hypoglycemia (<40) or hyperglycemia (>125-150)
Serum Na	135-145 mEq/L	Avoid hyponatremia (<130) or hypernatremia (>150)
Serum K	3.5-5.5 mEq/L	Avoid hypokalemia (<3) or hyperkalemia (>6)
Serum Cl	95-105 mEq/L	Avoid hypochloremia (<90) or hyperchloremia (>115)
Serum HCO_3	20-27 mEq/L	Avoid metabolic acidosis (<17) or alkalosis (>28)
Plasma Osmolarity	275-290 mOsm	Calculated osmolarity/osmolality may be less than measured – osmolal gap
Blood Urea Nitrogen	7-20 mg/dL	
Serum Creatinine	0.4-1.3 mg/dL	Postnatal 1-3 days values reflect maternal renal function
Urine Specific Gravity Urine Osmolarity	1.005-1.015 100-400 mOsm	
FENa Urinary Na and Creatinine are required to calculate FENa ; FENa = [(Urine Na × Plasma Cr)/(Plasma Na × Urine Cr)] × 100	1-2%	<1% suggests pre-renal factors reducing renal blood flow; >3% suggests acute renal failure, diuretic use, and occasionally in extreme prematurity
Urine Output Blood pH	1-3 ml/kg/hr 7.25-7.45	Capillary blood gas samples will have a slightly lower pH

Fluid and Electrolyte Management

The goal of neonatal fluid and electrolyte management is to permit normal postnatal changes in fluid and electrolyte balance to occur.[2] Fluid and electrolyte management is a balancing act between intake and output. Primary goals are to maintain the appropriate ECF volume, ECF and ICF **osmolality**, and ionic concentrations. It is necessary to allow the initial loss of ECF over the first week, as reflected by weight loss, while maintaining normal intravascular volume and tonicity, as reflected by heart rate, urine output, and electrolyte and pH values. Subsequently, one needs to maintain water and electrolyte balance while supplying requirements for body growth. However, conditions such as prematurity, renal failure, septicemia, etc. that occur in neonates cannot be considered as "normal" states.

Attempting to achieve normal postnatal changes during abnormal pathophysiologic states may lead to worse outcomes. It is therefore important to individualize fluid and electrolyte management depending upon the clinical situation. This individualized management plan requires an understanding of the pathophysiology underlying the infant's disease process, as well as the principles of basic physiology, biochemistry, and nutrition. The first step is to arrive at a diagnosis and then decide the management.

Fluid Requirement

Total fluid requirement equals maintenance requirements (IWL + urine + stool water) plus water required for growth (as 60-70% of new tissue is water). In the immediate postnatal period, IWL constitute the largest component of fluid losses. After the first few days, as renal solute load increases, the amount of water required to excrete the solute load also increases (80-120 cal/kg/d = 15-20 mOsm/kg/d, equivalent to 60-80 ml/kg/d required for urine output). Stool losses, in the absence of diarrhea, are usually 5-10 ml/kg/d. In addition, as 2/3rd of new tissue is water, an infant gaining 30 g of weight a day needs 20 ml/day for new tissues. In general, term infants nursed with clothes in a **thermoneutral environment** need about 60 ml/kg/day on the first and second day of life, and this increases to 150 ml/kg/day by the second to third postnatal week, and upto 200-250 ml/kg/

day for normal infants fed *ad libitum* at a month of age. Premature infants need more fluid, due to their higher IWL. Extremely low birth weight infants with very thin skin who are not cared for in humid micro-environments may need more than 150 ml/kg/day to avoid dehydration. A recent comparison of incubator care versus radiant warmer care has shown that radiant warmer care results in better temperature control, although with higher fluid requirements.[3] These results however need to be investigated in larger studies.

Electrolyte Requirement

Electrolyte-free fluids are recommended for the first few days of postnatal life. Additional electrolytes (sodium, potassium, or chloride) are usually added after the second postnatal day. By the end of the first week, needs are usually 1-3 mEq/kg/d for sodium and chloride and 1-2 mEq/kg/d for potassium. Extremely premature infants who have a tendency to develop metabolic acidosis may benefit from sodium acetate administration instead of sodium chloride. Subsequently, during active growth, the requirement for sodium and chloride increase to 3-5 mEq/kg/d and for potassium to 2-3 mEq/kg/d. Extremely low birth weight infants may have a very large requirement as high as 6-8 mEq/kg/d because of the decreased capacity of the kidneys to retain sodium, the need for growth, and the frequent use of diuretics in this population (Table 5.3).

Fluid and Electrolyte Requirement in Common Neonatal Conditions

Sick neonates may be preterm or term infants. Preterm infants are often further classified by birth weight as low birth weight (LBW; <2.5 kg), very low birth weight (VLBW; <1.5 kg), and extremely low birth weight (ELBW; < 1 kg) preterm infants. In addition, infants can be further classified as large for gestational age (LGA), appropriate for gestational age (AGA), or small for gestational age (SGA), on the basis of usual birth weight ranges for each gestational age stratum. Common problems involving preterm infants are those directly due to prematurity itself (e.g. increased IWL, thermoregulation, feeding problems due to poor sucking and swallowing etc.), and other defined entities such as

Table 5.3: Fluid and electrolyte requirements in the first week of life for a term or near-term infant

	Day 1	*Day 2*	*Day 3*	*Day 4*	*Day 5*	*Day 6*	*Day 7*	*2nd postnatal week onwards*
Fluids (ml/kg/day)	60	70	90	110	120	130	140	140-180
Na (mEq/kg/day)	0	0	1-2	1-3	1-3	1-3	1-4	2-5
Cl (mEq/kg/day)	0	0	1-2	2-3	2-3	2-3	2-4	2-5
K (mEq/kg/day)	0	0	1-2	1-2	1-3	1-3	1-3	2-3

respiratory distress syndrome (RDS), bronchopulmonary dysplasia (BPD), persistent ductus arteriosus (PDA), necrotizing enterocolitis (NEC), intraventricular hemorrhage (IVH), and infections. The common diagnostic categories involving term infants are asphyxia (hypoxic-ischemic encephalopathy: HIE), aspiration syndromes (e.g. meconium aspiration syndrome: MAS), infection (including septicemia, meningitis, tetanus and others), transient tachypnea of the newborn (TTNB), persistent pulmonary hypertension of the newborn (PPHN), and congenital malformations (Table 5.4).

HYPONATREMIA

Definition

Hyponatremia is usually defined as a serum sodium level <130 mEq/L, and is very common in infants admitted to neonatal intensive care units.

Etiopathogenesis

In the first week or so after birth, hyponatremia usually results from excessive free water intake. In extremely premature infants who are rapidly growing or in infants with increased sodium losses (e.g. orogastric drainage, diuretic therapy), inadequate sodium intake can contribute to hyponatremia. Chronic hyponatremia is usually not a cause for much concern until the serum sodium has dropped to <125 mEq/L.

Syndrome of inappropriate antidiuretic hormone (SIADH) secretion may lead to hyponatremia, but this syndrome is rare in the absence of other pathology. Hyponatremia may also result

Table 5.4: Changes in fluid and electrolyte requirements in common neonatal conditions

Condition	*Fluid requirements*	*Electrolyte requirements*	*Comments*
LBW	Variable	Variable	Different approach for LBW if term SGA or preterm AGA
VLBW	Increased with increased IWL	Increased during period of rapid growth	
ELBW	Increased with increased IWL	Increased during period of rapid growth	
LGA	Variable – infants of diabetic mothers may need additional glucose, and fluid restriction if respiratory distress	Infants of diabetic mothers may need additional calcium and magnesium	
SGA	Variable	Variable	
HIE	Decreased	Variable	Management of associated renal failure or syndrome of inappropriate anti-diuretic hormone (SIADH) secretion
MAS	Decreased	Variable	
TTNB	Decreased	Variable	
Sepsis	Increased	Usually increased	Management of hypotension
PPHN	Variable	Usually increased	Management of hypotension

Contd.

Contd.

Congenital malformations	Variable – depends upon malformation	Variable – depends upon malformation	
RDS	Decreased	Initially decreased	Fluid restriction is of benefit
PDA	Decreased	No change	Fluid restriction is of benefit
IVH	Variable	No change	Management of hypotension
NEC	Increased	Variable	Management of hypotension
BPD	Decreased	Variable	Fluid restriction is of benefit; Electrolyte intake depends upon diuretic usage

See text for abbreviations.

from appropriate ADH secretion in the setting of hypotension, when baroreceptor stimulation increases ADH. Very rarely, hyponatremia is the result of conditions such as congenital adrenal hyperplasia.

Clinical Features

Most infants with hyponatremia are asymptomatic. Some infants with hyponatremia may not have the anticipated postnatal weight loss, and may have other clinical features of fluid overload (e.g. eyelid puffiness). Sudden or marked decreases in serum sodium may occasionally cause seizures or lethargy, especially if the serum sodium is <120 mEq/L.

Investigations

Besides measurement of serum electrolytes, specialized laboratory investigations other than serum electrolytes are not usually required, unless conditions such as inappropriate ADH secretion or congenital adrenal hyperplasia are suspected. It is important to remember that blood samples obtained from arterial catheters are sometimes diluted by fluids being infused into the catheter, and hyponatremia may be misdiagnosed in such situations.

Management

This usually consists of fluid restriction if the etiology is excessive free water intake. If infants are symptomatic, an infusion of hypertonic saline (3% saline; usually 6 ml/kg given over 1 hour) can be administered to correct the serum sodium to 125 mEq/L.

Asymptomatic infants should have their hyponatremia corrected slowly (over 2-3 days) to avoid rapid increases in serum sodium.

Complications

These are rare in asymptomatic hyponatremia. Hyponatremia and extracellular fluid overload in the setting of respiratory distress syndrome in premature infants may be associated with an increased risk of BPD. However, central pontine and extrapontine myelinolysis as a consequence of hyponatremia has not been often described in infants.

Prognosis

This depends upon the etiology of the hyponatremia, and not usually upon the hyponatremia per se.

HYPERNATREMIA

Definition

Hypernatremia is defined as a serum sodium level >150 mEq/L. Most neonatologists closely monitor serum sodium if it is increasing rapidly as it may indicate dehydration, and are concerned if serum sodium level has risen to greater than 150-155 mEq/L.

Etiopathogenesis

Hypernatremia typically is seen in the first few days of life in ELBW infants and is most often the result of inadequate free water intake to compensate for very high IWL.

Very rarely, hypernatremia is the result of excessive sodium intake, such as following administration of sodium bicarbonate to infants with pulmonary hypertension in an effort to increase pH. In term infants, hypernatremic dehydration may occur in breast-fed infants who receive inadequate intake, usually in the first postnatal week.

Clinical Features

Infants with hypernatremia may present with dehydration and a weight loss of >10% from birth in term infants or >15-20% in preterm infants. In the initial stages of hypernatremia, term infants are usually vigorous and hungry. Complications of dehydration such as cerebral venous thrombosis may be occasionally noted.

Investigations

Specialized laboratory investigations other than serum electrolytes are not usually required.

Management

This is directed towards correction of dehydration, and achieving a slow decline (over 48-72 hours) in serum sodium by administration of increased amounts of free water. Rapid correction of hypernatremia may lead to seizures. Prevention and management of an insufficient milk intake in term infants is important.

Complications

These are usually secondary to dehydration, rather than of hypernatremia per se.

Prognosis

Hypernatremia in the setting of adequate hydration (e.g. in term infants with PPHN who have received excessive sodium intake) usually resolves without incident and the prognosis is good.

HYPOKALEMIA

Definition

Hypokalemia is usually defined as a serum potassium level <3.5 mEq/L, and is common in infants in NICUs. Blood samples obtained from arterial catheters are sometimes diluted by fluids being infused into the catheter, and hypokalemia may be misdiagnosed in such situations. Unless the infant is receiving digoxin, hypokalemia is rarely a cause for concern until the serum potassium level is <3.0 mEq/L.

Etiopathogenesis

Most of the potassium in the body is intracellular. Therefore, serum potassium levels often do not indicate total body potassium stores. Serum potassium levels also depend on blood pH levels, as pH affects the distribution of potassium between ICF and ECF compartments. A handy rule is that each 0.1 unit of pH change results in a 0.3-0.6 mEq/L change in the serum potassium level. The potassium level therefore increases with acidosis, and decreases with alkalosis.

Hypokalemia often results from chronic diuretic use and unreplaced electrolyte loss from nasogastric drainage or ostomies.

Clinical Features

Most infants with mild hypokalemia are asymptomatic. Severe

hypokalemia can produce **cardiac arrhythmias**, ileus, and lethargy. EKG manifestations of hypokalemia include a flattened T wave, prolongation of the QT interval, or the appearance of U waves.

Investigations

Specialized laboratory investigations other than serum electrolytes and an **EKG** are not usually required.

Management

When significant, hypokalemia is treated by slowly replacing potassium either intravenously with fluids containing 40-80 mEq/L of potassium or orally. Rapid administration of potassium is hazardous and should be done only in infants with severe or symptomatic hypokalemia (less than 2 or 2.5 mEq/L). This rapid partial correction is often done with 0.25 -0.5 mEq/kg of potassium chloride administered over 1 hour while the EKG is monitored.

Complications

These are usually the result of the underlying etiology rather than electrolyte abnormalities.

Prognosis

Hypokalemia uncomplicated by cardiac arrhythmia normally has a good prognosis.

HYPERKALEMIA

Definition

Hyperkalemia is often defined as a serum potassium level >6 mEq/L, measured in a nonhemolyzed specimen.

Etiopathogenesis

Causes of hyperkalemia include potassium release from damaged cells following IVH, trauma, and intravenous hemolysis. In addition, severe acidosis and decreased urinary potassium excretion such as in acute renal failure contribute to elevations in serum potassium. Finally, hyperkalemia may be one of the earliest manifestations of **congenital adrenal hyperplasia**.

Clinical Features

Hyperkalemia is of far more concern than hypokalemia, especially when serum potassium levels exceed 6.5 mEq/L or if EKG changes have developed. Mild hyperkalemia is usually asymptomatic. Severe hypokalemia may lead to cardiac rhythm problems. EKG manifestations of hyperkalemia are a progression from peaked T waves, as the earliest sign, to a widened QRS configuration, bradycardia, tachycardia, supraventricular tachycardia (SVT), ventricular tachycardia, and ventricular fibrillation.

Management

Significant hyperkalemia management may include the following:

1. All administration of potassium is discontinued.
2. Calcium gluconate 100-200 mg/kg (1-2 mL/kg of 10% solution) is administered as a slow IV infusion over 5-10 minutes.
3. Alkalinization is performed, either with hyperventilation or sodium bicarbonate 1-2 mEq/kg IV.
4. Insulin is administered to assist in driving potassium into the intracellular fluid compartment. Insulin must be administered with glucose as a combined infusion to avoid producing hypoglycemia.
5. Medications are administered to enhance potassium excretion, including furosemide 1 mg/kg IV or sodium polystyrene sulfonate (Kayexalate) 1 g/kg rectally (not recommended for ELBW infants). Several hours must pass before any effect is observed with either of these medications.
6. Dialysis or exchange transfusion may be used to assist in more rapidly removing potassium from the body.

Complications

These include ventricular fibrillation which may lead to significant mortality and morbidity.

Prognosis

In the absence of cardiac rhythm problems, prognosis usually depends upon the underlying etiology of the hyperkalemia (e.g. acute renal failure).

ACIDOSIS

Definition

Acidosis is generally defined as a low arterial blood pH. What is considered "low" varies by postnatal age as the normal pH in the first 24 hours after birth ranges from 7.27 to 7.43, and from 7.32 to 7.42 at 1 week of age. Acidosis can be either metabolic (low bicarbonate, usually <17 mEq/L), respiratory (high $PaCO_2$, usually >50 torr), or combined (mixed metabolic and respiratory). An arterial blood gas will help identify which disorder is present.

Etiopathogenesis

Respiratory acidosis is usually due to hypoventilation, and sometimes due to a severe ventilation-perfusion mismatch. An increase in alveolar minute ventilation is usually sufficient to increase $PaCO_2$ elimination and restore the pH to normal, although sometimes a moderately high $PaCO_2$ is tolerated ("permissive hypercapnia") in order to reduce volutrauma.

Metabolic acidosis can result either from accumulation of acid or loss of buffer. The difference between the sodium (cation) concentration and the sum of the chloride and bicarbonate anions is known as the anion gap, and indicates the unmeasured anions of the extracellular fluid. The anion gap is normally between 5 and 15 mEq/L (varying with albumin concentration), and an increase in the anion gap (>15) suggests an accumulation of acid (e.g. in acute renal failure, inborn errors of metabolism, lactic acidosis due to decreased tissue perfusion), while a normal anion gap (<15) in the presence of acidosis indicates a loss of bicarbonate (e.g. renal losses as in renal tubular acidosis or dysplasia, gastrointestinal losses, or dilutional acidosis).

Clinical Features

The infants with mild to moderate respiratory acidosis are usually asymptomatic. Infants symptomatic with metabolic acidosis, depending upon the underlying etiology, may have general (vomiting, dehydration, tachypnea, hypothermia) or specific (for example: neurological – hypotonia, seizures) manifestations.

Management

There is insufficient evidence from randomized controlled trials to determine whether infusion of base or fluid bolus reduces morbidity and mortality in preterm infants with metabolic acidosis.[4] There is also insufficient evidence to indicate that bicarbonate is useful in resuscitation of term infants. In general, many neonatologists attempt to keep bicarbonate levels at >15 mEq/L and the arterial pH >7.20 in sick infants. Therapy should be directed at the underlying cause of acidosis.

Complications

Moderate acidosis is generally well tolerated, although care must be taken to ensure that homeostasis is otherwise maintained – for example, a lower pH may increase serum potassium levels and ionized calcium levels and lead to secondary complications. Infants with severe respiratory acidosis and high $PaCO_2$ may have increased cerebral blood flow and an increased risk of IVH. Severe acidosis (<7.15) may also depress cardiac function, surfactant production, and increase pulmonary vascular resistance.

Prognosis

This depends upon the underlying etiology of acidosis.

ALKALOSIS

Definition

Alkalosis is generally defined as a high arterial blood pH, which is often considered as a pH >7.4 or >7.45. Alkalosis can be either metabolic (high bicarbonate, usually >28 mEq/L), respiratory (low $PaCO_2$, usually <35 torr), or combined (mixed metabolic and respiratory). An arterial blood gas will help identify which disorder is present.

Etiopathogenesis

Respiratory alkalosis is due to an increased alveolar minute ventilation, and may be secondary to excessive mechanical ventilation which may either be deliberate (e.g. for PPHN) or accidental (e.g. weaning not fast enough in resolving RDS), or may be due to spontaneous hyperventilation or crying. Respiratory alkalosis is often noted on blood gases obtained by arterial puncture in infants who are crying.

Metabolic alkalosis indicates retention of bicarbonate. The etiology of metabolic alkalosis can be determined by evaluation of urinary chloride. A low urinary chloride (<10 mEq/L) indicates retention of bicarbonate to compensate for chloride loss, such as may occur with chronic diuretic therapy, of gastrointestinal losses due to vomiting/nasogastric drainage/diarrhea. A high urinary chloride (>20 mEq/L) may occur with alkali administration, early in diuretic therapy, with Bartter's syndrome and excess of mineralocorticoids.

Clinical Features

The infants with mild to moderate respiratory alkalosis are usually asymptomatic. In infants with metabolic alkalosis, symptoms mostly depend upon the underlying etiology. The infant may have general (vomiting, failure to thrive) or specific (for example: palpable mass in the abdomen in cases of hypertrophic pyloric stenosis, characteristic facies with thin, triangular face, prominent forehead, large eyes, protruding ears, and drooping mouth in **Bartter's syndrome**) manifestations.

Management

Therapy of the underlying etiology usually controls metabolic alkalosis.

Complications

Metabolic alkalosis, if mild, is well tolerated, but if severe, may result in hypokalemia, hypocalcemia, and other complications.

Prognosis

This will depend upon the underlying etiology of the alkalosis.

REFERENCES

1. Hermansen MC, Buches M: Urine output determination from superabsorbent and regular diapers under radiant heat, Pediatrics 1988;81:428-431.

2. Lorenz JM. Assessing fluid and electrolyte status in the newborn, Clinical Chemistry 1997;43:205-210.
3. Meyer MP, Payton MJ, Salmon A, Hutchinson C, de Klerk A: A clinical comparison of radiant warmer and incubator care for preterm infants from birth to 1800 grams. Pediatrics 2001:108:395-401.
4. Lawn CJ, Weir FJ, McGuire W: Base administration or fluid bolus for preventing morbidity and mortality in preterm infants with metabolic acidosis. Cochrane Database Syst Rev 2: CD003215, 2005 April 18.

6 NUTRITION IN THE NEWBORN

Raghavendra Rao

INTRODUCTION

Nutrition management is an important aspect of neonatal care. In spite of recent advances, malnutrition remains a significant morbidity in the neonatal intensive care unit (NICU) and after discharge. Very low birth weight (VLBW, birth weight <1500 g) and small-for-gestational age (SGA) infants are particularly vulnerable to malnutrition and its adverse impact on growth and development. There is also concern regarding the potential impact of postnatal malnutrition on the cardiovascular health during adolescence and adulthood.

GOAL OF NUTRITIONAL MANAGEMENT [1-4]

The goal of nutrition in full term infants is to ensure successful transition from fetal growth to postnatal growth. The goal in preterm infants is to maintain the intrauterine growth rate until full term (40 weeks postmenstrual age) and to support catch-up growth thereafter. An additional goal is to mimic the body composition of the age-matched fetus and to maintain normal blood and tissue concentrations of nutrients.

NUTRIENT REQUIREMENTS [1-5]

The nutrient requirements are calculated based on a combination of fetal reference values, balance studies and the serum concentrations of the nutrient. With certain exceptions, breast milk meets the nutrient requirement of full term infants. The recommended enteral intake of nutrients for preterm infants is given in Table 6.1. Energy and protein are considered "**macro" nutrients** (daily requirements: g/kg), and minerals and vitamins, "**micro" nutrients** (daily requirements: mg to mg/kg). In practice, it is difficult to provide optimal nutrition to preterm infants due to physiological immaturity of the gastrointestinal system and metabolism, presence of multiple morbidities and lack of suitable formulas. Furthermore, region-specific intrauterine growth curves are currently not available in India.[6]

Water

Water constitutes upto 80% of body weight in full term infants and nearly 90% in preterm infants at birth. Water is necessary for growth, excreting waste products (e.g. as urine) and thermoregulation (e.g. heat dissipation). The main source of water is enteral and parenteral nutrition, with a small portion gained during oxidation. Water is lost in urine and stools, and evaporation through skin. Loss through the respiratory tract is minimal under conditions of adequate humidity and temperature. The osmolality in extracellular and intracellular compartments is approximately 270-300 mOsm/L.

Healthy full term infants will regulate their **daily water intake** on *ad libitum* breastfeeding or bottle feeding. An intake between 180 and 200 mL/kg d^{-1} is typical when lactation is well established. A 5%-10% loss of body weight during the first 5-10 days of life is normal in this population.

Fluid status should be closely monitored in preterm infants. An intake of 60-80 mL/kg is provided enterally or parenterally on postnatal day 1. The volume is increased 20-30 mL/kg daily until 150-160 mL/kg d^{-1} is reached between 5 and 7 days of age.[1] Gestational and postnatal ages, birth weight, presence of illnesses and their management determine the daily water requirements (Table 6.2). Fluid and nutritional needs should be managed with close monitoring of serum electrolytes and osmolality in these conditions. Fluid management of extremely low birth weight (ELBW, birth weight <1000 g) is further discussed in the perinatal nutrition section.

Table 6.1: Recommended enteral intake of nutrients for stable, growing preterm infants

Nutrient	*Requirements (Units/kg.d⁻¹)** *ELBW*	*VLBW*	*AAP-CON§ Recommendation*
Water	160-220	135-190	
Energy (kcal)	130-150	110-130	105-130
Carbohydrate (g)	9-20	7-17	10-14
Fat (g)	6.2-8.4	5.3-7.2	5.0-7.0
Protein (g)	3.8-4.4	3.4-4.2	3.5-4.0
Vitamin A (IU)	700-1500		90 – 270
Vitamin D (IU/d)	400		400
Vitamin E (IU)	6-12		> 1.3
Vitamin K (mg)	8-10		4.8
Ascorbate (mg)	18-24		42
Thiamine (mg)	180-240		> 48
Riboflavin (mg)	250-360		> 72
Pyridoxine (mg)	150-210		> 42
Niacin (mg)	3.6-4.8		> 0.3
Pantothenate (mg)	1.2-1.7		> 0.36
Biotin (mg)	3.6-6.0		> 1.8
Folic acid (mg)	25-50		40
Vitamin B_{12} (mg)	0.3		> 0.18
Sodium (mEq)	3-7		2-3
Potassium (mEq)	2-3		1.7-2.5
Chloride (mEq)	3-7		2-3
Calcium (mg)	100-220		210
Phosphorus (mg)	60-140		110
Magnesium (mg)	8-15		
Iron (mg)	2-4		2-3
Zinc (mg)	1000-3000		> 600
Copper (mg)	120-150		110
Selenium (mg)	1.3-4.5		
Chromium (mg)	0.1-2.25		
Manganese (mg)	0.7-7.5		> 6
Molybdenum (mg)	0.3		
Iodine (mg)	10-60		6

* Consensus recommendation from Tsang *et al.* (Eds): *Nutrition of the Preterm Infant: Scientific Basis and Practical Guidelines* (2nd Rev Ed), Cincinnati, Ohio, Digital Educational Publishing, 2005.

§ American Academy of Pediatrics—Committee on Nutrition, Nutritional Needs of the Preterm Infant, In: Kleinman RE (Ed): *Pediatric Nutrition Handbook*, 5th Ed, Elk Grove Village, IL, American Academy of Pediatrics 2004, pp 23-54.

Abbreviations: *ELBW*, extremely low birth weight (<1000 g); *VLBW*, very low birth weight (<1500 g).

Table 6.2: Conditions influencing fluid requirement during the neonatal period

Conditions with increased fluid requirement
Birth weight <1000 g
Gestational age <28 weeks
Increased ambient temperature (e.g. radiant warmer)
Excessive fluid loss through gastrointestinal tract (e.g. diarrhea and vomiting)
Abdominal wall defects (e.g. gastroschisis, omphalocele, bladder extrophy)
Increased third space losses (e.g. necrotizing enterocolitis, sepsis)
Extensive denudation of skin (e.g. ruptured myelomeningocele, staphylococcal scalded skin syndrome)
Osmotic and non-osmotic diuresis (e.g. hyperglycemia, diuretic phase of acute renal failure, diabetes insipidus)
Iatrogenic causes (e.g. phototherapy, gastrointestinal suctioning)
Conditions with decreased fluid requirement
Oliguric phase of acute renal failure
Congestive heart failure
Severe pulmonary disease
Inappropriate anti-diuretic hormone secretion (e.g. following hypoxic-ischemic encephalopathy).

ENERGY [1-5, 7-9]

Adequate energy supply is necessary for physiological homeostasis and to promote postnatal growth. Energy balance is represented as

Energy intake = Energy excreted + Energy expenditure + Energy storage

The estimated energy intake for low birth weight infants is 90-120 kcal/kg d^{-1}. Approximately 15 kcal/kg d^{-1} is excreted, predominantly as loss of fats in stools and small amounts of carbohydrates and amino acids in stools and urine. Malabsorption (e.g. due to cholestasis) will increase energy excretion. Energy expenditure is the sum of energy spent for homeostasis, thermoregulation, growth and activity. It accounts for 40-75 kcal/kg d^{-1}. Under thermoneutral conditions, approximately 90% of the energy expenditure will be for maintaining homeostasis and growth, since activity levels are low soon after birth. Beyond the immediate neonatal period, physical activity accounts for 20-25% of total energy expenditure. The energy cost of synthesis and storage is approximately 3-4.5 kcal/g of new tissue. Energy storage represents energy stored (typically as protein and fat) in newly formed tissue and accounts for 20-30 kcal/kg d^{-1}. Illnesses and interventions influence energy expenditure (Table 6.3).

Table 6.3: Factors influencing energy expenditure during neonatal period

Factors that increase energy expenditure
Temperature deviations
Enteral nutrition
Physical activity
Excessive crying
Prematurity
Weight gain
Postnatal age
Respiratory distress syndrome
Bronchopulmonary dysplasia
Sepsis
Congestive heart failure
Methylxanthines[1]
Surgery
Factors that decrease energy expenditure
Thermoneutral conditions
Human milk use
Parenteral nutrition
Respiratory interventions (nasal CPAP and assisted ventilation)
Conditions associated with decreased activity (e.g. neuromuscular diseases, use of paralytic agents)
Factors that are unlikely to affect energy expenditure
Phototherapy under thermoneutral conditions
Kangaroo care
Steroid use[2]

[1] Transient effect during the initial 48 hours of treatment.

[2] The lack of effect could be secondary to the transient growth retardation associated with steroid use.

Energy Requirements

Full Term Infants

An energy intake of 100-116 kcal/kg d^{-1} is recommended between 0-3 months of age.

Preterm Infants

An intake of 105-135 kcal/kg d^{-1} is recommended for stable, growing preterm infants. The energy requirements of ELBW infants, SGA and sick preterm infants have yet to be established. Even though these infants are likely to have higher energy needs secondary to their illnesses and greater rates of catch-up growth, the current recommendation is to provide similar energy as stable preterm infants.[7]

Energy Substrates

Glucose and amino acids are the major energy substrates *in utero*. Glucose and fatty acids are used as energy source postnatally. Absorption of enterally administered energy ranges between 80% and 90% depending upon gestational age, birth weight, postnatal age, type of milk, presence of illness and use of medications. The carbohydrates and fats in milk provide 3.95 kcal/g and 9.25 kcal/g, respectively. Amino acids are predominantly used for growth after birth. When energy needs cannot be met from carbohydrates and fats, amino acids are used as energy source and provide approximately 4 kcal/g, typically after conversion to glucose.[8]

Carbohydrates

Carbohydrates provide 40%-50% of the daily calories. D-glucose (dextrose) is the main carbohydrate used in parenteral nutrition. Lactose is the predominant carbohydrate source in breast milk and formula. Preterm infants <34 weeks have low lactase activity at birth. Although the activity matures faster *ex utero*, it may be prudent to limit lactose intake.[4] Conversely, glycosidase enzymes (glucoamylase) are adequate in preterm infants. Therefore, the carbohydrate mixture in preterm formulas typically contains 40%-50% lactose and 50%-60% glucose polymers. An additional benefit of adding glucose polymers to formula is their negligible effect on osmolarity.

Lipids

There is minimal oxidation of fatty acids before birth. Most of the fatty acids transported across the placenta are stored in tissues. **Lipids** are a major source of energy after birth; 50% of energy in human milk and 40%-50% in formula is from fats. The daily intake of lipids is 5-7 gm/kg at full enteral feedings and decreases to approximately 5.5 gm/kg/d at 2 months of age. At least 3% of energy should come from **essential fatty acids**, linoleic and α-linolenic acids.

Human milk lipids are well digested by preterm infants. Adding human milk improves absorption of formula lipids due to the presence of lipases in human milk. When compared with the full term infants, absorption of saturated long chain fatty acids is lower in preterm infants due to lower bile salt pools. Medium chain fatty acids, which do not need bile salts for absorption, are better tolerated.

Additional Considerations in Preterm Infants

Long Chain Poly-Unsaturated Fatty Acids (LCPUFA)

Docosahexaenoic acid (DHA) and arachidonic acid (AA) that are present in human milk are absent in cow milk-based formulas. Preterm infants do not have the ability to synthesize docosahexaenoic acid (DHA) and arachidonic acid (AA) in sufficient quantities from their precursors, linoleic and α-linolenic acids. Hence, LCPUFAs are often added to the cow milk-based formulas. Improved visual acuity has been demonstrated with LCPUFA supplementation in preterm infants. However, the benefits appear to be short-term.

PROTEIN[1-5, 10-14]

The total **amino acid** uptake *in utero* is 3.5-4.0 gm/kg/day. Postnatally, **protein** is required for linear body growth, tissue repair, metabolism (enzymes and co-factors) and fighting infection (immunoglobulins and cytokines). Withholding amino acids after birth results in catabolism of 1-2% of body protein stores daily and may have immediate and long-term adverse impacts on growth and development. Protein catabolism is inversely related to gestational age and is double in ELBW infants when compared with full term infants. Therefore, amino acid supplementation should commence as soon after birth as possible, preferably on the first postnatal day. At least 1.0-1.5 gm/kg d^{-1} of protein is necessary to prevent catabolism. Daily intake of 3-4 gm/kg of protein is well tolerated and results in positive **nitrogen balance**.

An additional benefit of early protein supplementation is improved utilization of non-protein calories due to the stimulatory action of certain amino acids (e.g. arginine and leucine) on insulin secretion.

The absorption of protein is similar in full term and preterm infants. The efficiency of protein utilization in preterm infants is approximately 70%. Nitrogen retention is better with higher protein and energy intakes. An energy intake of 30 kcal/g of protein (energy-protein ratio) is necessary for optimal utilization of proteins. Providing non-protein energy as carbohydrates results in better nitrogen retention than lipids. However, there is a ceiling effect beyond which additional protein or energy supplementation does not promote optimal growth and body composition. There is no advantage with >50-60 non-protein calories/g of protein. Fat deposition and low serum albumin concentration are the outcome, especially if protein intake is marginal. Similarly, protein supplementation beyond 4.5 g/kg d^{-1} is unlikely to have additional benefits. Furthermore, the long-term adverse effects of such supplementation are unknown. Finally, inadequate supply of other nutrients required for tissue synthesis (e.g. Na, K and P) also adversely effect protein utilization for growth.

Protein Requirements

Full Term Infants

Human milk meets the daily protein requirements of full term infants. The protein content of human milk decreases from 1.6 g/dL during early lactation to 0.9 g/dL at 6 months. Human milk proteins have greater bioavailability than those in formula. Provision of non-nutritive proteins (e.g. growth factors, IgA and lactoferrin) is additional benefit of human milk. When breastfeeding is contraindicated or not possible, currently available formulas designed for full term infants adequately meet the daily protein requirements (Table 6.4).

Table 6.4: Selected nutrients in human milk and commonly used preterm and full term formulas in India

Nutrient (per 100 mL)	Human milk			Preterm formulas[4]		Fullterm formulas[4]			
	Full term[1]	Preterm[2]	Preterm with HMF[3]	Lactodex LBW	Dexolac special care	Prelactogen	Dexolac1	Lactogen1	NAN1
Energy (kcal)	67	67	78	80	68	70	69	67	68
Protein (g)	1.4	2.4	2.0	2.0	1.7	1.9	1.6	1.7	1.4
Carbohydrate (g)	6.6	6.1	9.4	8.9	7.5	8.0	7.4	7.5	8.3
Fat (g)	4.0	3.8	4.2	4.0	3.5	3.4	3.6	3.3	3.2
Calcium (mg)	25	25	140	128	112	91	55	62	45
Phosphorus (mg)	13	14	70	64	56	45	40	47	22
Sodium (mEq)	1.1	2.2	1.6	2.1	1.2	1.0	1.1	1.3	0.7
Iron (mg)	0.5	0.5	0.3	0.9	1.4	0.8	0.9	0.8	0.8
Vitamin A (IU)	390	560	1700	240	175	210	236	200	180
Vitamin D (IU)	2	4	500	72	70	70	38	40	29

[1] Human milk 1 month after delivery.

[2] Human milk during the first month after delivery of a preterm infant (From: Schanler RJ, Enteral nutrition for the high risk neonate. In: Taeusch HW, Ballard RA, Gleason CA (Eds), *Avery's Diseases of the Newborn* (8th Ed). Philadelphia, PA. Elsevier Saunders 2005, pp 1043-1060.

[3] Human milk fortified with 4 g/100 mL of *Lactodex-HMF*. Modified from Agarwal *et al.*, *Indian Pediatr* 2004; 41: 63-67.

[4] Approximate composition based on the nutrient content of the powder and assuming formula preparation in accordance with manufacturer's recommendation.

Lactodex-HMF and Lactodex LBW are products of Raptakos, Brett and Co. Ltd., Worli, Mumbai, India; *Dexolac Special Care* and *Dexolac1* are products of Wockhardt Ltd., Bandra (East), Mumbai, India; *Prelactogen*, *Lactogen1* and *NAN1* are products of Nestle India, Gurgaon, Haryana, India.

Preterm infants

During the transitional period soon after birth, approximately 1.0-1.5 g/kg protein is needed daily to prevent catabolism. A higher intake (1.5-2.0 g/kg/d) may be necessary in infants with gestational age <26 weeks, birth weight <1200 g and those at risk of disease-induced tissue catabolism (e.g. surgery). During the stable-growing period, higher protein intakes are necessary (Table 6.5). These recommendations are based on postmenstrual age, instead of gestational age, and take into consideration gain in lean body mass. Since energy intake has a significant effect on efficient protein accretion, the optimal protein:energy ratio (g/100 kcal) is also provided. These recommendations are based on analysis of available studies and have yet to be prospectively evaluated in large controlled studies.

Table 6.5: Recommended protein intake for stable, growing preterm infants

Post-menstrual age	*Lean body mass gain (g/kg d-1)*	*Daily protein requirements (g/kg)*	
		Without need for catch-up growth	*With need for catch-up growth*
26-30 weeks	16-18	3.8-4.2 PER: ~3.3	4.4 PER: ~3.4
30-36 weeks	14-15	3.4-3.6 PER: ~2.8	3.8-4.2 PER: ~3.3
36-40 weeks	13	2.8-3.2 PER: 2.4-2.6	3.0-3.4 PER: 2.6-2.8

Modified from Rigo J. Protein, amino acid and other nitrogen compounds. In Tsang R *et al.* (Eds): Nutrition of the Preterm Infant: Scientific Basis and Practical Guidelines (2nd Rev Ed), Cincinnati, Ohio, Digital Educational Publishing, 2005, pp 45-80.

Abbreviation: *PER,* Protein Energy Ratio (g/100 kcal).

Additional Considerations in Preterm Infants

Due to their physiological immaturity, arginine, cysteine, glutamine, glycine, histidline, proline, taurine and tyrosine are considered conditionally essential amino acids for preterm infants. Carnitine (which is essential for fatty acid metabolism) and nucleotides are other nitrogen compounds that are considered essential in preterm nutrition.

MINERALS [1-5, 15-18]

Sodium, potassium, calcium, magnesium and phosphorus are "macro" **minerals** in newborn nutrition. Iron, zinc, copper, selenium, chromium, molybdenum, manganese and iodine are considered "micro" minerals (Table 6.1).

Sodium (Na) and Potassium (K)

The daily requirement of Na and K during the stable and growing period is 2 to 3 mEq/kg, each. Requirements are higher with chronic administration of diuretics. It is not unusual to have requirements of 8-10 mEq/kg d^{-1}. Chloride salts are typically administered; however, acetate salts may be used in presence of metabolic acidosis. Breast milk has low Na content. Combined with a higher fractional excretion of Na in urine and the frequent use of diuretics, this predisposes the preterm infant to hyponatremia. Persistent hyponatremia also may be a manifestation of total body K deficiency (e.g. due to prolonged diuretic usage). Even though serum K levels may be normal, supplementation of K, along with Na, is necessary to correct hyponatremia in this situation.

Calcium (Ca), Magnesium (Mg) and Phosphorus (P)

80% of the total body Ca, Mg and P is accreted during the third trimester. Therefore, preterm infants are at risk for osteopenia and should be periodically screened for the condition. It is not possible to meet the daily requirements of these minerals with unfortified human milk and formulas designed for full term infants. Bone mineralization is better with fortified human milk and preterm formulas.

IRON [15, 17-19]

Iron is a paradoxical element: both deficiency and excess are associated with adverse effects. **Iron** deficiency is more prevalent than iron excess. The iron concentration in human milk is low (approximately, 0.5 g/dL). However, it meets the daily requirements in full term infants due to better bioavailability. Therefore, additional iron supplementation is not necessary for breastfed full term infants, provided iron-rich food items are used during weaning.

Preterm infants who are exclusively breastfed, ELBW and who received few or no red blood cell (RBC) transfusions are at risk of iron deficiency. There is controversy about the dose, time of initiation and duration of iron supplementation. The current recommendation is to provide 2-4 mg/kg d^{-1} of iron to exclusively human milk-fed preterm infants from 1 month of age.[1,2] Supplementation is recommended until 12 months of age. An intake of 1 mg/kg d^{-1} is recommended for preterm infants receiving iron-fortified formula.[1] While some human milk fortifiers adequately meet the daily iron requirements, others do not. In such instances, additional iron supplementation is necessary. Infants receiving recombinant human erythropoietin require 6 mg/kg d^{-1} of iron.[1]

VITAMINS [1,4,15]

Water-Soluble Vitamins

Many water-soluble **vitamins** play essential roles in amino acid and carbohydrate metabolism. Human milk meets the daily requirements of full term infants. Supplementation is necessary for preterm infants due to their higher protein requirements, low body reserves and loss of vitamins during storage and handling of human milk. Supplementation can be achieved using vitamin-containing human milk fortifiers or supplementation with formula milk. Both full term and preterm formula have adequate levels of water-soluble vitamins.

Fat-Soluble Vitamins

Vitamin A

Preterm infants are at risk of vitamin A deficiency due to a combination of low reserves and inefficient absorption from the gastrointestinal tract. This can be ameliorated using human milk fortifiers or a preterm formula. Vitamin supplementation reduces the severity of bronchopulmonary dysplasia in VLBW infants with underlying vitamin A deficiency (serum level <20 µg/L). Therefore, we administer 5000 IU of vitamin A intramuscularly to infants with birth weight <1200 g, three times a week during the first month of life or until the establishment of full enteral feedings. We monitor serum retinol levels periodically, since hypervitaminosis A has detrimental effects.

Vitamin D

Unless the mother has deficiency, vitamin D deficiency is rare during the newborn period. A daily intake of 400 IU of vitamin D is recommended to human milk-fed preterm infants. Fortified human milk and commercial formulas have adequate vitamin D levels.

Vitamin E

Excess amounts of polyunsaturated fatty acids in the presence of vitamin E deficiency results in hemolytic anemia, especially if iron supplementation is also undertaken. An enteral intake of 6-12 IU/kg d^{-1} is recommended. There is no evidence that higher doses prevent oxidant-associated neonatal disorders, such as retinopathy of prematurity.

Vitamin K

Vitamin K deficiency results in hemorrhagic disease of the newborn. An intramuscular injection of 1 mg phylloquinone prevents this disorder in full term infants. Preterm infants are given half the dose. We add 1 mg of vitamin K to the intravenous solution twice a week in infants on total parenteral nutrition.

METHODS OF NUTRITION DELIVERY [1-5, 20-22]

Nutrition during the newborn period can be provided via enteral or parenteral route. Enteral nutrition is preferred due to its physiological benefits, safety and feasibility, and avoidance of parenteral nutrition-associated complications.

Enteral Nutrition

Early Enteral Nutrition (Trophic Feeding) [20, 23]

Initiation of early **enteral nutrition** promotes growth, maturation and function of the gastrointestinal tract. Direct contact with breast milk increases mucosal mass and improves local host defense. Gastrointestinal motility is better due to the stimulatory effect of milk on hormonal secretion. As a result, feedings are better tolerated and full volume feedings are reached sooner. The other advantages of early enteral nutrition are better weight gain, improved mother's milk supply, decreased parenteral nutrition-associated sepsis and cholestasis, and less need for photothearpy.

More importantly, these beneficial effects are achieved without an increased predisposition to necrotizing enterocolitis.

There is no uniform definition of trophic feeding (i.e. time of initiation, volume, frequency etc). Typically, <25 mL/kg d^{-1} (<20 kcal/ kg d^{-1}) of full strength human milk or half- or full-strength formula is started between 1 and 7 days after birth.[23] Feedings can be administered intermittently or continuously. The feeding volume is held constant for 5 days and the nutritional needs are met via parenteral nutrition.[23]

Necrotizing enterocolitis, significant ileus, gastrointestinal hemorrhage and intestinal obstruction are the few contraindications for early enteral nutrition. Trophic feeds can be safely used in the presence of low Apgar score, umbilical catheters, apnea and bradycardia, mechanical ventilation, CPAP, phototherapy, sepsis, steroid administration, maternal magnesium sulfate and low doses of vasoactive drugs. In our unit, we withhold trophic feedings during and for 24 hours after the last dose of indomethacin or ibuprofen administration for patent ductus arteriosus. However, this is not a universal practice.

Enteral Nutrition during the Stable-Growing Phase

The goal of nutrition during this phase is to meet the full energy and protein requirements of catch-up growth and achieve optimal body composition until discharge from the NICU.

Human Milk [5, 22-25]

Human milk is ideal for newborn nutrition. It is better tolerated than formula milk and full volume feedings are reached earlier. Human milk proteins have better bioavailability, are rich in tryptophan and cysteine and low in methionine and phenylalanine, when compared with cow milk-based formulas. The concentration of glutamine, which promotes intestinal development, also is higher in human milk. Human milk lipids are better absorbed than the cow milk lipids and vegetable oils. Oligosaccharides, LCPUFAs and nucleotides present in human milk have beneficial effects on neurodevelopment.

Use of own mother's milk protects against necrotizing enterocolitis, nosocomial infection, diarrhea and urinary tract infection in preterm infants. Similar protective effects are also seen in preterm infants receiving both human milk and formula, provided the intake of human milk is at least 50 mL/ kg d^{-1}. An additional benefit is lower incidence of atopy (e.g. cow milk protein allergy) in the infant.

There is a large variation in the nutrient composition of human milk, depending upon the stage of lactation (Table 6.4), collection and storage methods, and method of administration. Protein, Na and zinc content decrease from transitional period to mature milk. The content of Ca and P have less variability. Vitamins A and C and riboflavin decrease with storage.

Preterm infants fed human milk require close monitoring of their nutritional state. Compared with the mothers who have delivered full term infants, milk from mothers of preterm infants contains higher concentration of fat, protein and Na, but lower concentrations of lactose, Ca, and P during the first 2 to 3 weeks after delivery. Beyond that period, the composition is comparable to the milk from mothers of full term infants. After the commencement of growth, unfortified human milk does not adequately meet the protein, Ca, P, Mg, Na, copper, zinc, riboflavin, pyridoxine, folic acid, ascorbic acid, and vitamins D, E and K requirements of preterm infants.

Mothers of preterm infants should be encouraged to express their milk within the first 24 hours of delivery. Hind milk has higher fat content than fore milk. Therefore, when growth is suboptimal, exclusive use of hind milk may be attempted before considering formula. Infants can be fed freshly expressed or stored milk. Milk stored in the refrigerator at -4°C can be used upto 48 hours after collection. Milk stored at -20°C in freezer retains most of its immunological properties and vitamin contents for 3 months. Frozen milk should be thawed before feeding by holding in a basin of lukewarm water. Thawing in a microwave should be avoided since the method destroys immunoglobulin A and lysozyme activities.

Infants with coordinated sucking, swallowing and respiration may be allowed to breastfeed. Emptying of the milk from the breast during feeding promotes better milk production. Therefore, full term infants should be encouraged to breastfeed from predominantly one breast during a feeding. Preterm infants may tire with the effort involved with such feeding. Since milk output is greater during the initial phase of breastfeeding, feeding from both breasts at each feeding allows greater intake by preterm infants.

Donor Milk [25]

When own mother's milk is not available, **donor milk** may be used. However, this entails rigorous screening of the donor and/or donor milk for blood-borne pathogens, determining the nutrient composition and pasteurization of the donor milk. The collection and storage methods also affect the nutritive and anti-infectious properties of the donor milk. A centralized system for collecting and processing the milk is ideal. The donors are typically mothers of full term infants and the milk is obtained during later stages of lactation. Therefore, fortification is necessary.

Fortification of Human Milk [1,5,26]

Without fortification with a human milk fortifier (HMF) or supplementation with a preterm formula, human milk does not adequately meet the nutritional needs of preterm infants <34 weeks gestation. Exclusive use of unfortified, own mother's or donor milk is associated with lower rates of growth during stay in NICU that persists post-discharge. Compared with infants fed formula or fortified human milk, weight gain, length and skin fold thickness are lower in these infants. Head circumference is typically unaffected. Blood urea nitrogen, serum albumin, prealbumin, total protein and phosphorus concentrations are lower, and Ca and alkaline phosphatase levels higher in preterm infants fed unfortified human milk.

Fortification of human milk is recommended for VLBW infants when enteral feeding reaches 100 mL/kg d^{-1}. Fortification may be attempted early (e.g. at 50 mL/kg d^{-1}) when weight gain has been poor for extended period. Human milk fortified with energy and protein (Table 6.4) is associated with better weight gain, increments in length and head circumference. The beneficial effects are cumulative. Supplementation of Ca and P normalizes bone mineralization. Fortification does not diminish the anti-infectious properties of the human milk and is not associated with significant feeding intolerance.

Additional mineral and vitamin supplementations are not necessary when using HMF-fortified human milk with the exception of iron, which is absent in the HMF available in India (Table 6.4). Supplementation of 2-4 mg/kg d^{-1} iron is therefore necessary. Similarly, infants receiving diuretics long-term may need additional supplementation of Na, K and Cl. When human milk fortifiers are not available, vegetable oils may be used to enhance energy delivery to preterm infants.[26] However, additional protein, mineral and vitamin supplementation is necessary in such situations.

Formulas for Preterm Infants

The composition of commonly used **preterm formulas** in India is given in Table 6.4. Generally, these cow milk-based formulas contain higher concentration of protein and minerals than full term formulas and have lactose and glucose polymers as carbohydrate sources and medium-chain triglycerides as a significant source of lipids. Whey-predominant formulas are usually preferred, even though currently available casein-based formulas are well tolerated. Soy-based formulas are not recommended, as there is insufficient information on the absorption and utilization of energy and protein from these formulas. Hydrolyzed formulas are thought to reduce gastrointestinal disturbances. However, hydrolysis affects amino acid content and availability. The physical form (powder vs. liquid) also appears to affect the digestibility of the proteins in formulas.

Feeding Methods for Preterm Infants [5,21]

Gestational age, birth weight and clinical condition are taken into consideration while determining the type of feeding, method of delivery and rate of advancement (Figure 6.1). Stable infants who exhibit coordinated sucking and swallowing (generally ≥34 weeks) may be allowed to breastfeed or bottle-feed. Cup-feeding is also appropriate in this population. Infants <37-38 weeks' gestation should be closely monitored as their oral intake may be inadequate due to weak sucking and swallowing.

Tube Feeding (Gavage Feeding)

Premature infants <32-34 weeks' gestation and those who lack coordinated sucking, swallowing and breathing require feeding via nasogastric or orogastric tube. The former is easier to maintain

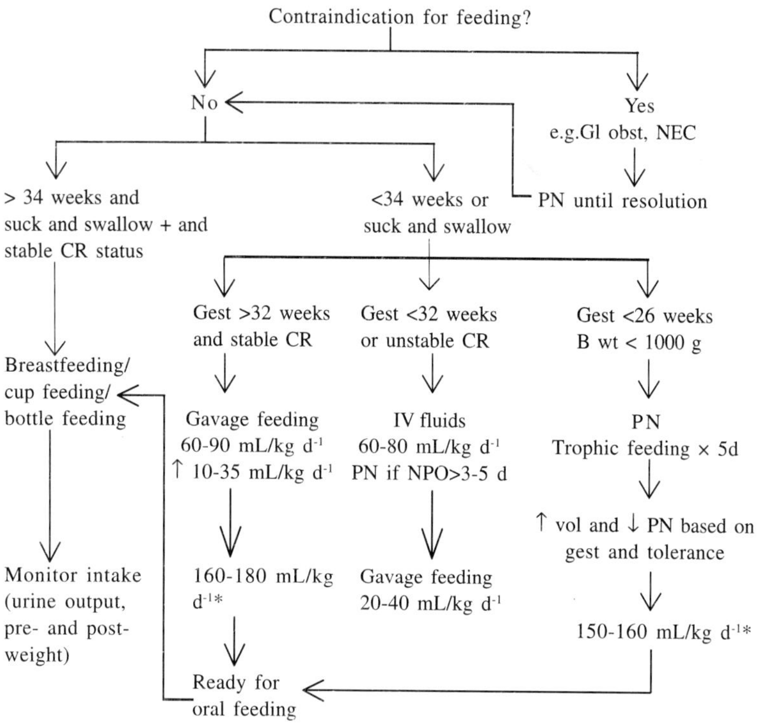

Fig. 6.1: Guidelines for nutrition management in the newborn infant. Stable CR status = Stable cardiovascular (normal perfusion, BP and heart rate) and respiratory (rate <60/min and absence of respiratory distress/apnea) status

*Consider fortification of human milk when feeding volume reaches 100 ml/kg/d.
BP: blood pressure, B wt: birth weight, Gest: gestational age, GI: gastrointestinal,
IV: intravenous, NPO: nil per os, NEC: necrotizing enterocolitis, PN: parenteral nutrition

long-term, but may increase upper airway resistance and work of breathing. Ensuring the correct position of the tube by checking for gastric aspirates or by auscultating over the stomach area after injecting a small amount of air is essential before giving the feeding.

Feedings can commence within 2-3 hours of birth in healthy preterm infants with birth weight >1500 g. A volume of 60-90 mL/kg d^{-1} is provided on first day after birth. Feedings can be provided as gravity-assisted bolus feedings or using a pump every 2 to 4 hours, depending on birth weight and gestation. Feeding is increased 10-35 mL/kg daily until 150-180 mL/kg d^{-1} is reached between 1 and 2 weeks. Providing non-nutritive sucking during tube feeding shortens the time to achieve sucking feedings.

Beginning oral feeding when the infant demonstrates readiness allows transition from gavage feeding at an earlier gestational age. Therefore, providers should be attentive to the infant's cues (e.g. rooting and sucking) during gavage feedings.

Smaller infants and those with feeding intolerance may require continuous feeding given using a pump. Feeding tolerance is better and energy expenditure lower with continuous feeding. However, continuous feeding results in loss of energy, protein and micronutrients in the milk. The milk fats separate and tend to rise to the top over time. Using shorter tubes and positioning the syringe upright during feeding ensures better delivery of fats. Another problem with continuous feeding is greater risk of bacterial contamination. In exceptional conditions (e.g. pulmonary aspiration) transpyloric (e.g. naso-jejunal) or gastrotomy feeding may be necessary. Transpyloric feeding is provided as continuous feeding using a pump; both continuous and intermittent feedings are possible via gastrostomy.

PARENTERAL NUTRITION [1,15,16,27]

Parenteral nutrition (PN) meets the fluid and nutrition needs of the infant when sufficient enteral nutrition is not expected for extended periods. PN can be used to support the complete nutritional needs (total PN) or supplement enteral nutrition (partial PN). VLBW infants who are not expected to receive enteral nutrition for >3 days and full term infants for >5 days are considered candidates for PN in the Indian context.[27] PN as the sole source of nutrition is rarely needed beyond 2 to 3 weeks in most infants. Even though long-term PN is feasible with appropriate fluids and delivery systems, it is expensive and associated with significant complications.

Composition of PN Solution

The goal of PN is to avoid dehydration or over-hydration, support growth and maintain stable osmolality and nutrient levels in the serum. Standardized or individualized formulations are used. A centralized location for preparing and dispensing PN solution is optimal.

Energy

Dextrose is the major energy source in PN. It has a caloric value of 3.4 kcal/g and 10% dextrose in water is typically used soon after birth. A **glucose infusion rate** (GIR) of 4-6 mg/kg/min is necessary to meet the cellular energy needs. An initial infusion rate ≥ 6 mg/kg/min may result in hyperglycemia (serum glucose >125 mg/dL) in ELBW infants. However, a steady daily increase of GIR by 2-4 mg/kg/min stimulates endogenous insulin secretion, and most infants tolerate a GIR of 11-12 mg/kg/min between 5 and 7 days. Administration of exogenous **insulin** may be necessary for hyperglycemia. The routine administration of insulin to improve glucose tolerance is considered investigational and is not recommended.

Intravenous lipid is another energy source in PN. Withholding lipids for an extended period results in essential fatty acid deficiency. Emulsions containing soyabean oil and/or safflower oil are commonly used. A 20% preparation is tolerated better than 10% preparation and has a caloric value of 2 kcal/mL. It has same osmolality as plasma and does not cause irritation of peripheral veins. Infusion is started at an initial dose of 0.5 to 1.0 g/kg/d and increased to a maximum of 3.0-4.0 g/kg d^{-1} over a period of 3 to 7 days. Infusion is given over a period of 16 to 24 hours.

Following infusion, the triglycerides are hydrolyzed to fatty acids and glycerol, which are further metabolized. If the rate of infusion exceeds the rate of hydrolysis, **serum triglyceride** concentrations increase. Lipid tolerance is determined by monitoring serum triglyceride levels, which should be kept <150 mg/dL. Addition of carnitine to PN solution may improve lipid tolerance by promoting oxidation of free fatty acids. However, since the data have been contradictory, carnitine supplementation should be considered in ELBW infants or when TPN is contemplated for >4 weeks. While serum fatty acid levels increase following lipid infusion, there is no data that these fatty acids would displace serum bilirubin from its binding sites. Therefore, lipids may be used during hyperbilirubinemia.

Amino Acids

Crystalline amino acids designed for infants should be used for PN. Compared with casein hydrolysates, metabolic acidosis, hyperaminoacidemia and hyperammonemia are rare with crystalline amino acids. Intravenous amino acids should be provided at 1-2 gm/kg d^{-1} within 24 hours of birth to avoid a catabolic state. To achieve positive nitrogen balance and achieve intrauterine rates of growth, an intake of 3-4 g/kg d^{-1} of amino acids and 80-120 kcal/kg d^{-1} of non-protein calories is necessary.

Electrolytes and Minerals

The recommended electrolyte and mineral intake for PN is given in Table 6.6. Intakes are adjusted subsequently based on serum levels. In the case of Ca and P, an additional goal is to prevent osteopenia. The pH of the solution affects Ca and P solubility. Addition of cysteine lowers the pH of the solution and allows greater amounts of Ca and P. Among the trace minerals, only zinc is necessary if TPN is needed for < 1 to 2 weeks. Selenium, copper, chromium and molybdenum are added if TPN is needed for more than 2-4 weeks. The iron requirements are typically met from the frequent RBC transfusions given to the preterm infants. During long-term PN, iron can be added to the PN solution or can be

Table 6.6: Recommended intakes of electrolyte and minerals for parenteral nutrition

Electrolytes and Minerals	*(Amount/kg day^{-1})*
Sodium (mEq)	3-4
Potassium (mEq)	2-4
Chloride (mEq)	3-4
Calcium (mg)	40-80
Magnesium (mEq)	0.25-0.5
Phosphorus (mMol)	0.5-1.5
Microminerals[1]	
Zinc (μg)	200-400
Copper (μg)	20
Selenium (μg)	2.0
Chromium (μg)	0.2
Manganese (μg)	1.0
Molybdenum (μg)	0.25
Iodide (μg)	1.0
Iron (μg)[2]	100

[1] Only zinc is necessary if parenteral nutrition is short-term (<1-2 weeks).

[2] Not necessary unless prolonged total parenteral nutrition.

intermittently administered as intramuscular injection of iron dextran 0.1 mg/kg.

Vitamins

A multivitamin preparation that provides optimal quantities of all vitamins to newborn infants is currently not available in India. Adult multivitamin preparation in a dose of 0.1 ml/kg is recommended.[27] Fat-soluble vitamins, especially vitamin A, adhere to plastic tubing during infusion. Administering vitamin mixture in lipid infusion overcomes this to some extent.

Routes of Administration

PN can be delivered using a peripheral or central vein. The solution should be infused at a constant rate using a pump.

Peripheral PN

PN through a peripheral vein is adequate for infants who are likely to receive sufficient enteral nutrition within 7-10 days. Intakes of 2.5-3.0 gm/kg d^{-1} of amino acids and lipids, each, can be safely delivered via this route. However, glucose concentration greater than 12.5% causes local irritation of peripheral veins. Combined with fluid restriction to 150 ml/kg d^{-1} that is often necessary, this limits the total energy intake to <80 kcal/kg d^{-1}, even with 3 gm/kg d^{-1} of intravenous lipids. Sloughing of the skin and subcutaneous tissue due to extravasation of hypertonic and Ca-containing PN solution and the relatively short life span of catheters in peripheral veins are other problems associated with peripheral PN. To prevent sloughing of the skin, the osmolality of the PN solution should be <1000 mOsm/L. Often this requires restricting amino acids and/or multivitamins in the PN solution.

Central PN

PN through a central vein allows >50% greater energy delivery than peripheral PN. PN solutions containing Ca and 20% to 30% dextrose can be infused. A catheter is placed surgically or inserted percutaneously and positioned in a central vein, such as superior or inferior vena cava. Silastic catheters are preferred over polyvinyl catheters, which tend to harden over time. Radiographic confirmation of the catheter is mandatory.

Strategies of PN

The endogenous nutritional state of the infant should be taken into consideration while determining PN therapy.

Infants with Birth Weight >1500 g

Most of these infants are stable and can be started on enteral feedings soon after birth (see above). Those who need PN are started on 60-80 mL/kg of 10% dextrose. In our unit we infuse a premixed "starter" parenteral solution containing 10% dextrose and crystalline amino acids. When infused at a volume of 60 ml/kg d^{-1} it provides a GIR of 4.2 mg/kg/min and 2 gm/kg d^{-1} of amino acids. Na, K and Cl are added to the fluid on the second day or third day. We also start intravenous lipids in a dose of 2 g/kg and vitamin supplementation on the second day. The fluid volume is increased by 20-30 mL/kg daily to a total intake of 150 mL/kg d^{-1} between 5 and 7 days of age. Amino acids and intravenous lipids are increased by 0.5-1.0 g/kg daily to a maximum of 3.0-3.5 g/kg d^{-1}, each. Enteral nutrition is started within 1-2 days of birth and PN beyond the first week of life is rarely needed for these infants. Therefore, other minerals and trace elements are not typically necessary and PN can be provided using a peripheral vein.

Infants with Birth Weight <1500 g

PN is the mainstay of nutrition for these infants due to the physiological immaturity of the gastrointestinal tract and cardiopulmonary instability. The fluid requirements are high during initial 5-7 days due to increased insensible and urinary losses and may be as high as 160-220 mL/kg d^{-1} in ELBW infants. Fluid administration should be tailored taking into consideration daily weight loss, urine output and serum electrolytes. Hypernatremia (serum sodium >150 mEq/L) is common due to excessive free water loss. Therefore, sodium is withheld until serum sodium is <140 mEq/L. Due to the potential for hyperglycemia, GIR should be increased gradually. Beyond first 1-2 days, these infants need Ca, Mg and P. Amino acids and intravenous lipids are infused as above. Once the stable growing phase is reached, 140-160 mL/kg fluid, 2-4 mEq/kg Na, K and Cl, and 3.5-4.0 gm/kg amino acid and intravenous lipids, each, are required to support growth. Carnitine (10-20 mg/kg) may be added to the solution if the infant is ELBW or PN is needed for >2-4 weeks. Minimal enteral feeding should be started as soon as possible. As increasing volumes of enteral feedings are tolerated, PN infusion rate is reduced. PN can be stopped when enteral intake reaches >100 mL/kg d^{-1}.

Complications of PN

The complications associated with PN can be classified as infusion-related complications and metabolic complications (Table 6.7).

Infusion-Related Complications

Infection is the most significant infusion-related complication. It is usually related to improper care of the insertion site and rarely due to contaminated PN solution. Proper asepsis during catheter

Table 6.7: Complications associated with parenteral nutrition

Infusion-related complications
Central TPN
Sepsis
Thrombosis of the vein
Malposition and dislodgement of catheter.
Peripheral TPN
Thrombophlebitis
Sloughing of the skin due to infiltration of the hypertonic solution.
Metabolic complications
Related to metabolic capacity of the infant
Hyperglycemia/hypoglycemia
Azotemia
Excess or deficiency of electrolytes and minerals.
Related to the infusate composition
Abnormal plasma aminograms
Hypercholesterolemia
Abnormal fatty acid pattern
Cholestasis.

insertion and meticulous monitoring for infection at the insertion site is mandatory. An antiseptic ointment should be applied to the insertion site and the dressing should be changed every other day. Avoiding the use of catheter for purposes other than nutrient delivery, such as blood draws and infusion of medications and blood products, also reduces the risk of infection. Risk of infection is less with peripheral PN than central PN.

Metabolic Complications

Metabolic complications could be related to infant's limited metabolic capacity, the infusate *per se* or non-participation of gastrointestinal system in nutrition. Disorders related to glucose, electrolytes and minerals are usually due to the provision of either too much or too little of the respective nutrient. Compared with the breastfed infant, the concentrations of many amino acids (e.g. cysteine and tyrosine) are lower in infants on PN. This is a reflection of the currently available amino acid mixtures. Similarly, fatty acid pattern may be abnormal due to the relatively low concentration of LCPUFA in the infusate and the inability of the preterm infants to synthesize them from their precursors. Clinical and histological evidence of cholestasis is seen in many infants maintained on TPN for long periods. The etiology of this condition has yet to be established. Minimal enteral feeding reduces this complication.

Many of the PN associated complications can be minimized using a monitoring schedule. Institutions should establish a monitoring schedule based on their patient demographics and hospital practices. The monitoring system used in our NICU and the one recommended for Indian nurseries is given in Table 6.8. We do not routinely check complete blood count (CBC) as a screen for sepsis. When sepsis is suspected, CBC and appropriate cultures are obtained. More frequent monitoring is necessary during the initial few days of PN. Checking for glycosuria and visual inspection of plasma for lipemia may be used to screen for glucose and lipid tolerance, respectively.

NUTRITIONAL MONITORING [4,6,11,27]

Growth Guidelines

Region- and population-specific, intrauterine and postnatal growth curves are currently not available in India.[6] The goal is to achieve a gain 10-20 g/kg d^{-1} in weight, 0.75-1 cm/week in length and 0.75-1 cm/week in head circumference. A day-to-day change in weight may be a reflection of fluctuating fluid balance and not linear growth *per se*. Persistent growth failure for >2-4 weeks, especially if associated with static head circumference requires additional nutritional rehabilitation. If full volume enteral feedings have yet to be established, increasing the volume should be the first step, as this would provide supplementation of all nutrients. Growth failure after the establishment of full volume feedings requires additional supplementation of protein (maximum: 4.5 g/kg d^{-1} from all sources) and energy (26-28 kcal/oz, maximum 30 kcal/oz from all sources).

Laboratory Monitoring

Blood urea nitrogen (BUN) and serum creatinine can be used as screening tools for adequacy of protein intake. In the absence of renal disease, low BUN reflects poor protein intake and creatinine,

Table 6.8: Suggested laboratory monitoring for infants receiving parenteral nutrition

Laboratory test	*Schedule practiced at University of Minnesota*	*Schedule recommended for Indian nurseries*[1]
Glucose and electrolytes	Daily during first week, then on alternate days	Daily (glucose)
Ca, Mg, P	On days 3 and 5 of first week of PN, then twice a week	
Triglycerides	On days 3 and 5 of first week of PN, then twice a week	Once a week
BUN, creatinine and HCO_3	Once a week	Once in 48-72 hours
Prealbumin	Once a week	
Bilirubin (total and direct)	Once a week	
Alkaline phosphatase	Once a week	
Liver function tests	When cholestasis is suspected	When cholestasis is suspected
Complete Blood Count	When sepsis is suspected	Once a week

[1] Tagare A, Vaidya U: *J Neonatology* 2007; 21: 186-188

the muscle mass. Weekly assessment of prealbumin (transthyretin), which indexes recent protein intake, is another serum marker for determining the need for protein supplementation. Serum alkaline phosphatase is an index of bone mineralization. Rapidly increasing alkaline phosphatase levels reflect osteopenia and need for Ca and P supplementation. Increased loss of P in urine is also seen in osteopenia. Higher alkaline phosphatase levels during NICU stay are associated with reduced linear growth lasting until 9-12 years of age. It is prudent to monitor hemoglobin weekly, since severe anemia may result in growth failure. As both iron deficiency and iron overload are common in preterm infants, serum ferritin should be monitored periodically (e.g. during postnatal erythropoiesis and catch-up growth, and before discharge) to determine the adequacy of iron supply.

Post-Discharge Nutrition of Preterm Infants

Fortification of human milk after discharge is neither practical nor desirable. Exclusive breastfeeding *ad libitum* will be sufficient for preterm infants >34 weeks' gestation and >2500 g birth weight. Poor growth, osteopenia and excessive fat deposition have been reported in preterm infants fed non-fortified human milk exclusively post-discharge. Formulas designed for full term are also inappropriate for preterm infants. Preterm infants, with a history of poor weight gain or abnormal nutrient indices, being discharged on breast milk may benefit from 1-2 feedings of a post-discharge enriched formula.

Supplementation is recommended until catch-up growth is achieved or until 9 months post-discharge, whichever is earlier. Post-discharge enriched formulas are also recommended for preterm infants whose mothers choose not to breastfeed.

Vitamin Supplementation Post-Discharge

Commercially available multivitamin preparations contain adequate levels of fat-soluble vitamins with the exception of vitamin K. Relatively few of the water-soluble vitamins are provided. We supplement exclusively breastfed full-term and preterm infants with a multivitamin preparation containing vitamin D and iron at the time of discharge and recommend supplementation until 1 year of age. Vitamin supplementation is not necessary for those receiving formula feeding.

ACKNOWLEDGEMENTS

The author is grateful to Drs. Praveen Kumar, Srinivas Murki, Naveen Jain and Jaikrishan Mittal, and Ana A. Sinha of Nestle India for providing composition of formula milks available in India, and to Caitlyn Nysted for assistance with manuscript preparation.

REFERENCES

1. American Academy of Pediatrics—Committee on Nutrition: Nutritional Needs of the Preterm Infant, In: Kleinman RE (Ed) *Pediatric Nutrition Handbook* (5th Ed), Elk Grove Village, IL, American Academy of Pediatrics 2004, pp 23-54.
2. Nutrition Committee, Canadian Pediatric Society: Nutrient needs and feeding of premature infants, *Can Med Assoc J* 1995; 152: 1765-1785.
3. Committee on Nutrition of the Preterm Infant, European Society of Paediatric Gastroenterology and Nutrition. Nutrition and feeding of preterm infants, Acta Paediatr Scand Suppl 1987;336:1-14.
4. Georgieff MK: Nutrition, In: MacDonald MG, Mullett MD, Seshia MMK (Eds): *Avery's Neonatology: Pathophysiology and Management of the Newborn* (6th Ed), Philadelphia, PA, Lippincott Williams and Wilkins 2005, pp 380-412.
5. Schanler RJ: Enteral nutrition for the high risk neonate, In: Taeusch HW, Ballard RA, Gleason CA (Eds): *Avery's Diseases of the Newborn* (8th Ed), Philadelphia, PA, Elsevier Saunders 2005, pp 1043-1060.
6. Bhat SR: Postnatal growth in VLBW neonates, *J Neonatology* 2007; 21: 203-207.
7. Hulzebos CV, Sauer PJ: Energy requirements, Semin Fetal Neonatal Med 2007;12: 2-10.
8. Kashyap S, Schulze KF: Energy requirements and protein-energy metabolism and balance in preterm and term infants, In: Thureen PJ, Hay WW (Eds), *Neonatal Nutrition and Metabolism* (2nd Ed), Cambridge, United Kingdom, Cambridge University Press 2006, pp 134-146.
9. Leitch CA, Denne SC: Energy, In: Tsang R, Uauy R, Koletzko B, Zlotkin SH (Eds): *Nutrition of the Preterm Infant: Scientific Basis and Practical Guidelines* (2nd Rev Ed), Cincinnati, Ohio, Digital Educational Publishing 2005, pp 23-44.
10. Reynolds RM, Bass KD, Thureen PJ: Achieving positive protein balance in the immediate postoperative period in neonates undergoing abdominal surgery, J Pediatr 2008;152:63-67.
11. Ridout E, Melara D, Rottinghaus S, Thureen PJ. Blood urea nitrogen concentration as a marker of amino-acid intolerance in neonates with birthweight less than 1250 g. J Perinatol 2005;25:130-33.
12. Rigo J: Protein, amino acid and other nitrogen compounds, In: Tsang R, Uauy R, Koletzko B, Zlotkin SH (Eds): *Nutrition of the Preterm Infant:*

Scientific Basis and Practical Guidelines (2nd Rev Ed), Cincinnati, Ohio, Digital Educational Publishing 2005, pp 45-80.
13. te Braake FW, van den Akker CH, Riedijk MA, van Goudoever JB: Parenteral amino acid and energy administration to premature infants in early life. Semin Fetal Neonatal Med 2007;12:11-18.
14. Thureen PJ, Melara D, Fennessey PV, Hay WW, Jr: Effect of low versus high intravenous amino acid intake on very low birth weight infants in the early neonatal period, Pediatr Res 2003;53(1):24-32.
15. Heird WC: Intravenous feeding, In: Thureen PJ, Hay WW (Eds): *Neonatal Nutrition and Metabolism* (2nd Ed), Cambridge, United Kingdom, Cambridge University Press, 2006, pp 312-331.
16. Poindexter BB, Denne SC: Parenteral nutrition, In: Taeusch HW, Ballard RA, Gleason CA (Eds): *Avery's Diseases of the Newborn* (8th Ed) Philadelphia, PA, Elsevier Saunders 2005, pp 1061-1070.
17. Rao R, Georgieff MK: Microminerals, In: Tsang R, Uauy R, Koletzko B, Zlotkin SH (Eds): *Nutrition of the Preterm Infant: Scientific Basis and Practical Guidelines* (2nd Rev Ed), Cincinnati, Ohio, Digital Educational Publishing 2005, pp 277-310.
18. Rao R, Georgieff MK: Iron in fetal and neonatal nutrition, Semin Fetal Neonatal Med 2007;12:54-63.
19. Siddappa AM, Rao R, Long JD, Widness JA, Georgieff MK: The assessment of newborn iron stores at birth: A review of the literature and standards for ferritin concentrations, Neonatology 2007;92:73-82.
20. Reynolds RM, Thureen PJ: Special circumstances: Trophic feeds, necrotizing enterocolitis and bronchopulmonary dysplasia, Semin Fetal Neonatal Med 2007;12:64-70.
21. Yu VH, Simmer K: Enteral nutrition: Practical aspects, strategy and management. In: Tsang R, Uauy R, Koletzko B, Zlotkin SH (Eds), *Nutrition of the Preterm Infant: Scientific Basis and Practical Guidelines* (2nd Rev Ed), Cincinnati, Ohio, Digital Educational Publishing 2005, pp 311-332.
22. Marinelli KA, Hamelin K: Breastfeeding and use of human milk in the neonatal intensive care unit, In: MacDonald MG, Mullett MD, Seshia MMK (Eds): *Avery's Neonatology: Pathophysiology and Management of the Newborn* (6th Ed), Philadelphia, PA, Lippincott Williams and Wilkins 2005, pp 413-444.
23. Neu J: Minimal enteral nutrition, In: Thureen PJ, Hay WW (Eds): *Neonatal Nutrition and Metabolism* (2nd Ed), Cambridge, United Kingdom, Cambridge University Press 2006, pp 369-376.
24. Heiman H, Schanler RJ: Benefits of maternal and donor human milk for premature infants, Early Hum Dev 2006;82:781-87.
25. Heiman H, Schanler RJ: Enteral nutrition for premature infants: The role of human milk, Semin Fetal Neonatal Med 2007;12:26-34.
26. Agarwal R, Singal A, Aggarwal R, Deorari AK, Paul VK: Effect of Fortification with Human Milk Fortifier (HMF) and other Fortifying Agents on the Osmolality of Preterm Breast Milk, Indian Pediatr 2004;41:63-67.
27. Tagare A, Vaidya U: Parenteral nutrition: Current guidelines: *J Neonatology* 2007; 21: 186-188.

7 RESPIRATORY DISTRESS SYNDROME

Deepak Chawla and
Ramesh Agarwal

DEFINITION

Respiratory distress syndrome (RDS) is a disorder of lung surfactant deficiency in preterm neonates. It is characterized by onset at birth or within first 6 hours of life in the form of tachypnea, grunting, chest retractions and need of progressively increasing respiratory support to maintain normal gas exchange.

EPIDEMIOLOGY

Incidence of RDS is inversely proportional to gestation at birth. The incidence is 60% at less than 30 weeks of gestation, but decreases with maturation to near zero by 39 weeks.[1] True incidences may be difficult to define in extremely preterm infants (gestation <28 weeks) who have structural lung immaturity and receive prophylactic surfactant at birth.

PATHOPHYSIOLOGY

Lung **surfactant** is synthesized by type II alveolar cells and covers the alveolar membrane at its gaseous interface. The surfactant coating consisting of phospholipids and surfactant proteins decreases surface tension, thereby reducing the pressure needed to inflate the lungs and preventing lung collapse at end-expiration. Normal lung surfactant pool size at birth is about 100 mg/kg of phospholipids.[2] In preterm neonates, the pool size is less than 25 mg/kg.[3] Surfactant deficiency leads to reduced compliance and alveolar collapse at end expiration. Due to reduced compliance, higher pressure is needed for a given increase in lung volume. This leads to increased work of breathing. Due to alveolar collapse **functional residual capacity (FRC)** is decreased. As a result of alveolar collapse, part of right ventricular output passes through the lungs without getting oxygenated (intrapulmonary right-to-left shunting). In addition, there may be extrapulmonary right-to-left shunting due to persistence of high pulmonary vascular pressure. Persistent hypoxemia leads to metabolic acidosis, myocardial depression and hypotension.

Findings at autopsy include atelectesis, congestion and edema. The lungs are airless and do not float in water. On histological examination, peripheral air spaces are collapsed. Respiratory bronchioles are filled with a hyaline membrane consisting of fibrin and cellular products.

RISK FACTORS

Prematurity is the single most important risk factor for the development of RDS.[1] But, all preterm neonates do not have RDS. There are a number of antenatal and perinatal factors, which increase or decrease the risk of development of RDS. Maternal diabetes, maternal malnutrition, cesarean section and male gender increase the risk.[4-6] Perinatal asphyxia and hypothermia increase severity of RDS.[7] In twin pregnancies, second twin is at higher risk to develop RDS.[8] Protective factors against RDS include antenatal corticosteroid administration, prolonged rupture of membranes and female gender.[9, 10]

CLINICAL AND LABORATORY FEATURES

Clinical signs characteristic of RDS include tachypnea, expiratory grunting and retractions of sternum, intercostals spaces and lower chest. Baby is cyanotic in room air and needs progressively increasing oxygen supplementation to maintain normal oxygen saturation. Onset of these signs is usually within first 4-6 hours of birth. Extremely preterm neonates may not develop these signs due to poor respiratory efforts and may need intubation immediately after birth. If untreated, disease reaches its peak between 24 and 48 hours of life. The magnitude of chest retractions, tachypnea, nasal alae flaring, grunting and oxygen requirement are markers of severity of RDS and can be used to monitor the disease progression.[11] Onset of apnea indicates respiratory decompensation.

If RDS course is uncomplicated, recovery starts after 48 hours of life and usually oxygen can be discontinued at end of first week of life. Improvement in respiratory condition is often associated with diuresis. Course of disease is markedly curtailed if exogenous surfactant replacement therapy is given soon after onset.

Chest radiograph shows diffuse **reticulogranular** opacification with **air bronchogram**. In severe form (Figure 7.1), there is complete opacification of lung fields and cardiac borders are not visible ('white-out' appearance). Asymmetrical involvement with more severe disease in right lung may be seen. Lower lobes may be involved more than upper lobes. Blood gas shows hypoxemia, hypercapnia and a combined metabolic and respiratory acidosis.

Shake test is a rapid bedside method of diagnosing surfactant deficiency.[12] 0.5 ml absolute alcohol is added to 0.5 ml of gastric aspirate in a 4 ml glass test tube-10.0 mm by 82.0 mm dimensions. The test tube is vigorously shaken for 15 seconds and allowed to stand for 15 minutes. Gastric aspirate is obtained within one hour of birth. Formation of stable foam indicates presence of surfactant.

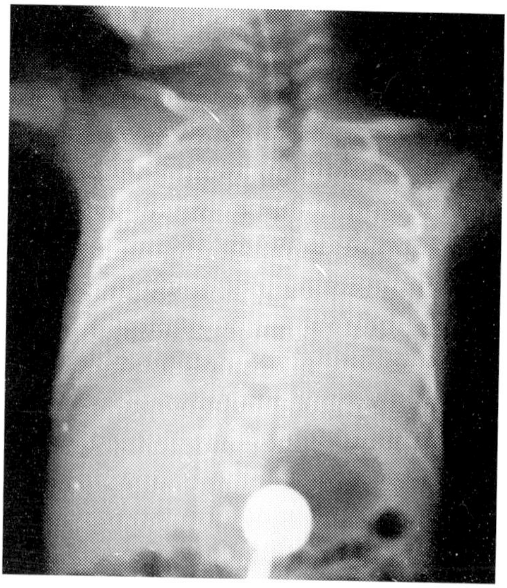

Fig. 7.1: Ground-glass appearance in X-ray chest of a neonate with RDS

Interpretation of test is shown in Table 7.1. Probability of RDS is around 60% if the shake test is negative or 1+ and 5% if shake test is 2+ or higher.[12]

Table 7.1: Interpretation of shake test [12]

Negative	
1+	Very small bubbles in meniscus extending one-third or less of distance around test tube
2+	Single rim of bubbles extending one-third to all around the test tube
3+	A rim of bubbles all the way around the test tube and a double row in some areas
4+	A double row or more of bubbles

DIFFERENTIAL DIAGNOSIS

Respiratory distress immediately after birth can be caused by a variety of pulmonary and extrapulmonary causes. Pulmonary causes include congenital pneumonia, transient tachypnea of newborn (TTNB), meconium aspiration syndrome, persistent pulmonary hypertension, air leaks or lung malformations. Extrapulmonary causes include congenital heart disease, neurological disorders, anemia and polycythemia. Most of these conditions can be diagnosed by good history and clinical examination accompanied by chest X-ray and sepsis screen. It may be difficult to differentiate between RDS and group B *Streptococcus* congenital pneumonia, as chest X-ray picture may be similar.

PREVENTION

As prematurity is the biggest risk factor of RDS, preventing prematurity can prevent RDS. However, pathophysiology of most of cases of premature labor is not known and therefore, most of prematurity burden is non-preventable. After onset of preterm labor, use of tocolytic agents can help in prolonging pregnancy for a short duration during which antenatal corticosteroids may be administered. Betamethasone or dexamethasone administered 24 hours to 7 days before preterm birth reduce the risk of RDS by about 60% and neonatal mortality by about 40%.[9] In addition, there is decrease in risk of intraventricular hemorrhage, periventricular leucomalacia and necrotizing enterocolitis.[9]

Guidelines for use of antenatal corticosteroids are summarized in Table 7.2.

Table 7.2: Guidelines for antenatal corticosteroid (ACS) prophylaxis

- All women with gestation between 24 and 34 weeks and at risk of preterm birth are candidates for antenatal corticosteroids (ACS).
- The decision to use ACS should not be altered by fetal sex, race or availability of surfactant therapy.
- Treatment options are two intramuscular doses of 12 mg of betamethasone given 24 hours apart or four intramuscular doses of 6 mg of dexamethasone given 12 hours apart.
- Optimal benefit is observed 24 hours to 7 days after initiation of therapy. But ACS treatment decreases risk of RDS and mortality even if duration between initiation of therapy and preterm birth is less than 24 hours.
- Gestational hypertension, diabetes and prolonged rupture of membranes in the absence of overt chorioamnionitis are not contraindications of ACS therapy.

MANAGEMENT

Optimal management of RDS starts immediately after birth in the delivery room with appropriate resuscitation, which is then followed by surfactant administration, ventilation and general supportive care.

Surfactant administration should be preceded by adequate stabilization of the infant. Intrapartum asphyxia can increase the severity of RDS. First few breaths of large tidal volume in a surfactant-deficient lung can also cause irreversible damage. Use of T-piece during resuscitation may limit the inadvertent delivery of high tidal volume breaths. Resuscitation of a preterm baby at risk of development of RDS needs a skilled team with expertise and experience in managing such babies.

A number of natural and synthetic surfactants are available.[13] Natural, animal-derived surfactant preparations are associated with lower risk of **pneumothorax** and mortality as compared to synthetic surfactants.[13] Although prophylactic surfactant administered within 10-15 minutes of birth decreases neonatal mortality, cost considerations has led to recommendation of this approach in babies born at gestation less than 29 weeks. For infants with gestation more than 28 weeks, early rescue approach can be followed. All babies of gestation less than 32 weeks needing intubation due to respiratory distress may be administered surfactant without delay, irrespective of extent of ventilator support required.

Nursing the neonate in thermoneutral environment and minimizing manipulations can minimize energy expenditure and oxygen demand. Oxygen therapy helps by increasing alveolar oxygen pressure and by causing pulmonary vasodilatation and therefore decreasing the right-to-left shunting. Early use of **continuous positive airway pressure (CPAP)** has been associated with decreased need of ventilation and decreased risk of chronic lung disease in observational studies.

Principals of pulmonary management in a baby with RDS include early administration of surfactant, maintenance of FRC with use of CPAP and avoiding or minimizing the duration of endotracheal intubation. A preterm baby with RDS or at risk of RDS can be managed by following treatment strategies:

1. For babies born at gestation less then 28-29 weeks prophylactic surfactant should be administered within 15 minutes of birth, if baby has not received ACS therapy or needs intubation during resuscitation. If baby does not need intubation at birth and has received ACS therapy, it is an option to start delivery room CPAP, follow the clinical course and give surfactant early if baby develops respiratory distress, irrespective of degree of respiratory support needed (early rescue).
2. Prophylactic surfactant may also be considered for babies born at gestation 29-31 weeks if they need intubation during resuscitation. Otherwise, nasal CPAP may be started if they develop RDS and given early rescue therapy if they need FiO_2 higher than 30-40%.
3. For babies with RDS born at 32 or more weeks of gestation, **INSURE** approach (intubation, surfactant and rapid extubation to nasal CPAP) can be followed.

Ventilation if needed should be initiated with synchronized intermittent mandatory ventilation (SIMV) or assist control (A/C) mode, if available. Preferred settings are a peak inspiratory pressure just enough to achieve chest rise, short inspiratory time (0.3-0.4 seconds), high rates (50-60 breaths per minute) and positive end-expiratory pressure of 5-6 cm H_2O. Rapid and watchful lowering of peak inspiratory pressure should follow surfactant

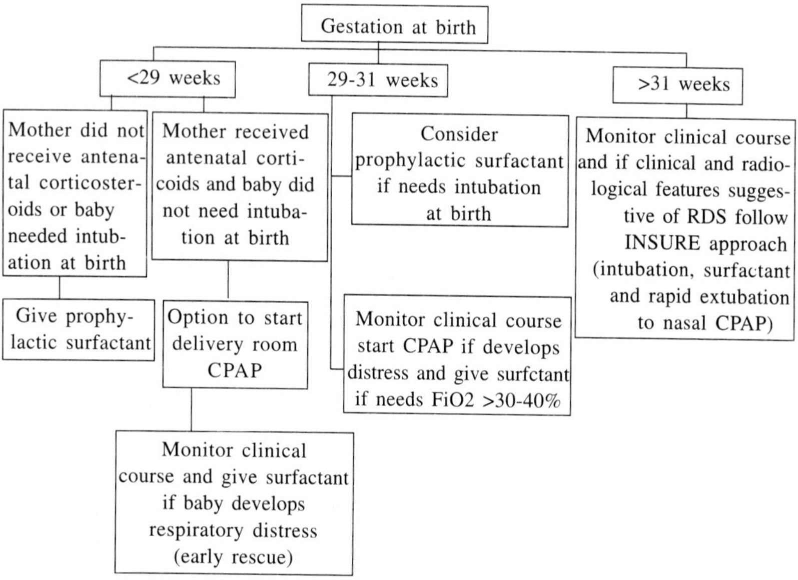

Fig. 7.2: Surfactant replacement therapy in RDS

administration and FiO_2 to prevent oxygen and volume induced lung injury.

High frequency ventilation (as primary modality to ventilate babies with RDS) is not better than optimal conventional ventilation, needs more experienced user and may be associated with slightly increased risk of intraventricular hemorrhage.[14]

COMPLICATIONS

Complications during management of RDS may be related to prematurity per se or to management practices. Pulmonary complications include **pulmonary interstitial emphysema**, pneumothorax, pulmonary hemorrhage, hospital-acquired pneumonia, subglottic stenosis and bronchopulmonary dysplasia. Air leaks are decreased with prophylactic or early rescue use of natural surfactant. Extrapulmonary complications include intraventricular hemorrhage, patent ductus arteriosus and retinopathy of prematurity.

PROGNOSIS

Mortality due to RDS is related to gestation and weight at birth,

ACS therapy, timing of surfactant administration, ventilation strategy, co-morbidities and complications during the management.

REFERENCES

1. Greenough A, Morley CJ, Roberton NRC: Acute respiratory distress in the newborn, Edinburgh: Churchill Livingstone; 1992.
2. Jobe AH: Pulmonary surfactant therapy, N Engl J Med 1993;328:861-868.
3. Hallman M, Merritt TA, Pohjavuori M, Gluck L: Effect of surfactant substitution on lung effluent phospholipids in respiratory distress syndrome: Evaluation of surfactant phospholipid turnover, pool size, and the relationship to severity of respiratory failure, Pediatr Res 1986;20:1228-1235.
4. Morrison JJ, Rennie JM, Milton PJ: Neonatal respiratory morbidity and mode of delivery at term: Influence of timing of elective caesarean section, Br J Obstet Gynaecol 1995;102:101-106.
5. Banias BB, Devoe LD, Nolan TE: Severe preeclampsia in preterm pregnancy between 26 and 32 weeks' gestation, Am J Perinatol 1992;9:357-360.
6. Farrell PM, Avery ME: Hyaline membrane disease. Am Rev Respir Dis 1975;111:657-688.
7. Thibeault DW, Hall FK, Sheehan MB, Hall RT: Postasphyxial lung disease in newborn infants with severe perinatal acidosis, Am J Obstet Gynecol 1984;150:393-399.
8. Hacking D, Watkins A, Fraser S, Wolfe R, Nolan T: Respiratory distress syndrome and birth order in premature twins, Arch Dis Child Fetal Neonatal Ed 2001;84:F117-121.
9. Roberts D, Dalziel S: Antenatal corticosteroids for accelerating fetal lung maturation for women at risk of preterm birth, Cochrane Database Syst Rev 2006;3:CD004454.
10. Bryan H, Hawrylyshyn P, Hogg-Johnson S, *et al.*: Perinatal factors associated with the respiratory distress syndrome, Am J Obstet Gynecol 1990;162:476-481.
11. Silverman WA, Anderson AH: A controlled clinical trial of effect of water mist in obstructive respiratory signs, death rate and necropsy findings in premature infants. Pediatrics 1956;17:1-9.
12. Evans JJ: Prediction of respiratory distress syndrome by shake test on newborn gastric aspirate, N Engl J Med 1975;292:1113-1115.
13. Moya F, Maturana A: Animal-derived surfactants versus past and current synthetic surfactants: Current status, Clin Perinatol 2007;34:145-77, viii.
14. Henderson-Smart DJ, Cools F, Bhuta T, Offringa M: Elective high frequency oscillatory ventilation versus conventional ventilation for acute pulmonary dysfunction in preterm infants, Cochrane Database Syst Rev 2007(3):CD000104.

8 AIR LEAK SYNDROMES IN THE NEWBORN

M. Jeeva Sankar and Ramesh Agarwal

Air leak syndromes are one of the dreaded complications of assisted ventilation in neonates. They occur following alveolar overdistension and are characterized by rupture of alveoli and subsequent escape of air into the surrounding tissue(s). Based on the site of escape, they are classified into various forms: **pneumothorax, pulmonary interstitial emphysema (PIE), pneumomediastinum, pneumopericardium, pneumoperitoneum**, and **air embolism**. Of these, pneumothorax and PIE are the two most common forms that occur in the neonatal period. Appropriate preventive measures, coupled with early diagnosis and interventions are crucial to reduce the significant morbidity and mortality associated with air leak syndromes.

INCIDENCE

Incidence varies depending upon the gestation, presence and severity of the underlying lung disease, and the need for respiratory support. Based on radiographic surveys, the overall frequency of spontaneous pneumothorax has been found to be about 1% of all live births. However, only 10% of these would be symptomatic.[1] The incidence as well as the odds of being symptomatic are much higher in infants with associated lung disease and/or on assisted ventilation. In 1970s, Kirkpatrick *et al.* reported that upto 40% of their infants with respiratory distress syndrome (RDS) had one or more of air leak syndromes.[2] With the advent of optimal ventilatory strategies and the use of postnatal surfactant, there has been a substantial decline in the incidence of air leaks. Data from Vermont Oxford Network for the period between 1991 and 1999 reveals an incidence of 5.0 to 8.7% in very low birth weight (VLBW) infants.[3] Similar data from eighteen level 3 neonatal units across India show an incidence of 1.21% (2002-03).[4]

ETIOLOGY

Air leaks can occur either spontaneously or secondary to an associated lung disease/assisted ventilation.

Spontaneous Pneumothorax

It occurs immediately after birth probably due to the transpulmonary pressure swings generated by the newborn during the first few breaths.[5] It is more common in term and postmature infants (compared to secondary air leaks which are more common in preterm infants). Familial spontaneous pneumothorax has been reported rarely in neonates.[6]

Pneumothorax Secondary to Lung Disease/Assisted Ventilation

The underlying lung diseases that usually result in pneumothorax are: **RDS**, meconium aspiration syndrome **(MAS)**, transient tachypnea of newborn **(TTNB)**, congenital malformations such as diaphragmatic hernia and **pulmonary hypoplasia**, and direct injury to the lung (e.g. perforation by suction / central venous catheters). During **assisted ventilation**, the following components of ventilatory support have been incriminated in the causation of air leaks:

- *Peak inspiratory pressure (PIP):* In pressure-limited ventilators, **PIP** is the primary factor that determines the tidal volume delivered to the lungs. A very high PIP (and hence a large tidal volume) stretches the lung tissue resulting in injury (*Barotrauma*). To minimize such injury, newer concepts such as 'Gentle ventilation' (avoiding higher pressures and using only sufficient pressure to allow adequate oxygenation while tolerating a relatively high $PaCO_2$) and 'permissive hypercapnia' (accepting a relatively high $PaCO_2$ provided the arterial pH does not fall below a preset value) have come into vogue.

However, these approaches have not yet been proved to reduce the incidence of air leaks.[7,8]

- *Continuous positive airway pressure (CPAP) / peak end-expiratory pressure (PEEP):* Unlike PIP, the relation between CPAP/PEEP and air leaks is relatively complex. Inappropriately high CPAP/PEEP could lead to over distension of the more compliant areas of the lung resulting in air leak syndromes. Studies from the pre-surfactant era have shown that **CPAP** when used as the primary ventilatory therapy for RDS might increase the incidence of air leaks. More recent trials of early CPAP, however, have not shown any significant increase in their incidence.[9] One should also note that early use of CPAP reduces the need for intubation and mechanical ventilation which are distinctly more harmful than CPAP alone. Like CPAP, high **PEEP** has also been traditionally implicated in the causation of air leaks. In conditions such as MAS where there is overdistension of the lungs due to air trapping, high PEEP could further aggravate the underlying condition. But in conditions where reduced compliance is the underlying pathology (e.g. RDS), often it is the *inadequate/low* PEEP (resulting in atelectasis and uneven ventilation) that causes more injury than a *high but optimal* end expiratory pressure. An optimal PEEP helps in recruiting the alveoli and improving the functional residual capacity in RDS resulting in better oxygenation with relatively *low* peak inspiratory pressures (PIP). However, once the lung compliance improves, PEEP should promptly be reduced; otherwise, it would lead to alveolar over distension and rupture (*see 'Pathogenesis'*).
- *Inspiratory time (Ti):* Long **inspiratory time** (>0.66 sec) during mechanical ventilation in preterm infants with poorly compliant lungs (e.g. RDS) has been associated with a significant increase in the incidence of pneumothorax.[10]
- *High flow rates:* Very high flow rate (>6 to 10 L/min) has been shown to increase the risk of air leaks.
- *Ventilation asynchrony ('fighting' the ventilator): Asynchrony* (infants' own spontaneous breaths out of phase with the mechanically delivered breaths) has also been shown to contribute to pneumothorax.

PATHOGENESIS

Air leaks are usually caused by a high intra-alveolar pressure that results in a pressure gradient from the affected alveoli to the adjacent tissue space(s). The gradient causes the rupture of the bases of alveoli that overlie capillaries (Figure 8.1).[11]

In immature lungs (e.g. in preterm infants with RDS), even the terminal airways have been found to rupture in addition to the alveoli.

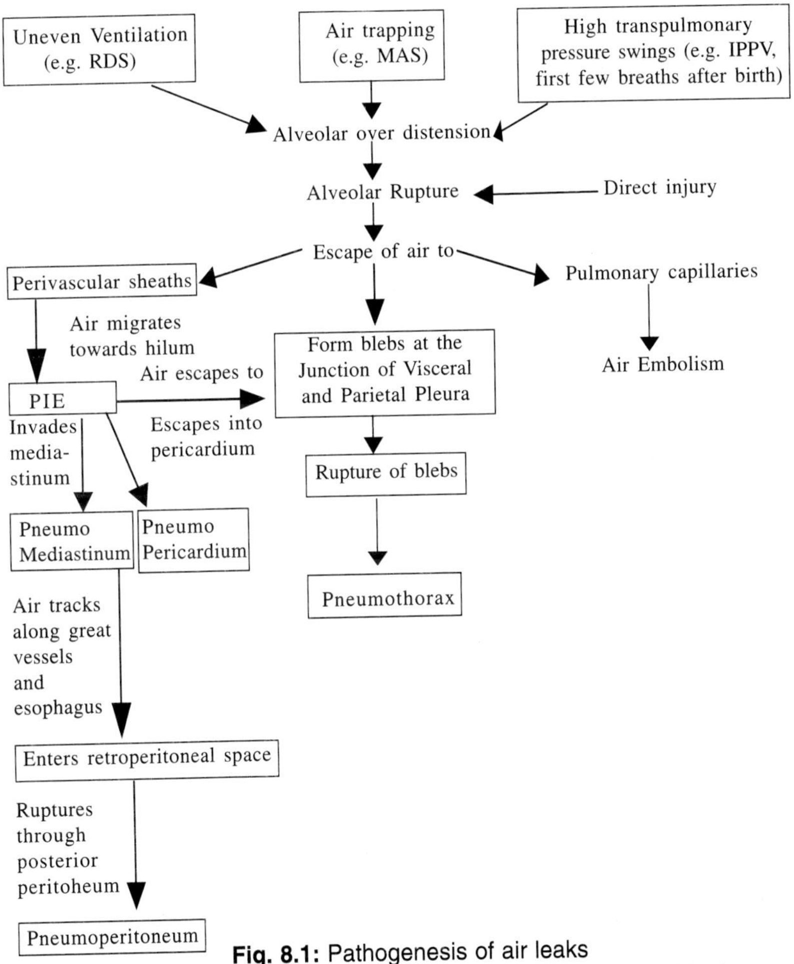

Fig. 8.1: Pathogenesis of air leaks
(RDS, respiratory distress syndrome; MAS, meconium aspiration syndrome; IPPV, intermittent positive pressure ventilation; PIE, pulmonary interstitial emphysema)

CLINICAL FEATURES

PIE

It usually develops in premature infants with RDS on ventilator support. Often clinically silent, the condition is suspected by increasing oxygen requirements with severe CO_2 retention. A chest X-ray would readily reveal the underlying pathology.

Pneumothorax

Manifestations depend generally on the size of the pneumothorax.

- Small pneumothorax (usually a spontaneous one) – asymptomatic
- Large pneumothorax—presents with respiratory distress (tachypnea, grunting, retractions and cyanosis)
- Tension pneumothorax—sudden deterioration of the clinical condition with pallor, shock and cyanosis. The signs include increased resonance on percussion and reduced air entry on the side of pneumothorax, mediastinal shift, and a positive transillumination test.

Pneumomediastinum

Usually asymptomatic; may present with tachypnea, cyanosis, bulging sternum, and muffled heart sounds in severe cases.

Pneumopericardium

Usually asymptomatic; severe cases might develop features of cardiac tamponade (cyanosis, fall in arterial blood pressure along with muffled heart sounds).

Pneumoperitoneum

Can result in abdominal distension; however, absence of tenderness and other abdominal signs will help in ruling out a significant gastrointestinal illness.

DIAGNOSIS

I. Radiology

X-rays remain the gold standard for diagnosing air leak syndromes

(Figures 8.2 to 8.4).The classical X-ray findings in various forms of air leaks are described in Table 8.1. It is not difficult to detect a large or tension pneumothorax in a traditional supine film; however, small pneumothoraces are often missed in this view because air collects *anterior* to the lung and hence free lung edge may not be visualized. In such instances, some signs might help in suspecting an anterior pneumothorax:

a. Increased lucency and size of the involved hemithorax; and
b. Increased sharpness of the ipsilateral mediastinal edge. If there is a suspicion in the supine view, a cross-table lateral or decubitus film should be obtained for confirmation.

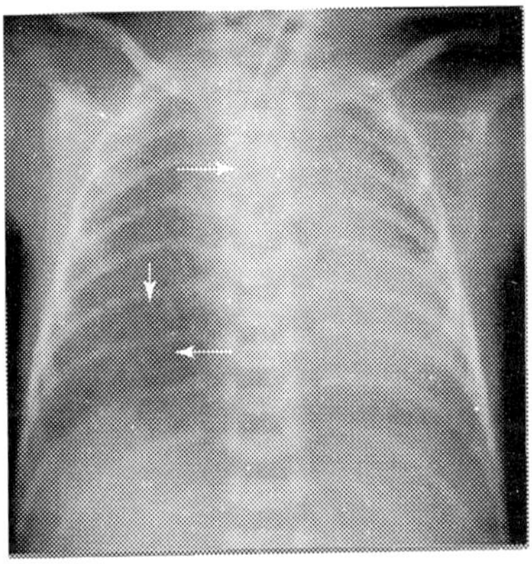

Fig. 8.2: Chest radiograph showing the cystic and linear translucencies of pulmonary interstitial emphysema (Rt. side); short arrow indicates cystic lesions while long arrow indicates linear translucencies. Note the incorrect position of the tip of endotracheal tube at T4 (arrow head)

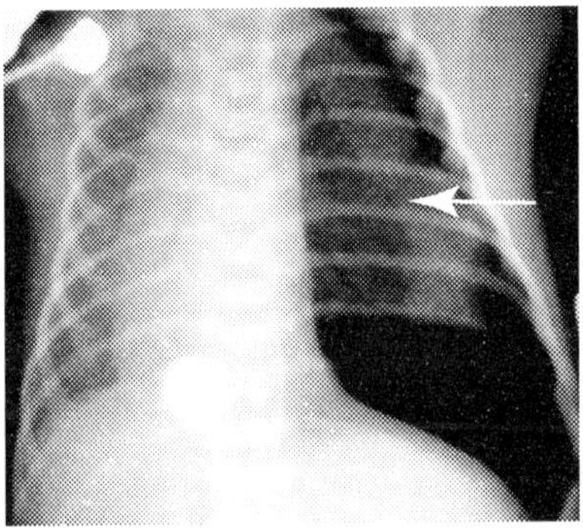

Fig. 8.3: Chest radiograph showing pneumothorax (Left side). Note the mediastinal shift to the opposite side; arrow indicates the collapsed left lung border

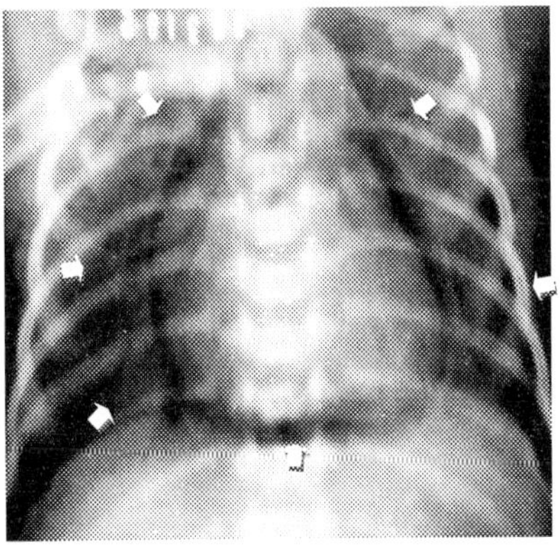

Fig. 8.4: X-ray chest showing pneumopericardium. Note the radiolucent halo completely surrounding the heart (arrows)

Table 8.1: Air leak syndromes: Radiographic features and differential diagnoses

Pathology	*X-ray findings*	*Differential diagnosis*
PIE	Characterized by 2 major forms of ***radiolucencies:*** *Linear and cystic.* *Linear translucencies:* vary in width, do not branch, and extend from hilum to periphery. *Cystic translucencies:* usually 1-4mm in size; are oval/lobulated and non-confluent (Fig. 8.2).	• Air-bronchogram *(smooth and branching radiolucencies)* • BPD *(larger, irregular cysts)* • Congenital cystic adenomatoid malformation (CCAM)
Pneumothorax	Radiolucent lung field(s) with absent lung markings and collapsed lung (Fig. 8.3); Mediastinal shift, bulging intercostal spaces, and diaphragmatic eversion (in tension pneumothorax)	• Congenital lobar emphysema *(lung markings are usually present)* • CCAM
Pneumomediastinum	*Lateral view:* Radiolucent area behind the sternum. *AP view:* A halo around the heart that does not extend to its inferior (diaphragmatic) border; lifting of thymus from the heart by the mediastinal air (*'Spinnaker sail'* sign)	• Pneumopericardium *(see below)*
Pneumopericardium	Broad halo completely surrounding the heart including the diaphragmatic surface (Fig. 8.4).	• Pneumomediastinum

Contd.

Contd.

Pneumoperitoneum	Air under diaphragm	• Gastrointestinal perforation secondary to necrotizing entero-colitis (NEC) and other illnesses *(other features such as dilated bowel loops, pneumatosis intestinalis etc. would be present)*
Air embolism	Intracardiac and intravascular air	

Other imaging techniques such as computed tomography (CT) of the chest are rarely needed for diagnosis of air leaks.

II. Transillumination

Increased transmission of light on the ipsilateral side (using fiberoptic 'cold' light) in cases of pneumothorax and extensive PIE (Figure 8.5).

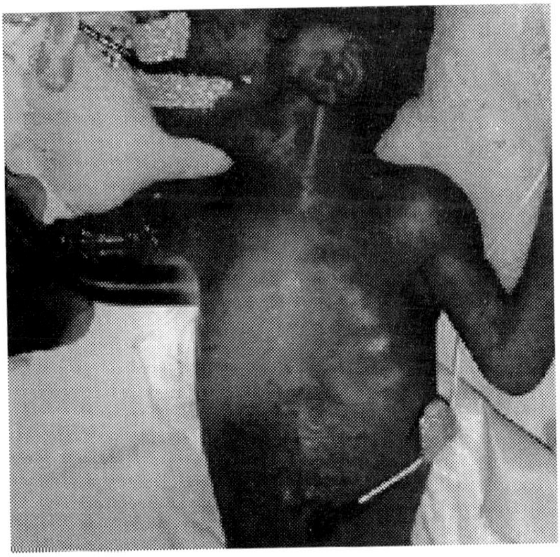

Fig. 8.5: Positive transillumination test in an infant with Rt. sided Pneumothorax

III. ECG

Reduced QRS voltage especially in pneumopericardium and pneumothorax.

MANAGEMENT

General Principles

1. Only conservative approach is needed for asymptomatic conditions. If symptomatic, early and often aggressive management is essential to prevent the high mortality and morbidities (see below).
2. It is of paramount importance to keep the ventilator settings at a minimum to prevent progression of the disease. PIP should be reduced to a minimum to accept a relatively high $PaCO_2$ of 45-55 mmHg (provided pH >7.25); mean airway pressure (MAP) is reduced to achieve a target PaO_2 of 40-70 mmHg and saturation of 88-93%. Increasing the rates (>60/min) would often improve ventilation and oxygenation thus allowing one to set relatively low PIP and MAP. Reducing the PEEP in an infant with air leak, accepted as the 'standard of care' not so long ago, is now contentious. A low PEEP, especially in preterm infants with RDS, results in more areas of atelectasis and uneven ventilation that could possibly cause overdistension of the 'normal' areas and further progression of air leak. Hence, PEEP should be reduced only if there is any evidence of overdistension of the lungs – either clinically or radiologically.
3. If there is significant asynchrony, then shifting to a patient triggered mode (such as SIMV or assist-control) might help. If the infant is already on a patient triggered mode, then analgesics/sedatives (e.g. morphine) can be used to reduce the asynchrony. It should be kept in mind that these strategies, though seem logical, have not been proved to be beneficial in clinical trials.[12]
4. **High frequency ventilation (HFV)** can be instituted *if* the *conventional ventilation fails* to maintain adequate *oxygenation* and *ventilation*. High frequency jet ventilation (HFJV) has been shown to accelerate resolution of PIE;[13] no such data are available with regard to other types of HFV.

Specific Management

a. *PIE:* Usually responds to conservative management. If the condition progresses, one should consider the following treatment options based on whether the condition is localized or diffuse: for localized/unilateral PIE, placing the infant with the diseased lung dependent in the lateral decubitus position, selective bronchial intubation, and creation of an artificial pneumothorax on the ipsilateral side. For diffuse/bilateral PIE, consider placing the infant on HFV; another approach is to do linear pleurotomies to create artificial pneumothoraces (on both sides).[14]

b. *Pneumothorax:* In term infants with mild respiratory distress, increasing the FiO_2 to 100% might help in rapid resorption of the extra-alveolar air; such an approach cannot be employed in preterm infants because of the increased risk of retinopathy of prematurity and other oxidant-mediated diseases.

   Symptomatic pneumothoraces (usually a large/tension pneumothorax in non-ventilated infants and any pneumothorax in a ventilated infant) must be drained using a **chest drain** (*see procedures in* ***Appendix A***). If the infant is unstable, needle aspiration using an 18G needle/catheter (inserted through the second intercostal space in the midclavicular line) can be performed until a chest tube is inserted. Once the tube is inserted, it should be connected to an underwater seal drain with suction of 5-10 cm H_2O. It should be left in-situ for at least 72-96 hours or for 24 hours after it stops bubbling.[15]

c. *Pneumomediastinum:* Only careful observation is needed in most of the cases. Unlike pneumothorax, a pneumomediastinum is very difficult to drain since the air is collected in numerous independent lobules.

d. *Pneumopericardium:* Only conservative management is needed for small, asymptomatic lesions. If symptomatic, needle aspiration should be performed via the subxiphoid route under strict cardiac monitoring (heart rate and blood pressure). Catheter drainage might be needed if air re-accumulates in the pericardial cavity.

e. *Pneumoperitoneum:* No treatment is necessary if the abdomen is soft and not tense. If the abdominal distension results in respiratory compromise, needle aspiration and /or catheter drainage may become necessary.

f. *Air embolism:* No beneficial treatment is available for an acute air embolism.

PREVENTION

The status of various modalities/strategies employed for prevention of air leak syndromes based on the current available evidence is depicted in Table 8.2. Some of these strategies are briefly discussed below:

- *Surfactant therapy:* Early and appropriate use of postnatal **surfactant** therapy in preterm infants with or at-risk for respiratory distress syndrome reduces the risk for pneumothorax. Estimates from various studies indicate that there is a 30 to 65% relative reduction in the risk of pneumothorax when compared to placebo or no therapy.[16]
- *High frequency ventilation:* In contrast to animal studies where HFV was shown to result in significantly less barotrauma, studies in preterm infants are not as convincing. While some have shown to reduce the incidence of new air leaks,[17] others have not reported any benefit. Indeed, *elective* use of HFV in

Table 8.2: Air leak: Preventive strategies and their current status[11-15]

Type	*Proven benefit*	*Potentially beneficial (but still unproven)*	*Controversial*
Ventilator mode/type	-	Patient triggered modes Volume targeted ventilation	High frequency ventilation
Ventilator strategies	-	Permissive hypercapnia Gentle ventilation Employing short Ti Using rapid rates	-
Pharmacologic	Postnatal surfactant (prophylactic as well as rescue therapy)	-	Muscle relaxants

preterm infants with RDS could lead to increased incidence of air leaks.[18]

- *Gentle ventilation and permissive hypercapnia:* Though conceptually attractive, these strategies have not yet been shown to be beneficial in preventing air leaks.[7, 8]
- *Use of neuromuscular blocking agents, analgesics and sedatives:* Breathing out of phase with the ventilator often increases the incidence of air leaks. Neuromuscular blockers can reduce the asynchrony by abolishing the spontaneous respiratory efforts. However, routine use of such agents has not been shown to reduce the incidence of pneumothorax and other air leak syndromes.[19] It can probably be used in those infants who continue to have active respiratory pattern despite an 'optimal' ventilatory strategy.

COMPLICATIONS

Acute

- Cardiorespiratory failure with bradycardia, hypoxia, hypercarbia, hypotension, cardiac arrest and even death. The mortality risk almost doubles in neonates with RDS and air leaks when compared to those without air leaks.[15]
- **Intraventricular hemorrhage (IVH)** because of the abrupt increase in cerebral blood flow velocity.
- Syndrome of inappropriate ADH secretion (SIADH).

Chronic/Long-Term

- Increased incidence of **bronchopulmonary dyspalsia (BPD)**.
- Adverse neurodevelopmental outcome, especially if the air leak results in severe IVH.

REFERENCES

1. Steele RW, Metz JR, Bass JW, Dubois JJ: Pneumothorax and pneumomediastinum in the newborn, Radiology 1971;98:629-32.
2. Kirkpatrick BV, Felman AH, Eitzman DV: Complications of ventilator therapy in respiratory distress syndrome, Am J Dis Child 1974;128:496.
3. Horbar JD, Badger GJ, Carpenter JH, Fanaroff AA, Kilpatrick S, LaCorte M, *et al.* Trends in mortality and morbidity for very low birth weight infants, 1991-1999, Pediatrics 2002;110:143-151.

4. National Neonatal Perinatal Database: Report for year 2002-03, National Neonatology Forum, India.
5. Vyas H, Field D, Hopkin IE, Milner AD: Determinants of the first inspiratory volume and functional residual capacity at birth, Pediatr Pulmonol 1986;2:189-93.
6. Engdahl MS, Gershan WM: Familial spontaneous pneumothorax in neonates, Pediatr Pulmonol 1998; 25:398-400.
7. Mariani G, Cifuentes J, Carlo WA: Randomized trial of permissive hypercapnia in preterm infants, Pediatrics 1999;104:1082-8
8. Woodgate PG, Davies MW: Permissive hypercapnia for the prevention of morbidity and mortality in mechanically ventilated newborn infants, Cochrane Database of Systematic Reviews 2001; 2: CD002061.
9. Thomson M: Early continuous positive airway pressure (nCPAP) with prophylactic surfactant for neonates at risk of RDS, The IFDAS multicentre randomized trial, Pediatr Res 2002;51:379A.
10. Kamlin COF, Davis PG: Long versus short inspiratory times in neonates receiving mechanical ventilation, Cochrane Database of Systematic Reviews 2003; 4: CD004503.
11. Macklin CC: Transport of air along sheaths of pulmonic blood vessels from alveoli to mediastinum: Clinical implications, Arch Intern Med 1939;64:913.
12. Greenough A, Dimitriou G, Prendergast M, Milner AD: Synchronized mechanical ventilation for respiratory support in newborn infants, Cochrane Database of Systematic Reviews 2008;1: CD000456.
13. Keszler M, Donn SM, Bucciarelli RL, Alverson DC, Hart M, Lunyong V, Modanlou HD, *et al.*: Multi-center controlled trial comparing high-frequency jet ventilation and conventional mechanical ventilation in newborn infants with pulmonary interstitial emphysema, J Pediatr. 1991;119:85-93.
14. Korones SB: Complications, In: Goldsmith JP, Karotkin EH *(eds)*, Assisted Ventilation of the Neonate, 4th edn, Philadelphia: Saunders 2003:361-77.
15. Greenough A, Milner AD: Acute respiratory disease, In: Rennie JM (*ed*), Roberton's Textbook of Neonatology, 4th edn, Elsevier 2005:487-96
16. Soll RF: Surfactant treatment of the very preterm infant, Biol Neonate 1998;74:35-42.
17. HiFO Study Group: Randomized study of high-frequency oscillatory ventilation in infants with severe respiratory distress syndrome, J Pediatr 1993;122:609-19.
18. Thome UH, Carlo WA, Pohlandt F: Ventilation strategies and outcome in randomised trials of high frequency ventilation, Arch Dis Child 2005;90:F466-73.
19. Shaw NJ, Cooke RW, Gill AB, Shaw NJ, Saeed M: Randomised trial of routine versus selective paralysis during ventilation for neonatal respiratory distress syndrome, Arch Dis Child 1993; 69:479-82.

9

APNEA IN NEWBORNS

Vishal Sondhi and Girish Gupta

The breathing movements of fetus have been discerned and they have been shown to change in character and frequency throughout gestation. The initiation of breathing at birth and normal control of postnatal breathing is dependent on the degree of maturation of breathing control attained *in utero*. This chapter initially discusses the physiologic aspects of breathing and thereafter addresses apnea.

BREATHING

Neurology of Breathing

The control and maintenance of normal breathing largely resides within the **respiratory control centers** of the bulbopontine region of the brainstem. The afferent inputs to this area are predominantly from central and peripheral chemoreceptors, pulmonary stretch receptors, and cortical and **reticuloactivating system (RAS)** neurons while the efferent output is directed to the respiratory and airway muscles and lungs (Figure 9.1). Sleep state can have a profound effect on respiratory pattern, possibly acting via the RAS. In the newborn infant and especially in the preterm infant, however, central responses are less well-organized and apnea is a common result of a disorganized response to multiple non-integrated afferent inputs.

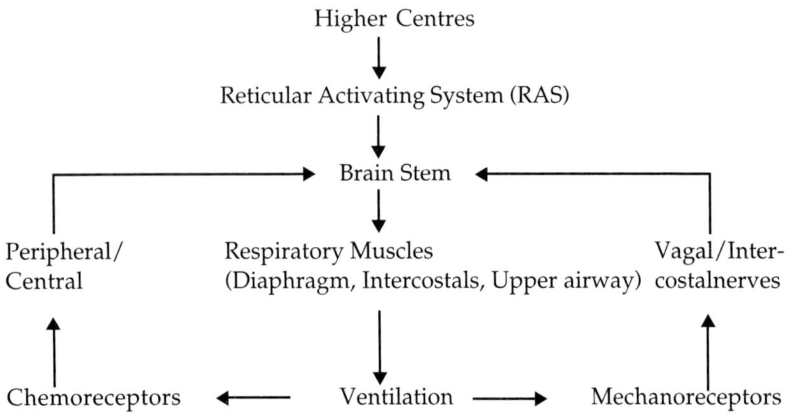

Fig. 9.1: Respiratory regulation

Periodic Breathing

Periodic breathing is defined as recurrent sequences of pauses in respiration lasting 5 to 10 seconds followed by 10 to 15 seconds of rapid respiration; occurring through three cycles of respiration in succession. This regular irregularity of respiration is so common that it is considered normal in preterm infants. Increasing environmental oxygen can abolish it, but because periodic breathing is considered harmless, this is **not recommended**.

Periodic breathing may be observed for 2-6% of the breathing time in healthy term neonates and as much as 25% of the breathing time in preterm neonates. The occurrence of periodic breathing is directly proportional to the degree of prematurity. Periodic breathing typically does not occur in neonates during their first 2 days of life. Though periodic breathing most frequently occurs during active sleep, it can also happen when neonates are awake or quietly sleeping.

APNEA

Definition

Apnea is defined as cessation of airflow; it is considered pathological if this cessation lasts for more than 20 seconds or for a shorter period of time but is accompanied by **bradycardia** (heart rate less than 100 bpm) and cyanosis or **pallor**. In preterm neonates,

cyanosis and bradycardia may set in even before 20 seconds of apnea; while apnea over 30 to 45 seconds may result in hypotonia and pallor.

Types of Apnea

Apnea has been classified depending upon presence or absence of inspiratory efforts accompanying the cessation of flow. Apnea is labelled as **Central** if the cessation of airflow is not accompanied by any inspiratory efforts. If inspiratory muscle activity is present without airflow, this is termed **Obstructive apnea**. Obstructive apneas (obstructed breaths) are also central in origin but are related to absence of neuromuscular control of upper airway patency rather than absence of inspiratory diaphragmatic stimulation. Hence, obstructive apneas are characterized by cessation of inspiratory airflow into the lungs despite persisting respiratory effort. **Mixed apneas** represent a combination of missed breaths (central apnea) and obstructed breaths (Figure 9.2).

In terms of relative frequency of each type, mixed apnea generally accounts for 53% to 71% of events, with obstructive apnea 12% to 20% and central apnea 10% to 25%.

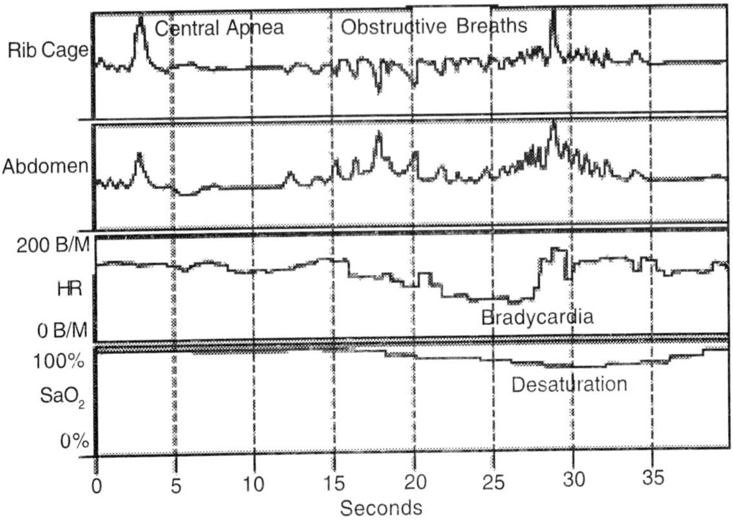

Fig. 9.2: Mixed apnea commencing by central component and prolonged by obstructive respiratory efforts (Note that desaturation and bradycardia are secondary to ineffective ventilation)

Epidemiology

- *Incidence:* The incidence of apnea increases with decreasing gestational age (GA). Studies have reported an incidence of 25% in infants born at a GA less than 34 completed weeks; this incidence increases to nearly 100% for infants born at GA less than 28 completed weeks.
- *Onset:* In majority of cases the onset of apnea occurs within first week of life. **Apnea of prematurity** (AOP) typically has a peak incidence between 5th to 7th postnatal days, while it is unlikely cause of apnea on first two days of life. Apnea due to other causes can occur depending upon occurrence of underlying pathology.
- *Duration:* Usually AOP tends to decrease with increasing GA and ceases at a GA of 37 weeks. In few infants, especially those born ≤28 weeks apneic episodes may continue to occur till term or even beyond term GA.

Etiology

Apnea is only a symptom and frequently occurs secondary to other disease processes. However, AOP is a specific diagnosis and also one of exclusion. Hence, every episode of apnea should be pursued to detect pathological processes (Tables 9.1 and 9.2) which can present with apnea, more so if the apnea progresses in severity, fails to respond to appropriate therapy, severe episodes occur on the first day of life, or it appears at a gestational age when it should not occur.

Pathogenesis[1-4]

- *Central respiratory regulation:* AOP is a direct consequence of immaturity of brainstem respiratory control centers. Vulnerability of the ventral surface of the medulla and adjacent areas in the brainstem to inhibitory mechanisms (hypoxia, hyperthermia, adenosine secretion) is the likely explanation for why apneic episodes occur in prematurely born infants (Figure 9.3). In addition, the respiratory responses to hypercarbia are diminished in preterm infants less than 33 weeks' GA. The slope of the CO_2 response curve (Figure 9.4) increases significantly in infants with apnea. The cause of this decreased sensitivity of central respiratory centers to CO_2 in

Table 9.1: Apnea: Causes with their clinical features and investigations

Causes	*Clinical features*	*Investigations*
1. Temperature instability	- Hyper or hypothermia	
2. Metabolic • Hypoglycemia • Hypocalcemia • Dyselectrolytemia • Acidosis • Inborn errors of metabolism (IEM)	- Lethargy - Jitteriness - Poor feeding - Irritability - CNS depression	- Blood sugar - Serum calcium, sodium, potassium - IEM profile if clinically indicated
3. Anemia/ Polycythemia	- Blood loss - IUGR - Infant of diabetic mother	- Hematocrit
4. Hypoxia	- Cyanosis - Tachypnea - Respiratory distress	- Arterial blood gases
5. Infection	- Temperature instability - Poor feeding - Lethargy	- CBC, ANC - CRP, micro ESR - Blood cultures, CSF
6. Drugs • $MgSO_4$ • Narcotics	- CNS depression - Hypotonia - Suggestive maternal history	-Serum levels of narcotics, magnesium
7. Intracranial abnormalities • Intracranial hemorrhage • Developmental abnormalities	- Seizures - Abnormal neurological examination	- Cranial ultrasound

Contd.

Contd.

8. Cardiovascular lesions • Patent ductus arteriosus • Congestive heart failure due to any cause • Hypotension • Hypertension	- Hyperdynamic chest - Hepatomegaly - Wide pulse pressure - Positive calf sign - Unexplained weight gain - Unexplained tachycardia	- Chest X-ray - ECHO
9. Gastroesophageal reflux	- Feeding difficulty	- Nuclear scan
10. Anatomical abnormalities (choanal atresia, micrognathia, macroglossia, tracheomalacia)	-Abnormal clinical examination - Respiratory distress	
11. Apnea of prematurity (AOP)	- Preterm, otherwise well	- Diagnosis of exclusion

Table 9.2: Causes of apnea based on postnatal age

- Day 1-2
  - Germinal matrix-Intraventricular hemorrhage
  - Sepsis
  - Hypoglycemia
  - Impending respiratory failure
  - Polycythemia
- Days 3-6
  - Sepsis
  - Impending respiratory failure
  - Patent ductus arteriosus
  - Massive intraventricular hemorrhage
  - Apnea of prematurity
- Late
  - Sepsis
  - Progressive post-extubation atelectasis
  - Inadequate dosing of theophylline/caffeine
  - Gastro-oesophageal reflux
  - Presenting symptom of respiratory syncytial virus (RSV) infection

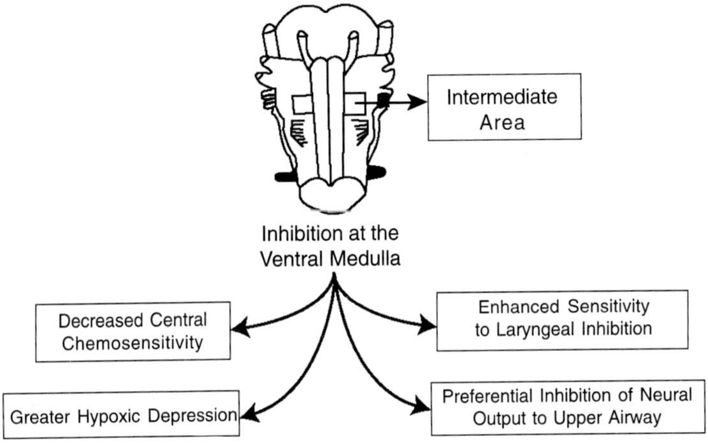

Fig. 9.3: Inhibition of intermediate area of ventral medullary surface results in characteristics exhibited by apneic infants

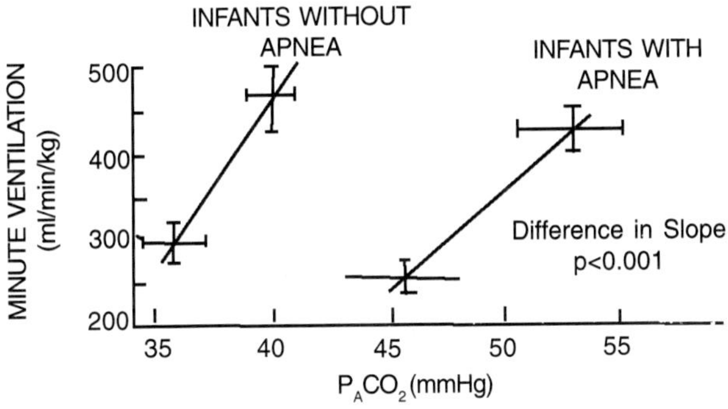

Fig. 9.4: Ventilatory response to carbon dioxide has a decreased slope in infants with apnea

preterm infants is related to central nervous system immaturity as indicated by decreased synaptic connections and incomplete dendritic arborization.

- *Sleep state:* Although determination of sleep state in infants younger than 34 weeks' gestation is controversial, apnea appears to occur predominantly during active (or **rapid eye movement or REM**) and indeterminate (or transitional) sleep in both preterm and term infants. It is uncommon for prolonged apnea to be observed during quiet sleep, when respiration is characteristically regular, with little breath-by-breath change in tidal volume or respiratory frequency. During active sleep, respiration is mostly paradoxical due to spinal motor neural inhibition of the activity of intercostal muscles. In extremely preterm infants, the paucity of quiet sleep, together with an extremely compliant rib cage, makes paradoxical chest-wall movements almost a constant phenomenon which may predispose the baby to apnea by decreasing functional residual capacity (FRC) and limiting oxygenation.

- *Peripheral chemoreceptors:* In contrast to the sustained hyperventilation in older infants in response to hypoxia, preterm infants have only a transient hyperventilation lasting 30 seconds to a minute. Subsequently, minute ventilation returns to baseline over several minutes and then progresses to ventilatory depression despite continued low inspired oxygen concentrations. It is thought that this transient hyperventilation is in response to peripheral chemoreceptor input that is subsequently overridden by depression of central respiratory centers by hypoxia, and the hypoxic ventilatory depression is secondary to descending inhibition from the upper brainstem, midbrain, or higher structures.
- *Peripheral mechanoreceptors:* Abnormal respiratory response can occur due to incoordination between inspiratory muscles and muscles of upper airway. The sensory afferent fibers in upper airway (pharynx, larynx) may get stimulated due to negative pressure while suctioning or with foreign body like nasogastric tube or feeds and this leads to inhibition of respiration. In addition, pulmonary stretch receptors send an afferent neural input to brain and mediate the Hering-Breuer reflex by means of the vagus nerve. Thereafter, they inhibit inspiration; prolong expiration, or both, while increasing lung volume.
- *Respiratory muscles:* Airway obstruction contributes to mixed and obstructive apneic episodes. The site of obstruction is usually upper pharynx (Figure 9.5), which is vulnerable due to poor muscle tone, especially in REM sleep. The pharyngeal obstruction may become more significant due to passive neck flexion spontaneously or during nursery procedures. Nasal obstruction can lead to apnea particularly in preterms that fail to switch to oral breathing after nasal occlusion.
- *Gastro-esophageal reflux (GER):* GER and apnea are common in preterm infants. There is significant controversy about the role

of GER in AOP. Monitoring studies demonstrated that, when a relationship between reflux and apnea is observed, apnea might precede rather than follow reflux.

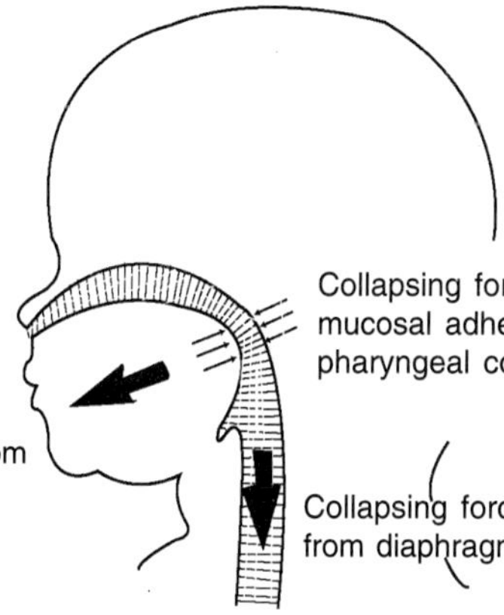

Fig. 9.5: Pharyngeal patency controlled by the balance of dilating and collapsing forces

Diagnosis

Clinical

Threshold criteria for diagnosis have not been objectively defined and there is no established diagnostic test. The identification of individual episodes of AOP is routinely based on detection of:

a. Central apnea lasting at least 20 seconds using standard impedance-based cardiorespiratory monitoring.
b. Bradycardia of less than 100 beats per minute; and
c. Arterial oxygen desaturation using a pulse oximeter (SpO_2).

These symptoms are typically associated with clinically observed cyanosis. To be certain that monitor alarms are clinically significant, episodes initially detected by the monitors need to be confirmed by visual observation. Since impedance-based cardiorespiratory monitors cannot detect obstructive apneas unless and until associated with bradycardia, heart rate should be monitored in addition to or, instead of respiration. If only one parameter can be monitored then it should always be heart rate and episodes of bradycardia should always alert the caretaker about a possible apneic episode.

AOP can be distinguished from periodic breathing by the presence of frequent swallow-like movements in the pharynx during the apnea. The etiology of swallows during apnea is unknown. They could be attributed to GER or possibly increased pooling of secretions in the pharynx. Because swallowing directly inhibits respiratory drive, such events could serve to prolong the apneic pause.

Criteria to classify the severity of apnea have not been well developed in clinical studies. The University of Washington published indications for different treatments based on the severity of AOP.[5] This classification for AOP (Table 9.3) uses the terms spontaneous, mild, moderate, or severe.

Investigations

The diagnosis of apneic episodes is clinical. Investigations are done to detect any underlying pathology presenting with apnea as a symptom. These investigations have been mentioned in Table 9.1.

Table 9.3: Types of apnea and indications for initiating methylxanthines

Definition of apneic event by type of intervention		*Indications for initiating methylxanthines*
Spontaneous/ No intervention required	• Event with minimal physiologic change • Self recovery • No intervention required	Frequent episodes associated with desaturations (SpO_2 <80%) and/or bradycardia (HR <80 bpm); e.g., one or more per hour over a long period of time such as 12-24 hours
Mild	• Light touch, stroke back • Associated with desaturations <80% and bradycardia <90/bpm	Multiple episodes; more than 6 over a 12- hour period or 12 over a 24-hour period
Moderate	• Move infant, i.e. Roll over, re-position, etc. • O_2 administered	More than 2 episodes in a 24-hour period
Severe	• Prolonged vigorous stimulus • Positive pressure ventilation with or without O_2	More than 1 episode in a 24-hour period

Management

Whenever a monitor alarm sounds, one should remember to **respond to the infant**, not the monitor. Most apneic episodes respond to tactile stimulation. Infants who fail to respond to stimulation or in whom these episodes are frequent or severe should be managed by nasal continuous positive airway pressure (CPAP) / ventilation or with pharmacotherapy as described below. The approach to an infant with apneic episode has been outlined in Figure 9.6. The various interventions/drugs, their mechanism of action and adverse effects have been highlighted in Table 9.4.

General Measures

The general measures which should be directed to every infant who has had an apneic episode include:

- Attempt should be made to identify underlying pathology and

Apnea alarm

↓

Check - Child breathing or not/Cyanosis/Bradycardia
- Pallor Hypotonia
- Airway Obstruction (check neck position)

↓

Tactile stimulation
Gentle oropharyngeal and nasal suction
Initiate oxygen (Use FiO_2 less than 0.4)

↓

Bag and mask ventilation
(Use FiO_2 less than 0.4 or what baby was already getting prior to apneic episode)

↓

Intubation and ventilation

Fig. 9.6: Algorithmic approach to apneic episode

Table 9.4: Drugs/ intervention for apnea: Mechanism of action and their adverse effects

Drug/ Intervention	*Mechanism of action*	*Adverse effects*
Avoid extreme flexion/ extension	• Prevents mechanical obstruction of airway	-
Reduce temperature of incubator to lower end of thermo-neutral zone	• Reduces metabolic and oxygen demands	• Monitor for hypothermia
Stopping oral feeds	• Prevents stimulation of mechanoreceptors	-
Packed RBC transfusion	• Increases oxygen carrying capacity of blood	• Transfusion associated infections/reactions
Methylxanthines	• Antagonize adenosine (a respiratory depressant) • Increase diaphragmatic function • Decrease muscle fatigue • Increase catecholamine activity	• Tachycardia • Jitteriness • Irritability • GER
Doxapram	• Analeptic	• Decreases cerebral blood flow
Nasal CPAP	• Increases FRC • Splinting of upper airway in open position	• Local trauma

specific therapy directed at the underlying cause should be initiated.

- The SpO_2 of the infant should be maintained between 88-92%, with supplemental oxygen if needed.
- Positions of extreme flexion and extension of neck should be avoided to reduce narrowing of anatomical space for air to traverse.
- Temperature of incubator/surroundings should be reduced to lower end of thermo-neutral zone.
- The reflexes, which may trigger apnea, should be avoided. This includes stopping of oral feeds and careful suctioning of pharynx.

- Though the role of blood transfusion in apnea is controversial, transfusion of packed red blood cells may be considered if the hematocrit is less than 25%.

Patency of Airway

Ensuring correct position and gentle suction of nasopharynx must ensure it.

Stimulation

Tactile stimulation is usually sufficient to terminate an isolated apneic event caused by central apnea. Stimulation akin to that used during neonatal resuscitation (e.g., a gentle tap to the sole of the foot or rubbing the back) is often enough to terminate a central apnea. However, if the upper airway is obstructed, repositioning the patient's head and neck or gently elevating the infant's jaw may alleviate the occlusion

Administration of Oxygen

Supplemental oxygenation or bag-mask ventilation is indicated in infants with signs of bradycardia or desaturation. Infants who fail to respond to tactile stimulation should be ventilated during spell with bag and mask, with fractional concentration of inspired oxygen (FiO_2) of under 0.40 or equal to FiO_2 prior to spell to avoid marked elevations in arterial oxygen pressures.

Pharmacotherapy

- *Methylxanthines:* **Methylxanthines** are central respiratory stimulants (by antagonizing adenosine, a respiratory depressant) causing increased CO_2 sensitivity and hence lead to improved tidal and minute volumes and blood gas values. They also increase diaphragmatic function, decrease muscle fatigue, and increase metabolic rate and catecholamine activity. These agents include aminophylline and caffeine. Table 9.5 reviews the recommended starting doses and dosing intervals for caffeine and aminophylline. The recommended therapeutic blood levels are 5 to 10 µg/mL for aminophylline and 8 to 20 µg/mL for caffeine. Methylxanthine side effects are secondary to catecholamine stimulation and include tachycardia,

Table 9.5: Methylxanthines: Dosing regimen

Drug	*Loading*	*Maintenance*
Aminophylline*	5-7 mg/kg IV over 30 minutes	1.5 to 2.0 mg/kg PO or IV every 6 to 8 hourly
Caffeine citrate**	20 mg/kg PO or IV over 30 min (equivalent to 10 mg/kg caffeine base)	5 to 8 mg/kg once daily (equivalent to 2.5 to 5.0 mg/kg caffeine base)

If apnea continues to occur after starting methylxanthines, give an additional dose of 50% of initial loading dose and increase maintenance by 20%.

* Start maintenance dose 8 to 12 hours after loading dose. If changing from IV to PO aminophylline, increase dose by 20%. If changing to PO theophylline, no change in dose is required.

** Start maintenance dose 24 hours after loading dose. Caffeine citrate may be given IV or PO.

jitteriness, and irritability. Direct comparisons of aminophylline and caffeine indicate similar efficacy at equivalent levels of central ventilatory stimulation. However, side effects are less with caffeine than with aminophylline. The treatment indications for starting methylxanthines have been depicted in Table 9.3.

- *Doxapram:* **Doxapram**, an intravenous analeptic agent, is excluded as a therapy for AOP because it is associated with reduced cerebral blood flow. It should be reserved for infants in whom appropriate methylxanthine therapy and CPAP fail to control severe apneic events. The intravenous loading dose for doxapram is 2.5 to 3.0 mg/kg over 15 minutes followed by a continuous infusion of 1.0 mg/kg titrated to the lowest responsive dose (maximum dose 2.5 mg/kg/hour).

Nasal CPAP

Some premature infants continue to have apnea while on theophylline therapy. A low CPAP of 4 to 5 cm H_2O, most simply administered via the nasal route, decreases the incidence of apnea in these infants. The main disadvantage of this technique is that it becomes cumbersome over a prolonged period. Apnea frequency can be reduced on CPAP by several mechanisms, including stabilization of Pao_2 by increasing FRC, alteration of the stretch receptor influence on respiratory timing, or splinting of the upper airway in an open position. The splinting hypothesis is suggested by the observation that CPAP specifically eliminates apneas that have an obstructive component and reduces supraglottic resistance in preterm infants.

If nasal CPAP, in conjunction with a methylxanthine, is not sufficient to prevent recurring episodes associated with bradycardia and intermittent hypoxemia, some investigators have suggested using nasal intermittent positive pressure ventilation (NIPPV). **NIPPV** may most likely be needed when episodes are related predominately to central apneas that are not being effectively eliminated by the NCPAP.

Intubation and Assisted Ventilation

If an infant is still having clinically significant episodes of apnea despite optimal pharmacologic and NCPAP/NIPPV, then endotracheal intubation and positive pressure ventilation is the treatment of last resort.

Prognosis and Follow-up

Apnea in premature infants exhibits a gradual decrease in frequency over the first 2 months of postnatal life. Apnea can persist for many weeks in very preterm infants born at less than 28 weeks GA, although resolution has typically occurred by 43 to 44 weeks' postmenstrual age. The dilemma faced by the infant's physician is to decide whether such events are potentially dangerous for the infant and whether home monitoring of such infants is necessary or useful.[6] The answers to these questions are still under debate. Most neonatologists allow a 5- to 7-day apnea-free period after discontinuing xanthenes therapy before sending a premature infant home without a monitor. If home monitoring is recommended for persistent cardiorespiratory events, it can usually be discontinued by 44 weeks' postmenstrual age. Routine **home monitoring** of asymptomatic preterm infants is not indicated. Continued use of xanthines may be helpful in infants whose spells recur when the drug is discontinued and in situations where home monitoring is not feasible. A repeat attempt to withdraw the drug can be made after a period of 4 to 8 weeks while closely monitoring the child.

Neurodevelopmental Outcome

Most reports have found little evidence of any neurodevelopmental risk directly attributable to history of apneic episodes. All of these AOP studies are limited due to nonstandardized criteria for diagnosis and for quantifying severity of apnea-related events. The researchers have found that infants with clinically significant AOP do not perform as well as prematurely born infants without recurrent apneas during neurodevelopmental follow-up testing. Nonetheless there is no consensus whether the apneic events and developmental delay are both the consequence of antecedent events occurring antenatally or in the postnatal period or the developmental delay is a direct result of apnea related to "decreased cerebral blood flow".

REFERENCES

1. Miller MJ, Martin RJ: *Pathophysiology of apnea of prematurity*, In: Polin RA, *et al.*, ed. *Fetal and Neonatal Physiology*, 3rd ed., Philadelphia: Saunders; 2004.
2. Finer NN, Higgins R, Kattwinkel J, Martin RJ: Summary proceedings from the apnea-of-prematurity group, Pediatrics 2006;117:S47-51.
3. Stark AR: Apnea, In: Cloherty JP, Eichenwald EC and Stark AR, ed, Manual of neonatal care, 5th ed, Lippincott Williams & Wilkins, 2004.
4. Martin RJ, Abu-Shaweesh JM: Control of breathing and neonatal apnea, Biol Neonate 2005;87:288-295.
5. Mayock DE: Apnea, Revised February 24, 2000, University of Washington Division of Neonatology Website, NICU-WEB.
6. Hunt CE, Baird T: The Collaborative Home Infant Monitoring Evaluation (CHIME) Study Group, *et al.*, Cardiorespiratory events detected by home memory monitoring and neurodevelopmental outcome at one year of age, J Pediatr 2004;145:465-471.

10 BRONCHOPULMONARY DYSPLASIA

Vineet Bhandari

DEFINITIONS

Older definitions include supplemental O_2 at 28 days of age, need for O_2 at 28 days with at least 21 days of O_2 supplementation and a consistent chest X-ray, and O_2 need at 36 weeks corrected postmenstrual age.[1] New criteria for diagnosis of **broncho-pulmonary dysplasia** (BPD) and its severity have been proposed.[2] These have been summarized in Table 10.1.

Epidemiology

In infants with birth weights 501-1500 grams, the overall incidence of BPD (using the 36 weeks definition) is 22%.[3] Using the physiologic definition, the incidence was 25% in a cohort of infants 501-1249 grams birth weight.[4] BPD is infrequent in infants with birth weights of >1200 grams and gestational ages of >30 weeks.[5] The incidence of BPD by birth weight has been summarized in Table 10.2.

Pathology

The histopathological lesions in "old" BPD consisted of severe airway injury and alternating sites of overinflation and fibrosis. In the "new" BPD, irrespective of whether infants have been treated with antenatal steroids and/or surfactant, the lungs show large, simplified alveolar structures, abnormal capillary morphology and an interstitium with variable cellularity/ fibroproliferation.[6]

Table 10.1: Diagnostic criteria for BPD*			
	Mild	*Moderate*	*Severe*
	Supplemental O_2 (for 28 days) and	Supplemental O_2 (for 28 days) and	Supplemental O_2 (for 28 days) and
< 32 weeks GA at birth	RA at 36 weeks corrected GA or at discharge	<0.3 FiO_2 at 36 weeks corrected GA or at discharge	≥ 0.3 FiO_2 +/- positive pressure support at 36 weeks corrected GA or at discharge
≥ 32 weeks GA at birth	RA by postnatal day 56 or at discharge	<0.3 FiO_2 by postnatal day 56 or at discharge	≥ 0.3 FiO_2 +/- positive pressure support by postnatal day 56 or at discharge

*Adapted from reference [2]. BPD: Bronchopulmonary dysplasia; FiO_2: Fraction of inspired oxygen; GA: Gestational age; RA: Room air.

Table 10.2: Incidence of BPD*		
Birth weight (grams)	*BPD***	*BPD****
501-750	90-100%	46-54%
751-1000	50-70%	33-34%
1001-1250	30-60%	14-20%
1251-1499	6-40%	6-10%

* Adapted from references [3, 7].

** Supplemental O_2 at 28 days.

***Supplemental O_2 at 36 weeks corrected postmenstrual age.

Pathogenesis

"Old" BPD is said to occur secondary to injury to the immature lung by *in utero* infection, and exposure to postnatal mechanical ventilation with high pressures and oxygen concentrations.[7,8] These processes initiate an inflammatory cascade leading to fibrosis and scarring of lung parenchyma.

"New" BPD is a consequence of resuscitation of extremely

immature lungs. It is hypothesized that the etiology of new BPD is the initiation of inflammatory mediators that cause impairment of **alveolarization** and vasculogenesis.[9] Deficient anti-inflammatory mediators in the premature neonate may be easily overwhelmed by the pro-inflammatory cascade. These neonates may also be particularly susceptible to infection that accelerates inflammation and lung injury. An imbalance in the release of pro- and anti-inflammatory cytokines, occurring as a result of ventilator trauma, oxidants, pulmonary edema, and/or sepsis, damages the immature lung. This is followed either by healing (resolution of injury) or repair of the lung (BPD). These may be modified by nutrition and stem cells. Cytokine release and the responses of the immature lung are determined by allelic differences of genes that create genetic susceptibility.[10] Differential interactions between genetic susceptibility and environmental factors create intermediate clinical phenotypes that would modify the degree of the final clinical outcome, as mild or moderate or severe. Figure 10.1 illustrates the possible pathophysiologic mechanisms underlying new BPD.

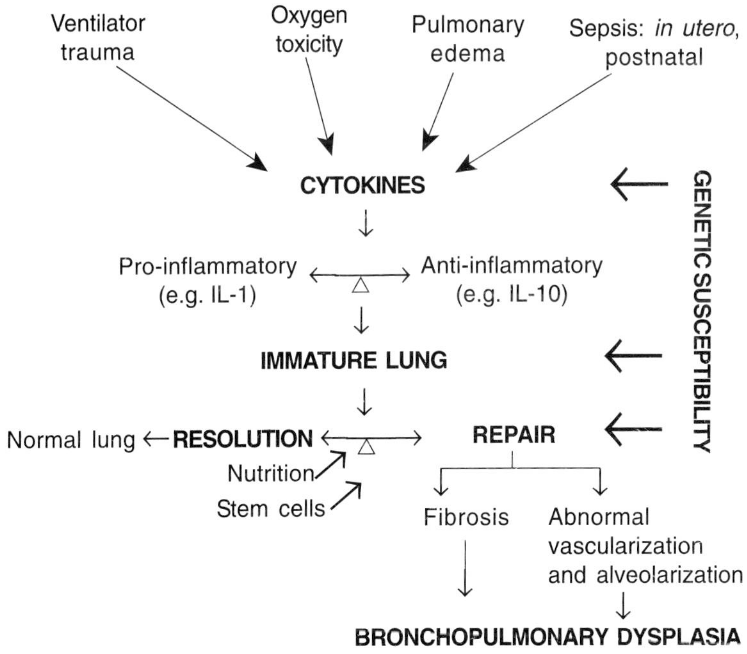

Fig. 10.1: Pathogenesis of BPD

Chapter 10

Clinical Features

Signs and symptoms include tachypnea, dyspnea, and chronic or intermittent crackles and wheezing. In children with subglottic stenosis secondary to prolonged intubation, there may be presence of a stridor on exam. Noisy breathing exacerbated with high airflow activities such as feeding and agitation may be heard in infants with tracheomalacia and bronchomalacia. BPD spells are episodes of tracheal obstruction associated with episodes of cyanosis and oxygen desaturations and bradycardia, usually occurring secondary to agitation, and are thought to be related to tracheomalacia and bronchomalacia. Cardiac complications of severe BPD include pulmonary hypertension and corpulmonale. Poor growth may be related to undiagnosed hypoxia, cardiac disease, gastroesophageal reflux and swallow dysfunction or recurrent aspiration.

Radiological findings: These are non-specific and include pulmonary edema, atelectasis, hyperinflation, and cystic areas. Some of these features are shown in Figure 10.2.

Diagnosis

The diagnosis of BPD is usually established clinically. The classical presentation in history of a premature infant with Respiratory

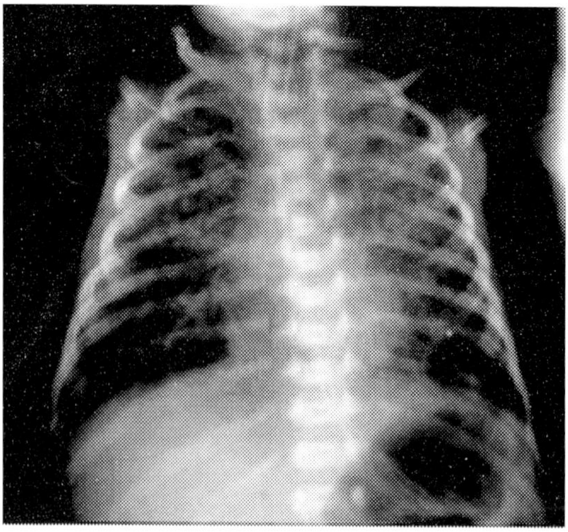

Fig. 10.2: Chext X-ray of an infant with established BPD

Distress Syndrome (RDS) who has been ventilated and exposed to supplemental **oxygen** for the first week of life or longer. Usually these infants experience bouts of postnatal sepsis and have inadequate nutritional intake. Over time, these infants fulfil the diagnostic criteria for BPD, as defined earlier. The *differential diagnosis* of BPD has been shown in Table 10.3.

Table 10.3: Differential diagnosis of BPD

Pneumonia
Congenital heart disease
Aspiration
Wilson Mikity syndrome
Surfactant protein deficiency
Pulmonary lymphangiectasia
Interstitial lung disease

Management

This has been summarized in Table 10.4.

Complications

Side effects of **diuretics** include electrolyte disturbances (hyponatremia, hypokalemia, hypocalcemia) and osteopenia, especially with furosemide. Increased incidence of neurological sequelae with early use (<96 hours) systemic glucocorticoids has been noted. Use of beta agonists may increase large airway instability in infants with tracheomalacia and bronchomalacia.

Prognosis and Follow-up

Pulmonary outcomes[11]: Infants with BPD have higher rates of rehospitalizations, with upto 50% of very low birth weight infants with severe BPD needing rehospitalization in the first year of life and 36% rehospitalized the second year of life. Most common reasons for rehospitalization were reactive airway disease, pneumonia, RSV infection and worsening BPD. Significant respiratory symptoms and greater utilization of asthma medications persist in 25% of adolescents and adults with BPD. In infants with BPD, lung mechanics normalize overtime whereas small airway abnormalities persist through adolescence and

Table 10.4: Management of BPD*

Intervention	*Mechanism of action*	*Comments*
Oxygen supplementation	Prevents development of pulmonary hypertension and corpulmonale	Maintain O_2 saturations between 85-93%.
Glucocorticoids	Decrease pulmonary inflammation	Dexamethasone effective in weaning off mechanical ventilation when used moderately late and late. Increased incidence of neurological sequelae with early use (<96 hours). No benefit from inhaled steroids.
Diuretics	Decreases pulmonary edema and improve lung compliance	Result in significant decrease in oxygen required though duration of oxygen requirement is not significantly decreased. Furosemide used as daily or every other day therapy in the short-term. Spirnolactone and thiazides used for chronic therapy.
Beta agonists	Provides bronchodilatation	Nebulized albuterol most commonly used.
Anticholinergics	Provides bronchodilatation	Used in conjunction with beta agonists; no clear benefit in BPD.
Nutrition	Promotes lung and somatic growth	Optimal weight gain of 15-20 g/day.
Immunization	Prophylaxis against RSV and influenza. Other immunizations should be as per chronological age	Decreases incidence of re-hospitalization and morbidity.

*Adapted from reference[5].

adulthood, thus reflecting dysnaptic growth and repair. In addition to tracheomalacia and bronchomalacia, other large airway problems commonly encountered are sub-glottic stenosis, airway granulomas and pseudopolyps and may require surgical intervention. Majority of survivors of BPD participate in various physical activities without any symptoms.

Neurodevelopmental outcomes[12]: Children with BPD exhibit low average IQ, academic difficulties, delayed speech and language development, visual-motor integration impairments, and behavior problems. There is some evidence that children with BPD also display attention problems, memory and learning deficits and executive dysfunction. BPD does not appear to be associated with a specific neuropsychological impairment but rather a global impairment.

Prevention

This is primarily dependent on the prevention of premature birth and lung immaturity. Recent use of progesterone in prevention of premature labor has shown promise, though the prolongation of gestation has yet to be shown to improve infant outcomes.[13] For lung maturation, antenatal **steroids** remain the single most effective strategy to date.

After the delivery of the premature baby, avoidance of the endotracheal tube with the use of **non-invasive ventilation** has shown benefit.[14] If endotracheal tube ventilation is essential, an approach favoring permissive hypoxemia and hypercapnia has been suggested.[15] Prevention, early diagnosis and treatment of sepsis and postnatal fluid/electrolyte[16] as well as nutritional management are other key areas for prevention of BPD. Use of vitamin A may be helpful. Understanding the **genetic** contribution to BPD will likely open up other avenues of research that may potentially impact on the management and prevention of BPD.[10]

REFERENCES

1. Shennan AT, Dunn MS, Ohlsson A, Lennox K, Hoskins EM: Abnormal pulmonary outcomes in premature infants: Prediction from oxygen requirement in the neonatal period, Pediatrics 1988;82:527-532.
2. Jobe AH, Bancalari E: Bronchopulmonary dysplasia, Am J Respir Crit Care Med 2001;163:1723-1729.
3. Fanaroff AA, Stoll BJ, Wright LL, Carlo WA, Ehrenkranz RA, Stark AR, Bauer CR, Donovan EF, Korones SB, Laptook AR, Lemons JA, Oh W,

Papile LA, Shankaran S, Stevenson DK, Tyson JE, Poole WK: Trends in neonatal morbidity and mortality for very low birthweight infants, Am J Obstet Gynecol 2007;196:147 e141-148.

4. Walsh MC, Yao Q, Gettner P, Hale E, Collins M, Hensman A, Everette R, Peters N, Miller N, Muran G, Auten K, Newman N, Rowan G, Grisby C, Arnell K, Miller L, Ball B, McDavid G: Impact of a physiologic definition on bronchopulmonary dysplasia rates, Pediatrics 2004;114:1305-1311.
5. Bhandari A, Bhandari V: Bronchopulmonary dysplasia: An update, Indian J Pediatr 2007;74:73-77.
6. Coalson JJ: Pathology of bronchopulmonary dysplasia, Semin Perinatol 2006;30:179-184.
7. Bhandari A, Bhandari V: Pathogenesis, pathology and pathophysiology of pulmonary sequelae of bronchopulmonary dysplasia in premature infants, Front Biosci 2003;8:e370-380.
8. Lyon A: Chronic lung disease of prematurity: The role of intrauterine infection, Eur J Pediatr 2000;159:798-802.
9. D'Angio CT, Maniscalco WM: The role of vascular growth factors in hyperoxia-induced injury to the developing lung, Front Biosci 2002;7:d1609-1623.
10. Bhandari V, Gruen JR: The genetics of bronchopulmonary dysplasia, Semin Perinatol 2006;30:185-191.
11. Bhandari A, Panitch HB: Pulmonary outcomes in bronchopulmonary dysplasia, Semin Perinatol 2006;30:219-226.
12. Anderson PJ, Doyle LW: Neurodevelopmental outcome of bronchopulmonary dysplasia, Semin Perinatol 2006;30:227-232.
13. Dodd JM, Crowther CA, Cincotta R, Flenady V, Robinson JS: Progesterone supplementation for preventing preterm birth: A systematic review and meta-analysis, Acta Obstet Gynecol Scand 2005;84:526-533.
14. Bhandari V: Non-invasive ventilation of the sick neonate: Evidence-based recommendations, Journal of Neonatology 2006;20:214-221.
15. Ambalavanan N, Carlo WA: Ventilatory strategies in the prevention and management of bronchopulmonary dysplasia, Semin Perinatol 2006;30:192-199.
16. Bhandari V, Brodsky N, Porat R: Improved outcome of extremely low birthweight infants with Tegaderm application to skin, J Perinatol 2005;25:276-281.

11 TRANSIENT TACHYPNEA OF THE NEWBORN

Dinesh Kumar Chirla
and Girish Gupta

DEFINITION

Transient tachypnea of the newborn (TTNB) is a self-limited disease presenting soon after birth. It is also known as "**wet lung disease**", "**newborn with retained fetal lung liquid**", and "**neonatal retained fluid syndrome**". The neonate usually presents with tachypnea and mild grunting within 2-3 hours of birth. Recovery usually is complete within 24-72 hours.

EPIDEMIOLOGY

The incidence is 4 to 5.7 per 1000 infants delivered at 37 to 42 weeks of gestation. Risk is equal in both males and females. TTNB does occur in preterm infants but co-existing problems like respiratory distress syndrome (RDS) may mask the presentation.

ETIOPATHOGENESIS

TTNB is the result of a delay in clearance of fetal lung liquid. Neonates born following elective cesarean section (i.e. without labor) are at a higher risk of TTNB. Low adrenaline levels, absence of anticipatory lung fluid clearance because of lack of appropriate catecholamine surge during labor and relative surfactant deficiency are contributing factors in the pathogenesis of TTNB. The end result is alveoli with retained fluid that inhibit gas exchange. Other reasons for TTNB have been enumerated in Table 11.1.

Table 11.1: Risk factors for TTNB

Elective caesarean section	Lack of catecholamine surge which causes fetal lung fluid absorption
	Relative surfactant deficiency
Maternal asthma	Genetic predisposition to β-adrenergic hyporesponsiveness
Na+ transport cell	Inability of immature fetal lung to switch from fluid secretion to fluid absorption

Clinical Features

The maternal history consists of caesarean delivery without labor or precipitous delivery. The symptoms and signs in the neonate are shown in Table 11.2.

Table 11.2: Symptoms and signs of TTNB

Symptoms	Respiratory distress immediately after birth (Respiratory rate can be as high as 100-120/minute)
	May be associated with grunting
	Cyanosis usually settles with oxygen
Signs	Tachypnea (usually "quiet" tachypnea)
	Nasal flaring, grunting, tachycardia, blood pressure is normal
	Chest barrel shaped; on auscultation crepitations are heard

Investigations

These are summarized in Table 11.3.

Table 11.3: Investigations in an infant suspected of TTNB

- Arterial blood gas (ABG): To ascertain the degree of gas exchange and acid-base balance
- Chest X-ray: The characteristic findings include (Fig. 11.1)
  - Prominent perihilar streaking
  - Fluid in the fissures
  - Small pleural effusions
  - Mild cardiomegaly
- Sepsis screen: CBC, CRP, blood culture. If respiratory distress is persistent after 4 hours or in presence of risk factors of sepsis.

Diagnosis

Most neonates present with respiratory distress immediately after birth or in first 2-3 hours. Improvement is usually noted within the first 24 hours of life.

Management

They should be transferred to nursery/neonatal intensive care unit for further monitoring and treatment. Initial steps of management are summarized in Table 11.4.

Table 11.4: Initial steps of management on transfer of an infant with TTNB to the nursery

- Keep baby warm.
- Monitor heart rate, respiratory rate, oxygen saturation and blood pressure. Pulse oximetry allows the clinician to adjust the level of oxygen support needed to maintain appropriate saturation.
- Head box oxygen: To maintain oxygen saturation 94-100% (term infant).

Further medical care is shown in Table 11.5.

Table 11.5: Further medical care of an infant with TTNB

- Mainly supportive. As the retained lung fluid is absorbed by the infant's lymphatic system, the pulmonary status improves.
- Intravenous fluids and gavage feedings until the respiratory rate has decreased enough to allow oral feedings (usually <60/minute).
- Supplemental oxygen to maintain adequate arterial oxygen saturation.
- Following blood cultures, a course of antibiotic therapy may be initiated and then terminated at 48 hours if cultures are negative and the clinical condition is improving.
- Repeat ABG if worsening of respiratory distress or increased oxygen requirement.
- Worsening respiratory distress may need continuous positive airway pressure (CPAP) or mechanical ventilation (uncommon).

Complications

Any infant who does not follow the typical course of TTNB and who develops worsening respiratory distress must be re-evaluated for alternate diagnosis or comorbidities, which confound respiratory distress. These include:

- Pneumonia.

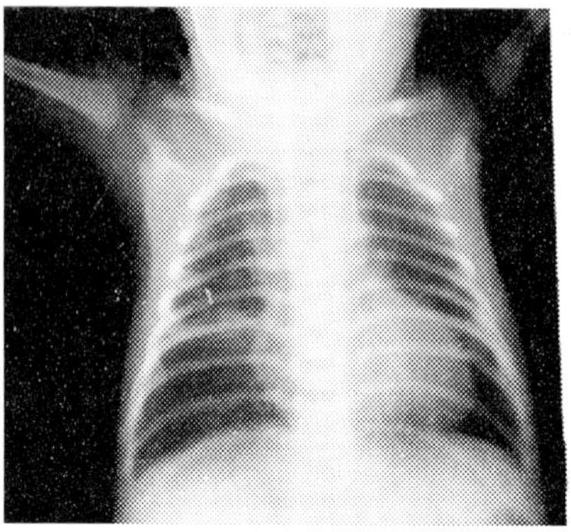

Fig. 11.1: Chest X-ray of an infant with TTNB

- Air leak syndromes.
- Metabolic abnormalities.
- Thermal abnormalities.
- Central nervous system disorders.
- Congenital abnormalities of the cardiorespiratory system.
- Hematological disorders.

Prognosis

TTNB is usually a self-limited disorder and is not life threatening. Recovery is usually complete without significant morbidity. There is some evidence that neonates with TTNB may later develop asthma.

12 MECONIUM ASPIRATION SYNDROME

Namasivayam Ambalavanan

INCIDENCE

Meconium staining of the amniotic fluid (MSAF) occurs in 6 to 25% (average 13%) of all deliveries. Of these infants, approximately 25% are "depressed" at birth with 1-minute Apgar scores $\leq$6. Between 5 to 12% of neonates born with MSAF, or about 0.5 to 1% of all deliveries develop meconium aspiration syndrome (MAS). In developed countries, only about 1 in 5-10 infants with MAS, or 1 in 500-1000 livebirths will require mechanical ventilation. The reduction in the incidence of MAS over the past three decades is generally considered to be due to a reduction in postmaturity, rather than due to any innovative advances in neonatal-perinatal medicine.

ETIOLOGY

Passage of meconium is normally after birth, but occasionally occurs *in utero*. MSAF may range from a clear, greenish-yellow tinged fluid to a thick "**pea-soup**" consistency fluid, depending upon the magnitude and timing of meconium passage. Fetal distress may lead to MSAF, but MSAF does not imply fetal distress in the absence of other evidence. Meconium-stained amniotic fluid was associated with lower fetal pulse oximetry values only when fetal heart monitoring showed a "non-reassuring" pattern. MSAF is usually seen in **term** or **post-term** gestation, and rarely in premature infants. It is generally considered that aspiration of the meconium occurs at or soon after delivery. However, **fetal gasping** movements may sometimes lead to meconium aspiration *in utero*. There is increasing evidence that a chronic *in utero* insult occurs in most cases of severe MAS. Vigorous infants who aspirate meconium at birth are usually at low risk for severe MAS. Risk factors for MAS in the setting of MSAF include "thick" meconium, no oropharyngeal suctioning at delivery, meconium present in the trachea, "depression" at birth, abnormal **fetal heart rate** (FHR) tracing, cesarean delivery, and oligohydramnios. Compared with healthy neonates with MSAF, those with MAS had higher rate of non-reassuring FHR tracing, thick meconium, and lower Apgar scores ($\leq$ 5 at 5 min).

PATHOLOGY

Once meconium is inhaled into the trachea and major bronchi, distal migration of meconium into the smaller bronchi and alveoli can occur with the onset of respiration. The pathophysiology of MAS includes: (a) mechanical airway obstruction by meconium and exudates, (b) pulmonary vasoconstriction and increased pulmonary vascular resistance, (c) surfactant inactivation by meconium, and (d) chemical pneumonitis. Areas of atelectasis occur due to total airway obstruction and surfactant inactivation, and areas of gas trapping occur due to a "ball-valve" phenomenon in areas of partial obstruction. The gas trapping predisposes to air leak syndromes such as **pneumothorax** and **pneumomediastinum**. Direct toxicity due to meconium constituents as well as release of chemical mediators of inflammation leads to a chemical pneumonitis. The ventilation-perfusion mismatch caused by these events leads to hypoxemia, hypercapnia and acidosis, which in turn lead to hypoxic pulmonary vasoconstriction and pulmonary hypertension. Antenatal pulmonary vascular remodeling secondary to chronic *in utero* hypoxemia may contribute to the altered pulmonary reactivity and pulmonary hypertension. **Persistent pulmonary hypertension of the newborn (PPHN)** hence is a major complication of MAS and the most frequent cause of a fatal outcome. PPHN is characterized by elevated pulmonary arterial pressures at or above systemic arterial level and by right to left or bi-directional shunting at the level of the foramen ovale or ductus arteriosus in the absence of structural heart disease. Unfortunately, the hypoxemia and acidosis noted in PPHN often further elevate the pulmonary pressures and right to left shunting, worsening further the hypoxemia and acidosis. This downward spiral may result in death if rapid intervention does not occur.

Clinical Features

The clinical features that are usually seen are **respiratory distress** with tachypnea, grunting, flaring, retractions and cyanosis. These features may not be present if the neonate also has severe hypoxic encephalopathy. Heterogeneous lung disease is classically seen, with alternating areas of **hyperinflation** and **atelectasis** which appear as diffuse asymmetric **patchy infiltrates** on the chest radiograph. It should be noted that many neonates have abnormal chest radiographs but a benign clinical course, and radiographic clearing may be slower than clinical resolution. The chest may appear hyperinflated and the abdomen scaphoid, due to the combination of lung hyperinflation and evacuated bowels. Some infants with MAS have pneumothorax, which may be secondary to resuscitative efforts, mechanical ventilation, or spontaneous strong respiratory efforts in the presence of "ball-valve" phenomena. **Hypoxemia** is usually noted, and hypocapnia may occur in milder cases due to hyperventilation, but severe cases of MAS usually present with **hypercapnia** and **acidosis**.

Cleary and Wiswell[1] have developed a severity classification for MAS: (1) mild MAS is disease that requires less than 40% oxygen for <48 hours; (2) moderate MAS is disease that requires >40% oxygen for >48 hours with no air leak; and (3) severe MAS is disease is that requires assisted ventilation for more than 48 hours and is often associated with PPHN. However, this classification is rather empirical and not generally used at the current time.

Diagnosis

The diagnosis is primarily a clinical diagnosis, with support from chest radiographs. An infant with history of MSAF and respiratory distress which cannot be otherwise explained, especially in combination with patchy lung infiltrates, may be presumed to have MAS.

Differential Diagnoses

If patchy infiltrates on the chest radiograph are not seen in a neonate with respiratory distress, and the lungs demonstrate either clear lungs or some vascular/interstitial markings, alternative diagnoses such as idiopathic PPHN, transient tachypnea of the newborn, or cardiac disease have to be considered. Some infants with spontaneous pneumothorax, lung malformations (e.g. congenital lobar emphysema, congenital cystic adenomatoid malformation) may also present with respiratory distress but the radiologic diagnosis is usually more evident.

Investigations

Chest radiographs and **arterial blood gases** are indicated. Hematocrit and complete blood counts/blood cultures are also routinely done, in order to ensure an adequate oxygen carrying capacity (adequate hematocrit) and absence of sepsis. Other investigations will depend upon the clinical presentation.

Management

During Labor

The presence of MSAF requires close monitoring of labor and fetal well-being. The combination of MSAF and abnormal FHR tracing is associated with a higher risk of MAS. **Amnioinfusion** for the prevention of MAS has been controversial, but recent reports indicate that amnioinfusion in the presence of moderate or thick MSAF is associated with a lower risk of MAS, especially in the setting of limited peripartum surveillance. It is not clear if amnioinfusion benefits by dilution of the meconium or by correction of oligohydramnios with consequent reduction of fetal heart rate abnormalities.

Higher rates of positive amniotic fluid cultures and clinical chorioamnionitis have been observed in the presence of MSAF, although without a concomitant increase in neonatal sepsis. The use of intrapartum antibiotics should therefore be considered.

During Delivery

The resuscitation team should be made aware of the impending delivery well in advance, and resuscitation equipment should be kept ready. Equipment for emergency management of a pneumothorax should also be available in close proximity.

Obstetrician may suction the infant's mouth and nose before delivery of the shoulders, with either a catheter or a bulb syringe. This used to be considered one of the preventive measures for MAS, although controlled trials for this intervention do not show any benefit.

There is no scientific evidence to support the practices of chest compression, placing a finger in the mouth, or cricoid pressure in an attempt to prevent meconium aspiration. These procedures may be hazardous and are not recommended.

Immediate Post-Delivery [2, 3]

New evidence from a large randomized controlled trial indicates that intubation and endotracheal **suctioning** of the infant born with MSAF who is vigorous (good respiratory effort, heart rate > 100/min and good tone) does not reduce MAS, and hence endotracheal suctioning is not indicated at delivery in these infants. Thin meconium, which is watery and non-particulate, is infrequently associated with neonatal problems and these infants are usually vigorous. All these infants require is additional suctioning of oral and nasal secretions followed by drying and observation.

It has been recommended that infants who are born "depressed" (not vigorous in the first 15-20 seconds after birth despite oral and nasal suctioning) need to be endotracheally suctioned, regardless of whether the meconium is thin or thick and particulate. However, the efficacy of this intervention has not been adequately investigated. Direct laryngoscopy should be performed and a 3.0 or 3.5 neonatal endotracheal tube inserted. The meconium aspirator attached to pressure-regulated wall suction (80 to 100 mm Hg pressure) is then attached to the endotracheal tube adapter, and suction applied as the endotracheal tube is withdrawn. Endotracheal suctioning takes less than 20 seconds for experienced resuscitators, and should be followed by tactile stimulation and drying. Visualization of the vocal cords for meconium followed by selective endotracheal suctioning (if meconium is present) is not recommended since meconium may be present in the trachea without any meconium in the pharynx or larynx. Re-intubation for suctioning is usually not required unless the tube is plugged with meconium or there is a very large amount of meconium in the tube. Unsuccessful multiple attempts at intubation should not be done, as subsequent resuscitation may be complicated. If the neonate continues to be "depressed" with inadequate respiratory effort or bradycardia following endotracheal suctioning and tactile stimulation, the infant should be re-intubated and positive pressure ventilation initiated. Sudden deterioration during the process of resuscitation, or lack of improvement, indicates the possibility of pneumothorax.

Care in the Nursery

Routine newborn care is usual for vigorous neonates born through thin MSAF. Infants born through thick MSAF and those "depressed" at birth need to be closely monitored for signs of respiratory distress or cyanosis. Continuous pulse oximetry is useful in the evaluation of hypoxemia in these neonates. Severely "depressed" neonates should also be observed for neurologic signs of hypoxic-ischemic encephalopathy. These "depressed" neonates may need evaluation and management of hypotension, renal function, and multi-organ system dysfunction. **Fluids** are usually restricted to 60 ml/kg/day in neonates with respiratory distress and in those with evidence of **hypoxic encephalopathy**, and **hypotension** is managed with inotropic support with dopamine and/or dobutamine. Blood glucose should also be monitored in the first few hours, as hypoglycemia (<40 mg/dL) is more frequent in neonates born through MSAF.

Prophylactic gastric lavage to clear the stomach of meconium has not been shown to improve feeding tolerance or other outcomes, and is therefore not recommended. Routine chest physiotherapy has also not been shown to be helpful, either in prevention or initial management of MAS.

Infants who have clear signs of MAS should be managed in a neonatal intensive care unit (NICU) and have arterial blood gases (ABGs) and a chest radiograph (CXR) rapidly evaluated. Infants who have respiratory distress are usually maintained on intravenous fluids at 60 ml/kg/day. Antimicrobial agents (often ampicillin and gentamicin, or antimicrobials based on local microbial isolates and sensitivities) are started after obtaining blood cultures as it is not often possible to differentiate between bacterial pneumonia and MAS. If blood cultures are negative, the antibiotics are usually discontinued after 48 hours.

Neonates who manifest hypoxemia despite good respiratory effort and without hypercapnia or acidosis should be administered oxygen, preferably by oxygen hood. It is important to prevent hypoxemia, which may contribute to pulmonary hypertension. Hypoxemia is prevented by elevation of the inspired oxygen concentration (FiO_2) to keep the PaO_2 in the 80-100 torr range. Infants with MAS are usually term or post-term infants and there is less concern with hyperoxia as compared to preterm neonates. If FiO_2 requirements are high (>0.6), a trial of continuous positive airway pressure (CPAP) may be tried, but with caution, as CPAP may increase gas trapping in the setting of MAS, and potentially increase the risk of pneumothorax.

Neonates who become hypoxemic (PaO_2 <50 torr) with severe respiratory distress, hypercapnia ($PaCO_2$ >60 torr), or acidosis (pH<7.25), and neonates who are apneic need to be mechanically ventilated. The goal should be to achieve adequate oxygenation with minimal additional lung injury. Again, hypoxemia should be prevented by maintaining the arterial PO_2 in the 80-100 torr range. **Ventilator management** is often difficult, due to the conflicting demands of areas of atelectasis and hyperinflation. A relatively rapid rate, the minimum effective peak inspiratory pressure (PIP), a low to moderate positive end expiratory pressure (PEEP), and an adequate expiratory time (usually 0.5 to 0.7 seconds) are required to prevent an increase in gas trapping or a pneumothorax. **Alkalosis** and **hyperventilation** are often attempted but there is little evidence to indicate their efficacy or safety (or lack thereof). Alkalosis, which is known to cause pulmonary vasodilation, is achieved by hyperventilation (to maintain arterial PCO_2 in the 30-35 torr range) and infusion of sodium bicarbonate (0.25-1 mEq/kg/h) to maintain a pH in the range of 7.45-7.55. It is important to avoid very low arterial PCO_2 in the <30 torr range as cerebral vasoconstriction may result. Most clinicians, however, prefer a more "gentle" approach to ventilation in order to diminish ventilator-associated lung injury and tolerate mild hypoxemia and/or hypercapnia. Many infants with MAS and possible PPHN are sedated with fentanyl or morphine, and may also be paralyzed with pancuronium if high ventilator settings are required or if the neonate "fights" the ventilator.

Constant vigilance for the presence of air leaks is necessary using clinical evaluation, transillumination, and chest radiographs. Pneumothoraces that occur usually need chest tube drainage.

Neonates with a large pre-ductal to post-ductal oxygen saturation difference indicative of ductal right to left shunting, and those with hypoxemia disproportionate to clinical signs, may have PPHN, and this diagnosis may be confirmed by echocardiography.

If hypoxemia or hypercapnia does not respond adequately to conventional mechanical ventilation, or if air leaks (pneumothorax or pneumomediastinum) are present, **high frequency ventilation** in the form of either high frequency oscillatory ventilation (HFOV) or high frequency jet ventilation (HFJV) is often used. There is no evidence to suggest that high frequency ventilation is superior to conventional ventilation in the setting of MAS.

Surfactant administration may improve oxygenation and reduce the need for **extracorporeal membrane oxygenation (ECMO)** in neonates with MAS. It is necessary to carefully monitor for dosing complications such as hypoxemia, bradycardia, or endotracheal tube occlusion.

Inhaled nitric oxide (iNO), a selective pulmonary vasodilator, may be administered in combination with high frequency ventilation or with conventional ventilators. Some neonatologists prefer to administer iNO before, rather than after, a trial of high frequency ventilation. Nitric oxide is usually started at an inhaled concentration of 20 parts per million (ppm) and subsequently weaned slowly, as long as oxygenation remains adequate. Higher concentrations of iNO (e.g. 40 and 80 ppm) may be attempted if there is inadequate response to 20 ppm, but these efforts are often unsuccessful and the risk of **methemoglobinemia** is higher with iNO>20 ppm. It should be noted that rapid discontinuation of iNO may result in rebound pulmonary hypertension. Unfortunately, the response to iNO is often less in MAS as compared to the response seen in idiopathic PPHN. It is important to realize that critically ill neonates with MAS requiring therapies such as high frequency ventilation and iNO may deteriorate rapidly and die during transport, and hence these therapies must be used with caution outside a neonatal intensive care unit with ECMO availability. Approximately 40% of infants with MAS treated with iNO fail to respond and need ECMO.

ECMO is normally considered an effective therapy of last resort for neonates with intractable reversible respiratory failure or PPHN, who persist with hypoxemia despite maximal ventilator support (and iNO, when available). Although mortality and morbidity are markedly improved compared to infants not offered ECMO, the incidence of adverse events due to ECMO (mainly intracranial bleeds) is still high.

Experimental Therapies

Diluted surfactant lavage has been promising in small pilot trials, but larger trials are required before this therapy can be recommended. **Liquid ventilation** with **perfluorochemicals** is another promising experimental therapy. Intratracheal pulmonary ventilation, a technique that decreases dead space ventilation, may enhance CO_2 elimination and thereby permit ventilation with lower pressures. Animal models of MAS have demonstrated elevated levels of endothelin-1 and other vasoactive mediators. Endothelin antagonists, and other vasoactive compounds such as **prostacyclin** have been shown to decrease pulmonary arterial pressures in animal models of PPHN. In animal models of MAS, methylprednisolone attenuates the pulmonary hypertensive response, and dexamethasone improves compliance and oxygenation. **Steroid** use for MAS in humans has not yet been investigated adequately.

Prognosis

The prognosis is good in the majority of neonates with MAS. The risk of mortality due to MAS in neonates requiring mechanical ventilation is usually less than 5% in developed countries. The short-term outlook depends upon the severity of clinical features. Infants with severe MAS and/or PPHN may require prolonged mechanical ventilation for a week or longer and may rarely develop chronic lung disease. Some of the morbidity and mortality observed in neonates with MAS may be due actually to prolonged *in utero* hypoxia that was associated with meconium passage rather than due to aspiration of meconium. The long-term outlook is also usually good unless the infant was also asphyxiated, although there is a small risk of chronic pulmonary function abnormalities or reactive airways disease. Neonates that exhibit signs of severe hypoxic-ischemic encephalopathy or require ECMO should have long-term neurological follow-up.

REFERENCES

1. Cleary GM, Wiswell TE: Meconium-stained amniotic fluid and the meconium aspiration syndrome, An update, Pediatric Clinics of North America 1998;45:511-529.
2. Wiswell TE, Gannon CM, Jacob J, Goldsmith L, Szyld E, *et al.*: Delivery room management of the apparently vigorous meconium-stained neonate: Results of the multicenter, international collaborative trial, Pediatrics 2000;105:1-7.
3. Walsh MC, Fanaroff JM: Meconium stained fluid: Approach to the mother and the baby, Clinics in Perinatology 2007;34:653-65.

13 PERSISTENT PULMONARY HYPERTENSION OF THE NEWBORN

Namasivayam Ambalavanan

INCIDENCE

The incidence of persistent pulmonary hypertension of the newborn (PPHN) is thought to be around 2-5 per 1000 live births in developed countries such as the United States.[1-4] In developing countries, due to the increased incidence of **meconium aspiration syndrome** (MAS), **pneumonia**, and other secondary causes of PPHN, the incidence of PPHN is higher, although there is a lack of adequate validated population data for reliable estimates.

ETIOLOGY

PPHN is characterized by systemic hypoxemia secondary to elevated pulmonary vascular resistance with shunting of blood (through persistent fetal channels such as the foramen ovale or the ductus arteriosus) from the pulmonary to the systemic circulation.[1-3] The four main causes of PPHN are shown in Table 13.1.

PATHOLOGY

The **pulmonary vascular resistance** in the normal late gestation fetus is high, and most of the right ventricular output shunts via the **ductus arteriosus** to the descending aorta. Much of the blood returning to the fetus via the umbilical vein shunts to the left atrium through the **foramen ovale**. This normal fetal circulation is supported by the hypoxic *in utero* environment (PaO_2 normally

Table 13.1: Causes of PPHN

Secondary to parenchymal lung disease in which the primary cause is alveolar hypoxia [e.g. meconium aspiration syndrome, pneumonia, respiratory distress syndrome (RDS), transient tachypnea of the newborn (TTNB)]
Secondary to lung hypoplasia (e.g. congenital diaphragmatic hernia, oligohydramnios sequence)
Secondary to systemic disorders (e.g. septicemia, asphyxia, hypothermia, hypoglycemia, hypocalcemia, hyperviscosity syndrome)
Associated with no obvious lung parenchymal disorder – this is usually termed idiopathic PPHN, and may be secondary to pulmonary vasoconstriction or remodelling due to intrauterine hypoxia or maternal use of medications (e.g., non-steriodal anti-inflammatory drugs (NSAIDs) such as ibuprofen, aspirin, naproxen; selective serotonin reuptake inhibitors (SSRIs) such as fluoxetine – risk of about 1%)

20-25 torr) which maintains pulmonary vasoconstriction (which occurs at a PaO_2 <40 torr) and ductal patency. In addition, there is some mechanical compression of lung blood vessels as the lungs are fluid-filled *in utero*.

At birth, the inflation of the lungs with air and the resultant increase in oxygenation normally leads to pulmonary vasodilation and ductal constriction. This leads to an increase in pulmonary blood flow, and increased pulmonary venous return to the left atrium. Removal of the low resistance placental circulation increases systemic vascular resistance, and does away with the umbilical venous return. The increase in left atrial pressure compared to right atrial pressure leads to functional closure of the foramen ovale. The right-to-left shunting through the ductus ceases and reverses (become left-to-right) as the systemic vascular resistance increases and the pulmonary vascular resistance falls. With complete ductal closure, this left-to-right shunting becomes passive.

PPHN results when there is an impairment of this process of normal transition.[2-4] After birth, the systemic resistance will increase following disconnection of the placenta, but if there is a persistent elevation of pulmonary vascular resistance such that it is higher than systemic vascular resistance, blood will continue to flow along the path of least resistance, and right-to-left shunts may persist at the level of the ductus or foramen ovale.

Clinical Features

PPHN may affect term infants, near-term infants [**respiratory distress syndrome** (RDS) or **transient tachypnea of the newborn** (TTNB) with PPHN], as well as post-term infants (MAS with PPHN). Very preterm infants with severe RDS may also have elevated pulmonary vascular resistance and right-to-left shunting, but are not usually labelled with the diagnosis of PPHN.

Infants with PPHN usually look normal, although infants with Down syndrome are at higher risk of PPHN. Infants with PPHN secondary to meconium aspiration or **diaphragmatic hernia** may have the other classic clinical features suggestive of such etiologies.

Cyanosis is usually noted, but pulse oximetry is often required to confirm low oxygen saturations as many neonates normally have acrocyanosis soon after birth and central cyanosis is difficult to appreciate without good perfusion and lighting.

Infants with PPHN may have extremely reactive pulmonary vascular resistance. Hence, such infants may be deeply cyanosed at one instant, but may become "pink" if the pulmonary vasodilation occurs in the next instant. Such a "flip-flop" phenomenon is often seen in infants with PPHN.

Tachypnea and mild retractions are common. Pulses and peripheral perfusion may be poor. Cardiac murmurs are not often heard as the ductal and foramen ovale shunting is quiet, although some infants have a murmur due to **tricuspid regurgitation**. The second heart sound (S2) is usually single due to an earlier P2, but this is difficult to evaluate at the high heart rates common in neonates (120-160/min).

Diagnosis

Neonates with a large pre-ductal to post-ductal oxygen saturation difference (>10-15%) indicative of ductal right to left shunting, and those with **hypoxemia** disproportionate to clinical signs, may have PPHN. This diagnosis should be confirmed by **echocardiography**, which can localize the site of shunting, and provide an estimate of the pulmonary pressures, if tricuspid regurgitation is present.

Differential Diagnosis [3, 4]

Cyanotic congenital heart disease is the main differential diagnosis.

The "**hyperoxia" test** or the "**hyperoxia-hyperventilation" test** may help make this diagnosis. The "hyperoxia test" consists of exposing the infant to 100% oxygen by oxygen hood for 10 minutes. A PaO_2 of <50 torr suggests a fixed right to left shunt such as in cyanotic congenital heart disease or PPHN, while a PaO_2 of >100 torr suggest parenchymal lung disease. A PaO_2 of between 50 and 100 torr may be seen with severe lung disease, cardiovascular disease, or PPHN. The "hyperoxia-hyperventilation" test consists of ventilation of the infant (manually or mechanically) with 100% oxygen at rates of 60-80/min for 10 minutes, so as to lower $PaCO_2$ (to around 25 torr) and induce respiratory alkalosis. Cyanotic congenital heart diseases will usually have a PaO_2 of <50 torr despite mechanical ventilation with 100% oxygen. In PPHN, oxygenation is typically labile, and a transient increase in PaO_2 of >100 torr is often noted with hyperventilation.

The other major differential diagnosis is pulmonary disorders without elevated pulmonary vascular resistance or right-to-left shunting. A simultaneous preductal and postductal arterial pressure gradient of >15 torr suggests right-to-left shunting at the ductal level. The difference may also be appreciated by **pulse oximetry** done simultaneously on the right upper limb (preductal) and on the lower limbs (postductal) which will demonstrate a higher preductal SpO_2.

Investigations [3, 4]

Chest radiographs and **arterial blood gases** are indicated initially. The chest radiograph may be normal or may demonstrate abnormalities consistent with RDS, MAS, diaphragmatic hernia etc. An echocardiogram is usually obtained upon presentation, and subsequently in the absence of clinical improvement, or if there is deterioration. Other investigations will depend upon the clinical presentation.

The frequency of arterial blood gases depends upon the clinical presentation. Sick infants usually require placement of arterial catheters, either umbilical arterial catheters or peripheral arterial catheters, in order to perform frequent (q 1-2 h) arterial blood gas estimations as well as obtain a continuous evaluation of arterial blood pressure.

A limited sepsis workup consisting of a complete blood count and blood cultures are usually done followed by institution of antibiotics (pending culture results) as pneumonia and/or septicemia is one of the causes of PPHN.

As most infants with PPHN are not fed in the first few days while being critically ill, close monitoring of fluid and electrolyte status is required.

Cranial ultrasound and evaluation of coagulation status is usually done in infants who meet **extracorporeal membrane oxygenation** (ECMO) criteria.

Management [3, 4] (Figure 13.1)

Neonates who manifest hypoxemia despite good respiratory effort and without hypercapnia or acidosis should be administered oxygen, preferably by oxygenhood. It is important to prevent hypoxemia, which may contribute to pulmonary vasoconstriction and thereby to pulmonary hypertension. Hypoxemia is prevented by elevation of the inspired oxygen concentration (FiO_2) to keep the PaO_2 in the 80-100 torr range. Infants with PPHN are usually term or post-term infants and there is less concern with hyperoxia as compared to preterm neonates. If FiO_2 requirements are high (>0.6), a trial of continuous positive airway pressure (CPAP) may be tried, but with caution, as CPAP may increase gas trapping in the some clinical situations associated with PPHN (e.g. MAS), and potentially increase the risk of **pneumothorax**.

It is important to maintain an adequate blood pressure, tissue perfusion, and urine output, but at the same time, it is necessary to avoid excessive fluid administration or over-zealous inotropic support.

Neonates who become hypoxemic (PaO_2 <50 torr or SpO_2 <90%) with severe respiratory distress, hypercapnia ($PaCO_2$ >60 torr), or acidosis (pH<7.25), and neonates who are apneic are usually mechanically ventilated. The goal should be to achieve adequate oxygenation with minimal additional lung injury. Again, hypoxemia should be prevented by maintaining the arterial PO_2 in the 80-100 torr range. A relatively rapid rate (40-60/min), the minimum effective peak inspiratory pressure (PIP) to produce chest expansion (usually 10-20 cm H_2O), a low to moderate positive

Current management

↓

Confirm diagnosis of PPHN

↓

Correct underlying abnormalities (hypothermia, acidosis, hypocalcemia, hypoglycemia, polycythemia); Oxygen by hood

↓

Conservative mechanical ventilation

↓

Trial of hyperventilation

↓

If low PO_2 trial of rescue therapies

↓

Metabolic Alkalosis	HFV	Surfactant	Vasodilators iNO, PGI_2, Tolazoline, Adenosine	ECMO

Fig. 13.1: Current management of PPHN

end expiratory pressure (PEEP; usually 3-5 cm H_2O), and an adequate expiratory time (usually 0.5 to 0.7 seconds) are generally sufficient. Alkalosis and hyperventilation are often attempted but there is little evidence to indicate their efficacy or safety. **Alkalosis**, which is known to cause pulmonary vasodilation, is achieved by hyperventilation (to maintain arterial $PaCO_2$ in the 30-35 torr range) and infusion of sodium bicarbonate (0.25-1 mEq/kg/h) to maintain a pH in the range of 7.45-7.55. Retrospective multicenter studies have suggested that the use of alkaline infusions (and not hyperventilation) is associated with an increased use of ECMO and oxygen at 28 days of age. It is important to avoid very low arterial $PaCO_2$ (<30 torr) as cerebral vasoconstriction may result. In addition, high ventilator settings in an attempt to hyperventilate may increase lung injury. Many infants with PPHN are sedated with fentanyl or morphine, if the neonate "fights" the ventilator. Some infants are also paralyzed with pancuronium or other muscle relaxants if high ventilator settings are required, but there is little evidence to show benefits or the absence of risk of this intervention. Hypoxemia-hyperoxemia swings should be avoided as much as possible.

In settings such as MAS, constant vigilance for the presence of air leaks is necessary using clinical evaluation, transillumination, and chest radiographs. Pneumothoraces that occur usually need chest tube drainage.

If hypoxemia or hypercapnia does not respond adequately to conventional mechanical ventilation, or if air leaks (pneumothorax or pneumomediastinum) are present, **high frequency ventilation** in the form of either high frequency oscillatory ventilation (HFOV) or high frequency jet ventilation (HFJV) is often used.

Surfactant administration may improve oxygenation and reduce the need for ECMO. It is necessary to carefully monitor for dosing complications such as hypoxemia, bradycardia, or endotracheal tube occlusion.

Inhaled nitric oxide (iNO), a selective pulmonary vasodilator, may be administered in combination with high frequency ventilation or with conventional ventilators.[5] iNO is usually used for infants with an oxygenation index (OI) >25 [OI = (Mean Airway Pressure × FiO_2 {usually close to 1.0} × 100)/Postductal PaO_2). iNO reduces the need for ECMO by approximately 40%. Some neonatologists prefer to administer iNO before, rather than after, a trial of high frequency ventilation. Nitric oxide is usually started at an inhaled concentration of 20 parts per million (ppm) and subsequently weaned slowly (20 to 10 ppm, then to 5 ppm, then in steps of 1 ppm until off), as long as oxygenation remains adequate. Higher concentrations of iNO (e.g. 40 and 80 ppm) may be attempted if there is inadequate response to 20 ppm, but these efforts are often unsuccessful and the risk of methemoglobinemia is higher with iNO>20 ppm. It should be noted that rapid discontinuation of iNO may result in rebound pulmonary hypertension. The response to iNO is often better in idiopathic PPHN as compared to the response in secondary PPHN such as in MAS. iNO probably does not reduce need for ECMO in congenital diaphragmatic hernia. It is important to realize that critically ill neonates with PPHN requiring therapies such as high frequency ventilation and iNO may deteriorate rapidly and die during transport, and hence these therapies must be used with caution outside a neonatal intensive care unit with ECMO availability. In resource-limited countries where iNO and/or high frequency ventilation is not available or readily available, **sildenafil** (1 mg/

kg orogastric every 6 hours for a few doses for infants with OI>25) may possibly be an option. However, the safety and effectiveness of sildenafil in neonates have not yet been established, and it is recommended that such use be preferably done in the setting of a randomized trial.

ECMO is normally considered an effective therapy of last resort for neonates with intractable PPHN, who persist with hypoxemia despite maximal ventilator support (and iNO, when available)[1, 3, 4]. ECMO is generally considered only for infants >34 weeks gestation (due to risk of intracranial bleeds) of sufficient weight (usually >2 kg birth weight), with reversible lung disease and no lethal congenital anomalies. Criteria for ECMO usually involve a combination of oxygenation variables and time (e.g. PaO_2 <40 torr for >2h; OI>40 for 4 hrs; $AaDO_2$ criteria >610 for 8 hrs etc.) which are associated with high mortality. Generally a risk of mortality of about 80% is considered to be the threshold at which ECMO is considered. Although mortality and morbidity are markedly improved compared to infants not offered ECMO, the incidence of adverse events due to ECMO (mainly intracranial bleeds) is still high (10-20%).

Experimental Therapies [1-3] (Table 13.2)

Vasodilators such as **tolazoline** have been used, either intravenously or intratracheally, but evidence as to their benefit compared to risks are not strong. Diluted surfactant lavage has been promising in small pilot trials in MAS, but larger trials are required before this therapy can be recommended. **Liquid ventilation** with perfluorochemicals is another promising experimental therapy. Intratracheal pulmonary ventilation, a technique that decreases dead space ventilation, may enhance CO_2 elimination and thereby permit ventilation with lower pressures. Animal models of PPHN have demonstrated elevated levels of endothelin-1 and other vasoactive mediators. Endothelin antagonists, and other vasoactive compounds such as **prostacyclin** have been shown to decrease pulmonary arterial pressures in animal models of PPHN. Prostacyclin has been used in human infants with PPHN, but may provide only small incremental benefit when combined with high frequency ventilation and iNO. In animal models of MAS, methylprednisolone attenuates the

Table 13.2: Experimental therapies for PPHN
Intratracheal pulmonary ventilation
Liquid ventilation
Diluted surfactant lavage
Prostacyclin
Steroids
Tolazoline

pulmonary hypertensive response, and dexamethasone improves compliance and oxygenation. **Steroid** use for MAS in humans has not yet been investigated adequately.

PROGNOSIS

Infants with PPHN who received ECMO are at higher risk for neurodevelopmental sequelae and are usually followed-up by developmental pediatricians or neurologists. In addition, an MRI or CT of the brain is often done near the time of discharge.

Infants with PPHN are at higher risk of hearing loss, and hearing screening is important.

Poor oral feeding is often a problem in infants recovering from PPHN, especially in those infants who required ECMO or prolonged mechanical ventilation, but this usually improves over a period of days to weeks.

Survival and long-term pulmonary and neurodevelopmental outcomes are usually excellent (>90% normal) in infants with idiopathic PPHN or MAS treated in centers with current neonatal intensive care. Infants who need ECMO have a 10-20% risk of mortality or morbidity. In countries without adequate neonatal intensive care, mortality rates may be very high. Infants with congenital diaphragmatic hernia have a higher risk of mortality and morbidity. There is some evidence that adults who had PPHN as infants may possibly be at higher risk for greater elevations in pulmonary pressure on hypoxic exposure (e.g. at high altitudes).

REFERENCES

1. Konduri GG: New approaches for persistent pulmonary hypertension of newborn, Clin Perinatol 2004;3:591-611.

2. Thérèse P: Persistent pulmonary hypertension of the newborn, Paediatr Respir Rev 2006;7:S175-6.
3. Steinhorn RH: Pulmonary Hypertension, Persistent-Newborn. http://www.emedicine.com/ped/topic2530.htm
4. Ostrea EM, Villanueva-Uy ET, Natarajan G, Uy HG: Persistent pulmonary hypertension of the newborn: Pathogenesis, etiology and management, Paediatr Drugs 2006;8:179-88.
5. Finer NN, Barrington KJ: Nitric oxide for respiratory failure in infants born at or near term, Cochrane Database Syst Rev 2006;(4):CD000399.

14 NEONATAL CARDIOVASCULAR DISEASE

Satyan Lakshminrusimha

PHYSIOLOGICAL PRINCIPLES [1]

Neonatal cardiac disease can present with the following derangements:

Decreased Cardiac Output

Cardiac output in a neonate is influenced by the following four factors (see Figure 14.1):

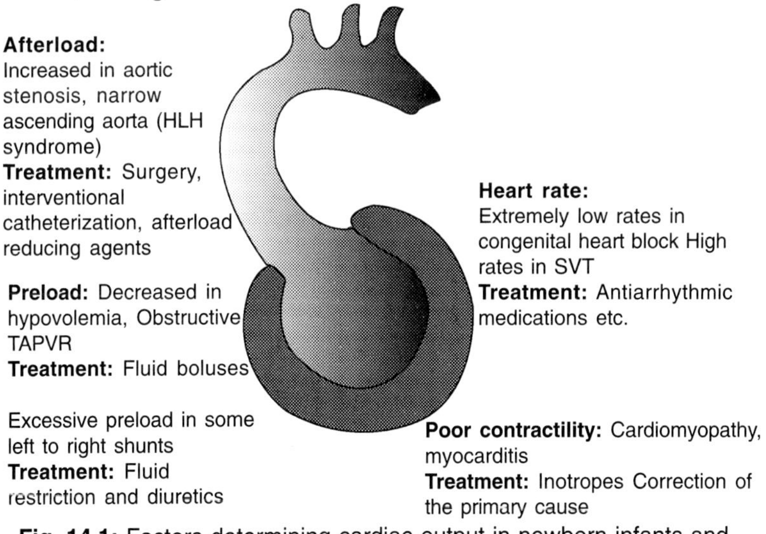

Fig. 14.1: Factors determining cardiac output in newborn infants and management principles

i. *Preload*–Defined as the volume at end-diastole that must be ejected from the ventricle (reflects venous return and intravascular fluid volume).

ii. *Afterload*–Defined as the force opposing ventricular resistance. Systemic and pulmonary vascular resistance (SVR and PVR) are important determinants of afterload.

iii. *Contractility*–Ability of myocardium to generate force – usually measured by echocardiogram as ejection fraction; the developing heart also has poor compliance compared to the adult heart.

iv. *Heart rate*–This is the *chief determinant of cardiac output in newborn infants*. Cardiac output = **stroke volume** × heart rate.

Decreased cardiac output can result from abnormalities of any of the above factors either alone or in combination.

Central Cyanosis and Hypoxemia

Cyanosis is defined as the bluish discoloration of skin or mucosa secondary to the presence of increased deoxygenated hemoglobin (usually > 3 to 5 g/dL). Various respiratory, metabolic and neurological conditions can present with central cyanosis in newborn infants. Cyanosis resulting from congenital heart disease (CHD) is usually due to one of the following hemodynamic derangements:

i. Decreased pulmonary blood flow (usually with a right to left shunt) – tetralogy of Fallot, severe **pulmonary stenosis, pulmonary atresia, tricuspid atresia.**

ii. Intracardiac shunt with admixture of pulmonary and systemic venous return (often with normal or increased pulmonary blood flow) – dextro-transposition of the great arteries (dTGA), hypoplastic left heart syndrome (HLH) and other conditions with single ventricle morphology, and total anomalous pulmonary venous return (TAPVR).

iii. Severe impairment of cardiac function resulting in poor output and pulmonary congestion (often without an intracardiac shunt) – coarctation of aorta (Co-A), cardiomyopathy, myocarditis, and supraventricular tachycardia (SVT).

Important Terms

i. *Oxygen saturation* – refers to the amount of oxygen actually combined with hemoglobin relative to the total amount of oxygen that could possibly be carried by the hemoglobin in a particular blood sample. This is easily measured by a pulse oximeter and expressed as a percentage.

ii. *Oxygen tension (pO_2)* – refers to the partial pressure of oxygen in the blood (mmHg). The relationship between oxygen tension and saturation is shown in the oxygen dissociation curve.

iii. *Oxygen content* – refers to the amount of oxygen in a given volume of blood (mL/dL).

iv. *Oxygen capacity* – refers to the total amount of oxygen (mL) that can possibly be taken up by blood (per dL).

Note: Infants with high hemoglobin levels (polycythemia) tend to present with cyanosis at higher oxygen saturation levels compared to infants who are anemic.

Abnormal Transition from Fetal Circulation

The fetal circulation differs from adult in many aspects (see Table 14.1).

PRESENTATION – ANTENATAL ULTRASOUND

With increasing frequency, neonates with CHD have been diagnosed before delivery by fetal echocardiography and are therefore born with a presumptive diagnosis into an expectant team of physicians and nurses. A four-chamber view during fetal echocardiography will accurately diagnose abnormalities such as septal defects, hypoplastic chambers. However, abnormalities of the great vessels such as TGA or isolated TAPVR may be difficult to visualize on an antenatal sonogram. Overall the diagnostic accuracy by fetal echocardiography is approximately 80 to 85% in the US.

APPROACH TO A NEWBORN INFANT WITH SUSPECTED CHD

History

1. *History of significant CHD in first-degree relatives carries a risk of 1 to 5% of recurrence*[1-4]

Table 14.1: The fetal circulation differs from adult circulation in the following aspects.

Structure	*Function during fetal life*	*Functional change at birth*	*Anatomical changes*	*Comments*
Placental circulation (low resistance, high flow circuit)	Nutrition, gas exchange, waste removal and hormonal production	Spasm and closure of umbilical vessels	Clamping or tying the umbilical cord and removal of placenta	Removal increases SVR
Pulmonary circulation (low flow, high resistance circuit in a fetus)	Only 8-10% of combined ventricular output enters the lung	Increase in pulmonary blood flow, drop in pulmonary arterial pressure	Flattening of the endothelium and reduced smooth muscle tone	Changes at birth mediated by oxygen, nitric oxide and prostaglandins
Ductus venosus (DV)	Channels oxygenated blood from the placenta to the right atrium (by-pass portal/ hepatic circulation)	Constriction and reduction of flow as umbilical venous flow decreases	Forms ligamentum venosum	Closure can worsen pulmonary venous obstruction in infra-diaphragmatic TAPVR
Foramen ovale	Shunts oxygenated blood from the inferior vena cava to the left atrium	Increased pressure in the left atrium (with increased	Anatomical closure results in formation of fossa ovalis (foramen ovale may remain patent in ~ 20% of adults)	Closure may result in poorer mixing in TGA, systemic venous obstruction in right heart obstruction and pulmonary venous

Contd.

Contd.

		pulmonary venous flow) closes the flap valve		obstruction in left heart obstruction
Ductus arteriosus (DA)	Blood flow from pulmonary artery (PA) to aorta to bypass the lungs and reach placental circulation	Increase in oxygen and decrease in prostaglandins result in ductal constriction (by 60 hours in 93% of term infants)	Forms ligamentum arteriosum (persistent patency causes major respiratory and other problems in preterm infants)	Closure results in marked deterioration of ductal dependent pulmonary or systemic circulations

a. More common defects occur more commonly (5% risk of recurrence of ventricular septal defect (VSD) in a sibling).

2. *Maternal conditions associated with CHD in the offspring*
   a. Maternal rubella – patent ductus arteriosus (PDA) and pulmonic stenosis (peripheral).
   b. Coxsackie B virus infection – myocarditis and severe heart failure.
   c. Systemic lupus erythematosus (SLE) – **congenital complete heart block.**
   d. Maternal diabetes – asymmetric septal hypertrophy and other defects such as aortic stenosis, d-TGA and VSD.
   e. Alcohol abuse – pulmonic stenosis, VSD.
   f. Maternal lithium use – Ebstein's anomaly.
   g. Aspirin or other non-steroidal anti-inflammatory drugs (NSAID) consumption – ductal closure and persistent pulmonary hypertension in the newborn (PPHN).
3. *Syndromes and chromosomal anomalies carry a high risk of CHD*
   a. Trisomy 21 – almost 40% have CHD (VSD, endocardial cushion defect, tetrology of Fallot, TGA, left ventricular (LV) outflow obstruction).
   b. Trisomy 18 – 85% risk of CHD (VSD, Co-A, valvular disease).
   c. Turner syndrome – 35% risk of CHD (Co-A, aortic valve lesions).
   d. Noonan's syndrome – 50% risk of CHD (pulmonic valve stenosis, cardiomyopathy, atrial septal defect (ASD)).
   e. CHARGE association – 80% risk of CHD (PDA, VSD, ASD).
   f. VACTERL association – 70% risk of CHD (VSD, tetralogy of Fallot).
   g. Williams syndrome – 75% risk of supravalvular aortic or pulmonic stenosis.
   h. DiGeorge syndrome – 85% risk of conotruncal anomalies (truncus arteriosus, interrupted aortic arch).

Examination

It is important that cardiovascular examination should be conducted when the baby is quiet, preferably prior to conducting procedures such as checking the red-reflex or hip clicks that are likely to make the infant cry.

1. **Inspection**
   a. *General condition and activity level:* hypoxemia results in reduced activity; an infant with congestive heart failure (CHF) may look tired during feeds or tachypneic.
   b. *Breathing:*
      i. Hyperpnea – deep, unlabored breathing at mildly elevated rates typically seen in conditions associated with decreased pulmonary blood flow.
      ii. Tachypnea – shallow, rapid, labored breathing associated with decreased lung compliance usually secondary to pulmonary parenchymal disease or pulmonary venous congestion and edema from LV failure.
      iii. Stridor associated with cardiovascular disease is secondary to upper airway compression from a vascular ring.
2. **Palpation**
   a. *Pulses* – Palpate both upper limb and lower limb pulses in all babies. The hallmark of aortic coarctation is the presence of palpable pulses in the upper extremities and diminished or absent femoral pulses. However, there are some exceptions:
      i. At times, a neonate with Co-A exhibits normal lower extremity pulses in the coarctation is the juxtaductal or preductal type and the descending aorta is perfused by right-to-left shunting through the the DA. In this case, although the femoral pulses are palpable, the lower limbs appear cyanotic (differential cyanosis) and have lower saturations by pulse oximetry.
      ii. If coarctation is associated with supravalvular aortic stenosis or aortic hypoplasia, the upper limb pulses may be asymmetric and weak also. In these cases it may not be easy to appreciate a radio-femoral difference in pulse volume.
   b. *Precordium* – Palpable cardiac impulses are common in hyperdynamic states.
   c. *Liver size* – Hepatomegaly is sometimes present in infants with heart failure.

d. *Skin temperature* – Cool skin temperature associated with mottling is a sign of poor peripheral perfusion. A delayed capillary refill is also suggestive of poor perfusion.

3. Auscultation

a. *Second heart sound* – It is difficult to appreciate changes in heart sounds and murmur because of the fast heart rate in newborn infant.

i. Single second heart sound with the absence of splitting is observed in atresia of either great vessel. In d-TGA, where the pulmonic valve is posterior, it is difficult to auscultate the pulmonic component of the second heart sound.

ii. Narrow split with loud S2 is a feature of left to right shunts with pulmonary hypertension.

iii. Wide split that does not change with respiration (fixed) is associated with large ASD and common atrium. Wide split may also be observed in Ebstein's anomaly and anomalous pulmonary venous return.

b. *Murmurs* – Most murmurs in the newborn period are transient and are related to the ductus arteriosus. Right to left shunts do not result in murmurs. Pulmonary hypertension with right to left shunt does not cause a murmur unless there is significant tricuspid regurgitation.

i. The loudest murmurs in neonates are often caused by tricuspid and mitral regurgitation. Tricuspid insufficiency is also noted commonly with perinatal asphyxia.

ii. Stenotic murmurs from aortic and pulmonary valves are harsh and ejection systolic and often associated with a click.

iii. Continuous murmurs are typical of PDA (although in proven cases of PDA in premature infants, the murmur is systolic in 60%, continuous in only 30% and absent in 10%).

Causes of continuous murmurs include:

a. Acyanotic (PDA, coronary A-V fistula, aorto-pulmonary window, peripheral pulmonic stenosis).

b. Cyanotic (truncus arteriosus, TAPVR with drainage

into right atrium or superior vena cava) and a to-and-fro murmur in absent pulmonary valve leaflet syndrome.

c. *Audible bruit* over the cranium in an infant with failure could be secondary to a vein of Galen malformation. Similar bruits can be auscultated over the liver in A-V fistulas.

4. **Pulse Oximeter:** It is very useful to check pulse oximeter readings in right upper (preductal) and lower (postductal) extremities. Low reading in both preductal and postductal regions is suggestive of many cyanotic CHD with intracardiac shunt. Lower oxygen saturations in the postductal regions is indicative of right to left shunt at the ductus. This is seen in PPHN.

LABORATORY STUDIES

1. **Arterial Blood Gas Analysis:**
   a. Oxygen levels: In cases of suspected cyanotic CHD, obtaining paired blood gas samples obtained in room air and 100% oxygen helps establishment of a fixed intracardiac lesions (hyperoxia test).
      i. A significant difference in the pre-ductal (right radial artery) and post-ductal (umbilical or posterior tibial artery) of > 20 mmHg suggests a right to left shunt at the level of the ductus arteriosus in cases of PPHN.
   b. In patients with CHD, the pH and pCO_2 values are usually normal. In fact, in patients with cyanotic CHD, with reduced pulmonary blood flow, increased ventilation results in mild respiratory alkalosis.
      i. Infants with CHF, alveolar hypoventilation results in retention of carbon dioxide.
      ii. Presence of respiratory acidosis in a cyanotic infant may also indicate poor pulmonary perfusion secondary to CHD or that the diagnosis may be PPHN secondary to a primary pulmonary parenchymal disease such as meconium aspiration or pneumonia.
      iii. Metabolic acidosis in an infant with CHD associated with left ventricular outflow obstruction with poor systemic perfusion. In infants with single ventricle

morphology, metabolic acidosis may be a sign of systemic hypoperfusion secondary to diversion of blood to the pulmonary circuit. The later situation is often secondary to excessive oxygen supplementation or overventilation resulting in a drop in pulmonary vascular resistance.

2. **Complete Blood Count:** A total and differential white cell count must be checked to rule out the possibility of a viral or bacterial infection. A high hematocrit in polycythemia may increase pulmonary vascular resistance and also give the appearance of cyanosis. A low platelet count may be a contraindication to the use of indomethacin in PDA.
3. **Basic Metabolic Profile (Electrolytes, blood urea nitrogen and creatinine):** Renal dysfunction may be a sign of systemic hypoperfusion secondary to left ventricular obstruction or indomethacin therapy. Low calcium levels may be associated with DiGeorge syndrome. Hypocalcemia may also have a negative inotropic effect. Hyponatremia and hyperkalemia may be a sign of adrenocortical insufficiency. Severe abnormalities of potassium metabolism may present with rhythm disturbances.
4. **Chest X-ray provides valuable information and is easily available**. The following information should be assessed:
   a. *The presence and position of various tubes* (endotracheal tube, orogastric tube) and lines (umbilical venous and arterial lines and percutaneous lines)
   b. *Cardiac silhouette* – A small cardiac shadow in a hypotensive patient may suggest hypovolemia. Cardiomegaly is common in myocarditis, cardiomyopathy, Ebstein's anomaly etc. A large thymic shadow is often present in healthy newborn children and should not be confused with cardiomegaly. An egg on a string appearance is suggestive of TGA and a boot shaped heart is seen in tetralogy of Fallot.
   c. *Position of the aortic arch* – Right sided arch is common with tetralogy of Fallot and truncus arteriosus. In VACTERL association with tracheo-esophageal fistula, the location of the aortic arch is important to decide the side of approach for fistula repair.
   d. *Pulmonary vascularity* – Low vascularity (pulmonary oligemia)

is a feature of right ventricular outflow obstruction (such as tetralogy of Fallot) and idiopathic PPHN. High pulmonary vascularity (pulmonary plethora).

5. **Electrocardiography (ECG):** The ECG of a newborn baby differs from that of an adult in several aspects. The rate is 120 to 140 beats/min. There is right ventricular dominance and QRS axis deviation to the right with an axis between 100 and 150 degrees with R wave dominance in the right precordial leads. The T waves are upright in right chest leads (V_1 to V_{4R}) on the first day of life but by 3 days, the T wave deflections are negative as pulmonary vascular resistance falls and right ventricular hypertrophy resolves.
   a. *Rate and Rhythm:*
      i. SVT is a common cause for a fast heart rate of 240 to 300/min. Often, but not always, p waves are absent. SVT can result in cardiac failure with a structurally normal heart and is a cause of hydrops when it occurs *in utero*. Prolonged SVT results in hypothermia, feeding intolerance leading on to poor perfusion and heart failure.

         Post-SVT ECG should be carefully examined for Wolff-Parkinson-White syndrome (WPW) characterized by a short P-R interval, slurred upstroke of R wave (delta wave) and wide QRS complex.
         a. An accessory pathway that can bypass the normal conduction route across the AV node exists in WPW syndrome.
         b. The management and prevention of SVT secondary to WPW syndrome is more complicated than isolated SVT. Digoxin should not be prescribed to infants with SVT secondary to WPW syndrome.
         c. WPW syndrome is commonly seen in CHD such as Ebstein's anomaly.
      ii. Congenital heart block results in a slow heart rate and cause heart failure (and hydrops *in utero*). The atria and ventricles are independently activated. The ventricular rate is the critical factor determining symptoms with rates below 40 to 45/min resulting in distress.

Chapter 14

1. The association between maternal SLE and congenital heart block is well established.
2. Complex CHD such as l-TGA, endocardial cushion defects and single ventricle may be associated with complete heart block. Ventricular rates of 60 to 70 beats/min are rarely associated with symptoms in isolated heart block but patients with complex CHD may be symptomatic even at these rates.
3. Cardiomyopathies are also associated with heart block.

b. *Axis:* In adults and older children, the QRS axis is in the lower left quadrant (0 to + 90 deg). In a normal newborn, the QRS axis is rightward (+90 to +180 deg) owing to RV hypertrophy *in utero*. Several CHD present with unique changes to QRS axis (see Figure 14.2).

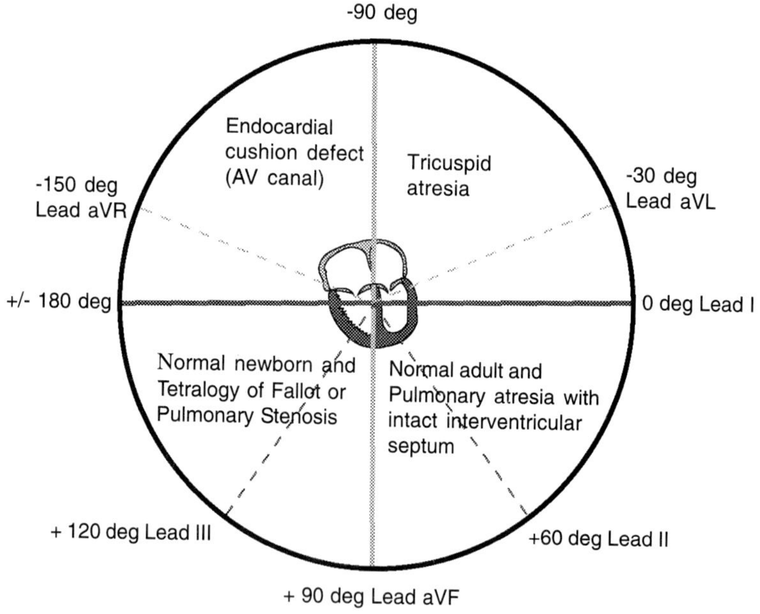

Fig. 14.2: QRS axis in CHD. Normal newborn QRS axis is located in the right lower quadrant and switches to the left lower quadrant later in life with left ventricular dominance

6. Echocardiography has become the principal tool for the diagnosis and assessment of CHD in neonates. Discussing the details of techniques and images is beyond the scope of this chapter.
7. Cardiac catheterization can be diagnostic or therapeutic. Given the present day echocardiographic capabilities, the need for diagnostic catheterization is uncommon. Therapeutic catheterization may be in the following situations in newborn infants with CHD.
   a. *Balloon septostomy* – TGA with restrictive foramen ovale.
   b. *Balloon dilatation of a stenotic valve or area* – Pulmonic or aortic valve stenosis.
   c. *Stenting techniques* – Stenting of DA is being explored as an initial palliative procedure of HLH syndrome.
   d. *Embolization of cerebral arterio*—Venous malformation (such as vein of Galen malformation) resulting in heart failure.

THERAPEUTIC PRINCIPLES

General principles of neonatal care including temperature control, electrolyte and acid base balance (especially glucose, potassium and calcium), prevention and treatment of infection and appropriate respiratory support are crucial in the management of a newborn infant with CHD. The main strategies in the management of CHD in newborn are usually under the following categories:

1. Promoting closure of ductus arteriosus especially in premature infants with PDA.
2. Maintaining ductal patency in ductal dependent CHD.
3. Management of congestive heart failure.
4. Anti-arrhythmia management.

CLOSURE OF DUCTUS ARTERIOSUS

See PDA below.

Maintaining Ductal Patency

1. *Avoiding excessive oxygen administration* – High oxygen levels promote ductal closure and also reduce PVR. This promotes a right to left ductal flow in patients with ductal dependent systemic flow.

2. Maintaining pCO_2 levels ≥ 50 mmHg and avoiding iatrogenic hyperventilation also helps in keeping pulmonary vascular resistance high in infants with ductal dependent systemic flow. These principles of avoiding hyperoxia and hypocarbia are useful in the management of patients with single ventricle physiology also (see Figure 14.3).

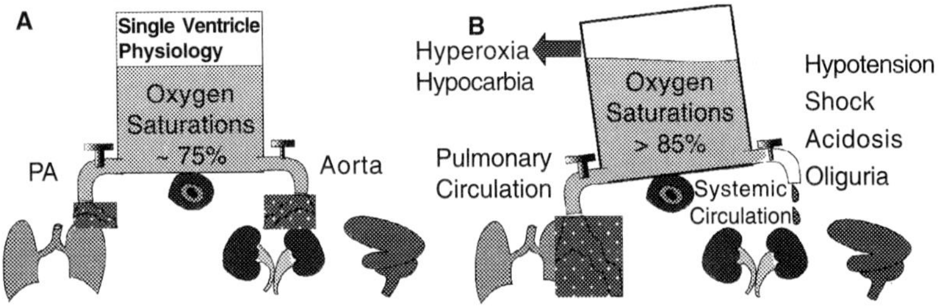

Fig. 14.3: (A) Single ventricle physiology explained using a double-faucet water tank on a fulcrum–a common chamber pumping to both plmonary and systemic circulations (B) Maintaining high oxygen saturation or low pCO_2 drops PVR resulting in preferential pumping into the PA resulting in poor systemic perfusion

3. *Prostaglandin E1 (PGE1)*[5]: This agent is used to promote dilation of ductus arteriosus in infants with ductal dependent CHD. In ductal dependent CHD, either the pulmonary flow or the systemic flow could be dependent on ductal patency (see Table 14.2).
   a. The *initial dose* is 0.05 to 0.1 mcg/kg/min by continuous infusion.
   b. *Maintenance dose:* Titrate to infant's response – look for improved oxygenation and echocardiographic evidence of ductal patency. Adverse effects are often dose dependent. *High initial doses are usually no more effective and have a high incidence of adverse effects.* Maintenance dose may be as low as 0.01 mcg/kg/min.
   c. *Route of administration:* Preferably a central venous catheter such as an umbilical venous line. PGE1 can also be administered by a high umbilical arterial catheter positioned near the DA (not preferred as it carries a theoretical risk of embolization to the cranial vessels).
   d. *Dilution:* One ampoule of PGE1 is 500 mcg/ml. Mix 500 mcg in 49 ml of D5W or normal saline to give a concentration of

10 mcg/ml. PGE1 is hyperosmolar (undiluted solution is 23,250 mOsm/kg) and should not be infused at a concentration higher than 20 mcg/ml.

e. *Delivery rate:* Infusion of the above-diluted solution at 0.6 ml/kg/hour provides a dose of 0.1 mcg/kg/min (a rate of 0.3 ml/kg/hour – 0.05 mcg/kg/min is the traditional initial dose).

f. *Monitor:* Cardiorespiratory status, oxygenation, temperature and the site of intravenous infusion for evidence of extravasation.

g. *Adverse effects:*

   i. Apnea is common and occurs with the initial doses (particularly high doses). Apnea can be prevented or treated with aminophylline or caffeine. Some patients may require intubation especially for transport.

   ii. Fever, leukocytosis, cutaneous flushing and bradycardia; some patients with temperature elevation may need cooling blankets.

   iii. Prolonged treatment is associated with gastric outlet obstruction and reversible cortical proliferation of long bones (Table 14.2).

Table 14.2
Ductal dependent CHD
Systemic flow – dependent on a patent ductus:
Coarctation of the aorta
Interrupted aortic arch
Critical aortic stenosis
Hypoplastic left heart syndrome with aortic atresia
Mitral atresia
Pulmonary blood flow – dependent on a patent ductus
Pulmonary atresia with intact ventricular septum
Tricuspid atresia
Critical pulmonary stenosis
Tetralogy of Fallot with severe pulmonary stenosis/atresia

Medical Therapy for CHF

1. A common cause for CHF in neonates is a large volume left to

right shunting. Impaired pulmonary function, wheezing, tachypnea and respiratory distress along with exhaustion with oral feeding are some features of CHF in neonates. Fluid restriction (by using calorie dense formulas – such as use of 80 kcal/dL instead of 67 kcal/dL) and pharmacologic agents such as diuretics and digoxin are helpful in management of CHF.

a. Furosemide is the most commonly used diuretic in neonates. It acts on the ascending limb of the loop of Henle and decreases absorption of chloride, sodium and potassium.
   i. *Initial dose* is 1 mg/kg IV, IM or PO. The dose may be increased to a maximum of 2 mg/kg IV or 6 mg/kg PO per dose.
   ii. *Dose interval:*
      1. Q 24 hours in preterm infants.
      2. Q 12 hours in term infants.
      3. Q 8 hours in full term infants > 1 month of age.
   iii. *Monitoring:* Urine output, body weight, serum electrolytes and serum calcium, phosphorus and bicarbonate. Monitor potassium carefully in patients on furosemide and digoxin.
   iv. *Adverse effects:* Hyponatremia, hypokalemia and hypochloremic metabolic alkalosis. Hypercalciuria and nephrocalcinosis occur with long-term therapy.

b. Bumetanide is 40 times more potent than furosemide. It is often used in patients who are refractory to furosemide. Its mechanism of action is similar to furosemide.
   i. Dose – 0.005 to 0.05 mg/kg per dose IV slow push, IM or PO.
   ii. Interval – Q 6 hours.
   iii. Monitoring and adverse effect profile similar to furosemide.

c. Chlorthiazide – is an alternative to furosemide and is preferred for chronic therapy by some physicians because of lower risk of nephrocalcinosis.
   i. Dose – 10 to 20 mg/kg per dose q 12 hours PO.
   ii. Adverse effects include hypokalemia, hyperglycemia and hyperuricemia.

d. Digoxin is the time-tested agent of choice to improve contractility. It is often administered orally. It can also be administered intravenously but extreme caution must be used because serious mistakes in dosing have frequently been committed through transcription or mathematical error. It is also useful in treatment of SVT, atrial flutter and atrial fibrillation.

   i. Dose – Loading dose (or 'digitalization') is generally used only when treating arrhythmias and acute CHF. This dose is administered over 24 hours in 3 divided doses. Typically, the first dose is ½ of the total loading dose and subsequent doses are ¼ administered in 6-8 hour intervals. Oral doses are 25% higher than IV doses. Do not administer IM. See Table 14.3 for loading and maintenance doses.

   ii. Monitor heart rate and rhythm by ECG. Monitor electrolytes and watch for decreased serum potassium and magnesium and increased calcium as these may predispose to digoxin toxicity.

   iii. Therapeutic serum concentration is 1 to 2 ng/mL.

   iv. Adverse effects include PR interval prolongation, sino-atrial block, feeding intolerance, vomiting, diarrhea and lethargy.

Table 14.3

Post menstrual age (PMA) in weeks	*Total loading dose (Digitalization) – Administer in 3 doses over 24 hours*		*Maintenance doses – titrate based on clinical response and signs of toxicity*		
	IV (mcg/kg)	*PO (mcg/kg)*	*IV (mcg/kg)*	*PO (mcg/kg)*	*Interval (h)*
≤ 29	15	20	4	5	24
30 to 36	20	25	5	6	24
37 to 48	30	40	4	5	12
≥ 49	40	50	5	6	12

Maintenance doses are begun 12 hours after the last loading dose

ANTI-ARRHYTHMIC THERAPY

Management of SVT

1. Prolonged SVT can cause significant cardiovascular compromise. In some cases it is secondary to the presence of an intravenous catheter (peripheral inserted long catheters such as PICC lines or umbilical venous catheter) in the right atrium. In such instances, these lines should be carefully withdrawn to superior or inferior vena cava to avoid irritation to the right atrium. In other cases, the following measures are used in the management of SVT.
   a. Neurogenic manipulation such as ice water application to the face stimulates vagal tone and induces bradycardia.
   b. In infants with normal peripheral perfusion, adenosine is the first drug of choice.
   c. Adenosine is used for the acute treatment of sustained paroxysmal SVT. ECG obtained during adenosine therapy may also aid in establishing the diagnosis of SVT.
      i. Adenosine acts by depressing sinus node automaticity and A-V node conduction.
      ii. Starting dose is 50 mcg/kg rapid IV over 1 to 2 seconds (increase dose in 50 mcg/kg increments every 2 minutes until return of sinus rhythm – maximum dose is 250 mcg/kg. Flush IV site with saline immediately and infuse as close to the IV site as possible.
      iii. Flushing, dyspnea, and irritability occur frequently along with transient arrhythmias but resolve spontaneously.
      iv. Recurrence of SVT occurs in approximately 30% of treated patients.
   d. However, if evidence of cardiovascular collapse exists, or if the disturbance has been present for an extended period, cardioversion with direct current countershock is indicated with a dose of 0.5 to 2 joules/kg.
   e. Preventive or maintenance therapy may be indicated to prevent recurrence. This therapy is based on whether evidence of WPW syndrome is present on the interval ECG.
      i. With WPW syndrome, oral propranolol is the drug of

choice (3 to 5 mg/kg/day in 3 to 4 divided doses).

In the absence of WPW syndrome, digoxin or propranolol may be used.

PREVENTION OF INFECTIVE ENDOCARDITIS

Prevention guidelines for bacterial endocarditis have been recently changed.

Indications for Prophylaxis

High-risk Patients

- Prosthetic heart valves (including homografts) or prosthetic material used for cardiac valve repair.
- Previous endocarditis.
- CHD:
  - Complex unrepaired cyanotic congenital heart disease (e.g., transposition of great vessels, tetralogy of Fallot, single ventricle), systemic-to-pulmonary artery shunts or conduits.
  - Repaired congenital heart defect with prosthetic material (surgery or catheter placed) during the first 6 months after procedure.
  - Repaired congenital defects with residual defects at the site or adjacent to the site of a prosthetic patch or prosthetic device (which inhibit endothelialization).
  - NOTE: Except for conditions listed above, antibiotic prophylaxis is no longer recommended for any other form of CHD.
- Cardiac transplantation if valvulopathy develops.

Negligible-risk Patients (prophylaxis not recommended)

- Isolated secundum ASD.
- Surgical repair of ASD, VSD or PDA (without residua and beyond 6 months after repair).
- Previous coronary artery bypass surgery.
- Functional heart murmurs.
- Previous Kawasaki disease or rheumatic fever without valve dysfunction.
- Cardiac pacemakers; implantable defibrillators.

Chapter 14

Antibiotic Regimen for Prevention of Bacterial Endocarditis** (Table 14.4)

Table 14.4

*Situation**	*Single dose administered 30 to 60 min before procedure*	
	Agent	*Dose*
Oral	Amoxicillin	50 mg/kg
Unable to take oral medication	Ampicillin	50 mg/kg IM or IV
	Or	
	Cefazolin or ceftriaxone	50 mg/kg IM or IV
Allergic to penicillin or ampicillin – oral	Cephelexin	50 mg/kg
	Or	
	Clindamycin	20 mg/kg
	Or	
	Azithromycin or clarithromycin	15 mg/kg
Allergic to penicillin or ampicillin – unable to take oral medication	Cefazolin or ceftriaxone (not recommended in an individual with history of anaphylaxis, angioedema, or urticaria with penicillin or ampicillin)	50 mg/kg IM or IV
	Or	
	Clindamycin	20 mg/kg IM or IV

* Patients with infections of the GI or GU tract may have intermittent or sustained enterococcal bacteremia. Prophylaxis for these procedures should include an anti-enterococcal antibody such as penicillin, ampicillin, piperacillin or vancomycin.

**If the patient is suspected or diagnosed to be infected with a resistant organism (such as MRSA), appropriate coverage to include these organisms should be provided during prophylaxis.

Procedures and Endocarditis Prophylaxis

Table 14.5

Prophylaxis indicated	*Prophylaxis not indicated*
DENTAL	DENTAL
All dental procedures that involve manipulation of gingival tissue or the periapical region of teeth or perforation of the oral mucosa	Routine anesthetic injections through noninfected tissue Dental radiographs Placement of removable prosthodontic or orthodontic appliances Adjustment of orthodontic appliances Placement of orthodontic brackets Shedding of deciduous teeth Bleeding from trauma to the lips or oral mucosa
RESPIRATORY TRACT	RESPIRATORY TRACT
Invasive procedure of the respiratory tract that involves incision or biopsy of the respiratory mucosa (such as tonsillectomy and adenoidectomy) Drainage of an abscess or empyema (add an antibiotic to cover S.viridans and S.aureus, if suspected)	Bronchoscopy (without incision of respiratory mucosa) Endotracheal intubation
GI OR GU TRACT	GI OR GU TRACT
Surgical operations involving intestinal mucosa Surgery of the biliary tract	Diagnostic esophagogastroduodenoscopy or colonoscopy Urethral catheterization through uninfected tissue Circumcision
SKIN	SKIN
Surgical procedure involving infected skin, skin structure or musculoskeletal tissue	Incision or biopsy of surgically scrubbed uninfected skin

Adapted from:

Dajani AS, Taubert KA, Wilson W, *et al.*: Prevention of bacterial endocarditis. Recommendations by the American Heart

Chapter 14

Association, *JAMA* 1997; 277:1794-1801 and Wilson W, Taubert KA, Gewitz M, *et al.*: Prevention of Infective Endocarditis—Guidelines from the American Heart Association, *Circulation* 2007;DOI:10.1161/circulationaha 106.183095.

CONGENTIAL HEART DISEASE IN THE NEWBORN [1-4]

Management of CHD in neonates includes the following three important steps:

1. Suspecting the presence of CHD.
2. Anatomic diagnosis of CHD and its functional classification.
3. Perioperative management.

The five most common diagnoses in the first month of life are:

a. D-TGA
b. HLH
c. Tetralogy of Fallot
d. Co-A
e. VSD.

These lesions can either present with cyanosis, cardiac failure or both.

ANATOMICAL LESIONS PRODUCING CYANOSIS

These conditions often involve right to left shunting at the level of foramen ovale. CHD involving abnormalities of right ventricular (RV) inflow tract (tricuspid atresia, Ebstein's anomaly) or RV outflow tract (pulmonary atresia or stenosis with intact interventricular septum). Tetralogy of Fallot represents similar right to left shunting at the ventricular level and will be discussed briefly in this chapter under specific lesions.

ANATOMICAL LESIONS PRODUCING CHF

A wide variety of conditions can present as cardiac failure in newborn infants. These can be classified based on abnormalities of the four factors determining cardiac output (see Figure 14.1).

i. *Increased preload (volume overload)* – Large left to right shunt (PDA), tricuspid or mitral regurgitation, arteriovenous fistula (including vein of Galen malformation) and intracardiac mixing lesions such as truncus arteriosus, TAPVR without obstruction.

ii. *Increased afterload (pressure overload)* – LV outflow obstruction such as aortic stenosis and Co-A.

iii. *Poor contractility* – Anomalous coronary artery (resulting in myocardial ischemia), myocarditis, cardiomyopathy and birth asphyxia.

iv. *Rhythm (heart rate) disturbances* – SVT and complete heart block.

LESIONS ASSOCIATED WITH COMBINED CYANOSIS AND HEART FAILURE

This list includes the following conditions:

1. TGA.
2. Double outlet right ventricle.
3. Single ventricle.
4. Truncus arteriosus.
5. Complete atrioventricular canal (endocardial cushion defect):
   a. Frequently associated with Down syndrome.
   b. Defects in the posterosuperior portion of the ventricular septum and the lower (primum) part of the atrial septum. Cyanosis results from intracardiac mixing at both atrial and ventricular levels.
   c. Heart failure results from atrioventricular valve regurgitation. Frequently, portions of mitral and tricuspid valves are joined, making a common leaflet which bridges across the crest of the ventricular septum.
   d. Partial atrioventricular canal refers to a combination of ostium primum ASD involving only the lowest part of the inter-atrial septum associated with a cleft in the mitral valve.
   e. ECG is characterized by an abnormal superior axis in patients with endocardial cushion defects (see Figure 14.2).
6. Anomalous pulmonary venous return: In this condition, saturated blood returning from the lungs follows an abnormal path and returns to the systemic venous pathway instead of returning to the left atrium. Infants may present with cyanosis or failure (especially if obstruction to the pulmonary venous

path is present). The point of return to the systemic veins could be:

a. Superior vena cava or one of its draining veins.
b. Inferior vena cava or portal system.
c. Coronary sinus.
d. Directly into the right atrium.

SPECIFIC CHD IN THE NEWBORN INFANT

Patent Ductus Arteriosus (PDA)

PDA is a critical feature of fetal circulation. The ductus is a principal conduit for the diversion of blood from the non-respiratory lungs to the systemic and umbilical circulation. During successful adaptation to extrauterine life, the DA undergoes closure, usually constricting nearly completely by 18 hours of life and closing permanently by 5 to 7 days. Following birth, the placental circulation is disrupted and pulmonary circulation is enhanced. Because the placenta is presumed to be a source for the dilating type prostaglandins and because the lungs are a site of their metabolism, these normal postnatal events lead to a fall in circulating, dilating prostaglandins. As alveolar ventilation improves, oxygenation is increased, and the relative ratio of SVR to PVR is increased, favouring left-to-right shunting across the ductus. Thus, the increase in oxygen tension that occurs in the ductus favours postnatal constriction. However, the ductus is more likely to remain patent in a preterm infant.

Patent Ductus Arteriosus in a Premature Infant

a. *Anatomical and Functional Defects:* A well-known complication of premature birth is the association of PDA with respiratory distress syndrome (RDS). Initially RDS results in higher PVR resulting in bidirectional shunt across the PDA. PDA remains open. Later on, with or without the use of surfactant, RDS improves and PVR decreases resulting in a large left to right shunt across the PDA. This shunt results in excessive pulmonary blood flow, left heart failure with pulmonary edema, and in some infants, need for prolonged mechanical ventilation. The heart is hyperdynamic because of increased preload (due to increased venous return to the left atrium) and decreased afterload because of left to right shunting of blood into a low resistance pulmonary circuit through the PDA (diastolic run-off). Changes in blood flow to the cerebral circulation increase the risk for intraventricular hemorrhage (IVH). Decreased blood flow through the descending aorta results in intestinal (increased risk for necrotizing enterocolitis) and renal ischemia (oliguria) (see Figure 14.4).

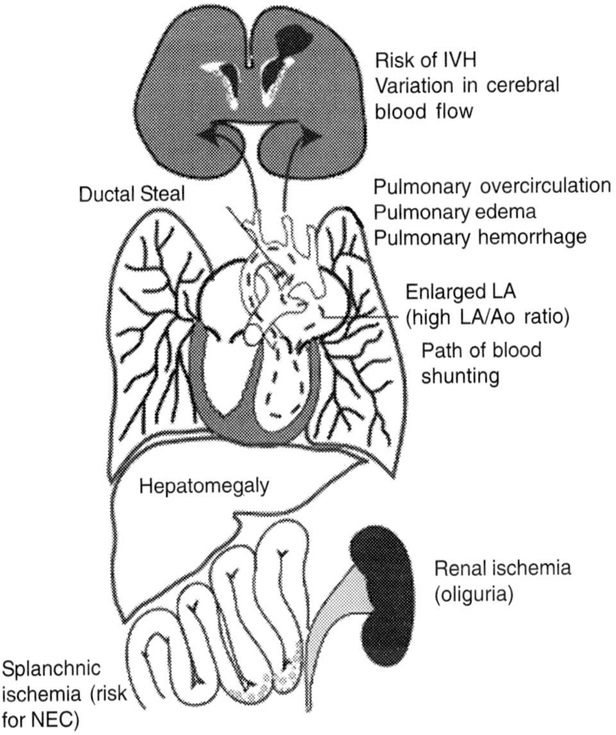

Fig. 14.4: Pathophysiological consequences of PDA in a premature infant

b. *Epidemiology and Incidence:*
   1. In 90% of term infants, ductal closure occurs by 60 hours of age.
   2. In preterm infants > 30 weeks gestation, by 4 days of age, 90% of PDA is closed.
   3. The rates of symptomatic PDA diminish with advancing gestational age and increasing birth weight.
      i. Rates of approximately 50% have been reported in premature infants with a birth weight of < 800 grams.

c. *Clinical Features:* (see Figure 14.5)

1. Murmur – often this murmur is systolic; although it can be continuous or even silent (especially with a large PDA). The murmur may not be clearly audible if the baby is on high settings on the ventilator.

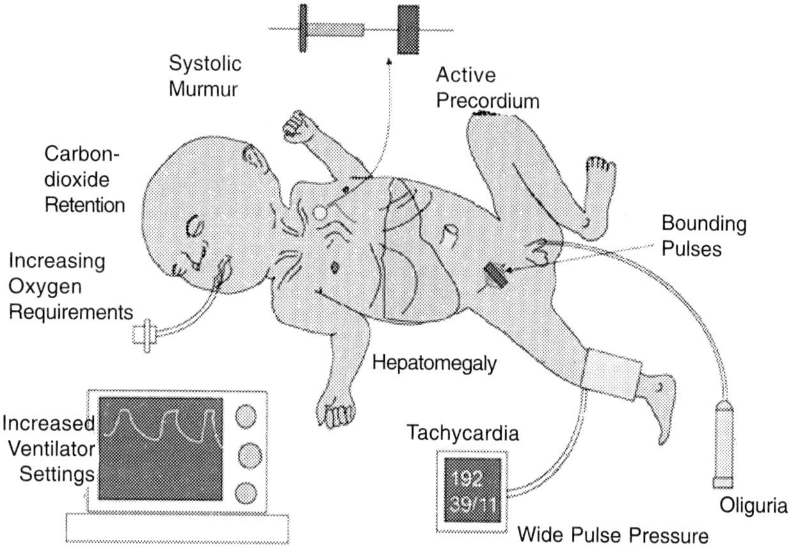

Fig. 14.5: Clinical features of PDA in a premature infant

2. Tachycardia.
3. Hyperdynamic precordium.
4. Bounding pulses – in normal preterm infants palmar and pedal pulses are not palpable. If these pulses are easily palpable, diastolic run-off should be suspected (as seen in PDA).
5. Wide pulse pressure (> 25 mmHg).
6. Increasing ventilator requirements and /or deteriorating blood gases.
7. Rarely PDA may present with acute pulmonary hemorrhagic edema (pink frothy secretions in the tracheal tube).

d. *Investigations:*

1. Chest X-ray (see Figure 14.6)
   - i. Cardiomegaly
   - ii. Increased pulmonary vascularity

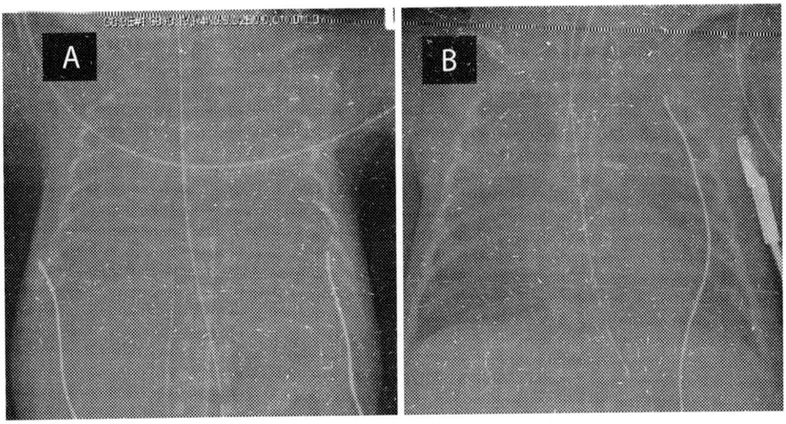

Fig. 14.6: (A) Typical chest X-ray findings in large symptomatic PDA in 26 weeks gestation premature infant at 5 days of age. Notice cardiomegaly and hazy vascular lung fields (B) Same patient's X-ray following ligation (notice the clip) and normal heart size and pulmonary vascularity.

2. Echocardiography
   - i. Indications:
     1. All patients with suspected PDA should have an echocardiogram to confirm the diagnosis, establish the size of the shunt and to rule out ductal dependent CHD.
     2. Presence of any of the clinical features described above (clinical examination is inaccurate in suspecting or confirming the diagnosis of PDA).
   - ii. Signs of significant PDA on echocardiography (see Figure 14.7):
     1. Predominant left to right shunt through the ductus.
     2. Ductal diameter > 1.5 mm.
     3. Enlarged left atrium (LA/Aortic root ratio > 1.3).
     4. Disturbed diastolic flow in the main PA.
     5. Reverse end-diastolic flow in the post-ductal aorta.

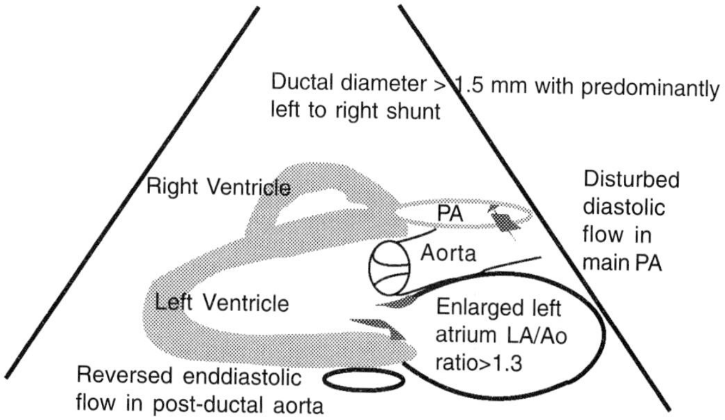

Fig. 14.7: Diagrammatic representation of echocardiographic findings in hemodynamically significant PDA

e. *Prevention*

1. Antenatal betamethasone administration (for lung maturation; decrease RDS).
2. Prophylactic indomethacin (to prevent IVH and PDA): 0.1 mg/kg/dose every 24 hours with the first dose administered within 6-12 hours of birth.

f. *Medical Treatment*[5]

1. Fluid restriction (usually 2/3 of maintenance).
2. NSAID: Ductal patency in maintained *in-utero* by prostaglandins. Inhibition of prostaglandin synthesis by NSAID results in promotion of ductal closure. An echocardiogram must be performed not only to confirm the presence of DA but to rule out the presence of a ductal-dependent CHD (such as Co-A) effectively prior to initiation of NSAID therapy for ductal closure.
   a. Intravenous indomethacin is the drug of choice in most centers and is given at a dose of 0.2 mg/kg/dose (see Table 14.6) over 30 minutes to minimize adverse effects

Table 14.6

Age at first dose	*First dose*	*Second dose*	*Third dose*
< 48 hours	0.2 mg/kg	0.1	0.1
48 hours – 7 days	0.2	0.2	0.2
> 7 days	0.2	0.25	0.25

on cerebral, gastrointestinal and renal blood flow velocities. Doses are repeated at 12 hours and 24 hours.

Prior to administration of each dose, the following list of contraindications should be reviewed:

Contraindications to the use of Indomethacin

1. Presence or suspicion of a ductal dependent cardiac lesion.
2. Decreased urine output (usually < 0.5 cc/kg/hour).
3. Elevated or rapidly increasing creatinine (> 1.8 mg/dL).
4. Thrombocytopenia (< 100,000 / cu. Mm).
5. Disturbances of coagulation.
6. The presence of active bleeding (including a large IVH).
7. Suspected or proven necrotizing enterocolitis (NEC).

i. Indomethacin course may be repeated for a second time. Some institutions prefer to use a prolonged course (0.2 mg/kg/dose q 24 hours × 5-7 doses). The persistence of a hemodynamically significant PDA after two courses of indomethacin (or the presence of contraindications to the use of indomethacin) warrants surgical ligation.

ii. Rapid infusion (< 5 min) of indomethacin is associated with reduction in organ (including cerebral) blood flow. So, this medicine should never be administered as a push. It should be given slowly as an infusion with a pump over at least 30 min.

iii. Concurrent treatment:
   1. Aminoglycosides and other renally excreted drugs: Consider prolonging the dosing interval.
   2. Gastrointestinal perforations occur frequently if indomethacin treatment is used concurrently with glucocorticoids (such as hydrocortisone).

iv. Some centers prefer to withhold feeds while on indomethacin therapy.

v. Indomethacin is also used to prevent IVH (and PDA) at a dose of 0.1 mg/kg q 24 hours for 3 doses beginning at 6 to 12 hours of age.

b. Ibuprofen lysine: This intravenous preparation is administered over 15 min by syringe pump as an alternative to indomethacin.

   i. Dose – 10 mg/kg first dose; 5 mg/kg second and third doses.

   ii. Monitor for decreased urine output (oliguria is less severe with ibuprofen compared to indomethacin).

   iii. Contraindications are similar to indomethacin and include:

      1. Preterm babies with active infection.
      2. Active bleeding.
      3. Thrombocytopenia and coagulation defects.
      4. Necrotizing enterocolitis.
      5. Significant renal dysfunction.
      6. Congenital heart disease with ductal dependent systemic or pulmonary blood flow.
      7. Ibuprofen may displace bilirubin from albumin and should be used carefully in patients with high levels of unconjugated bilirubin.
      8. Evidence of pulmonary hypertension.

   iv. Oral ibuprofen can be considered as an alternative to intravenous ibuprofen. However, data supporting the efficacy of oral ibuprofen is limited compared to the intravenous form.

g. *Surgical Treatment*

1. ***Indication:***

   a. 'Failure of medical management' – Usually persistent symptomatic PDA after two courses of medical therapy.

   b. Contraindications to medical management.

2. ***Procedure:*** Usually performed using a left thoracotomy and ligation or placing a clip to close the ductus arteriosus (see Figure 14.6B).

3. ***Complications:***

   a. Often infants deteriorate transiently following surgical ligation of PDA ('post-ligation syndrome').

b. Inadvertent ligation of the wrong vessel.
c. Rupture of the thoracic duct resulting in chylothorax.
d. Thrombosis of the great vessels.
e. Injury to the left recurrent laryngeal nerve resulting in stridor, secondary to vocal cord paralysis.
f. Recent data suggest long-term neurodevelopmental morbidity following surgical ligation of the ductus.

TRANSPOSITION OF GREAT ARTERIES (TGA)

1. **Definition and Anatomical Defects**
   a. Normally, aorta arises from the left ventricle and aortic valve is located to the right, inferior and posterior to pulmonary valve (Figure 14.8).
   b. In d-TGA, the aortic valve is still to the *right* (hence dextro- or 'd'), inferior but *anterior* to the pulmonary valve. In the classic simple version of d-TGA, PA arises from the left ventricle and the aorta originates from the right ventricle

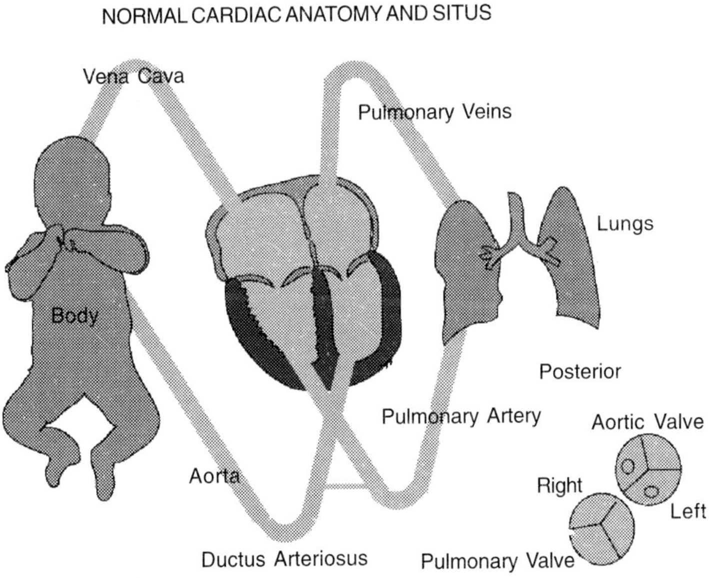

Fig. 14.8: Normal cardiac anatomy and relationship between aorta and pulmonary valves

(Figure 14.9). The only route for oxygenated blood returning to the left atrium to enter the aorta is through the PFO or PDA. Infants with TGA usually have increased pulmonary blood flow but are deeply cyanotic because oxygenated blood has only limited access to the systemic circulation.

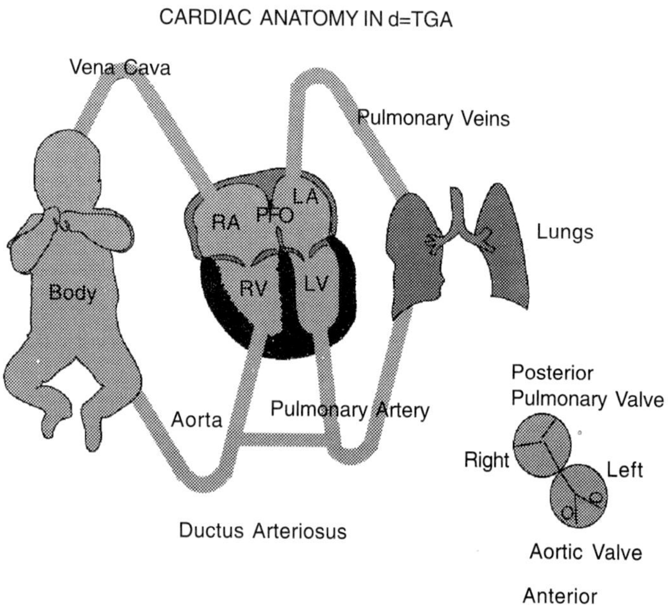

Fig. 14.9: Cardiac anatomy and relationship between aorta and pulmonary valves in dTGA

c. In L-TGA, aortic valve is located to the *left* (hence levo- or 'l') of pulmonary valve and aorta originates from the right ventricle. L-TGA is frequently seen in association with single ventricle conditions (in which there is often cyanosis and heart failure) and with 'corrected TGA', in which atrio-ventricular discordance is 'corrected' by TGA. Venous inflow patterns are reversed, with pulmonary venous blood draining into the right ventricle. The aorta arises from this malpositioned right ventricle and carries oxygenated blood to the systemic circulation (Figure 14.10).

2. **Further discussion in this section is limited to dTGA.**
3. **Functional Effects.**

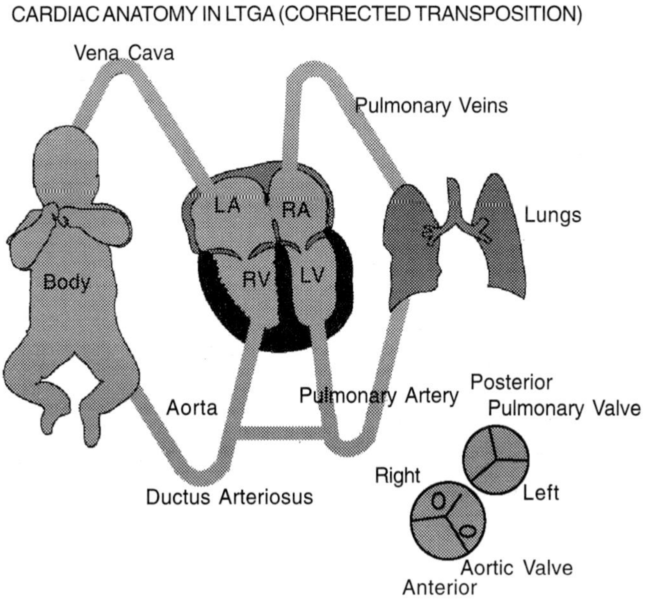

Fig. 14.10: Cardiac anatomy and relationship between aorta and pulmonary valves in L-TGA

Infants with dTGA have intense cyanosis and signs of cardiac failure. The degree of cyanosis or heart failure in TGA is dependent on:

a. Size and amount of shunt through the communications – PFO and PDA.
b. Presence of a VSD decreases the degree of cyanosis, but may increase the likelihood of heart failure.
c. Pulmonary arterial obstruction increases the degree of cyanosis.
d. Aortic obstruction (aortic stenosis or Co-A) increases the risk for heart failure.

4. **Epidemiology (Incidence)**
   a. D-TGA represents 5% of structural CHD.
   b. Rarely found in preterm infants. Most of the infants are born at term and appear otherwise healthy.
   c. Associated cardiac malformations include ASD, VSD, PDA, valvular and subvalvular pulmonary stenosis and Co-A.
   d. Rarely associated with extracardiac malformations or syndromes.

e. More often in males (3 times more common than females).

5. **Clinical Presentation**

It varies depending on the presence or absence of associated cardiac malformations.

a. Infants with dTGA without any shunts present early with cyanosis. The symptoms worsen with closure of DA.

b. The pulmonic component of the second heart sound may not be audible.

c. Marked pulmonary obstruction results in worse cyanosis, loud systolic murmur and pulmonary oligemia on chest X-ray.

d. Cases with large shunt lesions may present later. These patients may avoid metabolic acidosis if their ductal patency is maintained.

6. **Diagnosis**

a. Some cases of dTGA are missed on antenatal sonograms, especially if only a four-chamber view is visualized during fetal evaluation.

b. Chest X-ray:

   i. The classic description is that of an 'egg on a string' describing a narrow mediastinum (due to the orientation of aorta and PA).

   ii. Pulmonary oligemia suggests right ventricular outflow obstruction.

c. Echocardiogram shows the abnormal origin of the great arteries:

   i. Careful evaluation of associated defects (specifically, the presence of coarctation of aorta) is important.

   ii. Adequacy of shunt communication at the atrial level should be established.

   iii. Coronary artery anatomy must be clearly studied. If coronaries cannot be evaluated by echocardiogram, cardiac catheterization and angiography may be necessary.

7. **Management**

a. Intravenous PGE1 therapy (see above) to maintain ductal patency.

b. Often enlargement of the foramen ovale by balloon septostomy is necessary to obtain adequate entry of oxygenated blood into the right ventricle. This procedure may be done in the nursery by experienced cardiologists under echocardiographic guidance.

8. **Surgical Management**
   a. Arterial switch must be performed in the newborn period before left ventricular muscle has involuted (secondary to pumping into a low resistance pulmonary circulation), usually within the first three weeks of life.
   b. Associated anomalies such as coarctation should be repaired.

TETRALOGY OF FALLOT

1. **Anatomical Defect**
   a. This condition is a combination of VSD, malalignment and overriding aorta over the VSD so that blood from both RV and LV egress directly into the aorta, obstruction to RV outflow tract resulting in RV hypertrophy.
   b. The aortic arch is right sided in 20% of cases.
2. **Functional Effects**
   a. The degree of cyanosis is determined by intracardiac right to left shunting across the VSD and the amount of RV blood entering the ascending aorta.
   b. In cases of pulmonary atresia with VSD, all the blood from the RV enters the aorta resulting in cyanosis presenting in the immediate newborn period.
   c. In cases of mild pulmonary stenosis, cyanosis may not be apparent at birth and the baby may instead present with signs of cardiac failure following postnatal fall in PVR (pink Tetralogy of Fallot).
3. **Epidemiology and Incidence**

   Tetralogy of Fallot accounts for approximately 5-7% of major CHD.
4. **Clinical Presentation**

   It depends on the degree of RV outflow obstruction.
   a. Infants may have a prominent left parasternal impulse associated with a harsh systolic murmur along the left sternal border. The second heart sound is often single.

b. Infants with mild RV outflow obstruction may present with heart failure.

c. Newborn infants with severe RV outflow obstruction present with cyanosis soon after birth. Worsening cyanosis and circulatory collapse may occur after ductal closure.

d. Paroxysmal hypercyanotic attacks ('blue' or 'tet' spells) present with hyperpnea and increasing cyanosis. Vigorous crying usually precipitates these attacks. With decreasing flow across the RV outflow tract, the intensity of the murmur decreases. Prolonged spells result in loss of consciousness, stroke or convulsions.

   i. *Acute management of a 'tet' spell:*

      1. Calming the infant.
      2. Placement of the infant on the abdomen in a knee chest position.
      3. Avoid agitation (such as persistent and premature attempts to draw blood etc.).
      4. Administration of oxygen.
      5. Sedation.
      6. Correction of metabolic acidosis.

   ii. *Management of spells 'resistant' to conventional management:*

      1. Propranolol 0.1 mg/kg IV may be useful.
      2. Increasing SVR with phenylephrine may improve pulmonary blood flow.

5. **Investigations**

   a. Chest X-ray typically shows:

      i. Pulmonary oligemia with relatively black lung fields.
      ii. Concavity of the upper left heart border (area of PA).
      iii. RV hypertrophy results in a rounded uptilted apex above the diaphragm.
      iv. Cardiac silhouette resembles a boot or a wooden shoe ('coeur en sabot').

   b. ECG shows evidence of RV hypertrophy, right axis deviation and dominant 'R' wave in the right precordial leads.

c. Echocardiogram confirms the diagnosis. The side of the aortic arch and the presence of a PDA can be determined.

6. **Management**

Optimal management to avoid hypoglycemia, hypothermia and severe hypoxia.

a. *Medical Management:*

i. PGE1 infusion to maintain ductal patency in cases of severe RV outflow tract obstruction.

ii. Avoid dehydration and hemoconcentration.

iii. Oral propranolol 0.5 to 1 mg/kg/dose q 6 hours may be used to decrease the frequency and severity of 'tet' spells.

b. *Surgical Management:*

i. Palliative surgery – Modified Blalock-Taussig shunt consists of placing a Gore-Tex conduit anastomosing subclavian artery to the homolateral branch of the PA.

1. Complications include chylothorax, diaphragmatic paralysis and Horner syndrome.

2. Weak pulse on the side of the anastomosis and rare possibility of arm length discrepancy.

ii. Corrective surgery includes relieving RV outflow tract obstruction and patch closure of the VSD through a transatrial-transpulmonary approach.

7. **Complications**

Uncorrected Tetralogy of Fallot can result in several complications during infancy and early childhood.

i. Cerebral thrombosis.

ii. Polycythemia.

iii. Brain abscess.

iv. Bacterial endocarditis.

8. **Prognosis**

a. Total correction usually results in asymptomatic life style.

b. Patients may experience exercise intolerance, conduction disturbances and premature ventricular beats.

HYPOPLASTIC LEFT HEART SYNDROME (HLH)

1. **Anatomical Defect**

Underdevelopment of the left side of the heart results in a

group of anomalies that include one or more of the following anatomical defects:

a. Atresia or narrowing of the mitral orifice.
b. Small, non-functional or atretic left ventricle.
c. Atresia or stenosis of the aortic orifice.
d. Hypoplasia of the ascending aorta.

2. **Functional Effects**
   a. Pulmonary venous blood passes through the PFO and reaches the RV.
   b. Total mixing of pulmonary venous and systemic venous blood in the RV.
   c. RV ejects all the blood into the PA.
   d. Ascending aorta and coronaries are supplied by retrograde flow through the ductus.
   e. Systemic perfusion occurs through the PDA.
   f. If a VSD is present, RV pumps some blood into the LV and ascending aorta.
3. **Incidence**

   Approximately 1-3% of all major CHD.
4. **Clinical Presentation**
   a. Infants with HLH have a grayish-blue color and low pulse oximeter readings in the first day or two of life, but this feature may be missed in a busy nursery.
   b. With closure of the ductus, systemic hypoperfusion, shock and cardiac failure occur.
   c. A systolic murmur and a right parasternal lift are common.
5. **Investigations**
   a. *Chest X-ray:* Cardiomegaly and increased pulmonary vascularity.
   b. *ECG:* Signs of RVH and right atrial enlargement.
   c. Renal and head sonogram to look for anomalies.
      i. One-third of patients with HLH have a major or minor central nervous system (CNS) abnormality.
      ii. An ophthalmology and genetics consult is recommended.
   d. Echocardiogram confirms the diagnosis.

6. **Management**
   a. Maintenance of ductal patency with PGE1.
   b. Oxygen saturation should be maintained in the mid-70s to prevent systemic hypoperfusion (see Figure 14.3). In some patients, low oxygen concentrations (18% O_2 by blending nitrogen with air) may be necessary.
   c. Prevention of hypothermia, acidosis and hypoglycemia.
   d. Surgical therapy:
      i. Staged Norwood consists of the following procedures (Stage I):
         1. Division of the main PA.
         2. Closure of the distal segment of the main PA.
         3. Reconstruction of the ascending aorta using an allograft.
         4. Anastomosis of the proximal segment of the main PA to reconstructed ascending aorta.
         5. Atrial septectomy.
         6. Blalock-Taussig shunt (subclavian artery to homolateral PA).
      ii. Sano modification is similar to Norwood but instead of using a Blalock-Taussig shunt, it uses a RV to PA conduit.
      iii. Stage II Norwood procedure consists of:
         1. Glenn Anastomosis–Superior vena cava (SVC) to PA.
         2. Modified Fontan procedure–IVC to PA with an intraatrial or external baffle.
      iv. The old aortic root is attached to the neo-aorta to provide coronary perfusion.
   e. Cardiac transplantation–either as a primary procedure or following stage I Norwood procedure.
7. **Prognosis**
   Untreated patients usually die during the first or second week of life. The mortality of stage I Norwood is approximately 5-10% in the best centers.

VENTRICULAR SEPTAL DEFECT (VSD)

1. **Anatomical Defect**

   A defect in the ventricular septum can occur in different anatomical locations.

   a. Common membranous defects are located anterior to the septal leaflet of the tricuspid valve in the postero-inferior portion of the interventricular septum.

   b. Defects between the papillary muscle of the conus and crista supraventricularis are often associated with pulmonic stenosis.

   c. Supracristal lesions may cause aortic insufficiency.

   d. Defects at the apex of mid-portion of the interventricular septum are muscular and may be single or multiple (Swiss cheese septum).

2. **Functional Effects**

   The amount of shunt across the VSD is dependent on two factors:

   a. Size of the defect.

   b. The ratio of RV to LV pressure (or relative ratio of SVR to PVR).

   With large defects, once PVR falls after the immediate newborn period, pulmonary blood flow is increased resulting in pulmonary hypertension. With long standing VSD, pulmonary vascular disease develops resulting in severe pulmonary hypertension.

3. **Incidence**

   VSD is the most common cardiac malformation and accounts for 25% of CHD.

4. **Clinical Presentation**

   a. Most VSDs are asymptomatic at birth and a murmur may not be audible because of the higher right-sided pressure. A systolic murmur is typically audible after the first few days of life when the PVR and RV pressure decrease from the high fetal levels. This murmur is best heard at the lower left sternal border.

   b. In some cases of large defects, symptoms of cardiac failure may be delayed until the term infant is approximately 1 to 2 months of age. This is due to:

i. Fetal PVR is high and limits the left to right shunt because of high RV pressures. PVR gradually decreases over the first month resulting in increased pulmonary blood flow.

ii. A large shunt through the VSD may itself contribute to elevated pulmonary arterial pressures, thus further delaying the regression of PVR from fetal levels.

iii. High hematocrit at birth contributes to high PVR. The 'physiological anemia' of infancy noted at 6 to 8 weeks of age may result in lowered blood viscosity resulting in decreased PVR.

c. Note:

i. If symptoms of failure in an infant with VSD appear in the immediate newborn period, look for LV outflow tract obstruction especially Co-A. The increased LV afterload magnifies left to right shunt and hastens the onset of cardiac failure.

ii. Preterm infants have large left to right shunts early in life with VSD because of rapid regression of PVR presumably due to poor development of pulmonary vascular smooth muscle.

5. **Investigations**

a. Chest X-ray is often normal. In older infants with large lesions, cardiomegaly and increased pulmonary vascularity may be evident.

b. Echocardiogram with color Doppler will show the defects and the flow across the septum.

6. **Management**

a. Close observation for signs of heart failure and management of CHF (see above). Growth should be monitored closely as some infants with large defects fail to thrive.

b. One-third to half of the small defects close spontaneously. Muscular defects are more likely to close than membranous defects.

c. Indications for surgical closure of VSD:

i. Large defects with failure to thrive and symptoms of cardiac failure not responding to medical management (in infants of all age groups).

ii. Pulmonary arterial banding is indicated in some patients (especially premature infants with complicated health issues) for palliation followed by definitive repair at a later date.

iii. Defects with evidence of pulmonary hypertension (usually in infants 6-12 months of age).

iv. In older patients (> 2 years of age), persistent defects especially if associated with significant shunt (Qp/Qs > 2) need surgery.

d. Severe pulmonary vascular disease is a contraindication to closure of a VSD.

e. Use of occlusion devices during cardiac catheterization is being studied.

7. **Complications**

a. Residual VSD after surgery.

b. Heart block.

8. **Prognosis**

Long-term prognosis in the absence of post-operative complications is excellent.

COARCTATION OF AORTA (CO-A)

1. **Anatomical Defect**

There is narrowing of aorta in Co-A. The narrowing can be discrete or result in tubular hypoplasia. Although the site is variable, most cases, the site is below the origin of the left subclavian artery at the origin of the ductus arteriosus.

a. Bicuspid aortic valve is commonly seen in 50-70% of patients with Co-A.

b. Co-A may be a feature of Turner syndrome.

c. Shone complex – a group of left sided obstructive lesions occurring together (Co-A, mitral valve abnormalities, subaortic stenosis).

2. **Functional Effects**

The PDA serves to widen the juxtraductal area of coarctation limiting symptoms in the first few days of life. Blood flows through the ascending aorta and then traverses the narrow segment to reach the descending aorta. With more severe narrowing, descending aorta is supplied mainly through right to left shunt at the ductal level. Ductal closure results in hypoperfusion of the lower segment of the body.

3. **Incidence**

   Co-A accounts for 8% of CHD, with slight male preponderance.

4. **Clinical Presentation**

   The classic sign is disparity in pulsation and blood pressure (BP) in the arms and legs. The carotid, brachial and radial pulses are prominent and femoral pulses are weak. The BP in the legs is lower than that in the arms. It is important to measure BP in both the upper limbs as the left subclavian may sometimes be involved in the coarctation.

   a. A systolic ejection click and a murmur may be audible in cases with a bicuspid aortic valve.
   b. Hypoperfusion and low pulse oximeter readings in the lower body.
   c. Acidosis and severe heart failure occurs after ductal closure.

5. **Investigations**

   a. Chest X-ray is often normal in neonates with Co-A. The typical features such, as notching of the inferior border of the ribs from pressure erosion from enlarged collateral vessels is not evident until late childhood.
   b. ECG may show evidence of biventricular hypertrophy.
   c. Echocardiogram usually shows the area of narrowing but this can often be missed or underestimated in patients with an open ductus.
   d. Diagnostic catheterization may be required in some patients to delineate anatomical details.

6. **Management**

   a. *Medical:*
      i. Maintaining or establishing ductal patency with PGE1 will establish adequate blood flow to the lower segment.
      ii. Hypertension and cardiac failure may need to be addressed prior to surgery.

   b. *Surgical options include:*
      i. Excision of the area of coarctation and primary reanastomosis.

ii. Subclavian flap procedure – division of left subclavian artery and incorporation into the wall of the repaired coarctation.

iii. Patch aortoplasty using prosthetic material.

c. Primary angioplasty may be an option but is controversial.

7. **Complications**

a. Rebound hypertension – usually self-resolved.

b. Residual stenosis (more common with subclavian flap procedure).

8. **Prognosis**

a. Recoarctation is rare and can be treated with balloon angioplasty.

b. Watch for associated cerebrovascular disease.

c. Patients with subclavian flap procedure will have weak or absent pulses on the left upper extremity.

REFERENCES

1. Workbook in Practical Neonatology, 3rd edition; Polin RA, Yoder MC, Burg FD – Saunders/Elsevier, Philadelphia PA.
2. Residents Handbook of Neonatology, 3rd edition, Kirpalani H, Moore AM, Perlman M; B.C.Decker, Inc., Hamilton ON.
3. The Pediatric Cardiology Handbook, Park MK, Mosby.
4. Nelson Textbook of Pediatrics, 18th edition.
5. Neofax 2007 Editors–Young TE, Magnum B: Thomson Healthcare, Montvale NJ.

15

ANEMIA IN NEONATES

Hari B Srinivasan

DEFINITIONS: NORMAL HEMOGLOBIN LEVELS

Hemoglobin concentration undergoes constant physiologic change both during the fetal and neonatal period. A clear definition of the normal hemoglobin concentration is important for proper evaluation and management of anemia in the neonate.[1, 2]

Anemia is defined as a hemoglobin concentration 2 standard deviations (SD) below the mean for age. Table 15.1[3] shows the changes in **hemoglobin** and **hematocrit** concentration during fetal life and Table 15.2[4] shows changes during the neonatal period.

PHYSIOLOGIC ANEMIA OF INFANCY

After birth there is a transient increase in hemoglobin concentration as plasma moves extravascularly to compensate for the placental transfusion and an increase in red cell volume. Thereafter, the hemoglobin level gradually falls, to reach a nadir

Table 15.1: Normal (± SD) erythrocyte values during gestation

Weeks of gestation	*Hemoglobin (g/dL)*	*Hematocrit (%)*
18-21	11.7 ± 1.3	37.3 ± 4.3
22-25	12.2 ± 1.6	38.6 ± 3.9
26-29	12.9 ± 1.4	40.9 ± 4.4
>36	16.5 ± 1.5	51.0 ± 4.5

Table 15.2: Postnatal changes in erythrocyte values (mean ± SD) in term neonates

Age	*Hemoglobin (g/dL)*	*Hematocrit (%)*
Cord blood	16.2 ± 3.6	46.7 ± 5.1
12-18 hours	18.8 ± 2.8	49.0 ± 4.8
3 days	17.4 ± 3.0	46.9 ± 5.3
7 days	17.0 ± 2.4	45.0 ± 4.0
15 days	16.4 ± 2.2	43.4 ± 4.1
28 days	14.2 ± 2.4	42.1± 3.8

of 9.5-11 g/dL by 6-12 weeks of age. The reasons for this fall in hemoglobin concentration include:

- Decline in red cell production due to decreased erythropoietin production (*in utero* the fetal oxygen saturation is 45% and after delivery it rises to 95%, hence erythropoietin levels become undetectable).
- Shortened survival of neonatal erythrocyte.
- Rapid body growth.

ANEMIA OF PREMATURITY

This is an exaggeration of the normal physiological anemia. In preterm infants, the hemoglobin nadir of 6.5-9.0 g/dL is reached by 4-8 weeks of life. This can be attributed to the following reasons:

- Shortened red blood cell (RBC) survival compared to term infants.
- Relatively more rapid growth rate.
- Iatrogenic loss from blood sampling.
- Vitamin E deficiency.

Table 15.3[5] shows the hemoglobin nadir in babies during the first year of life.

ETIOPATHOGENESIS OF ANEMIA

Anemia in the neonate occurs as a result of one of the three processes:

A. Loss of RBC, or **hemorrhagic anemia;**

B. Increased destruction of RBC, or **hemolytic anemia;**

C. Underproduction of RBC, or **hypoplastic anemia**.

Table 15.3: Hemoglobin nadir in babies in the first year of life

Maturity at birth	*Hemoglobin level (g/dL) at nadir*	*Time of nadir (weeks)*
Term	9.5 - 11	6 - 12
Preterm (1200-1400 g)	8.0 - 10.0	5 - 10
Preterm < 1200 g	6.5 - 9.0	4 - 8

A. Hemorrhagic Anemia

1. *Antenatal period*
   a. Loss of placental integrity–placental abruption, placenta previa.
   b. Anomalies of umbilical cord or placental vessels—vilamentous insertion of the cord occurs in 10% of twin gestation, vasa previa and umbilical hematoma (1 in 5500 deliveries).
   c. Twin-twin transfusion.
2. *Intrapartum period*
   a. Feto-maternal hemorrhage. Occurs in 30-50% of all pregnancies. The risk is increased in instrumental deliveries and cesarean section.
   b. Traumatic rupture of umbilical cord.
   c. Obstetric trauma. Occult visceral and intracranial hemorrhage may occur.
3. *Neonatal period*
   a. Enclosed hemorrhage–caput succedaneum, cephalhaematoma (occurs in 2.5% of births and upto 5% of the infants may have non-displaced skull fractures), intracranial hemorrhage (subdural, subarachnoid or subependymal), visceral parenchymal hemorrhage (most commonly involves the liver).
   b. Defects in hemostasis–congenital coagulation factor deficiency, consumption coagulopathy, deficiency of vitamin K-dependent coagulation factors, thrombocytopenia.
   c. Iatrogenic blood loss.

B. Hemolytic Anemia

1. *Immune hemolysis*

a. Isoimmune hemolytic anemia (Rh and ABO incompatibility).
b. Autoimmune hemolytic anemia.

2. *Non-immune hemolysis*
   a. Bacterial sepsis.
   b. Congenital TORCH (Toxoplasmosis, Others, Rubella, Cytomegalovirus, Herpes simplex virus) infections.
3. *Congenital erythrocyte defects*
   a. Enzyme deficiency–Glucose-6-phosphate dehydrogenase (G6PD) and pyruvate kinase deficiency.
   b. Thalassemia (seen in homozygous α-thalassemia).
   c. Membrane defects–hereditary spherocytosis and elliptocytosis.
4. *Systemic diseases*
   a. Galactosemia.
   b. Osteopetrosis.
5. *Nutritional deficiency*
   a. Vitamin E deficiency.

C. Hypoplastic Anemia

1. *Congenital diseases*
   a. Diamond-Blackfan syndrome.
   b. Atransferrinemia.
   c. Congenital leukemia.
   d. Sideroblastic anemia.
2. *Acquired diseases*
   a. Infections – Rubella, Syphilis.
   b. Aplastic anemia.

Anemia in neonates can also be classified on the basis of mean corpuscular volume (MCV) as shown in Table 15.4.[6] Normal MCV in newborns is 95-121 fl.

DIAGNOSIS

History

Obstetric history should include information about vaginal bleeding during pregnancy, placenta previa, abruptio placenta, vasa previa

Table 15.4: Classification of anemia by mean corpuscular volume (MCV)

Macrocytic anemia	**Normocytic anemia**
Folic acid deficiency	**Low reticulocyte count**
Vitamin B_{12} deficiency	Infection
Organic aciduria	Transient erythroblastopenia of childhood
Diamond-Blackfan anemia	Chronic disease
Fanconi anemia	Immune hemolytic anemia
Aquired aplastic anemia	Mechanical hemolytic anemia
Drugs	Drugs
	Leukemia
Microcytic anemia	Hemoglobinopathy
Iron deficiency	
Lead poisoning	**Normal or High reticulocyte count**
Thalassemia	Blood loss
Chronic infection	Sequestration
	Red cell enzyme defect

and cesarean section. Additional questions should include: Was the birth traumatic? Was it multiple births? Did the cord rupture?

Family history: Information should be obtained about the ethnic origin and history of anemia in other family members or unexplained episodes of jaundice, cholelithiasis or splenectomy.

Age of onset is of significant diagnostic value. Marked anemia at birth is due to hemorrhage or severe isoimmunization. Anemia manifesting itself during the first 2 days of life is caused by external or internal hemorrhage; anemia appearing after the first 48 hours of life is most commonly due to hemolysis and is often associated with jaundice.

Clinical Examination

Physical examination may show the presence of associated anomalies as shown in Table 15.5 [6] and also provide clues regarding the etiology. Acute blood loss is associated with poor perfusion, cyanosis and metabolic acidosis, while chronic blood loss is associated with pallor, jaundice and hepatosplenomegaly.

Table 15.5: Morphological findings on the peripheral blood smear

Morphologic findings	*Etiology*
Hypochromia	Iron deficiency, lead poisoning, thalassemia
Target cells	HbC, S or E, thalassemia, abetalipoproteinemia
Sickle cell	Hb S disease and variants
Basophilic stippling	Iron deficiency, lead poisoning, thalassemia
Heinz bodies	Hemolytic anemia—due to enzyme defect
Howell-Jolly bodies	Postsplenectomy
Spherocytosis	Immune hemolytic anemia, G6PD deficiency
Elliptocytosis	Red cell membrane defect
Schistocytosis	Microangiopathic hemolytic anemia

Laboratory Studies

Complete blood count

Reticulocyte count (normal: 2-5%).

Peripheral blood smear: See Table 15.5.[6]

Coombs' test.

Serum bilirubin.

Apt test: To detect swallowed maternal blood.

Kleihaeur-Betke preparation: To detect fetomaternal transfusion.

Ultrasound of head and abdomen: To detect internal hemorrhage.

Studies to detect infection.

Bone marrow examination.

Figure 15.1 shows an algorithm to diagnose anemia in the neonate.

MANAGEMENT

In addition to specific treatment based on the etiology, guidelines for **blood transfusion** are as follows:

Simple Transfusion

The decision to transfuse must be made according to the infant's clinical condition and physiologic needs. The following are the red cell transfusion guidelines from the Unites States Recombinant Erythropoietin Trial.[7]

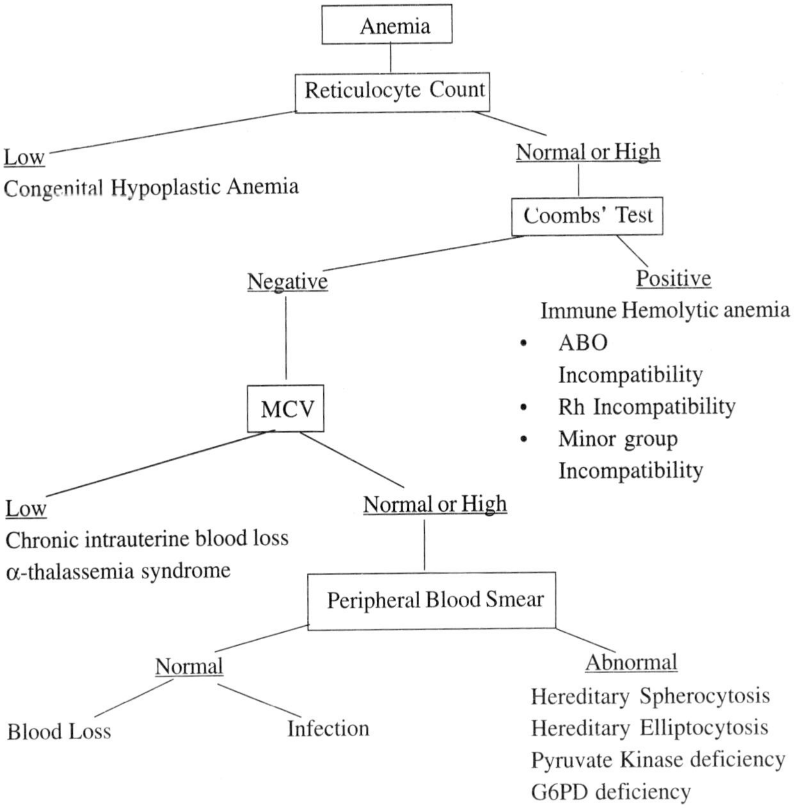

Fig. 15.1

Transfuse at hematocrit ≤35% in infants who are:

- Receiving >35% oxygen.
- Receiving continuous positive airway pressure (CPAP) or mechanical ventilation with mean airway pressure of 6-8 cm H_2O.

Transfuse at hematocrit ≤30% in infants who are:

- Receiving any supplemental oxygen.
- Receiving CPAP or mechanical ventilation with mean airway pressure <6 cm H_2O.
- Having significant episodes of apnea and bradycardia (>9 episodes in 12 hours or 2 episodes in 24 hours requiring bagging while receiving therapeutic doses of methylxanthines).

- Experiencing heart rates >180 beats/min or respiratory rates >80 breaths/min for 24 hours.
- Experiencing weight gain <10g/d over at least 4 days while receiving 100 kcal/kg per day.
- Undergoing surgery.

Transfuse at hematocrit £20% in infants who are:

- Asymptomatic with absolute reticulocyte count $<100\times10^9$/L.

The volume of transfusion can be calculated as follows:

$$\text{Weight} \times \text{blood volume in kg} \times \frac{\text{hematocrit desired-hematocrit observed}}{\text{hematocrit of blood given}}$$

The average newborn blood volume is 80 ml/kg; the hematocrit of packed RBC is 60-90%.

Irradiated RBCs are used for transfusion in premature infants weighing < 1200 grams, as premature infants are unable to reject foreign lymphocytes in transfused blood. Also blood from cytomegalovirus (CMV) negative donors is preferred for neonatal transfusions. As the concern for multiple exposure risk is high with repeated transfusion in extremely low birth weight infants, it is recommended to transfuse stored RBC from a single dedicated unit reserved for the infant.[8]

Exchange Transfusion

- Severe isoimmune hemolytic anemia.
- Chronic hemolytic anemia with elevated central venous pressure.
- Consumption coagulopathy.

Prophylaxis

Term infants do not require **iron supplementation** until 2 months of age. They should be discharged home on breast milk or iron fortified infant formula.[9]

Preterm infants require the following supplementation:

- Vitamin E – 25 IU daily until 2-3 months of age.
- Iron supplementation with 2 mg/kg/day of elemental iron is started at 6 weeks of age.

- Folic acid – 1-2 mg/kg/week.

Recombinant human erythropoietin (r-HuEPO) has been shown to increase neonatal erythropoiesis and decrease the need for transfusions beyond 2 weeks of age in preterm infants.[7] However, r-HuEPO treatment is of limited benefit in reducing the number of transfusions, if strict transfusion criteria are followed. Hence this therapy may have a role only in selected infants in whom it may be desirable to maintain a relatively high hematocrit. In these infants, r-HuEPO 750 U/kg/week subcutaneously is given in three divided doses. Iron supplementation at 2 mg/kg/day is started when oral feeds are tolerated and increased to 4 mg/kg/day when oral feeds reach 100 ml/kg/day.

REFERENCES

1. Nathan DG, Oski FA: Hematology of infancy and childhood, Philadelphia: WB Saunders, 1992.
2. Oski FA, Naiman JL: Hematologic problems in the newborn, 3rd ed, Philadelphia: WB Saunders, 1982.
3. Foristier F, Daffos F, Catherine N, *et al.*: Developmental hematopoiesis in normal human fetal blood, Blood 1991; 77:2360-2363.
4. Lokeswar MR, Singhal T, Shah W: Anemia in the newborn, Indian J Pediatr 2003; 70:893-902.
5. Glader B, Naiman JL: Erythrocyte disorders in infancy, Taeusch HW, Ballard RA, Avery ME, eds: Diseases of the newborn. Philadelphia: WB Saunders, 1991.
6. Fanaroff AA, Martin RJ: Diseases of the fetus and infant, 6th ed., St Louis: Mosby, 1997.
7. Shannon KM, Keith JF, Mentzer WC, *et al.*: Recombinant human erythropoietin stimulates erythropoiesis and reduces erythrocyte transfusions in very low birth weight preterm infants, Pediatrics 1995; 95:1-8.
8. Strauss RG: Blood banking issues pertaining to neonatal red blood cell transfusions, Transfus Sci 1999; 21:7-19.
9. Committee on Nutrition AAP: Iron-Fortified infant formulas, Pediatrics 1989; 84: 1114-1115.

16

POLYCYTHEMIA

Girish Gupta

DEFINITIONS

Polycythemia is defined as a central venous **hematocrit** of >65%.[1-3] The primary concern with polycythemia relates to hyperviscosity and its associated complications. Blood **viscosity** increases exponentially as hematocrit rises above 65%. Viscosity is measured using special viscometer e.g. a coaxial narrow-gap couette viscometer. Hyperviscosity is defined as a state with blood viscosity >14.6 centipoise at a shear rate of 11.5/sec as measured by a viscometer.

Epidemiology

Polycythemia occurs in 0.4-12% of neonates. It is more common in **small for gestational age (SGA)** (24%), and **large for gestational age** (LGA) infants. **Infants of diabetic mothers (IDM)** have a ~40% incidence, and those born to gestational diabetics have a ~30% incidence. Hyperviscosity has been found to occur in 0.4-5% of infants. However, it has been shown that only 47% of polycythemic infants exhibit hyperviscosity while only 24% of infants with hyperviscosity carry a diagnosis of polycythemia.

Hematocrit peaks 2 hours after birth and then declines until 6 hours of age at which time it equals cord blood hematocrit. Fewer than 40% of infants with a hematocrit >64% at 2 hours of age will still have a high value at 12 or more hours of age.

Etiology

It can occur because of the following reasons:

- *Increased Fetal Erythropoiesis Secondary to Fetal Hypoxia*
  - ***Placental insufficiency:*** Secondary to pre-eclampsia, eclampsia or primary renovascular disease, chronic or recurrent abruptio placenta, cyanotic congenital heart disease, post-dated pregnancy, maternal smoking or **intrauterine growth restriction (IUGR)**.
  - ***Endocrine abnormalities:*** Secondary to increased oxygen consumption resulting in fetal hypoxia which may be due to congenital thyrotoxicosis, congenital adrenal hyperplasia, Beckwith-Wiedemann syndrome or IDM.
  - ***Genetic disorders*** such as trisomy 13, trisomy 18 and trisomy 21 may also cause *in utero* hypoxia.[4]
- *Hyper Transfusion* [5]
  - Delayed **cord clamping** allows for an increased blood volume to be delivered to the infant. When cord clamping is delayed more than 3 minutes after birth, a 30% increase in blood volume is noted.
  - Gravity may also be a factor due to the lower position of the delivered infant in relation to the maternal introitus before cord clamping.
  - In the event of delayed cord clamping, blood flow to the infant will be enhanced by oxytocin.
  - **Twin-to-twin transfusion syndrome** occurs in approximately 10% of monozygotic twin pregnancies.[6]
  - Maternal-fetal transfusion
  - **Iatrogenic:** May be transfusion-related.
- *Dehydration:* Dehydration may be due to decreased plasma volume in relation to red cell mass.
- *Maternal Drug:* Propranolol; it is probably the condition for which drug is being given rather than the drug itself that causes polycythemia.
- *Maternal Smoking:* Term neonates of mothers who smoke during pregnancy require a partial exchange transfusion for neonatal polycythemia approximately two and a half times as often as neonates of mothers who do not smoke.[7,8]

Chapter 16

Pathophysiology

Cord hematocrit of > 56% is associated with polycythemia. Cord hyperviscosity is a more important determinant of later neurological function than polycythemia.[9]

Figure 16.1 summarizes the pathogenesis of polycythemia and its effects.

A. As the central hematocrit increases, viscosity increases. Blood viscosity is determined by multiple factors viz. plasma volume, plasma proteins, platelets, and endothelial factors. Factors unique to the neonate (e.g. increased red cell volume, decreased deformability of the fetal erythrocyte) also contribute to increased viscosity.
B. Blood viscosity is inversely proportional to red cell filterability. Newborn RBC has low filterability, and it further reduces in acidosis and hypoxia, producing hyperviscosity in neonates.
C. Changes in plasma osmolality and lipid contents have direct relation with blood viscosity.
D. Increased viscosity results in abnormal blood flow kinetics. This manifests as poor flow or sludging of blood, which

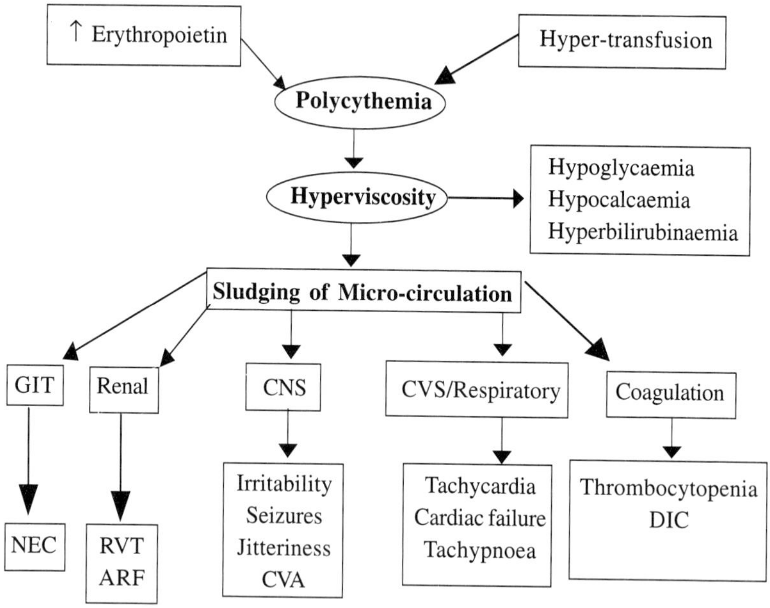

Fig. 16.1: Pathogenesis of polycythemia and its effects

predisposes the infant to an impairment of tissue oxygenation and decreased plasma glucose with a tendency to form microthrombi.

E. If these events occur in the cerebral cortex, kidneys, adrenal glands or other organs significant damage may result. Hypoxia and acidosis increase viscosity. Poor perfusion increases the possibility of thrombosis.

Clinical Features

The important symptoms are lethargy, irritability, jitteriness, tremors, seizures, cerebrovascular accidents, respiratory distress, cyanosis and apnea.

- The most obvious finding is plethora or ruddiness.
- Evaluate the infant for dehydration (e.g., sunken fontanelle, dry mucous membranes).
- Priapism may be observed in males.
- Central nervous system: CNS manifestations are the most common problems observed with polycythemia and hyperviscosity.
  - Symptoms include lethargy, irritability, jitteriness, tremors, seizures and cerebrovascular accidents (CVA).
- Cardiopulmonary system manifestations include respiratory distress, tachypnea, cyanosis, apnea and congestive heart failure.
- Gastrointestinal
  - Poor feeding is reported in over one half of all infants with polycythemia and hyperviscosity.
  - **Necrotizing enterocolitis (NEC)** is a rare but devastating complication of polycythemia/hyperviscosity. Term infants diagnosed with NEC have associated polycythemia upto 44% of the time.
- Renal manifestations include decreased glomerular filtration rates, oliguria, acute renal failure (ARF), hematuria, proteinuria, and renal vein thrombosis (RVT).
- Metabolic
  - Metabolic alterations are frequent.
  - **Hypoglycemia** is the most common metabolic derangement and is observed in 12-40% of infants with polycythemia.

  - **Hypocalcemia** is the next most common metabolic derangement and is found in 1-11% of neonates with polycythemia.
- Coagulation
  - Coagulation can be affected.
  - Thrombocytopenia may occur secondary to consumption with thrombosis.
  - Disseminated intravascular coagulation (DIC) is rare.

DIAGNOSIS

Method of Hematocrit Determination

The automated hematology analyzer gives a lower reading than values obtained on the same sample by centrifugation. This is due to inaccurate mean corpuscular volume (MCV) estimation because of poor neonatal RBC deformability. Therefore, in high risk cases hematocrit should be estimated by microcentrifugation method.

Methods of Blood Draw

Capillary hematocrit measurements are dependent upon regional blood flow and can vary widely from a central venous measurement.

A. Heel Stick Hematocrit

1. Hematocrits obtained from an unwarmed heel may not be reliable. Depending on perfusion to the heel, which varies greatly in the neonate, hematocrits from an unwarmed heel may be 5-20% higher than a central (venous) hematocrit.
2. A sample from a warmed heel (capillary blood) may more closely approximate a central venous hematocrit although it too is often higher than a central hematocrit.
3. A neonate may be screened with a heel stick sample but if the heel stick hematocrit is above 65% or the neonate is persistently symptomatic, a peripheral venous sample is recommended.

B. Venous Hematocrit (Central)

1. May be obtained from a peripheral venous sample.

2. If a central venous line or arterial line is already in place for other reasons, the hematocrit may be obtained from this site (after ensuring the sample is not diluted by the parenteral fluids running through the line).

Investigations

These have been shown in Table 16.1.

Table 16.1: Relevant investigations in polycythemia

Investigation	*Aim*
Central Hematocrit	Diagnostic
Blood Glucose	To exclude hypoglycaemia
Serum Calcium	To exclude hypocalcaemia
Serum Bilirubin	To treat early, if hyperbilirubinemia is present
Serum Sodium	For planning fluid therapy
Blood Urea Nitrogen	For planning fluid therapy
Urinary Specific Gravity	For planning fluid therapy
Arterial Blood Gas	For oxygenation and perfusion status
Platelet Count	To exclude DIC
X-ray Chest	To evaluate cardio-respiratory status
ECG	To evaluate myocardial function

Management

This has been summarized in Figure 16.2.

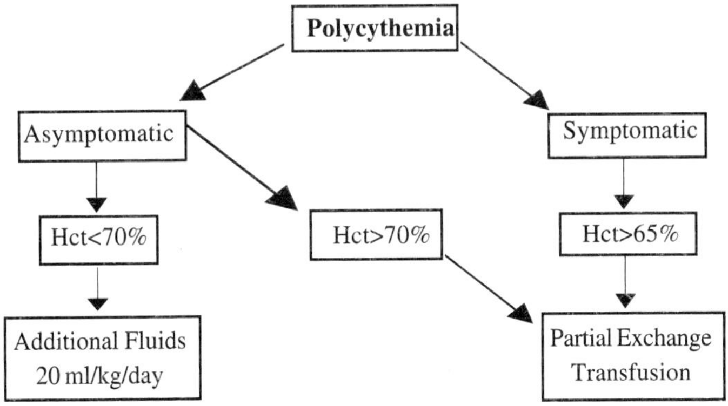

Fig. 16.2

- Therapy is based upon both the measured central hematocrit and the presence or absence of symptoms.[10]
- **Asymptomatic**
  - Hematocrit between 65-70%: Liberalise fluids (may increase fluid daily maintenance allowance by at least by 20ml/kg/day), follow hematocrits every 6 hours, and observe for symptoms.
  - Hematocrit greater than 70%: Partial exchange transfusion
- **Symptomatic**
  - Hematocrit between 60-65%: Consider alternative explanations for the symptoms. Although hyperviscosity may be the etiology of the symptoms, other causes for the symptoms need to be excluded.
  - Hematocrit greater than 65%: Partial exchange transfusion.
- **Partial exchange transfusion**
  - A partial exchange transfusion is performed, using either an umbilical arterial or venous catheter, in order to reduce the central hematocrit to 50-55%. The total blood volume that needs to be exchanged is determined using the following formula:

    (Blood volume) (Patient's hematocrit-desired hematocrit)/ (patient's hematocrit)

    Blood volume = (Patient's weight in kg) (90 cc/kg)

    Blood volume has an inverse relationship with birth weight and varies between 75 ml/kg for a baby with birth weight of 4.0 kgs to 110 ml/kg for baby weighing 1000 grams. Usually the volume exchanged is around 20 ml/kg. It is done in 3-5 ml/kg aliquots.
- Normal saline is the replacement fluid of choice for exchange transfusions, as it is effective and inexpensive. Alternatively plasmanate, 5% albumin or fresh frozen plasma and Haemaccel can be used.[11, 12] However, none of these are more effective than normal saline.[13,14]
- It is better to keep a lower desired hematocrit of 50% when crystalloids like normal saline or Ringer lactate are used for partial exchange transfusion so as to take care of possible rebound after 48 hours. Rebound is less significant when colloids are used for partial exchange transfusion. Partial exchange transfusion with Ringer solution may result in a

haemodilution comparable to partial exchange transfusion with serum.[15-18]

- Partial exchange transfusion requires sterile technique. There are two different ways in which an exchange transfusion can be performed, depending on the type of vascular access that is available:
  - If only a single umbilical arterial or venous catheter is in place, a push-pull technique should be used. With this technique, blood is alternately withdrawn and replacement fluid administered through the single catheter. No more than 5% of the patient's calculated blood volume should be removed in any single withdrawal.
  - If both an umbilical venous and arterial catheters are in place, then blood should be withdrawn from the arterial catheter while the replacement fluid is administered through the venous catheter. This is isovolumetric exchange and does not produce any hemodynamic disturbance. It is a desired method for any exchange transfusion in critically ill neonates.
    - ♦ The final option is to use an umbilical catheter (venous or arterial) for blood withdrawal, while a peripheral venous catheter is used simultaneously to provide a continuous infusion of the replacement fluid.
- Regardless of the method used, aliquots should not exceed approximately 5 mL/kg, delivered or removed over 2-3 minutes.
- The partial plasma exchange transfusion has a favourable effect for at least 24 hours on cerebral blood flow velocity in newborn infants with polycythemia.
- The increase in cardiac index demonstrates the acute hemodynamic benefits of partial exchange transfusion.

Monitoring and Follow-up

- Carefully monitor vital signs, bilirubin, glucose and electrolytes as needed.
- Feedings may be cautiously introduced only after some hours after completing the partial exchange transfusion so as to avoid development of NEC. Subsequently baby should be kept under long-term follow-up.

Complications

The complications of polycythemia include apnea, arrhythmia, vasospasm, air embolus, thrombosis, thrombocytopenia, hemolysis, hypoglycemia, hypocalcemia, intrahepatic hematoma and necrotizing enterocolitis.

Prognosis

- Infants are at increased risk for neurological deficits including speech abnormalities, fine motor delays and gross motor delays.
- There was no difference in developmental outcome of infants with neonatal polycythemia between the symptomatic and asymptomatic patients. No benefit of partial plasma exchange transfusion was noted in asymptomatic infants; only low birth weight and SGA infants were found to be risk factors for poor developmental outcome.[19]

Screening

The American Academy of Pediatrics does not recommend routine screening of hematocrits in the term neonates. However, high risk neonates like SGA, LGA, IDM, and twins should have at least one screening sample done at 6 hours from venous blood.

Medico-Legal Considerations

- Utilization of a blood product, such as albumin, in an exchange transfusion may result in transmission of infection. Blood product related infections can be avoided by use of normal saline, which is sterile, and has been shown to be as effective as albumin.
- Informed consent must be obtained as exchange transfusions have multiple risks.
- The question regarding the efficacy of partial exchange in improving neurological outcomes has not been answered. However, polycythemia and neurologic abnormalities have been linked. With this in mind, a symptomatic infant who has not been treated with partial exchange and subsequently develops neurologic abnormalities may be considered inadequately treated.

REFERENCES

1. Letsky EA: Polycythemia in the newborn, In: Textbook of Neonatology, 3rd edn., Eds Rennie JM, Roberton NRC, Chrchill Livingstone, London,1999; 834-38.
2. Oh W: Neonatal Polycythemia and hyperviscosity, Pediatr Clin North Am 1986;33:523-32.
3. Upadhyay A, Aggarwal R, Deorari AK, Paul VK: Polycythemia in the newborn, Indian J Pediatr 2002;69:79-82.
4. Henry E, Walker D, Wiedmeier SE, Christensen RD: Hematological abnormalities during the first week of life among neonates with Down syndrome: Data from a multihospital healthcare system, Am J Med Genet A 2007;143:42-50.
5. Hutton EK, Hassan ES: Late vs. early clamping of the umbilical cord in full-term neonates: Systematic review and meta-analysis of controlled trials, JAMA 2007;297:1241-52.
6. Lopriore E, Middeldorp JM, Oepkes D, Kanhai HH, Walther FJ, Vandenbussche FP: Twin anemia-polycythemia sequence in two monochorionic twin pairs without oligo-polyhydramnios sequence, Placenta 2007;28:47-51.
7. Narang A, Chaudhuri MK, Kumar P: Small for gestational age babies: Indian scene, Indian J Pediatr 1997;64:221-24.
8. Krishnan L, Rahim A: Neonatal Polycythemia, Indian J Pediatr 1997;64:541-46.
9. Drew JH, Guaran RL, Cichello M, Hobbs JB: Neonatal whole blood hyperviscosity: The important factor influencing later neurologic function is the viscosity and not the polycythemia, Clin Hemorheol Microcirc 1997;17:67-72.
10. Pappas A, Delaney-Black V: Differential diagnosis and management of polycythemia, Pediatr Clin North Am 2004;51:1063-86.
11. de Waal KA, Baerts W, Offringa M: Systematic review of the optimal fluid for dilutional exchange transfusion in neonatal Polycythemia, Arch Dis Child Fetal Neonatal Ed 2006;91:F7-10.
12. Dempsey EM, Barrington K: Crystalloid or colloid for partial exchange transfusion in neonatal polycythemia: A systematic review and meta-analysis, Acta Paediatr 2005;94:1650-55.
13. Acunas B, Celtik C, Vatansever U, Karasalihoglu S: Thrombocytopenia: An important indicator for the application of partial exchange transfusion in polycythemic newborn infants? Pediatr Int 2000;42:343-47.
14. Rothenberg T: Partial plasma exchange transfusion in polycythemic neonates, Arch Dis Child 2002;86:60-62.
15. Supapannachart S, Siripoonya P, Boonwattanasoontorn W, Kanjanavanit S: Neonatal polycythemia: Effects of partial exchange transfusion using fresh frozen plasma, Haemaccel and normal saline, J Med Assoc Thai 1999;82:S82-86.
16. Wong W, Fok TF, Lee CH, Ng PC, So KW, Ou Y, Cheung KL: Randomised controlled trial: Comparison of colloid or crystalloid for partial exchange

transfusion for treatment of neonatal Polycythemia, Arch Dis Child Fetal Neonatal Ed 1997;77:F115-18.

17. Deorari AK, Paul VK, Shreshta L, Singh M: Symptomatic neonatal Polycythemia: Comparison of partial exchange transfusion with saline versus plasma, Indian Pediatr 1995;32:1167-71.
18. Roithmaier A, Arlettaz R, Bauer K, Bucher HU, Krieger M, Duc G, Versmold HT: Randomized controlled trial of Ringer solution versus serum for partial exchange transfusion in neonatal Polycythemia, Eur J Pediatr 1995;154:53-56.
19. Dempsey EM, Barrington K: Short and long-term outcomes following partial exchange transfusion in the polycythaemic newborn: A systematic review, Arch Dis Child Fetal Neonatal Ed 2006;91:F2-6.

17

BLEEDING DISORDERS IN THE NEWBORN

Zubair H Aghai

COAGULATION DISORDERS

Coagulation disorders in neonates and infants can be congenital or acquired. Acquired coagulation disorders are more common in neonates than congenital. While congenital defects are seen in healthy infants, excessive bleeding in sick infants indicates acquired coagulation disorders. The results of common laboratory tests used to diagnose coagulation disorders in neonates should be interpreted with caution. Prothrombin time (PT) in full term and preterm infants are slightly higher than the normal adult range of 12-14 seconds. The **activated partial thromboplastin time (aPTT)** is much higher in premature (57±10.5 seconds) and full term infants (51±10 seconds) compared to adults (42±4 seconds).

CONGENITAL COAGULATION DISORDERS:

Infants with congenital coagulation disorders can present with prolonged **bleeding** after circumcision, oozing from venous or arterial puncture sites, bleeding from umbilicus, scalp hematomas (cephalhematoma, subgaleal hematoma) or intracranial **hemorrhage**.

Hemophilia A (factor VIII deficiency) and **Hemophilia B** (factor IX deficiency) are the most common congenital coagulation disorders. Both are X-linked recessive disorders and predominantly affect males. Only 15-33% of infants with hemophilia present with bleeding during infancy.[1,2] Hemophilia

A is 5-6 times more common than hemophilia B. Bleeding symptoms may be present from birth or occur *in utero* as neither factor VIII nor factor IX crosses the placenta.

Activated partial thromboplastin time (aPTT) is prolonged and prothrombin time (PT) is normal in both hemophilia A and B. The levels of factor VIII and IX are lower during the neonatal period and aPTT can be physiologically prolonged. Milder forms of hemophilia A and B are difficult to diagnose during the neonatal period. However, moderate and severe deficiencies can be reliably diagnosed by measuring the levels of factor VIII and IX.

Therapeutic options include **ε-aminocaproic acid** (Amicar) for limited oral bleeding in both factor VIII and IX deficiency, 1-deamino-8-D-arginine vasopressin (desmopressin or **DDAVP**) or **recombinant factor VIII** (20 U/kg) for mild to moderate bleeding in hemophilia A and **recombinant factor IX** (20 U/kg) for mild to moderate bleeding in hemophilia B. Higher doses of factor VIII (50 U/kg) and IX (80 U/kg) are required to control severe or life-threatening bleeding in hemophilia A and B, respectively. **Fresh frozen plasma (FFP)** can also be used in both disorders if recombinant factors are unavailable or diagnosis is uncertain. Cryoprecipitate can also be used to replace factor VIII in hemophilia A.

Hemophilia C (factor XI deficiency) is a milder form of congenital coagulation disorder, inherited as an autosomal recessive manner. Most of the neonates and infants with hemophilia C are asymptomatic but may manifest with prolonged bleeding after circumcision or surgery. Treatment includes FFP. Factor XII deficiency can cause prolonged aPTT without clinical signs or symptoms.

Factor XIII is responsible for the cross linking of fibrin and stabilization of fibrin clot. Factor XIII deficiency can cause mild bruising, prolonged bleeding from the circumcision wound, hemorrhage from the umbilical cord stump or intracranial hemorrhage. PT, aPTT and thrombin time are normal in infants with factor XIII deficiency. Factor XIII deficiency can be diagnosed by measuring its level in blood or instability of the infant's blood clot in 5M urea solution. Bleeding due to factor XIII deficiency can be controlled by infusing FFP, cryoprecipitate or factor XIII concentrates.

ACQUIRED COAGULATION DISORDERS

Prolonged bleeding in a sick infant is likely to be due to acquired coagulation disorders.

HEMORRHAGIC DISEASE OF THE NEWBORN

Vitamin K, a fat-soluble vitamin is required for the modification of coagulation factors II, VII, IX and X and anticoagulant proteins C and S. Hemorrhagic disease of the newborn (HDN) is a deficiency of vitamin K which results in the production of abnormal coagulation factors leading to uncontrolled bleeding.

Incidence

Approximately 2% of infants develop classical HDN if vitamin K is not given at birth.

Etiology

Several factors contribute to the deficiency of vitamin K in neonates.

a. The level of vitamin K is low in newborn infants as placental transfer of vitamin K is poor.
b. The normal gastrointestinal flora synthesizes Vitamin K. The gastrointestinal (GI) tract is sterile at birth and the colonization of vitamin K-producing bacterial flora occurs only after feeding is instituted.
c. Breast milk is a poor source of vitamin K.
d. Broad-spectrum antibodies can eliminate vitamin K-producing bacterial flora.

Clinical Features

Infants who are exclusively breastfed, those who are not fed orally or treated with broad-spectrum antibiotics are more likely to develop HDN.

HDN is classified into the following three types:

1. *Early onset HDN:* Seen in infants born to mothers treated with oral anticoagulant or anticonvulsants (interferes with vitamin K function). Infants are symptomatic within the first 24 hours of birth. Intracranial hemorrhage is common in early onset HDN.

2. *Classic HDN:* Seen in infants who did not receive vitamin K prophylaxis at birth. Manifests at 1-7 days of life with cutaneous, nasal, GI tract, circumcision wound and intracranial hemorrhage.
3. *Late Onset HDN:* Presents with bleeding after 7 days of age. Late onset HDN is associated with exclusive breastfeeding, broad-spectrum antibiotics, chronic diarrhea or diseases associated with fat malabsorption (biliary atresia, cystic fibrosis, neonatal hepatitis and α-1 antitrypsin deficiency).

Diagnosis

In vitamin K deficiency PT, aPTT is prolonged with normal fibrinogen and platelet counts. Treatment with vitamin K will improve bleeding symptoms and coagulation profiles within 24 hours. Measurement of specific factors (II, VII, IX and X), **protein induced by vitamin K absence (PIVKA)** and vitamin K levels may aid in confirming the diagnosis but are usually not required. Swallowed maternal blood (during delivery or from fissure in mother's nipples) can cause bloody stools on 2nd or 3rd day of life and may be confused with HDN or other bleeding disorders. An Apt test can be performed to differentiate maternal and fetal (alkaline resistant) origin of blood in the stool.

Treatment

Infants with HDN are treated with slow intravenous infusion of vitamin K1 (1 to 5mg). Intramuscular injection is avoided due to the risk of bleeding. FFP 10-20 ml/kg can be used for serious and life-threatening hemorrhage.

Prevention

HDN can be prevented by single IM vitamin K1 (1mg) given to all newborns immediately after birth. Oral vitamin K (2-3 mg) is effective in raising vitamin K levels, but not as effective in prevention of late onset HDN.[3-5] Infants treated with prolonged broad spectrum antibiotics, those on total parenteral nutrition (TPN) and those with chronic malabsorption should be treated with vitamin K. Mothers of infants at high risk of early onset HDN (mothers on anticonvulsants) should receive vitamin K before the delivery.[6]

HEPATIC DISEASE

Coagulation factors II, V, VII, IX and X are synthesized in the liver. **Hepatic dysfunction** can result in decreased production of coagulation factors and excessive bleeding. Vitamin K is converted into its active form by liver microsomes. Hepatic injury not only suppresses the activation of vitamin K, but also decreases its absorption due to cholestasis. Coagulopathy due to hepatic dysfunction can be managed with vitamin K supplementation, FFP and cryoprecipitate.

DISSEMINATED INTRAVASCULAR COAGULATION (DIC)

DIC is an acquired syndrome characterized by the intravascular activation of haemostatic system and generation of activated coagulation factors as well as accelerated fibronolysis. Infants with DIC may present with bleeding or thrombosis or both. Some infants may only have laboratory evidence of DIC. In neonates, DIC can be initiated by infection, hypoxia, acidosis, hemorrhage, tissue necrosis, or liver disease. Most cases of DIC in neonates are caused by cardiovascular collapse (cardiac arrest, profound hypotension or perinatal asphyxia). DIC is diagnosed by clinical findings consistent with DIC, thrombocytopenia, prolonged PT and aPTT, low levels of coagulation factors, protein C, protein S, AT III, fibrinogen and the presence of fibrin degradation product and D-dimers.

In infants with DIC, the most important therapeutic intervention is to treat the underlying cause. Supportive treatments include FFP and cryoprecipitate to replace clotting factors and platelet transfusion for thrombocytopenia. However, use of anti-coagulants and exchange transfusion are controversial in neonates.

The differences between the three common acquired coagulation disorders (HDN, hepatic disease and DIC) are described in Table 17.1. In infants with prolonged PT and aPTT, measurement of factor V and VIII can help in differentiating the three disorders. Factor V is synthesized in the liver but is not vitamin K-dependent. Factor VIII is neither synthesized in the liver nor vitamin K-dependent. Low levels of both factor V and VIII is seen in DIC. Factor V is low and factor VIII is normal in liver disease. Both factor V and VIII are normal in vitamin K deficiency.

Table 17.1: Differences between the three acquired bleeding disorders

	Vitamin K deficiency	*Liver disease*	*DIC*
aPTT	Prolonged/Normal	Prolonged	Prolonged
PT	Prolonged	Prolonged	Prolonged
Fibrinogen	Normal	Normal/Low	Prolonged
Platelet	Normal	Normal/Low	Low
D-dimer	Normal	Normal	Increased
Factor V	Normal	Low	Low
Factor VIII	Normal	Normal	Low

THROMBOCYTOPENIA

Definitions

Normal platelet counts in term and preterm newborn infants are in the range of 150,000 to 450,000/µL. Thrombocytopenia is defined as a platelet count of less than 150,000/µL. Some healthy newborns may have platelet counts between 100,000 and 150,000/µL without a clinical disease. Persistent or severe thrombocytopenia (platelet count <50,000/µL) in a neonate requires further evaluation.

Epidemiology

The incidence of thrombocytopenia in the general newborn population is less than 1%.[7, 8] In contrast, the incidence of thrombocytopenia in neonates admitted to the Neonatal Intensive Care Unit (NICU) may be as high as 22%.[9]

Etiology

The causes of thrombocytopenia can be classified as disorders of either increased platelet destruction or decreased production (Table 17.2). In certain disorders, a combination of two mechanisms may be seen (sepsis, necrotizing enterocolitis (NEC)). In neonates, thrombocytopenia due to increased platelet destruction is more common than decreased production.[9]

Clinical Features

History and physical examination is very important in the diagnosis and management of neonates with thrombocytopenia.

Table 17.2: Causes of thrombocytopenia

A. **Increased Platelet Destruction:**
   a. Neonatal alloimmune thrombocytopenia
   b. Autoimmune thrombocytopenia
   c. DIC
   d. NEC
   e. Infection
   f. Thrombosis (renal vein thrombosis)
   g. Kasabach-Merritt syndrome
   h. Hypersplenism
   i. Drug induced (heparin, penicillin)

B. **Decreased Platelet Production:**
   a. Thrombocytopenia absent radius (TAR) syndrome
   b. Chromosome abnormalities (Trisomies 13, 18 and 21, Turner syndrome)
   c. Wiskott-Aldrich syndrome
   d. Infiltrative disorders (leukemia, neuroblastoma, histiocytosis or storage diseases)
   e. Congenital infection
   f. Fanconi anemia (rare in neonates)
   g. Maternal Pre-eclampsia
   h. Drugs (anticonvulsant, sulfa)

C. **Both Decreased Production and Increased Destruction:**
   a. Congenital infections (TORCH)
   b. Sepsis
   c. NEC

D. **Uncertain Etiology:**
   a. Maternal Pre-eclampsia
   b. Birth asphyxia
   c. Hypothermia

A sick looking neonate with thrombocytopenia may have different etiology (sepsis, DIC and NEC) than the infant who looks healthy (maternal pre-eclampsia, iso and autoimmune thrombocytopenia). Some relevant history and examination details to be elicited in a case of neonatal thrombocytopenia have been enumerated in Table 17.3. Transient or little increase in platelet count after transfusion suggests increased destruction whereas sustained and significant increase in the count indicates decreased production.

Table 17.3: Relevant history and examination in neonatal thrombocytopenia

History/Exam finding	*Comments*
Family history	History of thrombocytopenia or intracranial bleed in a previous sibling suggests iso-immune or autoimmune thrombocytopenia. History of maternal thrombocytopenia suggests autoimmune thrombocytopenia. Family history of eczema, recurrent infection and thrombocytopenia in male relatives suggest Wiskott-Aldrich syndrome. History of maternal preeclampsia.
Small for gestational age	Suggestive of congenital infection
Hepatosplenomegaly	Suggestive of congenital infection, congenital leukemia or hypersplenism
Absent radius	TAR syndrome
Giant hemangioma	Kasabach-Merritt syndrome
Dysmorphism	Trisomies 13, 18 and 21, Turner syndrome
Microcephaly, Chorioretinitis, Cholestasis	Suggestive of congenital infection
Abdominal distension, bloody stool	NEC
Hematuria, abdominal mass, hypertension	Renal vein thrombosis

Thrombocytopenia is mild to moderate in autoimmune disorders and in neonates born to pre-eclamptic mothers whereas, it is moderate to severe in neonates with iso-immune thrombocytopenia, sepsis, DIC and NEC.

Diagnosis

Low platelets seen on capillary samples should be confirmed from venous or arterial samples. The presence of a blood clot in a sample can falsely decrease the platelet count. Thrombocytopenia diagnosed on an auto-counter should be confirmed by a manual count on peripheral smears. The initial investigation should include a complete blood count to evaluate for anemia and neutropenia as well as a maternal platelet count to rule out autoimmune thrombocytopenia. Platelet size is normal or smaller in disorders with decreased platelet synthesis but larger in size if thrombocytopenia is due to increased destruction.

Infants at risk for infection or appearing ill should be evaluated for sepsis. Consider coagulation studies (PT, aPTT, fibrinogen concentration, fibrin split products and D-dimers) in infants at risk for DIC. Depending upon the clinical presentation, evaluation for congenital infection or genetic testing may be indicated.

In healthy infants with moderate to severe thrombocytopenia an immune cause of thrombocytopenia should be considered (vide infra). If initial investigations are inconclusive and thrombocytopenia is due to decreased production, bone marrow studies can be performed.

Management

Treatment of the underlying cause is the mainstay of the management of thrombocytopenia in neonates and infants.

PLATELET TRANSFUSION

Infants should be transfused with platelets in severe thrombocytopenia or in the presence of clinical bleeding. A platelet transfusion should be performed if the platelet count is <20,000/µL in a full term infant.[10] In preterm infants or term infants who are unstable or have risk factors for hemorrhage, a transfusion should be administered if the platelet count is <50,000/µL. Platelet transfusion can be considered at a higher level if the infant is actively bleeding, in the presence of DIC or if the infant is receiving a drug that can cause platelet dysfunction (indomethacin or nitric oxide). Random donor platelets (10-15 ml/kg) of standard dilution will increase the platelet count by 50,000 to 100,000/µL. Volume reduction may cause platelet dysfunction. Consider using cytomegalovirus (CMV) negative and irradiated preparations. When considering platelet transfusion in infants with isoimmune thrombocytopenia, the platelets should be obtained from antigen-compatible donors. If this condition is anticipated, the mother's platelets can be collected prior to delivery and used for transfusion.

ISOIMMUNE (ALLOIMMUNE) THROMBOCYTOPENIA

Definitions

Isoimmune (alloimmune) thrombocytopenia occurs when fetal platelets (antigen positive) enter into maternal circulation and produce anti-platelet antibodies (IgG class). These antibodies then cross the placenta and destroy fetal platelets, resulting in fetal and neonatal thrombocytopenia. This condition is analogous to isoimmune hemolytic anemia (Rh hemolytic disease of the newborn).

Epidemiology

The incidence of isoimmune thrombocytopenia is approximately 1 in 1000 to 5000 births.[11] Unlike Rh hemolytic disease, isoimmune thrombocytopenia can develop in the first pregnancy.

Etiology

In isoimmune thromboctytopenia, fetus inherits human platelet antigen (HPA) from the father. Mother has no HPA on her platelets. HPA-1a is the most common antigen expressed on the platelets. Incompatibility for the HPA-5b is the next most common cause.

Clinical Features

Isolated low platelets at birth in otherwise healthy neonate suggest isoimmune thrombocytopenia. The degree of thrombocytopenia can be moderate to severe with platelets counts often lower than 10,000/μL. The neonate usually presents with mucocutaneous bleeding (petechiae, bruise). The infants are also at increased risk for intracranial hemorrhage.

Diagnosis

Isoimmune thrombocytopenia is often a clinical diagnosis. Isoimmune thrombocytopenia should be considered in healthy neonates with isolated thrombocytopenia. Platelet antigen typing (HPA-1a) of the mother, father and occasionally the newborn can be performed. Maternal or fetal serum can also be examined for antiplatelet antibody (anti-HPA-1a).

Management

Consider intravenous gamma-globulin (IVIG) (400 mg/kg per day for three to four days or 1 gm/kg per day for one to three days)[12,13] or methylprednisolone (2 mg/kg/day) or both. The risk of recurrence in subsequent pregnancy is very high (75-90%).[12] Thrombocytopenia is more severe in second or subsequent affected sibling. Prenatal management includes monitoring of fetal platelet counts, *in utero* platelet transfusion, and maternal IVIG and/or steroid therapy. Elective cesarean section at the time of fetal maturity is a safer mode of delivery for infants at risk.

AUTOIMMUNE THROMBOCYTOPENIA

Definition

Neonatal thrombocytopenia resulting from maternal immune thrombocytopenia. It is seen in infants with maternal idiopathic thrombocytopenic purpura (ITP), systemic lupus erythematosus (SLE) and other autoimmune disorders.

Epidemiology

Autoimmune thrombocytopenia is milder than isoimmune thrombocytopenia and only 3% of infants drop their platelet counts to less than 50,000 /μL.

Etiology

Maternal antibodies that react with both maternal and infant platelets mediate thrombocytopenia. Maternal antibodies cross the placenta and destroy fetal platelets, resulting in fetal and neonatal thrombocytopenia.

Clinical Features

Only 10% of infants with maternal ITP are thrombocytopenic. Infants are otherwise healthy. Neonates may present with petechiae, bruising or bleeding. The platelet count in the neonates usually falls after birth reaching the nadir at 2-5 days. The risk of thrombocytopenia in neonates correlates with the severity of ITP in the mother. The risk of thrombocytopenia is increased in neonates with history of maternal splenectomy, mother's platelet count < 50,000 /μL during the pregnancy or history of neonatal thrombocytopenia in previous siblings.

Diagnosis

Autoimmune thrombocytopenia should be considered in healthy infants with isolated thrombocytopenia whose mother is also thrombocytopenic. History of maternal ITP, SLE and other autoimmune disorder support the diagnosis.

Management

Consider IVIG and/or steroids in infants with platelet count lower than 40,000 to 50,000/μL. Antenatal monitoring and therapy is not justified in infants with autoimmune thrombocytopenia as the cord blood platelet count is rarely below 50,000/μL and intracranial bleeding is rare.

REFERENCES

1. Ljung R , Lindgren AC, Patrini P, *et al.*: Normal vaginal delivery is recommended for hemophilia carrier gravidae, Acta Paediatr 1994;83:609-611.
2. Chambost H , Gaboulaud V, Coatmelec B, *et al.*: What factors influence the age at diagnosis of hemophilia? Results of a French cohort study, J Pediatr 2002;141:548-552.
3. Sann L, Leclercq M, Guillaumont M, Trouyez R, Bethenod M, Bourgeay-Causse M: Serum vitamin K1 concentrations after oral administration of vitamin K1 in low birth weight infants. J Pediatr. 1985;107:608-611.
4. Hathaway WE, Isarangkura PB, Mahasandana C, Jacobson L, Pintadit P, Pung-Amritt P, Green GM: Comparison of oral and parenteral vitamin K prophylaxis for prevention of late hemorrhagic disease of the newborn, J Pediatr 1991;119:461-464.
5. von Kries R: Neonatal vitamin K, BMJ 1991;303:1083-1084.
6. Blayer WA, Skinner AL: Fetal neonatal hemorrhage after maternal anticonvulsant therapy, JAMA 1976;235:626.
7. Burrows, RF, Kelton, JG: Fetal thrombocytopenia and its relation to maternal thrombocytopenia, N Engl J Med 1993;329:1463.
8. Sainio, S, Jarvenpaa, AL, Renlund, M, Riikonen, S: Thrombocytopenia in term infants: A population-based study, Obstet Gynecol 2000; 95:441.
9. Castle, V, Andrew, M, Kelton, J, *et al.*: Frequency and mechanism of neonatal thrombocytopenia, J Pediatr 1986;108:749.
10. Calhoun, DA, Christensen, RD, Edstrom, CS, *et al.*: Consistent approaches to procedures nad practices in neonatal hematology, Clin Perinatol 2000; 27:733.

11. Bussel, JB, Zabusky, MR, Berkowitz, RL, *et al.*: Fetal alloimmune thrombocytopenia, N Engl J Med 1997; 337:22.
12. Ouwehand, WH, Smith, G, Ranasinghe, E: Management of severe alloimmune thrombocytopenia in the newborn, Arch Dis Child Fetal Neonatal Ed 2000; 82:F173.
13. Kaplan, C, Daffos, F, Forestier, F, *et al.*: Management of alloimmune thrombocytopenia: Antenatal diagnosis and in utero transfusion of maternal platelets, Blood 1988; 72:340.

18 NEONATAL HYPERBILIRUBINEMIA

Vineet Bhandari

DEFINITIONS

Clinical diagnosis of neonatal **jaundice** is usually obvious when the total serum bilirubin (TSB) is >5 mg/dl. The diagnosis of neonatal **hyperbilirubinemia** is based on a bilirubin nomogram in relation to postnatal age (in hours) and the percentile level, as defined for healthy infants (Figure 18.1).[1] It is important that such normative data be developed and validated for use in specific populations for local use.

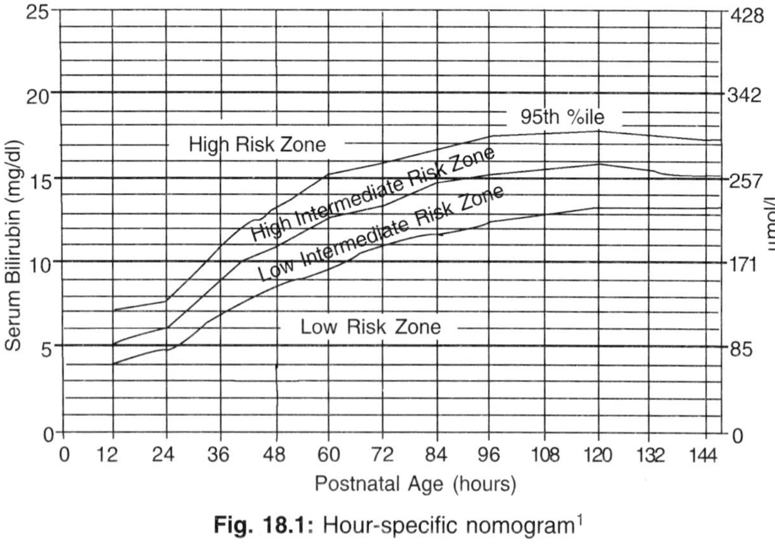

Fig. 18.1: Hour-specific nomogram[1]

Neonatal jaundice is classified into physiologic and pathologic jaundice. Physiologic jaundice is usually noted at postnatal day 2, peaks on days 3-5 and then decreases. Any jaundice in the first 24 hours of life is considered pathologic. In addition, TSB levels exceeding 95th percentile, as per the nomogram, are further subdivided into unconjugated and conjugated hyperbilirubinemia.

Epidemiology

In a hospital nursery in India, 8.92% of all live born babies had physiological jaundice.[2] The incidence of neonatal hyperbilirubinemia (>15 mg/dl; NNF India National Neonatal Perinatal Database Network 2002-03 report) was 3.3% for intramural deliveries and 22.1% for outborns. In very low birth weight (VLBW) neonates, the incidence of significant jaundice (requiring phototherapy and/or exchange transfusion) was 76.6%, with 37.3% requiring an exchange transfusion.[3]

Etiopathogenesis

Bilirubin is the final product of heme catabolism, derived mostly from hemoglobin. The hemoglobin in the red blood cells (RBCs) is broken down to heme and accounts for 75% of the source for bilirubin. Heme can also be derived from breakdown of other proteins such as myoglobin, cytochromes and nitric oxide synthases (25% of source of bilirubin). In the reticuloendothelial system, heme is further catabolized by heme oxygenase (rate-limiting step for bilirubin production) to biliverdin. This is acted upon by biliverdin reductase to form bilirubin. Bilirubin is then bound to serum albumin in the plasma and is transported to the liver. Bilirubin dissociates from albumin, and with the help of carrier proteins such as ligandins, is taken up into the hepatocytes. Bilirubin is then conjugated by the uridine diphosphoglucoronyl transferase (UDPGT) enzyme in the hepatocytes. Bilirubin glucuronide reaches the intestines via the gall bladder and common bile duct. In the intestines of the newborn, most of the bilirubin glucuronide is unconjugated by beta glucuronidase. Some of this unconjugated bilirubin is reabsorbed and gets into the enterohepatic circulation. The rest of the conjugated bilirubin reaches the colon, where the bacteria break it down to urobilinogen which is then excreted.

Unconjugated bilirubin is a cellular poison in the brain and is preferentially taken up by the basal ganglia, globus pallidus, putamen and caudate nuclei. It is said to disrupt the energy metabolism of the cells by affecting mitochondrial function.

The causes of physiologic and pathologic jaundice have been shown in Tables 18.1 and 18.2 (A and B) respectively.

Table 18.1: Causes of physiologic jaundice

A. **Increased bilirubin load secondary to**
   i. Increased red blood cell (RBC) volume
   ii. Decreased RBC life span
   iii. Increased enterohepatic circulation

B. **Decreased uptake by the liver**
   i. Decreased ligandins
   ii. Binding of ligandins to other anions

C. **Decreased conjugation in the liver**
   i. Decreased uridine diphosphoglucuronyl transferase (UDPGT) activity

D. **Decreased excretion into bile.**

Clinical Features

Some common risk factors for neonatal jaundice have been shown in Table 18.3. Initial visual assessment of the extent of dermal jaundice may provide a gross estimate of TSB (Table 18.4).

Some relevant history and examination details to be elicited in a case of neonatal jaundice have been enumerated in Table 18.5.

Diagnosis

The diagnostic approach focuses on confirmation of the visual appearance of jaundice with objective TSB measurements, differentiation of unconjugated and conjugated hyperbilirubinemia and finding out the specific etiology.

If a visual assessment suggests presence of neonatal jaundice, the following steps need to be followed. If age of the child is < 24 hours or transcutaneous bilirubin measurement is increased, TSB should be measured. If TSB > 12 mg/dl or >95th percentile for age (in hours), the Coombs' test should be done. If the **Coombs' test** is positive, mother's and infant's ABO and Rh blood groups

Table 18.2A: Causes of pathologic jaundice: Unconjugated hyperbilirubinemia

1. HEMOLYTIC ANEMIAS: These disorders result in increased destruction of RBCs, with resultant increased heme which gets converted to excess unconjugated bilirubin and the immature liver is unable to handle the excess load.
   - (i) Blood group incompatibility: Rh, ABO
   - (ii) RBC enzyme defects: Glucose-6-Phosphate Dehydrogenase (G6PD) deficiency; Pyruvate Kinase deficiency
   - (iii) RBC membrane defects: Hereditary spherocytosis; Infantile pyknocytosis
   - (iv) Thalassemia: Alpha; Delta-beta
   - (v) Drug induced: Vitamin K, Sulfonamides, Nitrofurantoin, Anti-malarials, Penicillin
   - (vi) Sepsis.
2. EXTRAVASATION OF BLOOD: These conditions lead to sequestration of blood in cavities with resultant increased bilirubin load. Examples include: Cephalhematoma, intracranial/pulmonary/gastrointestinal hemorrhage, large hemangiomas, excessive ecchymoses or petechiae.
3. POLYCYTHEMIA: Increased number of RBCs lead to increased production of bilirubin.
4. INCREASED ENTERO-HEPATIC CIRCULATION: These conditions lead to increased bilirubin due to delayed transit in the gastrointestinal tract. Examples include: Intestinal atresia/stenosis, Pyloric stenosis, Hirschprung's disease, Meconium ileus/plug syndrome.
5. DEFECTIVE CONJUGATION:
   - A. Congenital deficiencies of UDPGT enzyme include:
     - (i) Crigler-Najjar Syndrome Type I: Severe deficiency, Autosomal recessive.
     - (ii) Crigler-Najjar Syndrome Type II: Moderate deficiency.
     - (iii) Gilbert Syndrome: Mild deficiency, Autosomal dominant.
   - B. UDPGT enzyme inhibition:
     - (i) Drugs: Novobiocin
     - (ii) Lucey-Driscoll syndrome
6. METABOLIC CONDITIONS: Galacotosemia, Hypothyroidism, Tyrosinosis, Hypermethionemia, Maternal Diabetes.
7. BREAST MILK JAUNDICE.
8. DECREASED BINDING OF BILIRUBIN TO ALBUMIN: These factors increase the availability of the free (unconjugated) bilirubin to cross the blood-brain barrier. Examples include: Drugs (sulfonamides, penicillin, gentamicin); acidosis; asphyxia; free fatty acids; hypothermia; increased osmolality; hypoglycemia.

Table 18.2 B: Causes of pathologic jaundice: Conjugated hyperbilirubinemia (direct bilirubin >2.0 mg/dl)

1. HEPATOCELLULAR DISEASE:
   A. *Metabolic/Genetic Defects:* Examples include:
      (i) Alpha-1-antitrypsin deficiency
      (ii) Cystic fibrosis
      (iii) Zellweger's syndrome
      (iv) Dubin-Johnson syndrome
      (iv) Rotor syndrome
      (vi) Galactosemia.
   B. *Infection:* Examples include: Rubella, cytomegalovirus, herpes, syphilis, hepatitis A and B, toxoplasmosis, E. coli urinary tract infection.
   C. Total parenteral nutrition-associated.
   D. *Miscellaneous:* Examples include, neonatal hemochromatosis, idiopathic neonatal hepatitis, shock.
2. INTRAHEPATIC BILIARY DISEASE:
   (i) Alagille's syndrome (arteriohepatic dysplasia), Autosomal dominant.
   (ii) Inspissated bile syndrome.
3. EXTRAHEPATIC BILIARY DISEASE:
   (i) Biliary atresia
   (ii) Choledochal cyst
   (iii) Bile duct stenosis
   (iv) Cholelithiasis.

Table 18.3: Risk factors associated with neonatal hyperbilirubinemia
East-Asian race
Maternal diabetes
Maternal drugs: Oxytocin, sulfonamides, anti-malarials
Previous sibling with hyperbilirubinemia
Male gender
Low birth weight and decreasing gestational age
Decreased caloric intake and weight loss
Breastfeeding
Jaundice noted on the first postnatal day
Known blood group incompatibility (Coombs' positive) or other hemolytic disease
Extravasation of blood (cephalhematoma, bruising)

Table 18.4: Visual assessment of jaundice

Specific body site	*TSB (mg/dl)*
Face	4-8
Upper thorax	5-12
Lower thorax and thighs	8-16
Upper and lower extremities	11-18
Palms and soles	>15

Table 18.5: Relevant history and exam in neonatal jaundice

History/exam finding	*Comments*
Family history of jaundice	Along with anemia, splenectomy, early gall-bladder disease suggests hereditary hemolytic anemia or a metabolic/genetic etiology of jaundice. History of jaundice in a previous sibling suggests blood group incompatibility, breast milk jaundice or G6PD deficiency
Small for gestational age	Suggestive of congenital infection
Hepatosplenomegaly	Suggestive of hepatocellular disease
Microcephaly	Suggestive of congenital infection
Chorioretinitis	Suggestive of congenital infection
Plethora	Suggestive of polycythemia
Petechiae	Suggestive of congenital infection, sepsis
Clay colored stools	Suggestive of conjugated hyperbilirubinemia.

have to be checked. If no set-up, minor blood group antigens incompatibility (Kell, etc.) should be considered. If negative, direct bilirubin has to be checked.

If direct bilirubin is > 2 mg/dl, various causes of conjugated hyperbilirubinemia such as hepatocellular disease secondary to infections/metabolic or genetic causes, extrahepatic biliary diease need to be considered. Detailed guidelines for the evaluation of cholestatic jaundice in neonates are beyond the scope of this chapter, but are available.[4]

If direct bilirubin is < 2 mg/dl, causes of unconjugated hyperbilirubinemia (such as hemolytic anemias, extravasation of blood, causes of increased enterohepatic circulation or conjugation defects) should be checked. If hematocrit is >65%, polycythemia needs to be considered. This should be confirmed with a venous or arterial sample. If hematocrit is normal or decreased, reticulocyte count and peripheral smear are checked. If reticulocyte count is increased, causes of hemolytic anemia (blood group incompatibility, RBC enzyme deficiencies) have to be considered. If blood smear is abnormal, specific RBC membrane defects have to be looked for.

Investigations

These have been summarized in Table 18.6.

Table 18.6: Relevant investigations in neonatal jaundice

Name of test	*Result of test*	*Comments*
Transcutaneous bilirubinometer	"Physiologic" or increased levels	Needs confirmation by measurement of TSB if transcutaneous measurement value is >12 mg/dl.
End-tidal carbon monoxide	Normal or increased levels	An equimolar amount of carbon monoxide is produced for every molecule of bilirubin made from heme degradation. Can be detected via a breath analyzer. Increased levels need confirmation by TSB.
Total serum bilirubin	Increased TSB. Specific value as per age (hour)-specific nomogram	Gold standard test to confirm clinical impression. Collect blood and keep away from strong light sources; send for processing to the lab as soon as possible. TSB >12 mg/dl should be investigated further.
Direct serum bilirubin	Direct and/or indirect fractions are increased, depending on etiology	Gold standard test. Direct fraction > 2 mg/dl needs a focused work up for conjugated jaundice.

Contd.

Contd.

		Indirect bilirubin is the unconjugated fraction, derived by subtracting the direct bilirubin value from the TSB.
Hematocrit	Hemolytic anemia should be suspected if <45%. Polycythemia, if the value is >65%	Capillary samples usually suffice. Needs "central" (venous or arterial) to confirm polycythemia.
Complete blood cell count	High or low WBC or platelet counts	High or low (neutropenia) WBC count can suggest sepsis. Thrombocytopenia can suggest sepsis.
Reticulocyte count	Normal or increased	Increased counts are suggestive of hemolysis.
Peripheral blood smear	Normal or abnormal RBC shapes/size	Evidence of hemolysis. May aid in the diagnosis of hereditary spherocytosis.
Blood groups	ABO and Rh status	If mother is O and the neonate A or B, suggests ABO incompatibility. Rh negative mom with Rh positive neonate is suggestive of Rh incompatibility.
Direct Coombs test	Positive or negative	To diagnose ABO or Rh isoimmunization.
G6PD screening	Normal or decreased enzyme levels	Should be done after a couple of weeks to avoid false negative due to higher enzyme levels in younger RBCs in the circulation.
Osmotic fragility test	Positive or negative	Positive in hereditary spherocytosis.
Blood culture	Positive or negative	Gold standard. Positive in sepsis.
Liver function tests	Normal, increased or decreased	Decreased albumin levels may be helpful to evaluate bilirubin binding capacity and risk of bilirubin toxicity. Liver enzymes may be increased in congenital infections.

Contd.

Contd.

Urine for reducing substances	Present or absent	Present in galactosemia, if neonate is receiving galactose-containing feeds.
Urine culture	Positive or negative	Positive in urinary tract infection
Abdominal ultrasound	Normal or abnormal	Abnormal in specific cases of hepatocellular disease or obstructive causes of conjugated jaundice.
Percutaneous liver biopsy	Normal or abnormal	Abnormal in paucity of intrahepatic bile ducts, metabolic and storage disorders, infection.

Management

The main goal of treatment for unconjugated hyperbilirubinemia is to prevent bilirubin toxicity, specifically **bilirubin encephalopathy** and **kernicterus**. Specific treatment consists of providing **phototherapy** to decrease bilirubin levels. If the risk of kernicterus is considered high, an exchange transfusion is performed. Other and/or supportive management includes maintaining adequate hydration, albumin infusion (usually prior to exchange transfusion), and use of tin-mesoporphyrin.

Phototherapy: Phototherapy works by the use of light energy to cause photochemical reactions to transform bilirubin into isomers that are less lipohilic and more easily excretable and making breakdown products that do not require conjugation in the liver. Guidelines for initiation of phototherapy have been shown in Figure 18.2. The onset of action is immediate with the switching on of the phototherapy light. The most effective wavelengths are from 425-490 nm. Double-light phototherapy works better than single-light phototherapy.[5] Fibreoptic phototherapy is probably a safe alternative to conventional phototherapy in term infants with physiological jaundice.[6]

Special blue compact fluorescent lamp phototherapy had no superiority over special blue standard length tube lights phototherapy in terms of efficacy and adverse effects on the neonate and effects on nursing staff.[7]

Exchange Transfusion: Guidelines for doing an **exchange transfusion** have been shown in Figure 18.3. Continue

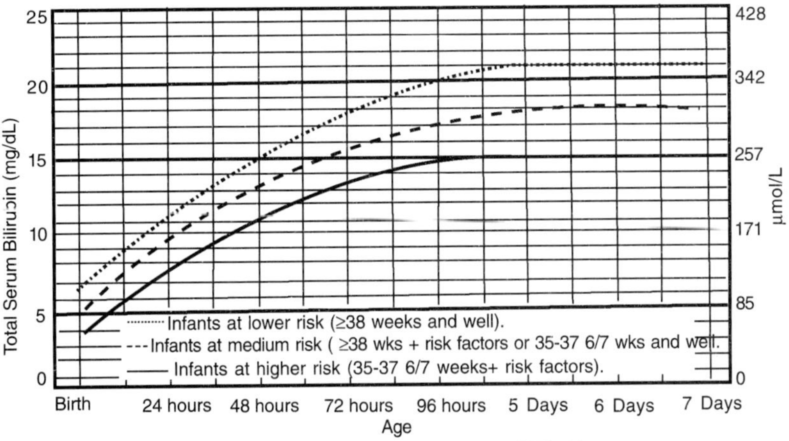

- Use total bilirubin. Do not subtract direct reacting or conjugated bilirubin.
- Risk factors = isoimmune hemolytic disease, G6PD deficiency, asphyxia, significant lethargy, temperature instability, sepsis, acidosis, or albumin < 3.0 g/dL (if measured).
- For well infants 35-37 6/7 weeks can adjust TSB levels for intervention around the medium risk line. It is an option to intervene at lower TSB levels for infants clsoer to 35 weeks and at higher TSB levels for those closer to 37 6/7 weeks.
- It is an option to provide conventional phototherapy in hospital or at home at TSB levels 2-3 mg/dL (35-50 mmol/L) below those shown but home phototherapy should not be used in any infant with risk factos.

Fig. 18.2: Guidelines for initiation of phototherapy[14]

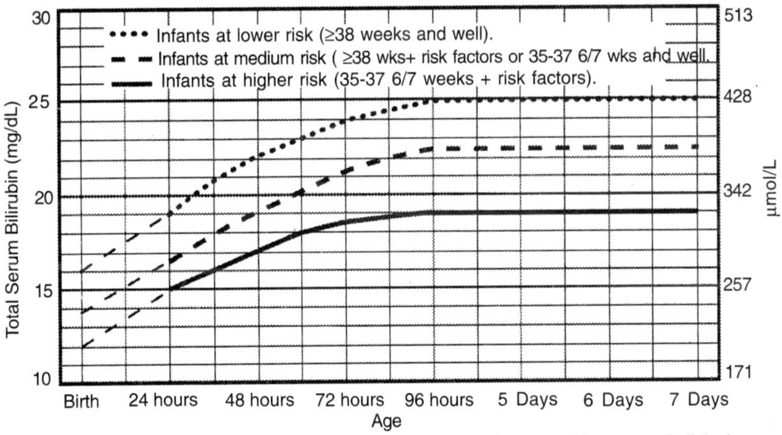

- The dashed lines for the first 24 hours indicate uncertainty due to a wide range of clinical circumstances and a range of responses to phototherapy.
- Immediate exchange transfusion is recommended if infant shows signs of acute bilirubin encephalopathy (hypertonia, arching, retrocollis, opisthotonos, fever, high pitched cry) or if TSB is ≥5 mg/dL (85 mmol/L) above these lines.
- Risk factos-isoimmune hemolytic disease, G6PD deficiency, asphyxia, significant lethargy, temeprature instability, sepsis, acidosis.
- Measure serum albumin and calculate B/A ratio (See legend).
- Use total bilirubin. Do not subtract direct reacing or conjugated bilirubin.
- If infant is well and 35-37 6/7 weeks (median risk) can individualize TSB levels for exchange based on actual gestational age.

Fig. 18.3: Guidelines for exchange transfusion[14]

phototherapy while waiting to start the procedure. The rationale is to remove the unconjugated bilirubin by doing a double-volume exchange transfusion, which should allow the bilirubin to move out of the brain tissue and hence, decrease the risk of neurological toxicity. An exchange transfusion will also remove antibodies responsible for hemolytic anemia. In severe cases of erythroblastosis and/or hydrops, it will correct anemia. Some recommend use of 5% albumin (0.5-1 g/kg; intravenous infusion; single dose) prior to the exchange transfusion in an attempt to bind unconjugated (free) bilirubin. Intravenous gamma globulin (500-1000 mg/kg, to be given slowly intravenously over at least 2 hours; can be repeated every 12 hours, if necessary, until TSB levels stabilize) has been shown to reduce the need for exchange transfusion in neonatal hyperbilirubinemia secondary to ABO and Rh hemolytic disease.

The recommended guidelines for initiating phototherapy and considering exchange transfusion for VLBW infants have been shown in Table 18.7.

Table 18.7: Guidelines for initiating phototherapy and considering exchange transfusion in VLBW infants[15]

Birth weight (grams)	*Initiate phototherapy: TSB (mg/dl)*	*Consider exchange transfusion: TSB (mg/dl)*
500-750 g	5-8	12-15
751-1000 g	6-10	>15
1001-1250 g	8-10	16-18
1251-1500 g	10-12	17-20

Phenobarbital: The mechanism of action is possible stimulation of hepatic UDPGT activity. The response to **phenobarbital** treatment differentiates Crigler-Najjar syndrome type I, in which there is no response (as there is complete absence of the UDPGT enzyme), from Crigler-Najjar syndrome type II. Initiation of this therapy usually results in a reduction of the bilirubin level of at least 20%, regardless of the initial TSB values. Best response noted with phenobarbital levels of at least 20 mg/dl. It has been found to be effective when given to mothers in the last weeks of pregnancy by reducing severe hyperbilirubinemia and need for exchange transfusion.[8] It has been found to decrease the duration of phototherapy.[9] However, it was not found effective in G6PD-deficient neonates.[10] The antenatal dose is 1g/day orally at bedtime for the last few weeks of pregnancy. The postnatal dose is 2-10 mg/kg/day, oral administration. It is recommended for use in populations with high risk of severe neonatal jaundice, or scarcity of resources for the management of neonatal jaundice with phototherapy and exchange transfusion.[11]

Tin-Mesoporphyrin (Stannosoporfin): It is a competitive inhibitor of heme oxygenase, the first and rate-limiting step in the metabolic pathway for the formation of bilirubin. It has been found to be effective in decreasing or eliminating the need for phototherapy as well as decreasing/preventing exchange transfusions.[12] The dose is 4 mg/kg birth weight, intramuscular, single dose.

Interruption of Breastfeeding: In breast-milk jaundice, interruption of breastfeeding for 48 hours does lead to a fall in TSB levels by 2-6 mg/dl. Resumption of breastfeeding after this period does lead to some increase in TSB levels, but usually not to very high levels. TSB monitoring still needs to be done.

The management of *conjugated hyperbilirubinemia* is dependent on its etiology. Babies with metabolic/genetic defects and clinical syndromes need a team approach to manage their varied clinical problems in addition to conjugated hyperbilirubinemia. Infants with conjugated hyperbilirubinemia secondary to infectious hepatitis need specific treatment, where available. Babies with extrahepatic biliary atresia need surgical treatment.

Ursodeoxycholic Acid: It is a hydrophobic bile acid that decreases the secretion of cholesterol from the liver and its intestinal absorption. It can be used (10-15 mg/kg/dose; oral administration; every 12 hours) in cholestatic jaundice associated with parenteral nutrition, biliary atresia and cystic fibrosis.

Complications

Side effects of phototherapy are generally mild and include insensible water loss, loose stools, skin rash and potential retinal damage. These can be prevented by maintaining adequate hydration and having the baby wear eye shields during phototherapy.

The major potential complications of exchange transfusion

include electrolyte disturbances, bleeding, infection, cardiac arrhythmias, thrombosis with embolization, necrotizing enterocolitis and graft versus host disease.

Phenobarbital can lead to somnolence. Tin-mesoporphyrin can cause mild, transient erythema in some treated babies.

Prognosis and Follow-up

Early bilirubin-induced neurologic toxicity can be detected by measuring brain stem auditory evoked responses. It is presumably due to specific entry of bilirubin into the neural cells of the auditory pathway. In jaundiced infants, there is absence or prolonged wave peak latencies and inter peak latencies.[13] Treated babies showed a tendency towards recovery in their auditory evoked responses.

If untreated, neonatal hyperbilirubinemia can result in *acute bilirubin encephalopathy*. The *initial phase* is characterized by lethargy, hypotonia and poor sucking with a high-pitched cry. In the *intermediate phase*, the infant is irritable, with variable tone and high-pitched cry. In the *advanced phase*, the infant goes into deep stupor to coma, with hypertonia (retrocollis and/or opisthotonus). *Kernicterus* is a clinico-pathologic entity characterized by yellow staining of specific parts of the brain (see above). The clinical manifestations of stage 1 are similar to initial and intermediate phases while stage 2 is similar to advanced phase of acute bilirubin encephalopathy. If the infant survives to stage 3, spasticity is somewhat decreased at around 1 week of age. Stage 4 incorporates the late sequelae–spasticity, athetosis, sensori-neural deafness, mild mental retardation, paralysis of upward gaze, and dental dysplasia. Stages 3 and 4 are also referred to as *chronic bilirubin encephalopathy*.

Neonates treated for unconjugated hyperbilirubinemia should be followed for monitoring of TSB and hematocrit levels, as appropriate. For the infants with hemolytic anemia (secondary to blood group incompatibility), polycythemia and extravasation of blood, monitoring for hematocrit levels are important to exclude late-onset anemia and any ongoing problems in normal bilirubin conjugation and excretion. Hearing and neurodevelopmental assessments should also be done, to check for any residual effects of bilirubin encephalopathy.

Surgical causes of increased enterohepatic circulation need follow-up with the pediatric surgeons to ensure proper excretion of bile is occurring. Babies with partial specific enzymatic conjugation defects need to have their TSB levels monitored periodically to ensure sustained high values do not occur. Neonates with conjugated hyperbilirubinemia need monitoring dictated by its etiology.

REFERENCES

1. Bhutani VK, Johnson L, Sivieri EM: Predictive ability of a predischarge hour-specific serum bilirubin for subsequent significant hyperbilirubinemia in healthy term and near-term newborns, Pediatrics 1999;103:6-14.
2. Basu K, Das PK, Bhattacharya R, Bhowmik PK: A new look on neonatal jaundice, J Indian Med Assoc 2002;100:556-560, 574.
3. Narang A, Kumar P, Kumar R: Neonatal jaundice in very low birth weight babies, Indian J Pediatr 2001;68:307-309.
4. Moyer V, Freese DK, Whitington PF, Olson AD, Brewer F, Colletti RB, Heyman MB: Guideline for the evaluation of cholestatic jaundice in infants: Recommendations of the North American Society for Pediatric Gastroenterology, Hepatology and Nutrition, J Pediatr Gastroenterol Nutr 2004;39:115-128.
5. Holtrop PC, Ruedisueli K, Maisels MJ: Double versus single phototherapy in low birth weight newborns, Pediatrics 1992;90:674-677.
6. Mills JF, Tudehope D: Fibreoptic phototherapy for neonatal jaundice, Cochrane Database Syst Rev 2001:CD002060.
7. Sarin M, Dutta S, Narang A: Randomized controlled trial of compact fluorescent lamp versus standard phototherapy for the treatment of neonatal hyperbilirubinemia, Indian Pediatr 2006;43:583-590.
8. Valaes T, Kipouros K, Petmezaki S, Solman M, Doxiadis SA: Effectiveness and safety of prenatal phenobarbital for the prevention of neonatal jaundice, Pediatr Res 1980;14:947-952.
9. Kumar R, Narang A, Kumar P, Garewal G: Phenobarbitone prophylaxis for neonatal jaundice in babies with birth weight 1000-1499 grams, Indian Pediatr 2002;39:945-951.
10. Murki S, Dutta S, Narang A, Sarkar U, Garewal G: A randomized, triple-blind, placebo-controlled trial of prophylactic oral phenobarbital to reduce the need for phototherapy in G6PD-deficient neonates, J Perinatol 2005;25:325-330.
11. Valaes TN, Harvey-Wilkes K: Pharmacologic approaches to the prevention and treatment of neonatal hyperbilirubinemia, Clin Perinatol 1990;17:245-273.
12. Drummond GS, Kappas A: Chemoprevention of severe neonatal hyperbilirubinemia, Semin Perinatol 2004;28:365-368.

13. Bhandari V, Narang A, Mann SB, Raghunathan M, Bhakoo ON: Brain stem electric response audiometry in neonates with hyperbilirubinemia, Indian J Pediatr 1993;60:409-413.
14. Subcommittee on Hyperbilirubinemia: Management of hyperbilirubinemia in the newborn infant 35 or more weeks of gestation, Pediatrics 2004;114:297-316.
15. Cashore WJ: Bilirubin and jaundice in the micropremie, Clin Perinatol 2000;27:171-179, vii.

19

PERINATAL ASPHYXIA

Pankaj B. Agrawal and
Muhammad Aslam

DEFINITION

Perinatal asphyxia is defined as a condition of impaired gas exchange during the first and second stages of labor with resultant hypoxemia and hypercarbia. Common synonyms include perinatal depression and **hypoxic-ischemic encephalopathy (HIE)**. The American Academy of Pediatrics (AAP) and American College of Obstetrics and Gynecology (ACOG) have published guidelines to define HIE. All of the following must be present for the designation of HIE:

1. Profound metabolic or mixed acidemia (pH <7.00) in an umbilical artery blood sample, if obtained.
2. Persistence of an Apgar score of 0-3 for longer than 5 minutes.
3. Neonatal neurologic sequelae (e.g. seizures, coma, hypotonia).
4. Multiple organ involvement (e.g. kidney, lungs, liver, heart, intestines).

INCIDENCE

Incidence of perinatal asphyxia is high in developing countries. The incidence is inversely related to gestational age and the birth weight. According to World Health Organization (WHO) approximately 1 million children worldwide die from birth asphyxia, and about the same number may survive with significant long-term neurological disability. It occurs in 0.5% of live born infants > 36 weeks gestational age and accounts for 20% of perinatal deaths. The disease is common in term infants but preterm infants can also suffer HIE with slightly different clinical manifestations. A higher incidence of HIE is seen in infants of diabetic mothers, term infants with maternal toxemia, infants with intrauterine growth restriction, breech presentation, and postdate infants.

ETIOLOGY

In term infants, 90% of asphyxial events occur during antepartum or intrapartum periods. A small number of events occur in the postpartum period secondary to pulmonary, cardiovascular or neurologic abnormalities.

Risk factors for perinatal asphyxia include maternal hypoxemia, decreased placental blood flow, impaired gas exchange at the level of placenta or fetal tissues, and increased fetal oxygen requirement. The major etiologic factors for perinatal asphyxia are summarized in Table 19.1.

Table 19.1: Etiologies of perinatal asphyxia
1. Maternal factors: Hypertension, Hypotension, Infections, Diabetes, Vascular diseases, Drug use, Shock.
2. Placental infarction, Fibrosis, Abruption or Hydrops.
3. Uterine rupture.
4. Umbilical cord prolapse, True knots or Compression.
5. Fetal factors: Anemia, Infection, Cardiomyopathy, Hydrops, Shock.
6. Neonatal factors: Cyanotic congenital heart disease, Shock.

PATHOPHYSIOLOGY

During normal course of labor, a number of events lead to decreased oxygen reserves in the baby. These include decreased placental blood flow from uterine contractions, maternal dehydration and alkalosis from hyperventilation, decreased oxygen delivery to the fetus, and increased oxygen utilization in the mother and the fetus. If a labor is complicated by hypoxia-ischemia the following changes may take place:

1. If the asphyxia is brief:
   a. Heart rate increases transiently and then decreases.
   b. Mild increase in blood pressure and central venous pressure.
   c. Redistribution of cardiac output to essential organs (brain, heart and adrenal glands).

2. If the asphyxia is prolonged:
   a. Loss of cerebral autoregulation and dependency on systemic blood pressure to maintain brain perfusion.
   b. Decrease in cardiac output leads to decrease in cerebral blood flow with resultant anaerobic metabolism and depletion of intracellular glucose, glycogen and adenosine triphosphate (ATP) and build up of lactate.

During the early phases of brain injury, brain temperature drops and local release of the neurotransmitters such as gamma-aminobutyric acid transaminase (GABA) increases. These changes reduce cerebral oxygen demand, transiently minimizing the impact of asphyxia. There is diminished ATP production due to decreased oxidative phosphorylation. This results in ion channel pumps failures with increased intracellular accumulation of sodium, chloride, water and calcium and extracellular potassium. If the insult continues, it results in an increase in excitatory neurotransmitters like glutamate and aspartate.

Failure of **oxidative phosphorylation** occurs in two phases: An initial primary phase lasting upto six hours and can be reversed with administration of oxygen and substrates (glucose), and a delayed secondary phase occurring 6-24 hours after the initial insult. The duration of the delayed phase is not known precisely in the human fetus and newborn but appears to increase over the first 24-48 hours and then start to resolve thereafter. Cell death is either immediate or delayed and apoptotic or necrotic. Immediate neuronal death is from intracellular edema due to osmotic load generated by intracellular sodium and chloride.

Delayed cell death is secondary to uncontrolled activation of catalytic enzymes. Reperfusion of ischemic areas results in the formation of oxygen free radicals (superoxide, hydrogen peroxide, hydroxyl, singleton oxygen) which further complicate neuronal injury. These free radicals can overwhelm the endogenous scavenger mechanisms resulting in damage to cellular lipids, proteins and nucleic acids. The already premature blood brain barrier suffers further damage as well. All these results in an influx of neutrophils that along with microglia release injurious cytokines (interleukin -1, tumor necrosis factor-alpha) causing further damage.

CLINICAL FEATURES

Clinical manifestations and course vary depending on severity of perinatal asphyxia. Common clinical scenarios include a post-term infant with asphyxia, meconium aspiration, pulmonary hypertension, pneumothorax or birth trauma.

Mild Perinatal Asphyxia

If the asphyxial event is short, the recovery is quick. There may be a slight increase in muscle tone and brisk deep tendon reflexes in first few days of life. Transient behavioral abnormalities, such as poor feeding, irritability, or excessive crying or sleepiness, may be observed. These findings become normal by 3-4 days of life.

Moderately Severe Perinatal Asphyxia

The infant is lethargic with significant hypotonia and diminished deep tendon reflexes. Neonatal reflexes like Moro, sucking and rooting are either sluggish or absent. Periods of apnea and seizures may occur within the first 24 hours of life. If appropriate care is given full recovery can occur within 1-2 weeks and long-term outcome is better.

Continued monitoring especially within first 2 weeks is essential as an initial period of well-being or mild asphyxia may be followed by sudden deterioration, suggesting ongoing brain cell dysfunction, injury and death. During this period, seizures intensity increases and neurologic examination findings worsen.

Severe Perinatal Asphyxia

The infant may not respond to any physical stimulus and may have irregular breathing requiring ventilator support. Generalized hypotonia and depressed deep tendon reflexes are common. Stupor or coma is typical. Neonatal reflexes (e.g., sucking, swallowing, grasping, Moro) are absent. Disturbances of ocular motion, such as a skewed deviation of the eyes, nystagmus, bobbing, and loss of "doll's eye" (i.e., conjugate) movements may be revealed by cranial nerve examination. Pupils may be dilated, fixed, or poorly reactive to light.

Seizures occur early and are often resistant to conventional treatments. The seizures are usually generalized, and their frequency may increase during the 24-48 hours after onset, correlating with the phase of reperfusion injury. As the injury progresses, seizures subside and the EEG becomes isoelectric or shows a burst suppression pattern. At that time, wakefulness may deteriorate further, and the fontanelle may bulge, suggesting increasing cerebral edema. Irregularities of heart rate and blood pressure are common during the period of reperfusion injury, as is death from cardiorespiratory failure.

Infants who Survive Severe HIE

The level of alertness improves by days 4-5 of life. Hypotonia and feeding difficulties persist, requiring tube feeding for weeks to months.

Involvement of Multiple Organs Besides the Brain is a Hallmark of HIE

Cardiac involvement in HIE may include reduced myocardial contractility, severe hypotension, passive cardiac dilatation, and tricuspid regurgitation. Severe pulmonary hypertension may be a manifestation of lung involvement requiring appropriate management including assisted ventilation. Renal failure presents as oliguria and, during recovery, as high-output tubular failure, leading to significant water and electrolyte imbalances. Intestinal injuries may not be apparent in the first few days of life. Poor peristalsis and delayed gastric emptying are common; necrotizing enterocolitis may also occur. Liver may be affected and present as elevated liver enzymes and coagulation disturbances.

The staging system proposed by Sarnat and Sarnat in 1976 is often useful in classifying the degree of encephalopathy. **Stages I, II and III** correlate with the descriptions of **mild, moderate, and severe encephalopathy** described above (Table 19.2).

DIAGNOSIS

Anticipation of HIE can prevent or decrease the incidence and severity of the disease. Assessment of perinatal risk factors should be performed routinely in all deliveries. Maternal, placental and fetal risk factors should be identified and appropriate actions taken as necessary. Ultrasonographic evaluation, biophysical profile, and non-stress test can provide valuable information on the placental

Table 19.2: Sarnat and Sarnat clinical stages of perinatal hypoxic ischemic brain injury[1]

	Stage 1	*Stage 2*	*Stage 3*
Level of Consciousness	Hyperalert	Lethargic or obtunded	Stuporous
Neuromuscular Control			
Muscle tone	Normal	Mild hypotonia	Flaccid
Posture	Mild distal flexion	Strong distal flexion	Intermittent decerebration
Stretch reflexes	Overactive	Overactive	Decreased or absent
Segmental myoclonus	Present	Present	Absent
Complex Reflexes			
Suck	Weak	Weak or absent	Absent
Moro	Strong; low threshold	Weak; incomplete; high threshold	Absent
Oculovestibular	Normal	Overactive	Weak or absent
Tonic neck	Slight	Strong	Absent
Autonomic Function	Generalized sympathetic	Generalized parasympathetic	Both systems depressed
Pupils	Mydriasis	Miosis	Variable; often unequal; poor light reflex
Heart Rate	Tachycardia	Bradycardia	Variable
Bronchial and Salivary Secretions	Sparse	Profuse	Variable
Gastrointestinal Motility	Normal or decreased	Increased; diarrhea	Variable
Seizures	None	Common; focal or multifocal	Uncommon (excluding decerebration)
Electroencephalogram Findings	Normal (awake)	Early: Low-voltage continuous delta and theta	

Contd.

Contd.

		Later: Periodic pattern (awake) Seizures: Focal 1- to 1-Hz spike-and-wave	Early: Periodic pattern with isopotential phases Later: Totally isopotential
Duration	<24 hours	2-14 days	Hours to weeks

and fetal status. In most cases the diagnosis is clinical, based on the typical risk factors and clinical features. Laboratory tests are useful in following the disease course.

Laboratory Evaluation

No specific laboratory test can always confirm or exclude a diagnosis of HIE and the results of the various tests should be interpreted in conjunction with the clinical history and the findings from physical examination.

A baseline complete blood count and frequent arterial blood gas monitoring is desirable in all cases. Blood glucose should be measured frequently to prevent hypoglycemia and progression to ischemic damage. In severe HIE cases, daily assessment of serum electrolytes are needed until the infant's status improves. Markedly low serum sodium, potassium, and chloride in the presence of reduced urine flow and excessive weight gain may indicate acute tubular damage or syndrome of inappropriate antidiuretic hormone (SIADH), particularly during the initial 2-3 days of life. Similar changes during recovery, with increased urine flow, might indicate ongoing tubular damage and excessive sodium loss relative to water loss. A full-scale hearing test is mandatory because of an increased incidence of deafness among infants with HIE that require assisted ventilation. Retinal and ophthalmic examination may be valuable, particularly as part of an evaluation for developmental abnormalities of the brain.

Specific laboratory tests to determine the effects of asphyxia include the following:

1. Cardiac troponin I (cTNI) and cardiac troponin T (cTNT) are specific cardiac proteins involved in calcium mediated cardiac contractility and are markers of myocardial damage. Normal

values in neonates are troponin I = 0-0.28 ± 0.42 μg/L and troponin T = 0-0.097 μg/L. Elevated levels of these proteins in infants correlate with the presence of asphyxia.

2. Elevated levels of serum creatine kinase cardiac fraction (CK-MB) of > 5-10% may indicate myocardial injury.
3. Elevated levels of serum creatine kinase brain fraction (CK-BB) are usually seen in the asphyxiated infants within 12 hours. This test is non-specific as the elevated levels do not correlate with long-term neurodevelopmental outcome and CK-BB is also found in placenta, lungs, gastrointestinal tract and kidneys.
4. Lumbar puncture to rule out intracranial infections.
5. Liver function should be monitored frequently to determine the hepatic damage and also to review the synthetic ability and coagulation profile.
6. Blood urea nitrogen (BUN) and creatinine elevations are typically seen 2-4 days after asphyxia. Renal failure may develop as well.

Imaging Studies

1. Cranial sonogram is less useful than other high resolution imaging studies. The advantages of ultrasound include easy availability, performed as portable at bedside and immediate answers regarding presence or absence of intracranial hemorrhage.
2. Computed tomography (CT) is useful in defining the extent of cerebral edema, especially when performed 2-4 days after the insult. It is also useful in the determination of subtle midline shift, superficial cortical or posterior fossa hemorrhage and ventricular compression.
3. Magnetic resonance imaging (MRI):
   a. Standard MRI may not detect hypoxic-ischemic changes during the first few days after the insult.
   b. T1- and T2-weighted MRI is considered the best modality for imaging of the neonatal brain. High signal on T2-weighted images indicate vasogenic edema.
   c. Diffusion-weighted images (DWI) can show abnormalities in the brain within hours of insult and can be used for prognostic purposes.
4. Magnetic resonance spectroscopy (MRS) measures the

concentrations of various metabolites within the brain substance. Elevated lactate level, high choline to total creatine ratio, and high N-acetylaspartate to total creatine ratio signifies hypoxic-ischemic insult to the brain.

5. Renal ultrasound to determine renal anatomy and structural damage.
6. Echocardiogram will determine the structure and function of the heart and evidence of pulmonary hypertension.

Electroencephalography (EEG)

EEG is used to define seizures as well as abnormal background neuronal activity such as burst suppression, continuous low voltage or isoelectric patterns. Amplitude integrated EEG (aEEG) can be used if expertise in neonatal EEG is not available. It is simple but less specific.

DIFFERENTIAL DIAGNOSIS

In most cases the diagnosis of perinatal asphyxia is obvious and further confirmed by laboratory and imaging tests. Differential diagnosis is limited and includes the following:

- Infections.
- Inherited metabolic disorders.
- Developmental defects.
- Brain tumors.

MANAGEMENT [2,3]

Management includes two broad categories of intervention:

- Supportive management.
- Therapeutic hypothermia.

SUPPORTIVE MANAGEMENT

1. Maintain Adequate Cardiorespiratory Status

Maintain adequate systemic arterial blood pressure as cerebral perfusion depends on it. Treat hypoxemia with supplemental oxygen and/or ventilation. Avoid hyperoxia as it may cause decreased cerebral blood flow and also exacerbate free radical injury. Maintain CO_2 in normal range, as hypercapnia is associated with cerebral acidosis and vasodilatation. This also results in steal phenomenon with increased flow to the injured areas and decreased flow to the normal areas.

2. Maintain Normal Metabolic Status

Maintain a tight control of blood glucose to avoid hypo- or hyperglycemia. Hyperglycemia can increase lactate level in the brain with damage to cellular integrity. Hypoglycemia on the other hand can potentiate excitotoxic amino acids induced injury. Hypocalcemia is common after HIE and can lead to compromised cardiac contractility and seizures. Maintain temperature in the normal range and avoid hyperthermia as it exacerbates HIE. Avoid fluid overload as volume retention is common after HIE. It can result from SIADH and oliguria secondary to acute tubular necrosis.

3. Control Seizures

Metabolic abnormalities of sodium, glucose and calcium should be corrected before starting anticonvulsants. Abrupt changes in heart rate, blood pressure and oxygenation may be a predictor for seizures.

- Phenobarbital is the initial drug of choice and is administered in a loading dose of 20 mg/kg IV. If the seizures continue, a second loading dose of 10-20 mg/kg IV can be given. Closely monitor the respiratory status as it can lead to severe respiratory depression. A maintenance dose of 3-5 mg/kg/day PO/IV divided BID is started 12-24 hours after the loading dose. Monitor the phenobarbital levels to keep in therapeutic range of 20-40 mg/dL.
- If the seizures are refractory to phenobarbital treatment with total loading dose of 40 mg/kg, phenytoin is considered. It is administered in a loading dose of 15-20 mg/kg IV followed by a maintenance dose of 4-8 mg/kg/day. Therapeutic serum levels are around 20 mg/dL. Phosphenytoin is used in many centers in place of phenytoin. In the body it is metabolized to phenytoin and the dose is calculated as phenytoin equivalents. Its advantages include less hypotension than the parent drug.
- Benzodiazepines are considered third line drugs and the agent

of choice is lorazepam given at a dose of 0.05-0.1 mg/kg/dose IV.

- Weaning of anticonvulsants should be started when there are no clinical and EEG seizures. In case of multi-drug regimen phenobarbital should be weaned last and tapered over several weeks.

THERAPEUTIC HYPOTHERMIA [4-7]

Initial evidence of the beneficial effects of therapeutic hypothermia in HIE neonates was noted by the CoolCap study where a pre-specified subgroup analysis found that head cooling was associated with improved outcome among infants with moderate, but not severe, EEG abnormalities. Subsequently, The Neonatal Research Network (NRN) trial of whole body cooling found that initiating the cooling within six hours of birth and continued for 72 hours reduced the risk of death or disability at follow up at mean age of 20 months.[8] Cooling was well tolerated and was not associated with any increase in death or serious adverse events. Since then, smaller studies have also suggested benefit for therapeutic hypothermia although not without mild to moderate systemic side effects. A small trial found that head cooling for 72 hours was associated with reduced incidence of moderate to severe cerebral edema on head CT at five to seven days of age compared with controls.

Whole body cooling is used as a modality of treatment for babies with HIE in our NICU at Children's Hospital Boston.[9] The inclusion criteria include: Gestational age=36 weeks and birth weight=2000g, and to be < 6 hours of age upon initiation of cooling.

Evidence of fetal distress as evidenced by at least two of the following:

a. History of acute perinatal event (e.g. placental abruption, cord prolapse, severe fetal HR abnormality, late decelerations).
b. Biophysical profile < 6/10 (or 4/8) within 6 hours of birth.
c. Cord pH ≤ 7.0 or base deficit = 16 mEq/L.

AND

Evidence of neonatal distress as evidenced by at least one of the following:

a. Apgar score ≤ 5 at 10 minutes.
b. Postnatal blood gas pH at < 1 hour=7.0 or base deficit ≥16 mEq/L.
c. Continued need for ventilation initiated at birth and continued for at least 10 minutes.

AND

Evidence of neonatal encephalopathy by physical examination as determined by neurology.

AND

Abnormal Cerebral Function Monitor (CFM), with minimum of 20 minutes recording, one of the following:

a. Severely abnormal: Upper margin <10μV.
b. Moderately abnormal: Upper margin >10μV and lower margin < 5μV.
c. Seizures identified by aEEG.

We use a cooling blanket and monitoring of the esophageal temperature via a probe. Total duration of cooling is 72 hours. Infant is placed on the cooling blanket and the target esophageal temperature goal during cooling is 33.5°C with acceptable range of 32.5-34.5° C. We record esophageal temperature hourly for 12 hours then every 4 hours for 72 hours. Record heart rate (anticipate bradycardia) and BP hourly for 12 hours and then every 4 hours for 72 hours. Check skin condition every 4 hours for areas of skin breakdown. At the end of 72 hours the infant is re-warmed no more than 0.5°C every 2 hours on the cooling unit. Once the infant has re-warmed to 36.5° C, cooling unit is stopped and the radiant warmer is turned on and infant returns to standard care. Avoid more rapid re-warming.

Safety Monitoring of Infants

During hypothermia and rewarming:

1. Monitor skin and esophageal temperature continuously and record every 15 minutes × 4 hours, hourly for the next 8 hours, and every 4 hours thereafter.
2. Monitor arterial blood gas at baseline, then at 4, 8, 12, 24 and 72 hours of age and more frequently if clinically indicated.

3. Monitor heart rate and blood pressure at baseline and then hourly for 12 hours and then every 4 hours for 72 hours.
4. Monitor glucose, serum electrolytes, serum calcium, blood urea nitrogen and creatinine, aspartate transaminase (AST) and alanine transaminase (ALT) at baseline and then at 24, 48 and 72 hours.
5. Monitor prothrombin time (PT), activated partial thromboplastin time (aPTT), international normalized ratio (INR), fibrinogen (Coagulation profile) and platelet count daily and as clinically indicated. Treat coagulopathy per routine, but keep platelet count above 100,000/microL as there is decreased platelet function while being cooled.
6. Draw complete blood count (CBC) and blood culture and start antibiotics (ampicillin and cefotaxime, avoid gentamicin due to concern for decreased renal function while being cooled). If the culture is negative and no risk factors and clinical features of sepsis identified, stop antibiotics at 72 hours.
7. Neurology consult at admission, cerebral function monitoring throughout 72 hours of cooling, 20 lead EEG, neurology examination at baseline and then daily for 72 hours, MRI within 24 hours or as clinically indicated and MRI at discharge or day of life 10, whichever comes first.

Management of Other Target Organ Injury

1. Cardiac dysfunction is common with HIE and can be managed with correction of hypoxemia, acidosis, hypoglycemia and avoidance of volume overload. Diuretics should be avoided due to concern for hypotension and concomitant renal impairment. Monitor mean systemic arterial pressure, central venous pressure and urine output. Consider inotropic agents like dopamine for blood pressure support as cerebral blood flow depends on adequate systemic blood pressure. To maintain adequate perfusion afterload reducing agents like milrinone can be used.
2. Renal dysfunction is monitored via measurement of urine output along with urinalysis, serum electrolytes and BUN and creatinine. If oliguria or anuria is present, give a normal saline bolus at 10-20 ml/kg as a volume challenge and if no improvement in urine output is seen, limit volume overload

by adjusting intake to insensible water losses plus urine output. May consider low dose dopamine infusion (<5 mcg/kg/min) for renal perfusion.

3. Avoid hypoglycemia and monitor glucose infusion rate. Avoid large changes in the infusion rate at one time. If renal failure necessitates volume restriction, use high concentration glucose infusion via a central line.
4. Hold enteral feedings until good bowel sounds are heard and stool is free of blood and reducing substances.
5. Monitor coagulation profile and blood counts. May need to correct anemia with packed red blood cell transfusions, thrombocytopenia with platelet transfusions and coagulopathy with cryoprecipitate and fresh frozen plasma.
6. Liver function should be monitored and drugs that are metabolized through the liver or are hepatotoxic should be avoided until liver function is normal.

OUTCOME IN PERINATAL ASPHYXIA [10-12]

Overall mortality rate is 10-30% and the frequency of neurodevelopmental sequelae in survivors is approximately 15-45%. The risk of cerebral palsy (CP) is 5-10% compared to 0.5% in general population. It is important to note that most CP is not related to perinatal asphyxia and most perinatal asphyxia does not cause CP. Only 3-13% of infants with CP have evidence of intrapartum asphyxia. Specific outcome depends on the level of encephalopathy, presence or absence of seizures, EEG results and neuroimaging findings. Stage 1 HIE has normal neurologic outcome in 98-100% infants with mortality of less than 1%. Stage 2 HIE results in abnormal neurologic outcome or death in 20-37% infants. Stage 3 HIE results in 50-90% mortality with severe neurodevelopmental sequelae in survivors. The presence of seizures increased CP risk by 50-70 fold. Mortality is high if seizures started in first 12 hours of life. Extreme burst suppression on EEG is a poor prognostic factor with mortality or neurologic sequelae in 85-100% of those infants. Normal DWI/MRI between 2-18 days is a good prognostic factor whereas abnormal DWI/MRI is associated with 60-80% risk of neurologic sequelae.

REFERENCES

1. Sarnat HB, Sarnat MS: Neonatal encephalopathy following fetal distress: A clinical and electroencphalographic study, Arch Neurol 1976; 33: 696-705.
2. Glass HC, Ferriero DM: Treatment of hypoxic-ischemic encephalopathy in newborns, Curr Treat Options Neurol 2007;9:414-23.
3. Chalak L, Kaiser J: Neonatal guideline hypoxic-ischemic encephalopathy (HIE), J Ark Med Soc 2007;104:87-89.
4. Barks JD: Current controversies in hypothermic neuroprotection, Semin Fetal Neonatal Med 2008;13:30-34.
5. Gluckman PD, Wyatt JS, Azzopardi D, *et al.*: Selective head cooling with mild systemic hypothermia after neonatal encephalopathy: Multicentre randomised trial, Lancet 2005;365:663-70.
6. Gunn AJ, Wyatt JS, Whitelaw A, *et al.*: Therapeutic hypothermia changes the prognostic value of clinical evaluation of neonatal encephalopathy, J Pediatr 2008;152:55-58.
7. Sarkar S, Barks JD, Donn SM: Should amplitude-integrated electroencephalography be used to identify infants suitable for hypothermic neuroprotection? J Perinatol 2008;28:117-22.
8. Shankaran S, Laptook AR, Ehrenkranz RA, *et al.*: Whole-body hypothermia for neonates with hypoxic-ischemic encephalopathy, N Engl J Med 2005;353:1574-84.
9. Manual for Therapeutic Hypothermia Protocol, Neonatal ICU Practice Guidelines, Children's Hospital Boston.
10. Abend NS, Licht DJ: Predicting outcome in children with hypoxic ischemic encephalopathy, Pediatr Crit Care Med 2007;8:1-8.
11. Ambalavanan N, Carlo WA, Shankaran S, *et al.*: Predicting outcomes of neonates diagnosed with hypoxemic-ischemic encephalopathy, Pediatrics 2006;118:2084-93.
12. Spitzmiller RE, Phillips T, Meinzen-Derr J, *et al.*: Amplitude-integrated EEG is useful in predicting neurodevelopmental outcome in full-term infants with hypoxic-ischemic encephalopathy: A meta-analysis, J Child Neurol 2007;22:1069-78.

20 NEONATAL SEIZURES

Vasanth H. Kumar

EPIDEMIOLOGY

Seizures are common in the newborn period than at any other time period. Seizures are common in the first day of life and about 70% are noted by day 4 of life. Neonatal seizures occur in the first 28 days in term infants or 44 weeks corrected age in preterm infants with a reported incidence of 2-3 per 1000 live births. The incidence of seizures is higher in preterm and very low birth weight infants compared to term infants. Majority of seizures in term infants have an underlying cerebral or biochemical abnormality. Prognosis of neonatal seizures depends on the etiology, neurological exam and electro encephalogram (EEG) results.[1] Seizure manifestations differ in the newborn compared to older children and adults. The neonate's susceptibility to seizures is partly explained by the excess of excitatory glutamate synaptic activity and delayed maturation of neuron-inhibitory system favoring neuro-excitation. Lack of myelin in the neonatal brain prevents conduction of epileptic activity throughout the brain in a generalized fashion.

CLINICAL CLASSIFICATION [2]

Neonatal seizures are generally brief and subtle in clinical appearance making it difficult for the clinician to make an accurate diagnosis. Certain behaviors of the neonate may be influenced by prematurity, intercurrent illness or state-specific behaviors.

Therefore, confirmation of the clinically suspected seizure is strongly recommended by a coincident EEG recording. Random suspicious clinical activity which may be missed by routine EEG recordings, are more likely to be captured by continuous video EEG recordings done over a longer time frame. Subtle seizures are the most common type of neonatal seizures followed by clonic seizures.

Subtle Seizures

They are the most commonly observed category of neonatal seizures. They occur with a relatively higher frequency in premature infants compared to term infants. This includes ocular phenomena such as staring, blinking, eye deviation and eye opening; oral phenomena such as mouthing, chewing, sucking and smiling; autonomic phenomena such as blood pressures and/or heart rate changes, pallor, increased secretions or central apnea and fragmentary body movements such as limb posturing, swimming or pedaling movements. Normal motor behaviors suggestive of subtle seizures are also noted commonly in premature and encephalopathic infants. These behaviors are less stereotyped, suppressed by restraints and triggered by stimulation. Subtle seizures are clinically difficult to confirm and a routine EEG misses them most often. A continuous video EEG recording best captures them, which demonstrate rhythmic epileptiform activity in a majority of subtle seizures.

Clonic Seizures

Involves rhythmic movements of a group of muscle in a focal distribution. They may be unifocal or multifocal involving face, trunk or limbs. EEG may be focally or diffusely abnormal. Sometimes jitteriness may be confused for clonic seizures. Jitteriness is symmetric tremors of equal amplitude, which are provoked by stimulus and aborted by restraining the limbs. Jitteriness is neither associated with abnormal eye movements nor autonomic changes that are seen in a seizure. They are seen in normal infants but may be associated with biochemical or neurological abnormality. Jitteriness per se does not cause any abnormality in an EEG.

Myoclonic Seizures

Myoclonic jerks may be focal, multifocal or generalized in origin.

Unlike clonic seizures, they involve a relatively more rapid movement of muscle groups with a predilection to flexor muscle groups. Generalized and mixed seizure types are associated with EEG seizure discharges and may persist into infancy.

Tonic Seizures

They are the least common form of neonatal seizures. They involve tonic posturing of limbs and/or trunk or eyes. These seizures may be associated with apnea, cyanosis and abnormal EEG background. Ictal discharges in EEG are common. Symmetric tonic postures are rarely true seizures. Most of them represent decerebrate or decorticate postures with EEG background being severely abnormal with poor outcome.

ETIOLOGY

Table 20.1 summarizes the causes of neonatal seizures. Among the many causes of neonatal seizures, only a few of them account for a majority of neonatal seizures. These include hypoxic-ischemic encephalopathy, intracranial hemorrhage and biochemical abnormalities such as hypoglycemia and hypocalcemia.

Table 20.1: Selected etiology of neonatal seizures

I. CNS
- Hypoxic-ischemic encephalopathy
- Intracranial hemorrhage
  - Subarachnoid hemorrhage
  - Subdural / Epidural hemorrhage
  - Intraventricular hemorrhage
- Cerebrovascular Accidents
  - Cerebral Infarction – Arterial thrombosis/occlusion
  - Cerebral vein thrombosis
- Infection
  - Bacterial meningitis
  - Viral encephalitis – herpes
  - Congenital infections

II. Biochemical
- Hypoglycemia
- Hypocalcemia

Contd.

Contd.

- Hypomagnesemia
- Hyponatremia
- Hypernatremia

III. Inborn Errors of Metabolism
- Amino acid disorders (maple syrup urine disease, phenylketonuria, isovaleric acidemia)
- Urea cycle disorders
- Non-ketotic hyperglycinemia
- Pyridoxine dependency
- Peroxisomal/mitochondrial disorders

IV. Developmental Defects
- Cerebral dysgenesis
- Cerebral malformations
- Neuro-cutaneous/Epileptic syndromes

V. Drugs
- Narcotic withdrawal (heroin/morphine/methadone/cocaine)
- Theophylline, propylene glycol, local anesthetics

VI. Miscellaneous
- Polycythemia
- Genetic syndromes

DIAGNOSIS

Every infant with seizures does not need an extensive work up to arrive at a diagnosis. Diagnostic evaluation must begin with a careful history and physical examination. Table 20.2 summarizes the diagnostic workup for neonatal seizures. Any infant with suspected seizure activity should get a bedside blood glucose test and also have a serum specimen sent to the lab for estimation of blood glucose. Initial work up should also include serum

Table 20.2: Diagnostic workup for neonatal seizures

I. Complete blood count (CBC), Blood cultures, CSF analysis–Bacterial / herpes.
II. Serum electrolytes including sodium, calcium, magnesium, potassium and phosphorus levels; serum glucose.
III. Urine/meconium toxicology.
IV. Head imaging studies such as cranial ultrasound, Head CT or MRI.
V. EEG – routine/Video EEG.
VI. Workup for metabolic disorders.

electrolytes and calcium. Blood should be sent for complete blood count for any evidence of infection. If infection is suspected then we need a blood culture and lumbar puncture to rule out bacterial meningitis. Hypoglycemia and infection are two of the important causes that need to be recognized and treated promptly. Suspicion of herpes infection should be confirmed by sending surface cultures for herpes virus and cerebrospinal fluid (CSF) for culture or polymerase chain reaction (PCR), whichever is available. Infant should be started on acyclovir pending herpes cultures. Imaging studies of the head will provide vital information regarding the gross central nervous system (CNS) pathology leading to neonatal seizures. It is better to start with head ultrasound in preterm infants and a computed tomography (CT), with or without contrast, in term infants. For cerebrovascular lesions, evolving lesions and for a better anatomic delineation of any CNS pathology, magnetic resonance imaging (MRI) of the head is most useful. Serum ammonia, lactate and pyruvate should be sent in infants with metabolic acidosis. Presence of dysmorphic features should alert one to the possibility of genetic syndromes.

EEG is an important tool in the diagnosis of suspected seizures. Most often it is done to confirm a clinically suspected seizures or to define interictal background abnormalities. A random half or an hour EEG is often not accompanied by clinical seizures. Video EEG or polysomnographic recordings can help in distinguishing epileptic from non-epileptic events. It is important to bear in mind that more than half of electrographic seizures are not accompanied by clinical seizures, more so in premature infants. Hence it is important to have a high degree of suspicion for any seizure activity in the newborn. There is an association between the amount of electrographic seizure activity and subsequent morbidity and mortality in at risk infants in general and in infants with perinatal asphyxia in particular. The major EEG correlates of neonatal seizures include focal or multifocal spikes or sharp waves or both and focal monorhythmic discharges. These ictal discharges occur on a background EEG activity, which is important for determining outcome. The background activity may be normal or abnormal. The severity of background abnormalities may vary from mild (voltage asymmetry) to severe (markedly low voltage, electrocerebral silence or burst suppression pattern).

PYRIDOXINE DEPENDENCY

This is a rare defect in pyridoxine metabolism causing severe seizures refractory to all therapy. It may begin *in utero* (hiccups) or as clonic seizures soon after birth. EEG is non-specific with burst suppression pattern or other generalized epileptiform activity. Diagnosis is established by demonstrating normalization of EEG (within minutes to hours) following 100 mg of pyridoxine intravenously (IV). Any suspicion of the disorder should lead to a therapeutic trial with pyridoxine.

Some of the benign seizure syndromes occurring in the neonatal period are summarized in Table 20.3.

Table 20.3: Benign seizure syndromes in the newborn

I. Benign Neonatal Sleep Myoclonus
- Not a seizure.
- Myoclonic movements occur only in sleep [non-rapid eye movement (REM) sleep].
- Not accompanied with any EEG abnormalities.
- Gets worse with restraint.
- Occurs in healthy infants and resolve in 2-3 months.
- Neurological outcome–Normal.

II. Benign Familial Neonatal Seizures
- Seizures are noted on the 2nd or the 3rd postnatal day.
- Resolves by 2-6 months of age with normal neurological development.
- Autosomal dominant inheritance.
- Defect in the voltage gated potassium channel.

III. Benign Idiopathic Neonatal Seizures

"Fifth day fits".
- 90% by day 4-6 of life.
- Multifocal, clonic, apneas.
- Normal healthy appearing infant.
- EEG is abnormal.
- Diagnosis of exclusion.
- Usually resolve within days.
- ?risk of minor neurological impairment.

MANAGEMENT [3]

Infant with seizures should be treated with anticonvulsants to prevent the potential effects of seizures on ventilation, circulation and brain metabolism. It is important to remember that treatment of clinical seizures does not guarantee elimination of electrographic seizures. Follow-up EEGs following treatment with anticonvulsants is necessary to ensure that seizures are adequately controlled. Hypoglycemia should be ruled out in any neonate with suspected seizure and should be treated promptly. In the absence of hypoglycemia, seizure should be controlled by anticonvulsants. Table 20.4 summarizes the management of neonatal seizures. Monitoring of plasma drug levels is essential for appropriate management of neonatal seizures more so following multiple loading doses, use of more than one anticonvulsant or recurring seizures. Most commonly used anticonvulsants include phenobarbital and phenytoin. In one study midazolam rapidly controlled electrographic seizures in all infants not responding to phenobarbital or phenytoin and correlated with significantly improved long-term neurodevelopment.[4]

It is important to establish normal electrolytes, calcium and magnesium levels prior to aggressive use of anticonvulsants. Routine use of calcium or magnesium in the treatment of neonatal seizure is not advisable. It is important to document hypocalcemia or hypomagnesemia as the cause of seizure, unless it is not practical to do these labs on an urgent basis. Any suspicion of pyridoxine dependency should lead to therapeutic trial of pyridoxine IV, if the infant is convulsing and has an abnormal EEG or oral (100 mg or more for several days) if seizures are intermittent. It may be difficult to differentiate pyridoxine deficiency from dependency. Both these disorders need to be treated with high doses for two weeks followed by a trial of withdrawal at 6 months of age.

Duration of therapy of the infant with seizures in the newborn period relates principally to the likelihood of recurrence of seizures if the drugs are discontinued. The risk of epilepsy in survivors varies from 10–30%. Discontinuation of anticonvulsant therapy (ACT) depends on infant's neurological exam, cause of neonatal seizure and the EEG. If the neurological exam is normal in the newborn period prior to discharge, then discontinue ACT. Similarly it is safe to discontinue anticonvulsants in the absence of seizure activity on EEG prior to discharge. Some infants may need to be discharged home on anticonvulsants secondary to abnormal neurological exam and/or abnormal EEG. Infants discharged home

Table 20.4: General management principles and acute therapy of neonatal seizure

1. Optimize ventilation, blood pressures; serum electrolytes and pH; intravenous access/fluids; treat infection.
2. Hypoglycemia-Glucose 10% solution–2 mL/kg IV followed by continuous infusion of glucose at 6-8 mg/kg/min.
3. Anticonvulsant Therapy.
   I. Phenobarbital – 20 mg/kg over 10-15 minutes; If no response repeat 5-10 mg/kg for a total of 40 mg/kg loading dose (LD); Maintenance dose (MD) – 3-5 mg/kg/day; Serum levels–15 to 40 µg/mL. Sedation occurs at serum levels of > 40 µg/mL and respiratory depression at levels > 60 µg/mL.
   II. Phenytoin-fosphenytoin–20 mg/kg LD; MD–4 to 8 mg/kg/day; Infuse at 0.5 – 1mg/kg/min; Serum levels–10 to 20 µg/mL. Phenytoin is highly unstable in any IV solution; Fosphenytoin – same dose as phenytoin; High water solubility; Ease of preparation; pH closer to neutral; Safe IM injection; No tissue injury with IV infiltration. Monitor for bradycardia, arrhythmias and hypotension during infusion.
   III. Lorazepam–0.05 – 0.1mg/kg over 2-5 minutes IV; repeat doses based on clinical response.
   IV. Midazolam– 0.05 – 0.2 mg/kg/dose IV over 5 minutes. Repeat Q2–Q4. May be given intramuscularly (IM). Serum concentrations increased by erythromycin/effects antagonized by theophylline/effects reversed by flumazenil. Can be used as an infusion for status – 1 to 10 µg/kg/min. Monitor blood pressure and respiratory status closely especially when concurrently used with narcotics.
   V. Lidocaine – 2 mg/kg IV over 10 minutes, followed immediately by maintenance of 6 mg/kg/hour. Begin to taper after 12-24 hours, as drug accumulation will occur. Used in treatment of severe recurrent or prolonged seizure that does not respond to first line therapies. Do not use concurrently with phenytoin. Stop infusion immediately if significant cardiac arrhythmia occurs.
   VI. Diazepam – 0.1-0.3 mg/kg IV; *Not recommended in neonatal period* as it is a poor drug for maintenance and contains sodium benzoate which may interfere with binding of bilirubin to albumin. Acts synergistically with phenobarbital to cause respiratory arrest.
4. Other therapies (as indicated)
   I. Calcium Gluconate–2 mL/kg of 10% calcium gluconate diluted in equal volume of water; injected slowly over 5-10 minutes with heart rate monitoring.
   II. Magnesium Sulfate–0.2 mL/kg of 50% magnesium sulfate, once daily.
   III. Pyridoxine – 50 to 100 mg IV under EEG control.

on anticonvulsants need to be on only one medication such as phenobarbital. Phenobarbital can be discontinued at follow-up as and when the infant has a normal neurological exam or has a normal EEG. Recurrent seizures, severely abnormal neurological exam or an abnormal EEG favor continued treatment with anticonvulsants.

PROGNOSIS [5]

The prognosis for infants with seizures has improved over the past two decades secondary to improvements in obstetric and neonatal intensive care. Mental retardation and motor deficits are more common than seizures as sequelae from a perinatal neurological insult. Overall outcome of seizures varies as a function of gestational age. The most premature infants with the most serious, life threatening illness have poorer outcomes. In one study variables associated with poor prognosis were Sarnat III or equivalent severe encephalopathy, cerebral dysgenesis, complicated intraventricular hemorrhage, infection in preterm infants, abnormal neonatal EEG and the need for multiple drugs to treat neonatal seizures. Poor prognosis for premature infants with seizures is reflected in high rates of subsequent long-term disability and mortality. *The severity and timing of the pathological process and EEG characteristics are the major determinants of neurodevelopmental outcome in infants with neonatal seizures.* The interictal EEG is of value in establishing prognosis of infants with seizures. Thus when the EEG correlates of seizures occur on a background that is normal, neurological sequelae are unusual. Severe background abnormalities e.g., burst suppression pattern, marked voltage suppression and electrocerebral silence are associated with neurological sequelae in more than 90% of infants. Moderate abnormalities, which account for 15 to 30% abnormalities, are associated with neurological sequelae in about 50% of infants.

About half of the infants with hypoxic encephalopathy and seizures have normal development. 50% of neonates with bacterial meningitis, early onset hypocalcemia and hypoglycemia have normal development. Newborns with primary subarachnoid hemorrhage and late onset hypocalcemia have good prognosis. In infant with developmental disorders, the severity and the type of disorder influence outcome. All infants with neonatal seizures need to be followed up regularly from a neurological and developmental standpoint, as this would ensure early intervention and appropriate services for optimal growth and development.

REFERENCES

1. McBride MC, Laroia N and Guillet R: Electrographic seizures in neonates correlates with poor neurodevelopmental outcome, Neurology 2000;55:506-514.
2. Neonatal seizures: In textbook of *Neurology of the Newborn* by Volpe JJ, 4th edition, Saunders, 2000, pp 178-214.
3. Neonatal seizures: By Scher MS (Chapter 55) in textbook of *Intensive Care of the Fetus and Neonate* by Alan R Spitzer, 2nd edition, Elsevier 2005; p817-852.
4. Castro Conde JR *et al.*: Midazolam in neonatal seizures with no response to Phenobarbital, Neurology 2005;64:876-879.
5. Ronen GA, Buckley D, Penny S and Streiner DL: Long-term prognosis in children with neonatal seizures, a population based study, Neurology 2007;69:1816-1822.

21 INTRAVENTRICULAR HEMORRHAGE AND PERIVENTRICULAR LEUKOMALACIA

Praveen Ballabh and
Vineet Bhandari

GERMINAL MATRIX-INTRAVENTRICULAR HEMORRHAGE

Definition

The periventricular **germinal matrix (GM)**, located in the region of the thalamostriate groove beneath the ependyma, is densely packed with neuroblasts and glioblasts, and is richly supplied with capillaries.[1] It undergoes progressive decrease in size from a width of 2.5 mm at 24 weeks to 1.4 mm at 32 weeks and disappears by 36 weeks of gestational age. The capillaries in the GM bleed underneath the ependymal lining of the lateral ventricle and a large hemorrhage is attended by rupture of the ependyma resulting in an intraventricular hemorrhage.

Incidence

Germinal matrix hemorrhage-intraventricular hemorrhage (GMH-IVH) continues to be a major problem of premature infants because survival rates are increasing in this group and a large number of these infants develop **neurodevelopmental delay**, **cerebral palsy**, **hydrocephalus** and mental retardation. The frequency of IVH is inversely related to the birth weight and gestational age of infants. In infants <1,000 g, the incidence of IVH is 50%-60%, and in infants 1,000-1,500 g, the incidence is 10%-20%.[2,3] Among the affected infants, about 50% develop IVH in the first 8 hours and about 90% in the first 24 hours of life.[4,5]

Pathophysiology

The pathogenesis of GMH-IVH is usually attributed to vascular wall weakness of the GM vasculature and fluctuation of **cerebral blood flow** in unstable preterm newborns. Vascular wall weakness is ascribed to a relative paucity of pericytes in the GM vasculature resulting from a rapid angiogenesis accompanied by high levels of vascular endothelial growth factor and low levels of transforming growth factor-β1 in the GM.[6,7] Well-recognized factors associated with fluctuation of cerebral blood flow include respiratory distress syndrome (RDS), hypoxia, hypercarbia, **pneumothorax**, **patent ductus arteriosus**, **chorioamnionitis**, **sodium bicarbonate** administration, volume expansion and seizures.

Table 21.1: Factors influencing development of GMH-IVH

Factors	*Comments*
INTRA-VASCULAR	
Cerebral autoregulation	Impaired. "Pressure -passive"
Cerebral blood flow	Fluctuating secondary to systemic blood pressure changes
Cerebral blood flow	Increased secondary to rapid volume expansion, hypercarbia
Cerebral venous pressure	Increased with pneumothorax
Hypotension	Secondary to blood loss
Reperfusion injury	
Coagulation disturbances	Increased prothrombin time in preterm infants
VASCULAR	
Germinal matrix	Poorly supported capillaries; vulnerable to hypoxia—ischemic insults
Arterial structure	Acute transition from large vessels to capillary network without gradual arborization
Venous drainage	"Hairpin" loops susceptible to outflow obstruction
EXTRA-VASCULAR	
Fibrinolytic activity	Increased in preterm infants
Cerebral tissue	Poor vascular support in preterm infants
Hypoxia-ischemia	Increased vulnerability in immature brains

Grades of IVH

In most neonatal intensive care units, severity of IVH is graded based on Papile's classification (Table 21.2):[8]

Table 21.2: Grades of GMH-IVH

Grades	*Description*
1	Subependymal GM hemorrhage
2	Intraventricular hemorrhage without ventricular dilatation
3	Intraventricular hemorrhage with ventricular dilatation
4	Intraventricular hemorrhage with parenchymal extension (Fig. 21. 1)

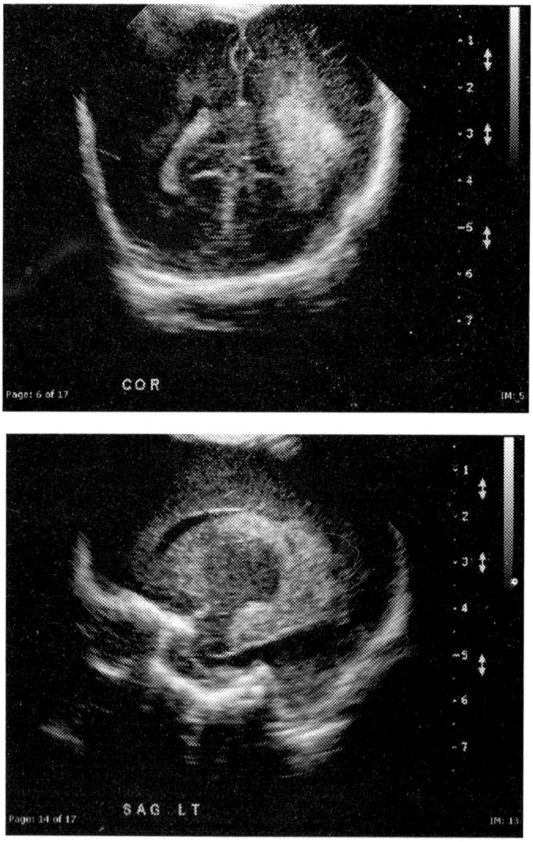

Fig. 21.1: Coronal (top) and sagittal (bottom) views of a head ultrasound of a premature infant with Grade 4 IVH on the left

Clinical Presentation

These infants are usually asymptomatic. However, severe IVH might manifest with bulging fontanelle, reduced hematocrit, apnea, bradycardia, acidosis, seizures and change in level of consciousness. A **catastrophic syndrome**, described as rapid onset coma, decerebrate posturing, weakness in extremities and fixed pupil, is seen more commonly with infratentorial hemorrhages and are not typically seen in IVH. Usually localizing signs on motor examination are seen later in the course or after infancy.

Table 21.3: Clinical presentation of GMH-IVH

Clinical presentation	*Comments*
Asymptomatic	Detected on routine ultrasound
Mild to moderate **("saltatory")** symptoms	Sudden fall in hematocrit, pallor, respiratory signs, acidosis, hypotonia, altered consciousness
Severe ("catastrophic") symptoms	Rapid onset coma, decerebrate posturing

Diagnosis

All infants less than 32-34 weeks of gestation are screened for IVH by performing head ultrasound. A number of neonatal intensive care units in the USA perform head ultrasound on days 1, 3, 7 and 30 to diagnose IVH. However, a head ultrasound on day 3 seems reasonable to perform and subsequent head ultrasounds could be performed if infants have either cardio-respiratory events such as pneumothorax, cardiac arrest, severe respiratory acidosis or in cases of drop in platelets (<20K) and presence of coagulation disorders. Spinal tap to evaluate cerebrospinal fluid (CSF) is not indicated in IVH. CT and MRI scans are expensive alternatives. All infants with grade 2-4 IVH need follow up ultrasounds to evaluate progression of IVH and the development of **post-hemorrhagic hydrocephalus (PHH)**.

MANAGEMENT

Prevention

1. **Prenatal steroids** to prevent RDS: National Institute of Health, Bethesda, USA recommends use of prenatal betamethasone or

dexamethasone in preterm labor for mothers of 24-34 weeks gestational age to prevent RDS and GMH-IVH.[9] It is not known whether the decrease in the incidence of IVH on prenatal steroid use is secondary to a decrease in the occurrence of IVH or resulting from direct effect of steroid on the vasculature of GM.

2. Prevent cardiorespiratory events and **gentle ventilation**: Prevention of hypoxia, hypercarbia, and pneumothorax reduces the incidence of IVH. Use of smaller mean airway pressure in mechanical ventilation might also reduce the risk of IVH.
3. Adequate management of patent ductus arteriosus, maternal chorioamnionitis also reduces risk of IVH.
4. Sodium bicarbonate administration and volume expansion should be slow, to prevent IVH.
5. Use of muscle relaxants including pancuronium in the first 2 days of life might reduce the risk of IVH. However, this is not the standard of care in view of the adverse effects associated with these medications.
6. **Indomethacin,** an inhibitor of the prostaglandin synthetic pathway, has been shown in multiple single-center studies to decrease the incidence of IVH in preterm infants.[10,11]

Treatment

Unfortunately, there is no optimal treatment of IVH and neuroprotective strategies to prevent brain damage in IVH have not yet been established. The infants with IVH need serial head circumference measurements and head ultrasounds to diagnose PHH.

PHH can be communicating or non-communicating (obstructive). The former is usually secondary to decreased absorption of CSF due to obstruction of arachnoid villi by blood debris. Obstructive hydrocephalus develops secondary to a blockade in the CSF circulation. Mild PHH usually arrests and does not need neurosurgical intervention. However, moderate to severe obstructive hydrocephalus eventually needs shunt surgery; temporizing measures include doing a ventriculostomy and placement of a subcutaneous Ommaya reservoir.[12]

Prognosis

Mortality from moderate to severe (grade 3 and 4) IVH is 27-

50%. An inverse relationship between extent of hemorrhage and survival exists. Mild to moderate (grade 1 and 2) IVH usually does not increase the mortality risks of the premature infants. Among the survivors of moderate to severe IVH, 50-80% develops PHH and other sequelae including cerebral palsy, learning disabilities, mental retardation, cognitive problems and seizures. Mild to moderate IVH is also associated with impaired cortical development and neurologic sequelae. About one-quarter of infants with moderate and severe IVH (grade 3 and 4) were noted to have motor deficits at about 5 years of age (Table 21.4).

Table 21.4: Prognosis of IVH

Grade	*Mortality (%)*	*Progressive Ventricular Dilatation (%)*	*Neurological Sequelae (%)*
1	5	5	5
2	10	20	15
3	20	55	35
4	50	80	90

PERIVENTRICULAR LEUKOMALACIA (PVL)

Definition

It is an ischemic injury to the immature brain. It is classically manifested as presence of echogenic cysts (as detected by cranial ultrasound) in the periventricular area of the brain. Another form of PVL, characterized by diffuse cerebral white matter injury in the periventricular region, is also commonly being recognized. This is more appropriately referred to as diffuse **periventricular white matter injury (PWMI)**.

Epidemiology

The group of highest risk for PVL is infants <32 weeks of gestation. As detected by cranial ultrasound, the incidence of **"cystic" PVL** has been reported to be 3-16%.[13, 14, 15] If both cranial ultrasound appearances of PVL (i.e. "**flares**" and "cystic") are included, the incidence has been reported to be 32% in very low birth weight (VLBW) neonates.[16] The autopsy incidence of PVL, however, is much higher, from 20-75%.[14]

Recent studies suggest that "cystic" PVL lesions are decreasing, whereas diffuse cerebral PWMI is emerging as the predominant lesion.[15, 17]

Pathology

The macroscopic pathology of PVL consists of necrotic foci in the periventricular white matter (within 1-2 cm of the ventricular wall), usually at the level of the trigone and occipital horn, and the parieto-occipital lobe (including the optic radiations). Cavitation takes a few weeks.[14]

The microscopic pathology consists of an initial phase of coagulative necrosis, followed by infiltrating macrophages and reactive astrocytes and microglia. Within a few weeks, resorption of necrotic tissue results in the appearance of periventricular cysts.[14]

Pathogenesis

Factors associated with PVL are listed in Table 21.5.

Table 21.5: Risk factors for PVL [15, 18]

Factors	*Comments*
Prematurity	The immature brain is more vulnerable to hypoxic-ischemic insults
Maternal PIH with IUGR	Hypoxia-ischemia to the developing brain
Maternal chorioamnionitis	Fetal exposure to endotoxins or cytokines can cause white matter injury via vasoactive mechanisms resulting in cerebral ischemia
Maternal cocaine abuse	Cerebral ischemia
Perinatal asphyxia	Cerebral ischemia
Apnea and bradycardia episodes	Cerebral ischemia
Hypotension	Cerebral ischemia
Marked hypocarbia	Cerebral ischemia

The development of PVL is linked to the loss of arterial blood supply to the deep white matter. **Vascular end zones** exist in the cerebral white matter, which are supplied by long or short penetrating arteries that arise from the pial arteries. Severe or persistent ischemia in these areas may account for "cystic" PVL while less severe or brief episodes of ischemia leads to diffuse PWMI.[15] Hypoxia-ischemia and reperfusion injury involve preoligodendrocyte injury and activation of microglia. The factors involved in these processes include excitotoxicity (glutamate), free radicals (reactive oxygen species) and inflammatory mediators (cytokines).[19]

Clinical Features

Most preterm infants are asymptomatic. Clinical signs are subtle and include: irritability, apnea/bradycardia spells, poor feeding, decreased tone in lower limbs, increased tone in neck extensors, pseudobulbar palsy and seizures. **Seizures** may occur in 10-30% of infants.

Diagnosis

This is usually made by using different imaging techniques.

Cranial ultrasound can be done at the bedside in most instances. During the first week following the injury, echogenic foci in the periventricular white matter are noted secondary to local necrosis with congestion and/or hemorrhage. This is followed by the appearance of echolucent "cysts" over the next 2 weeks (Figure 21.2). By 2-3 months, ventriculomegaly appears, often coincident with the disappearance of the "cysts". This is secondary to deficient myelin formation and/or gliosis with collapse of the "cysts".[20]

CT scans are not recommended as the scanning modality of choice. If done, however, it can delineate the extent and severity of PVL.

In general, it is useful to obtain T1-weighted, T2-weighted, T2*-weighted (sensitive to hemorrhage) and diffusion MRI images around term equivalent to evaluate myelination.[20] MRI scanning appears to be more sensitive than cranial ultrasound for detection of diffuse PWMI, though "cystic" PVL can be detected by either modality.[20] A marked reduction in cerebral cortical gray matter has been noted in infants with prior evidence of PVL.[20]

Management

Avoidance of the risk factors listed in Table 21.5, as much as

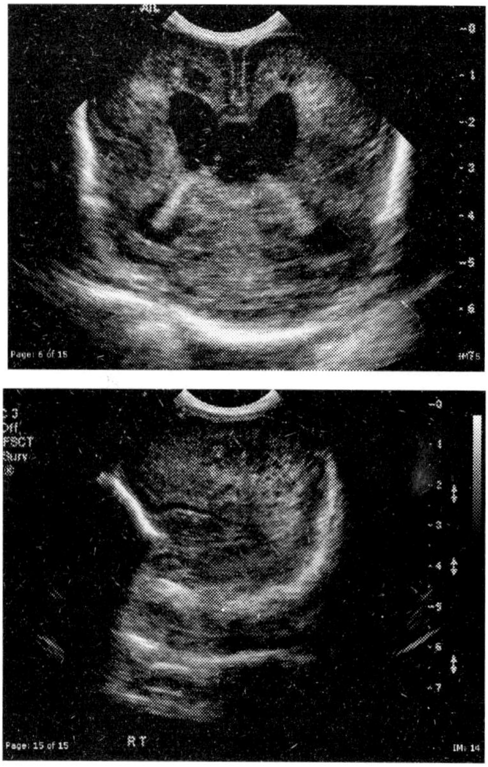

Fig. 21.2: Coronal (top) and sagittal (bottom) views of a head ultrasound of a premature infant with PVL. Note the cystic lesions in the anterior aspects of the lateral ventricles

possible, should be done. Once PVL develops, there is no specific treatment.

PROGNOSIS AND FOLLOW UP

Premature infants with PVL and diffuse PWMI require close follow up because of the increased risk of developmental delay and cerebral palsy. Abnormalities noted by MRI consistent with PVL showed moderate correlation with **cognitive and motor deficits** at ages 8 and 15 to 17 years.[20] Findings of PVL and widespread infarction were associated with **adverse neurological outcome** at 1 year.[20] Presence of signal abnormalities in white matter of former preterm infants evaluated at 15 years of age was associated with reduced white matter volume. Increased lateral ventricular size was associated with cognitive and motor deficits; sensorimotor and midtemporal cortices volumes were associated positively with full-scale, verbal and performance IQ scores.[20]

REFERENCES

1. Volpe JJ: Intracranial hemorrhage: Germinal matrix-intraventricular hemorrhage of prematue infants, In Neurology of Newborn, Ed 3, Philadelphia, WN Saunders,1995.
2. Courtney SE, Durand DJ, Asselin JM, Hudak ML, Aschner JL: Shoemaker CT; Neonatal Ventilation Study Group. High-frequency oscillatory ventilation versus conventional mechanical ventilation for very-low-birth-weight infants, N Engl J Med 2002;347:643-52.
3. Horbar JD, Badger GJ, Carpenter JH, Fanaroff AA, Kilpatrick S, LaCorte M, Phibbs R, Soll RF; Members of the Vermont Oxford Network: Trends in mortality and morbidity for very low birth weight infants, 1991-1999, Pediatrics 2002;110:143-51.
4. Beverley DW, Chance GW, Coates CF: Intraventricular haemorrhage—Timing of occurrence and relationship to perinatal events, Br J Obstet Gynaecol. 1984;91:1007-1013.
5. Perlman JM, Volpe JJ: Intraventricular hemorrhage in extremely small premature infants, Am J Dis Child 1986;140:1122-1124.
6. Ballabh P, Xu H, Hu F, Braun A, Smith K, Rivera A, Lou L, Ungvari Z, Goldman S, Csiszar A, and Nedergaard M: Angiogenic Inhibition Reduces Germinal Matrix Hemorrhage, Nat Med 2007;13:477-485.
7. Braun A, Xu H, Hu F, Kocherlakota P, Siegel D, Chander P, Ungvari Z, Csiszar A, Nedergaard M, Ballabh P. Paucity of pericytes in germinal matrix vasculature of premature infants, J Neurosci 2007;27:12012-12024.
8. Papile LA, Burstein J, Burstein R, Koffler H: Incidence and evolution of subependymal and intraventricular hemorrhage: A study of infants with birth weights less than 1,500 gm, J Pediatr 1978;92:529-534.
9. Consensus development conference on effect of corticosteroid for fetal maturation on perinatal outcomes, JAMA 1995;273:413.
10. Bada HS, Green RS, Pourcyrous M, Indomethacin reduced the risk of severe intraventricular hemorrhage, J Pediatr 1989;115:631-637.
11. Banstra ES, Montalvo BM, Goldberg RN, Prophylactic indomethacin for prevention of intraventricular hemorrhage in premature infants, Pediatrics 1988; 82:533-542.
12. Peretta P, Ragazzi P, Carlino CF, Gaglini P, Cinalli G: The role of Ommaya reservoir and endoscopic third ventriculostomy in the management of post-hemorrhagic hydrocephalus of prematurity, Child's Nerv Syst 2007;23:765-771.
13. Fanaroff AA, Stoll BJ, Wright LL, Carlo WA, Ehrenkranz RA, Stark AR, Bauer CR, Donovan EF, Korones SB, Laptook AR, Lemons JA, Oh W, Papile LA, Shankaran S, Stevenson DK, Tyson JE, Poole WK; NICHD

Neonatal Research Network. Trends in neonatal morbidity and mortality for very low birthweight infants, Am J Obstet Gynecol 2007;196:147.e1-8.
14. Folkerth RD: Periventricular leukomalacia: Overview and recent findings, Pediatr Dev Pathol 2006;9:3-13.
15. Back SA, Rivkees SA: Emerging concepts in periventricular white matter injury, Semin Perinatol 2004;28:405-414.
16. Maria A, Gupta A, Aggarwal R, Sreenivas V, Paul VK, Deorari AK: Incidence of periventricular leucomalacia among a cohort of very low birth weight neonates (< 1500 g), Indian Pediatr 2006;43:210-216.
17. Back SA, Riddle A, McClure MM: Maturation-dependent vulnerability of perinatal white matter in premature birth, Stroke 2007;38:724-730.
18. Okumura A, Hayakawa F, Kato T, Itomi K, Maruyama K, Ishihara N, Kubota T, Suzuki M, Sato Y, Kuno K, Watanabe K: Hypocarbia in preterm infants with periventricular leukomalacia: The relation between hypocarbia and mechanical ventilation, Pediatrics 2001;107:469-475.
19. Brunssen SH, Harry GJ: Diffuse white matter injury and neurologic outcomes of infants born very preterm in the 1990s, J Obstet Gynecol Neonatal Nurs 2007;36:386-395.
20. Neil JJ, Inder TE: Imaging perinatal brain injury in premature infants, Semin Perinatol 2004;28:433-443.

22 THYROID DISORDERS IN NEONATES

Shruti Gupta and Manoj Biniwale

INTRODUCTION

Thyroid hormones are critical determinants of brain and somatic development in infants, and of metabolic activity in adults; they also affect the function of virtually every organ system. **Thyroid hormones** are constantly available through large stores in the circulation and in the thyroid gland to perform these functions. Furthermore, thyroid hormone biosynthesis and secretion are maintained within narrow limits by a regulatory mechanism that is very sensitive to small changes in circulating hormone concentrations.

EMBRYOGENESIS

Thyroid gland develops from a median endodermal thickening in the primitive pharyngeal floor towards the back of the future tongue and is identifiable in a 17-day embryo. With the descent of the heart, the thyroid gland descents caudally and reaches its final position in front of second to sixth tracheal ring by 45-50 days gestation. The bilobed thyroid gland is evident by 7 weeks gestation. Ectopic thyroid gland, persistent thyroglossal duct or cysts result from abnormalities in thyroid descent. By 11th week of gestation thyroid gland histogenesis is complete and a single layer of endothelial cells surrounds the follicular lumen. By 78 days gestation **thyroxine (T4)** is detected in serum of a fetus. By early second trimester fetal thyroid is capable of secreting thyroid hormone.[1]

At the same time, the pituitary and the hypothalamus are developing as well and hence **thyroid stimulating hormone (TSH)** can be detected in the blood by 10-12 weeks gestation and **thyrotropin releasing hormone (TRH)** is found in hypothalamus by 9 weeks gestation. Maturation of the hypothalamic-pituitary-thyroid axis occurs during second half of gestation but normal feedback relationships are not mature until one to two months of postnatal life.[2]

PLACENTAL ROLE IN THYROID HORMONE REGULATION

Placenta produces estrogens that increase **triiodothyronine (T3), thyroxine (T4) and thyroxine binding globulin (TBG)**. In addition placenta also produces **human chorionic gonadotropin (hCG)**, which induces maternal T3 and T4 production as hCG is structurally similar to TSH. TSH does not cross the placenta but TRH does. Transfer of T4 across the placenta in the first trimester is greater than later on in gestation and this helps protect a hypothyroid fetus in a euthyroid mother. This suggests that fetus brain development is dependent on maternally derived T4 and hence maternal hypothyroidism during early gestation can lead to neurologic deficits in the fetus. Although T4 transfer later in pregnancy occurs only to a small extent, it is enough to protect a hypothyroid fetus with complete inability to produce thyroid hormones.[3]

Iodine deficiency does contribute to maternal and fetal hypothyroidism as iodides do cross the placenta readily. Excess iodine causes transient inhibition of T4 synthesis by its effects on thyroidal auto regulation. Hence iodine given to mother in large quantities, even topically as povidone-iodine, can cause **goiter** in the fetus. Also anti-thyroid drugs can cross the placenta and result in fetal goiter. Maternal thyroid stimulating immunoglobulin and TSH binding inhibitory immunoglobulins also cross the placenta.

THYROID HORMONE LEVELS IN FETUS AND NEONATE

Serum TSH concentrations rise gradually from 12 weeks gestation to term. But at birth there is a rapid TSH surge within 30-60 minutes after birth and this rise is associated with exposure of the infant to a colder environment and clamping of the umbilical cord. The serum TSH concentration then decreases rapidly 24 hours after delivery as shown in Figure 22.1[3, 4] and becomes normal by 3-5 days after birth. This initial TSH surge does stimulate T4 secretion and hence free and total T4 concentration also peak at 24-36 hours after delivery. Serum T3 concentrations also raise at the same time, which results in increases in both thyroidal secretion and conversion of T4 to T3 in peripheral tissues. Serum T4, T3 gradually fall off in the first four weeks of life and then level off at slightly higher levels than in adults.[5]

In preterm infants cord serum total and free T4 concentrations are proportional to gestational age. At birth, preterm infants

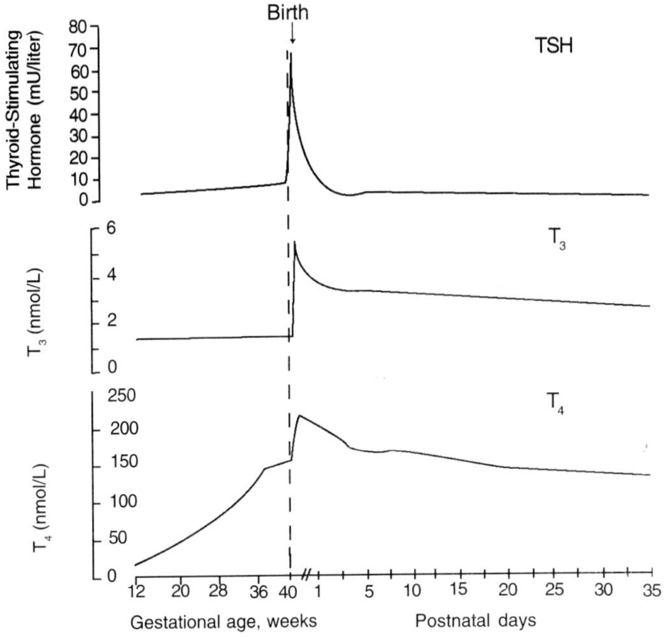

Fig. 22.1: Levels of thyroid hormones during gestation and immediately after birth

Normal patterns of change for TSH, total T4, and total T3 are depicted for the fetus (beginning at twelve weeks gestation) and continuing for the first five weeks of life in the newborn. *Data from Thorpe-Beeston, JG, Nicolaides, KH, Felton, CB, et al., N Engl J Med 1991;324:532, and Brown RS, Huang SA, Fisher, DA. Thyroid physiology in the perinatal period and during childhood. In: Werner's and Ingbar's The Thyroid:* A Fundamental and Clinical Text, *Braverman, LE, Utiger, RD (Eds), Lippincott-Raven,* Philadelphia,*PA 2005:1013-1028.*

undergo changes in serum TSH, T4 and T3 similar to in term infants. However, these changes are quantitatively smaller, most likely due to immaturity of the **hypothalamic-pituitary-thyroid axis**. Other factors that influence thyroid status of preterm infants are outlined in Table 22.1.[6] As in term infants, T4 concentrations fall in the first week of life and then after the first week there is a slow rise so that by six weeks of life preterm hormone values overlap those in term infants.[4]

Table 22.1: Factors influencing thyroid status of preterm infants

- Immaturity of the hypothalamic-pituitary-thyroid axis.
- Sudden interruption of maternal-fetal transfer of T4.
- Immaturity of thyroid hormone metabolism.
- Effects of neonatal diseases.
- Insufficient iodine intake.
- Iodine excess (use of povidone-iodine and other radio-opaque agents).
- Sudden requirement of thyroid hormone for thermogenesis, cardiac function, skeletal muscle action and other organ functioning.

THYROID HORMONE FUNCTION

Thyroid hormone maintains the **basal metabolic rate** and stimulates both anabolic and catabolic pathways and hence helps in normal growth. In thyroid hormone deficiency dental eruption, linear growth and skeletal maturation are retarded. Thyroid hormone does have effects on carbohydrate, calcium and vitamin D metabolism as well. The effects of thyroid on lipid metabolism are seen in the increased serum total cholesterol and low-density lipoprotein cholesterol concentrations in hypothyroidism.[7] Thyroid hormone increases heart rate, contractility of heart and cardiac output. T3 promotes the neural differentiation of stem cells and also affects genes involved in neural migration. Maturation of retina, cochlea and brain in general are dependent on thyroid hormone. Hence, in untreated hypothyroidism, mental retardation occurs. The degree of retardation is related to severity and duration of the hypothyroid state of the infant whose brain is developing. Thyroid hormone also affects peripheral nerves. Hence, sympathetic and autonomic responses may be sluggish in hypothyroidism and exaggerated in hyperthyroidism.[8]

LABORATORY TESTS

Table 22.2 illustrates laboratory tests used for diagnosis of thyroid disorders and assessment of thyroid function in infancy and childhood.[9, 10]

Table 22.2: Thyroid function tests

Serum Tests
- Thyrotropin Stimulating Hormone (TSH)
- Thyroid Hormones: Thyroxine (T4), free T4, Tri-iodothyronine (T3)
- Thyroid Binding Globulin (TBG)
- Thyroid Auto Antibodies: TSH receptor antibodies, thyroperoxidase (microsomal) antibodies, thyroglobulin antibodies
- Thyroglobulin (TG)

Imaging Tests
- Thyroid Scan
- Thyroid Ultrasound

Other Tests
- Bone age assessment by radiographs
- Thyrotropin releasing hormone (TRH) stimulation test
- Thyrotropin stimulating hormone (TSH) stimulation test
- Urinary iodine secretion

CONGENITAL HYPOTHYROIDISM

Neonates who are born with **congenital hypothyroidism (CH)** may have no overt clinical signs as a result of limited dependence of fetal peripheral tissues on thyroid hormone for development until late third trimester. Also maternal hormones acquired by transplacental transfer may mask the signs of hypothyroidism. However, it is extremely important to diagnose it as early as possible due to central nervous system effects of thyroid hormone. Failure of early replacement of thyroid hormone in a neonate can lead to irreversible brain damage or **cretinism.**[11, 12] Since 95% of hypothyroid infants don't have any signs or symptoms at birth it is extremely important to have an early universal screening process. Most newborn screening programs measure an initial T4 level and then 10% of the samples with lowest values are measured for TSH. Since this can still miss some infants, no neonate should be excluded from a formal screening based on normal newborn screening results, if hypothyroidism is suspected clinically.

ETIOPATHOGENESIS

Table 22.3 describes the causative disorders for congenital hypothyroidism and their incidences.

THYROID DYSGENESIS

This includes infants with ectopic or hypoplastic thyroid glands as well as total thyroid agenesis. This occurs in 1in 4000 live born infants and is twice as common in females compared to males. Although most cases are sporadic, some familial cases have been described. Loss of function mutations of the TSH receptor gene may lead to hypoplasia of the thyroid gland and elevations of TSH. Mutations in transcription factors may be responsible for some cases. Sixty to 80% of these infants may have some residual thyroid tissue in normal or ectopic position; hence, there is a spectrum of disease severity depending on how much residual thyroid tissue is present. Most of these infants are asymptomatic at birth. They have low serum T4 and high TSH concentrations in

Table 22.3: Thyroid disorders and their approximate incidences in the neonatal period

Disorder	*Incidence*
Thyroid Dysgenesis	1/4000
• Agenesis	
• Hypogenesis	
• Ectopia	
Thyroid Dyshormonogenesis	1/30,000
• TSH receptor defect	
• Iodide trapping defect	
• Organification defect	
• Iodotyrosine deiodinase deficiency	
• Defect in thyroglobulin	
Transient Hypothyroidism	1/40,000
• Drug Induced	
• Maternal Antibody Induced	
• Idiopathic	
Central Hypothyroidism	1/100,000
• Hypothalamic-pituitary anomaly	
• Panhypopituitarism	
• Isolated TSH deficiency	

the cord blood. Some infants may however have normal T4 with elevated TSH possibly secondary to the residual thyroid. Ectopic tissue can be seen on thyroid scan in these infants and circulating levels of thyroglobulin may be present as well. Infants with thyroidal dysgenesis may have ospteopenia as well due to abnormalities in thyroidal C cells and its effects on calcitonin levels.[1, 10]

THYROID DYSHORMONOGENESIS

The incidence of thyroid dyshormonogenesis is 1 in 30,000 live births. These disorders usually have an autosomal recessive inheritance pattern. Symptoms are same as in any other cause of CH. Enlargement of thyroid gland may develop at birth or later in life. The defects include:

- A decreased thyroid response to TSH.
- Decreased thyroid iodide trapping.
- Defective iodinification of trapped iodides.
- Defective deiodinification of trapped iodides.
- Abnormalities in thyroglobulin synthesis, storage or release.

TRANSIENT CONGENITAL HYPOTHYROIDISM

Transient congenital hypothyroidism usually occurs with an incidence of 1 in 40,000 live births and persists for a variable period after birth depending on the quantity and length of exposure of the causative agent during pregnancy. It can occur due to:

- Maternal ingestion of goitrogens; most common being iodide which is present in expectorants[13] or may be absorbed when povidone-iodine is used topically. Other substances include anti-thyroid drugs, sulphonamides and hematinic preparations, which contain cobalt.
- Transfer of maternal TSH receptor blocking antibodies in women who have autoimmune thyroid disease.
- Some cases of transient CH are idiopathic.

HYPOTHALAMIC-PITUITARY DEFECTS

Hypothyroidism due to central causes is present in 1 in 100,000 live births. These infants may have low thyroid hormone due to secondary (pituitary) or tertiary (hypothalamic) causes. These infants have low T4 and low TSH values and depending on the location of the defect they respond to TSH or TRH. These disorders are extremely rare and may be autosomal recessive in the inheritance pattern. Midline facial, cranial or intracranial defects like septo-optic dysplasia may cause the altered functioning of the hypothalamo-pituitary axis.

Clinical Features

Signs and symptoms of CH may be subtle or severe. Infants may present with **prolonged jaundice** (more than 7 days), birth weight more than 4 kgs, poor feeding, transient hypothermia, large posterior **fontanelle** (>1cm in diameter), **macroglossia, umbilical hernia, difficulty in feeding**, failure to thrive in infancy, lethargy, mottled skin, hoarse cry, distended abdomen and sometimes goiter (seen in CH due to thyroid dyshormonogenesis). Long-term sequelae include delayed bone and body growth, mental retardation (cretinism) and delayed puberty.

Diagnosis

Infants with CH are born with subtle signs of hypothyroidism. Hence, diagnosis based on clinical features alone is extremely difficult. Even though most countries have a newborn screening program that includes hypothyroidism screening, newborn screening may miss many infants, depending on the time and technique of testing. As mentioned earlier, during the first 24-48 hours after birth there is a TSH surge, hence a sample obtained during this time may result in false positive results.[14] The diagnosis of CH must be confirmed by measurement of serum T4 and TSH concentrations. After 7 days of age serum T4 <6 µg/dl and TSH >50µIU/ml confirms primary hypothyroidism. Values close to the above numbers are considered equivocal; hence repeat testing is warranted in those cases. A low serum T4 concentration with a normal TSH value characterizes central hypothyroidism. A poor TSH response to TRH confirms pituitary TSH deficiency, which may or may not be associated with other pituitary hormone deficiencies. If TSH levels normalize after TRH stimulation then hypothalamic TRH deficiency is likely. Table 22.4 illustrates T4 and TSH values in different diseases causing CH.[10, 15]

Table 22.4: Laboratory tests used for diagnosis of congenital hypothyroidism

Disease	*T4*	*TSH*	*Other*
Thyroid Dysgenesis	Low or normal	High	RAIU can detect ectopic tissue
Thyroid Dyshormonogenesis	Low	High	Low thyroglobulin and increased RAIU
Thyroid hormone resistance	High	Normal or High	Autosomal dominant or sporadic
TSH deficiency	Low	Low	Low cortisol and low growth hormone may be seen in panhypopituitarism
TRH deficiency	Low	Low	
Transient Hypothyroidism	Low or normal	Variably High	TSH receptor antibodies can be measured in disease due to maternal autoimmune disease
Sick Euthyroid	Low or normal	Normal	Low T3; normal or high free T4

RAIU: radioactive iodine uptake

Management

The treatment of CH is essentially replacement of thyroid hormone in the form of sodium-L thyroxine, which has good uniform potency and reliable absorption. The dose is 10-15 μg/kg/day. Adequacy of treatment is tested by periodic measurements of circulating levels of T4 and TSH. Infants with transient hypothyroidism secondary to goiterogenic drugs do not require any treatment unless high serum TSH persists beyond 2 weeks. Hypothyroidism due to TSH receptor blocking antibody may require treatment for 2-5 months.

Treatment of CH should restore any growth deficits within the first few months of treatment. Bone age is a sensitive indicator of adequacy of treatment as it may be delayed in inadequate treatment when all other signs have disappeared. However, excessive treatment for prolonged periods may cause craniosynostosis, advancement of bone age, tachycardia, excessive sweating, nervousness and disturbed sleep patterns.

Formal developmental and psycho-neurological evaluations should be considered in all infants with CH. Such evaluations are especially important in children whose treatment was delayed or inadequate.

Prognosis

Early diagnosis and treatment of CH prevents severe mental retardation and other neurologic complications. Even with early treatment, some children demonstrate mild delays in areas such as reading comprehension and arithmetic in third grade. As might be expected, infants with delayed bone age at diagnosis have poorer outcomes. Although continued improvement in IQ has been documented in treated patients through adolescence, some cognitive problems may persist. These may include problems in visuospatial, language, and fine motor function. Defects in memory and attention may also be present.[16]

NEONATAL THYROTOXICOSIS

Incidence

Congenital hyperthyroidism is extremely rare due to low incidence of thyrotoxicosis in pregnancy (1-2/1000 pregnancies). Of these, neonatal disease actually develops in only about 1-5% of thyrotoxicosis pregnancies.[17]

Etiology

It occurs in infants of mothers who have **Graves' disease**, which leads to transplacental passage of TSH receptor stimulating and TSH receptor-blocking antibodies. Depending on the ratio of stimulating to blocking antibodies the neonate may have transient hyperthyroidism or hypothyroidism. Sometimes blocking antibodies may mask the effects of stimulating antibodies for about 4-6 weeks leading to a late-onset neonatal Graves' disease.

Clinical Features

Clinical features in intrauterine life include fetal tachycardia, growth restriction, goiter, advanced bone age or craniosynostosis, preterm birth. Fetal goiter may be detected on ultrasonography by 27 weeks and may be associated with polyhydramnios due to possible compression of the esophagus by the enlarged thyroid gland. Postnatally, they may present with goiter, exopthalmos, tachycardia, bounding pulses, arrhythmias, irritability, hypertension, congestive heart failure, and poor weight gain. Thrombocytopenia, prolonged jaundice, hepatosplenomegaly and hypoprothrobinemia have also been reported. These symptoms may persist for 3-12 weeks, as the half-life of thyroid stimulating antibodies is four weeks.

Diagnosis

Diagnosis is confirmed by measuring high T4, freeT4 and T3 in blood postnatally. Serum TSH is low if measured after 2-5 days. Thyroid stimulating antibodies can also be measured in the neonatal serum.

Management

Management includes close monitoring of fetal tachycardia, fetal growth *in utero*. Mother may need to be treated with propylthiouracil if there is evidence of fetal hyperthyroidism. Postnatally, neonates' thyroid function tests should be monitored every 1-2 weeks for the first 4-6 weeks of life to check if elevated TSH-receptor antibody titers are present. Treatment includes iodide (Lugol's solution), which rapidly inhibits thyroid hormone release and decreases vascularity of thyroid gland. Propylthiouracil (PTU) may be used which inhibits organification and blocks conversion of T4 to T3. Beta-blockers like propanolol and digitalis are used to control tachycardia. Glucocorticoids in anti-inflammatory doses can be used in severe hyperthyroidism to decrease thyroid hormone secretion and inhibit conversion of T4 to T3. In extremely rare cases where hyperthyroidism is due to mutation in TSH receptor, near-total thyroidectomy with radioiodine ablation may be required.

Prognosis

Majority of infants will improve in 3-12 weeks as the titer of maternal antibodies in the neonatal serum decreases. There is a

15% mortality rate in severe cases of hyperthyroidism. Long-term sequelae include poor growth, craniosynostosis and intellectual impairment.

REFERENCES

1. Rose SR: Thyroid Disorders in Martin RJ, Fanaroff AA, Walsh MC (Eds), Neonatal Perinatal Medicine: Diseases of the fetus and infant 8th ed, Elsevier Mosby, Philadelphia, PA 2006:1526-1550.
2. Martin CR: Thyroid disorders in Cloherty JC and Stark AR (Eds); Manual of Neonatal Care 6th ed, Lippincott-Raven, Philadelphia, PA 2007:19-27.
3. Brown RS, Huang SA, Fisher, DA: Thyroid physiology in the perinatal period and during childhood in: Braverman, LE, Utiger, RD (Eds); Werner's and Ingbar's The Thyroid: A Fundamental and Clinical Text, Lippincott-Raven, Philadelphia, PA 2005:1013-1028.
4. Thorpe-Beeston JG, Nicolaides KH, Felton CV, Butler J, McGregor A: Maturation of the secretion of thyroid hormone and thyroid-stimulating hormone in the fetus, N Engl J Med 1991;324:532-536.
5. Williams Fl, Simpson J, Delahauty C, Ogston SA *et al.*: Developmental trends in cord and postpartum serum thyroid hormones in preterm infants, J Cli Endocrinol Metab 2004;89:5314-5320.
6. Van Wassenaer AG, Kok JH: Hypothyroxinaemia and thyroid function after preterm birth, Seminars in Neonatology 2004;9: 3-11.
7. Duntas LH: Thyroid disease and lipids, Thyroid 2002;12:287-293.
8. Van Wassenaer AG, Kok JH: Thyroid function and thyroid hormone requirements of Very preterm infants, Neoreviews 2000;1: e116-e121.
9. Baloch Z *et al.*: Laboratory medicine practice guidelines: Laboratory support for the diagnosis and monitoring of thyroid disease, Thyroid 2003;13:3-3.
10. Polk DH, Fisher DA: Disorders of thyroid gland in Taeusch HW, Ballard RA, Gleason CA eds; WB Saunders: Avery's diseases of the newborn 8th edn Philadelphia, PA 2005;1399-1409.
11. Bernal J, Guadaño-Ferraz A, Morte B: Perspectives in the study of thyroid hormone action on brain development and function, Thyroid 2003;11:1005-1012.
12. Bongers-Schokking JJ: Pre- and postnatal brain development in neonates with congenital hypothyroidism, J Pediatr Endocrinol Metab (Suppl 6) 2001;14:1463-1468.
13. Bostanci I, Sarioìlu A, Ergin H, Aksit A it A *et al.*: Neonatal goiter caused by expectorant usage, J Pediatr Endocrinol Metab 2001;14:1161-1162.
14. American Academy of Pediatrics, Rose SR, American Thyroid Association, Brown RS *et al.*: Update on Newborn screening for congenital hypothyroidism: Recommended guidelines, Pediatrics 2006;117:2290-2303.
15. Mitchell ML, Walraven C, Rojas DA, McIntosh KF, Hermos RJ: Screening very-low-birth weight infants for congenital hypothyroidism, Lancet1994;343:60-61.

16. Den Ouden AL, Kok JH, Verkerk PH, Brand R, Verloove-Vanhorick SP: The relation between neonatal thyroxine levels and neurodevelopmental outcome at age 5 and 9 years in a national cohort of very preterm and/or very-low-birth weight infants: Pediatr Res 1996; 39:142-145.
17. Buckingham B: The Hyperthyroid fetus and infant, Neoreviews 2000;1:e103-e109.

23 AMBIGUOUS GENITALIA IN THE NEONATE

Zubair H Aghai

DEFINITION

Any infant whose gender cannot be determined by the appearance of the external genitalia is said to have ambiguous genitalia.

NORMAL SEXUAL DIFFERENTIATION

The gonadal development starts at the 3rd week of gestation. Until the 7th week of gestation, the gonads are bi-potential and can differentiate either into ovaries or testes (Figure 23.1). In the presence of **SRY gene** (sex determining region of the Y chromosome), indifferent gonads develop as testes.[1] The fetal testes produce two hormones, testosterone and Mullerian inhibiting factor or anti-Mullerian hormone (AMH).[2] Testosterone is produced by the Leydig cells and directly stimulates the differentiation of the **Wolffian ducts** (mesonephric ducts). The Wollfian ducts give rise to the epididymides, vasa differentia, seminal vesicles and ejaculatory ducts. Testosterone is also converted to dihydrotestosterone (DHT) in the target organs by 5α-reductase. DHT is responsible for the differentiation of the external male genitalia. **Anti-Mullerian hormone (AMH)** is secreted by the Sertoli cells which regress the **Mullerian ducts** (paramesonephric ducts).

In the absence of the testes, the development of phenotype sex is female. The Wolffian ducts are regressed due to the lack of testosterone and the Mullerian ducts proliferate in the absence of

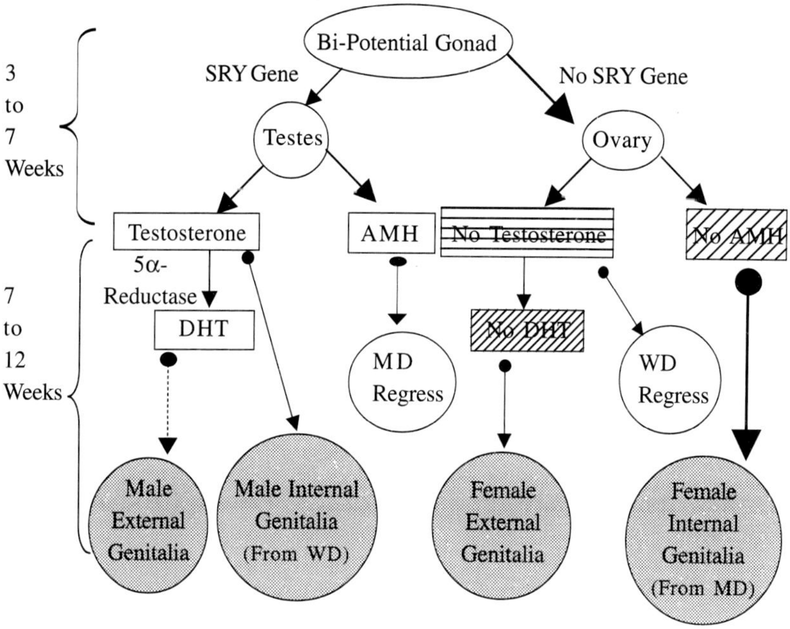

Fig. 23.1: Normal sexual differentiation

AMH. The Mullerian ducts give rise to the fallopian tubes, uterus and the upper vagina. In the absence of DHT, the external genitalia differentiate into the female phenotype.

PATHOPHYSIOLOGY

Ambiguous genitalia are seen in the disorders of gonadal differentiation or the disorders of differentiation of internal and external genitalia.

A. Disorders of Gonadal Differentiation

1. True **hermaphroditism**: In true hermaphroditism, both the testicular and the ovarian tissues are present, either in same or in opposite gonad. About 70% of infants with true hermaphroditism have a 46,XX karyotype; 10% 46, XY and 20% 46, XY/46XX mosaicism.
2. Gonadal dysgenesis
   a. Pure **gonadal dysgenesis**: Presence of streak gonad bilaterally (complete gonadal dysgenesis) or unilaterally

(partial gonadal dysgenesis). The streak gonads in an infant with Y chromosome carry a significant risk for tumor development.

b. **Mixed gonadal dysgenesis:** Presence of functioning testes on one side and streak gonad on the other side. All infants have a Y chromosome and increased risk for gonadal malignancy.

c. **WAGR syndrome** (*W*ilm's tumor, *a*niridia, *g*enitourinary malformation, *r*etardation and ambiguous genitalia).

d. **Camptomelic syndrome** (short limb dysplasia and ambiguous genitalia).

e. **Denys-Drash syndrome** (nephropathy, Wilm's tumor and ambiguous genitalia).

B. Disorders of Differentiation of Internal and External Genitalia

In the female fetus, exposure to androgens during the development of internal and external genitalia will lead to ambiguous genitalia (female pseudohermaphroditism). Whereas, the male fetus will develop ambiguous genitalia if there is an inadequate androgen production or incomplete end-organ response to androgen (male pseudohermaphroditism).

I. Exposure to androgens in female (Female pseudohermaphroditism)

This is the most common mechanism for the development of ambiguous genitalia. The neonates have a 46,XX karyotype and the gonads are ovaries, but the external genitalia are virilized due to androgen exposure. The source of the androgens could be either maternal or fetal.

1. **Fetal sources of androgens:**

a. Congenital adrenal hyperplasia (CAH)

i. 21-hydroxylase (OH) deficiency

ii. 11-OH deficiency

iii. 3-beta hydroxysteroid dehydrogenase (βHSD) deficiency.

b. Fetal tumors.

c. Placental aromatase deficiency (aromatase converts

androgen to estrogen, aromatase deficiency leads to increased androgen levels).

2. **Maternal sources of androgens:**
   a. Tumors (ovarian or adrenal).
   b. Exogenous androgens.

II. Androgen deficiency or unresponsiveness in male (Male pseudohermaphroditism)

This is the less common mechanism for the development of ambiguous genitalia and caused by either inadequate androgen synthesis or incomplete end organ response to the androgens. The neonates have a 46, XY karyotype, gonads are testes but infants are inadequately virilized.

1. **Decreased testosterone synthesis**
   a. Congenital adrenal hyperplasia (CAH)
      i. 17α-OH deficiency
      ii. 3β-HSD deficiency
      iii. 17,20 lyase deficiency
      iv. 17-HSD.
   b. Testicular unresponsiveness to human chorionic gonadotropin (hCG) and luteinizing hormone (LH) (mutation in LH receptor).
   c. Lipoid adrenal hyperplasia {20-22 desmolase deficiency, mutation in steroidogenic acute regulatory protein (StAR)}.
   d. Leydig cell aplasia.
   e. Anorchia.
2. **Defect in DHT synthesis** (5α-reductase deficiency).
3. **Decreased endorgan responsiveness to androgen:**
   a. Complete androgen insensitivity syndrome (**Testicular feminization**): Infants have a 46, XY karyotype, bilateral testes and female appearing external genitalia.
   b. Partial androgen insensitivity syndrome (**Reifenstein syndrome**): Infants have a 46, XY karyotype, bilateral testes but incomplete masculinization of external genitalia.
4. **Persistent Mullerian duct syndrome (Uterine hernia syndrome):**
   a. Gene mutation AMH.

b. Receptor defect AMH: Isolated AMH deficiency or AMH receptor defects results in regression of the Mullerian ducts. Infants have a 46, XY karyotype, bilateral testes, male appearing external genitalia with bilateral fallopian tubes and a uterus.

CLINICAL FEATURES

A careful history and physical examination are very important in the evaluation and the management of neonates with ambiguous genitalia. Some relevant history and examination details to be elicited in a case of ambiguous genitalia have been enumerated in Table 23.1. Physical examinations should include the measurement of penile or clitoral size, careful palpation to ascertain the size and the position of the gonads and careful inspection of the site of the urethral opening. In infants with male appearing genitalia, presence of micropenis, **hypospadias**, impalpable or small gonads, or inguinal mass requires further evaluation. In infants with female appearing genitalia, presence of clitoromegaly, posterior labial fusion, palpable gonads, or inguinal hernia or mass requires further work up.

Micropenis (penile length < 2 cm in full term neonate[3]) is seen in testosterone deficiency (second or third trimesters), partial androgen insensitivity and growth hormone (GH) or LH deficiency. Micropenis with accompanying hypospadias is suggestive of partial androgen insensitivity as hypospadias is rare in GH or LH deficiency. Bilateral non-palpable gonads in neonates with ambiguous genitalia may suggest CAH in genetic female and anorchia in genetic male. A single opening at the base of the phallus may be a hypospadias or urogenital sinus. Gentle insertion of catheter can help to differentiate between the two. The opening is the urogenital sinus if the tip of the catheter can be palpated beneath the perineal skin while directed towards the anal opening. The catheter cannot be palpated beneath the skin in perineal area in hypospadias.

An anogenital ratio (distance between the anus and posterior fourchette divided by the distance between the anus and the base of the clitoris) of >0.5 suggests virilization with posterior labial fusion.[4] The anogenital ratio is independent of gestational age and the body size.

Table 23.1: Relevant history and examination in infants with ambiguous genitalia

History/Exam finding	*Comments*
Family history	*Consanguinity* (increased autosomal recessive disorders e.g CAH, 5α-reductase deficiency) *Unexplained neonatal deaths* (CAH) Female relatives with amenorrhea and *infertility* (male pseudohermaphrotidism) *Maternal virilization in pregnancy* (placental aromatase deficiency) *Maternal ingestion or topical use of androgens e.g., testosterone, danazol or progesterones)* (female pseudohermaphrotidism)
Dehydration, hypotension	Suggestive of CAH
Hypertension	Suggestive of CAH
Dysmorphic features	Chromosomal abnormalities or syndromes e.g. Smith Lemli Opitz syndrome (microcephaly, micrognathia and syndactyly), WAGR syndrome, Camptomelic syndrome (short limb dysplasia), Denys-Drash syndrome (nephropathy, Wilm's tumor)
Hyperpigmentation	Congenital lipoid adrenal hyperplasia (20,22 desmolase deficiency)
Palpable gonads below inguinal ligaments	Testes (true or male pseudohermaphroditism)
Asymmetry of gonads	True hermaphroditism or gonadal dysgenesis
Urogenital sinus	Female with CAH
Palpable uterus on rectal examination	Suggestive of female pseudohermaphrotidism or AMH deficiency in male
Micropenis	Partial androgen insensitivity
Clitoromegaly	Androgen exposure (CAH, maternal androgen, gonadal dysgenesis, true hermaphroditism)
Inguinal mass	Persistent Mullerian duct syndrome, dysgenetic testes

Infants with true hermaphroditism may have varying forms of ambiguous genitalia to almost normal male or female external genitalia.

DIAGNOSTIC STUDIES

The important initial diagnostic studies in the evaluation of neonates with ambiguous genitalia should include, chromosome analysis (sex determination), abdominal/pelvic ultrasound and retrograde urethrogram (evaluate adrenal, pelvic structure and internal anatomy) and serum chemistry and adrenal steroids (CAH). If the uterus is not seen on pelvic US, it suggests the presence of testicular tissue producing AMH. Absence of uterus indicates bilateral ovaries, dysgenetic gonads that failed to produce AMH or AMH receptor defect. Additional studies will depend on the results of the karyotype and abdominal and pelvic US results. A suggested approach to an infant with ambiguous genitalia is described in Figures 23.2 and 23.3.

I. Female (46 XX) (Figure 23.2)

Female karyotype with ambiguous genitalia indicates exposure

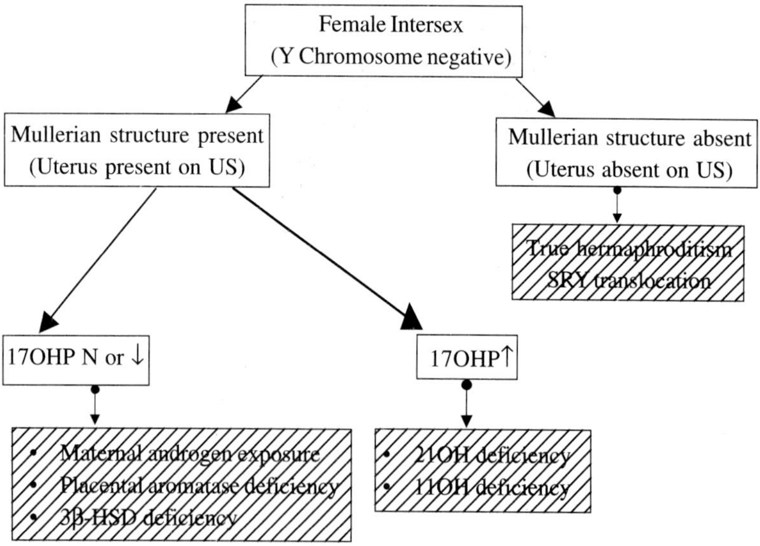

Fig. 23.2: Approach to infants with female intersex (Y chromosome absent)

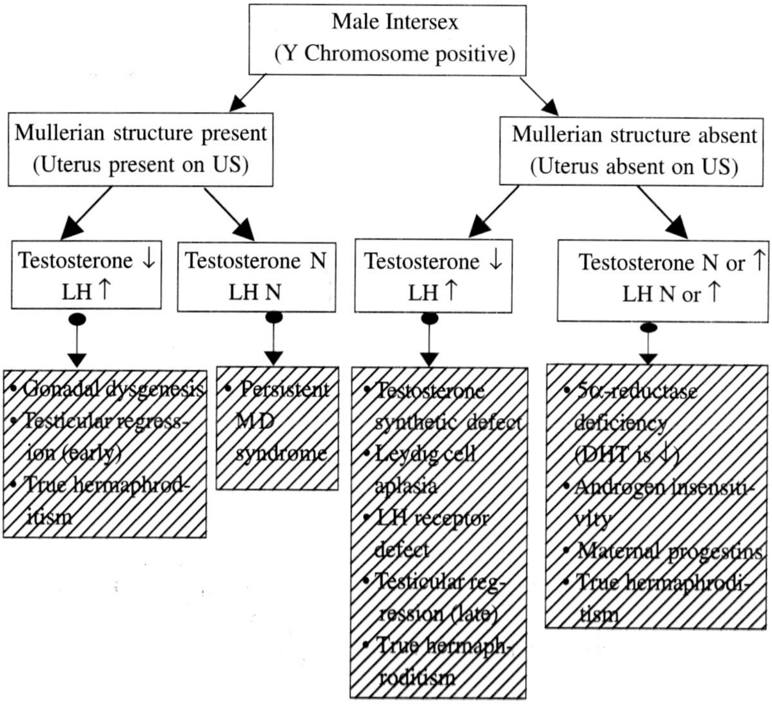

Fig. 23.3: Approach to infants with male intersex (Y chromosome present)

to excessive maternal or fetal androgens. The differential diagnosis includes:

1. CAH.
2. Exposure to maternal androgen or synthetic progestational agents.
3. Placental aromatase deficiency.
4. SRY translocation.
5. True hermaphroditism.

CAH is the most common diagnosis in infants with ambiguous genitalia and 46 XX karyotype. Maternal virilization during pregnancy suggests placental aromatase deficiency.[5]

Serum Adrenal Steroids

Serum 17-hydroxyprogesterone (17-OHP) level will be increased in infants with 21-hydroxylase deficiency and 11-hydroxylase deficiency. In infants with 3β-HSD deficiency, serum dihydroepiandrostenedione (DHEA) and 17-hydroxyprenenolone levels are markedly increased.

Serum Electrolytes

Monitoring of serum chemistry is very important in infants with ambiguous genitalia and suspected CAH. Infants with 21-hyroxylase or 3β-HSD deficiency are typically salt losers with underproduction of mineralocorticoids. Classic serum electrolyte pattern (**hyponatremia, hyperkalemia** and **metabolic acidosis**) may not be evident during the first 3-4 days of life.

Serum Testosterone and AMH

Once maternal androgen exposure and CAH is excluded, serum testosterone and AMH level can be measured. Elevated testosterone level suggests SRY translocation, true hermaphrotidism or fetal testosterone producing tumors.

SRY Translocation

The diagnosis of SRY translocation can be made by fluorescence *in situ* hybridization (FISH) with SRY specific probe.

II. Male (46 XY) (Figure 23.3)

The differential diagnosis and the diagnostic evaluation of infant with ambiguous genitalia and 46 XY karyotype are extensive and complex. The causes for under-virilized genetic male include:

1. **Abnormal testicular activity:**
   a. Pure XY gonadal dysgenesis (streak gonad, female external genitalia and intact Mullerian duct).
   b. Testicular regression syndrome (loss of testis in early development, female phenotype, atrophic Mulerian duct).
   c. Vanishing testes syndrome (loss of testis in late development, female phenotype, absent Mullerian structures and agonadism).
   d. AMH gene mutation (persistent Mullerian duct syndrome).
2. Defect of testosterone synthesis.
3. Defect in conversion of testosterone to DHT.
4. End organ resistance (androgen insensitivity syndrome).

Serum Testosterone, DHT and AMH Levels

Testosterone level is low in defects in testosterone synthesis and male pseudohermaphroditism. The testosterone-DHT ratio is increased in **5-α-reductase deficiency**. Serum concentration of AMH has been shown to correlate with functional testicular tissue. The levels are low in anorchia and gonadal dysgenesis.

Serum LH

In LH receptor defects, serum testosterone level is low despite an elevated concentration of LH.

hCG Stimulation Test

hCG stimulation test is performed in genetic male infants with ambiguous genitalia. The results from hCG stimulation test can help to distinguish between the various categories of causes of ambiguous genitalia in genetic male infants.[6] The basal LH, FSH, testosterone and DHT levels are measured. hCG (1500 units/m^2) is administered on days 1 and 3. Androstenedione, testosterone and DHT levels are measured on days 3 and 6. A rise in testosterone level confirms the presence of testicular tissue. In testosterone synthesis defects and LH receptor defects, hCG stimulation does not increase testosterone level. In testosterone synthesis defects, precursors of testosterone (androstenedione) are increased after hCG stimulation but not in LH receptor defects. In 5α-reductase deficiency testosterone, DHT is increased after hCG stimulation. A normal basal and hCG stimulated androgenic response in a genetic male infant with ambiguous genitalia implies androgen insensitivity syndrome.

Adrenocortico-Trophic Hormone (ACTH) Stimulation Test

ACTH stimulation test can be performed when a defect in testosterone synthesis is identified and the diagnosis cannot be made on basal steroid levels. Failure of steroidogenic response, after ACTH stimulation, suggests StAR mutation.

III. Mixed Sex Chromosome Pattern

Mixed chromosomal pattern can be seen in true hermaphroditism (XX/XY karyotype) or mixed gonadal dysgenesis (45 X/46 XY).

The presence of Y chromosome in infants with mixed gonadal dysgenesis increases the risk for gonadoblastoma.

MANAGEMENT

The management of infants with ambiguous genitalia requires attention to both medical and psychosocial issues. The most important and immediate medical concern in an infant with ambiguous genitalia is the possibility of adrenal crisis with CAH.

Medical Management

All infants with suspected CAH require early diagnosis and replacement therapy to prevent adrenal crisis and vascular collapse. Medical management of infants with suspected CAH is described in the following section (*vide infra*).

Psychosocial Issues

The birth of an infant with ambiguous genitalia is a psychosocial emergency for the family. The physician should meet and talk to the family as soon as the abnormality is noted. The parents should be told that the genitalia of their baby are not being fully formed and this condition is uncommon but biologically understandable. The discussion should help parents in understanding abnormal development of genitalia. Until the gender assignment of the baby is made, no name should be given and no birth announcement describing gender be distributed. The use of gender specific nouns should be avoided until the gender is assigned. The infant can be addressed as baby or child. The parents may feel guilty that they are in some way responsible for the abnormal genital development. This issue should be discussed openly and parents should be counseled that they are not responsible for the genital malformation.

Gender Assignment

The decision for gender assignment for infants born with the ambiguous genitalia is complex and should be postponed till the final diagnosis is made. As per American Academy of Pediatrics practice guidelines,[7] the decision for gender assignment and sex rearing of a baby born with ambiguous genitalia should include:

1. *Fertility potential:* All female infants with ambiguous genitalia

due to CAH or maternal androgen exposure are potentially fertile and should be raised as girls. In most of the other causes of ambiguous genitalia, the fertility is either reduced or absent.

2. *Capacity for normal sexual function:* One of the important issues in gender assignment is surgical reconstruction of external genitalia. It is simpler to construct a vagina than a satisfactory and functional penis. When considering a male gender for rearing, the size of the phallus and its potential to develop as a functional penis is important. A trial of testosterone injections should be given in equivocal cases when assessing the potential for penile growth.
3. *Endocrine function:* The ability of the gonads to produce appropriate hormones for sex rearing is also an important factor in gender assignment.
4. *Malignant change:* The potential for malignant degeneration in a retained gonad with a Y chromosome and testes with dysgenetic features on biopsy must be considered in the decision of the gender assignment.
5. *Testosterone imprinting:* The testosterone imprinting of the fetal brain may play a role in determining male sexual orientation. Caution should be exercised in recommending rearing gender if it differs from the chromosomal sex. In this situation, individual consideration and psychological counseling of affected individual and their parents may be beneficial.

Surgery

Infants raised as girls usually require clitoral reduction. In girls with CAH, surgery can be performed once hormone replacement therapy has begun. Reconstruction surgery can be deferred until 1 year of age or later. The testes should be removed soon after birth in infants with partial androgen insensitivity or testicular dysgenesis and those who have a small phallus and will be reared as a female.

Follow Up

Continuous psychosocial support and ongoing counseling of the parents and the affected child are important in the management of infants with the ambiguous genitalia. There are suggestion that the gender assignment and the surgical treatment of newborns with the most extreme forms of genital ambiguity can be delayed to a later time thereby allowing the affected person to participate in the gender assignment.[8]

CONGENITAL ADRENAL HYPERPLASIA (CAH)

Definition

Congenital adrenal hyperplasia refers to a group of autosomal recessive disorders relating to the adrenal glands. It is characterized by a complete or partial deficiency of an enzyme involved in cortisol or aldosterone synthesis, leading to a deficiency in these hormones. In addition to this deficiency, there may also be an overproduction of androgens in CAH.

Clinical Features

The clinical characteristics of CAH depend on the specific enzyme deficiency on steroids synthesis pathway (Figure 23.4). The most common enzyme deficiency is **21-hydroxylase** and accounts for 90% of the cases of CAH. The prevalence based on neonatal screening studies has been estimated to be about one in 14,200 live births. Newborn screening programs, originally designed to test for phenylketonuria and hyperthyroidism, are now increasingly testing for 21-hydroxylase deficiency. The deficiency of 21-hydroxylase leads to inadequate serum aldosterone and cortisol levels. The lack of negative feedback to the hypothalamus and pituitary by inadequate cortisol level leads to excessive ACTH stimulation, adrenal hyperplasia and excessive production of adrenal androgens. In the female fetus, exposure to adrenal androgens during the development of internal and external genitalia (7-12 weeks of gestation) will lead to ambiguous genitalia (female pseudohermaphroditism). The female neonates with CAH are virilized (clitoral enlargement, labial fusion and formation of a urogenital sinus). In male neonates with CAH, genitalia are normal at birth but if left untreated may manifest with precocious puberty. Depending upon the associated relative or absolute aldosterone deficiency, the neonate may present with simple virilizing form (25%) or salt-loosing form (75%). In relative

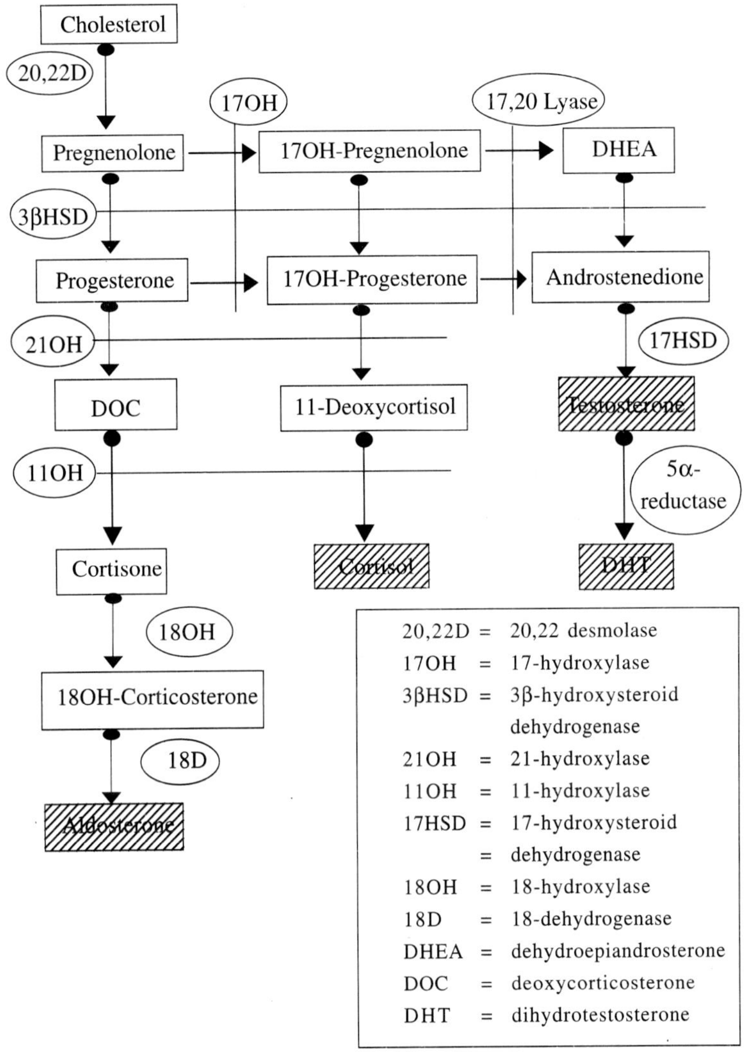

Fig. 23.4: Steroids biosynthesis pathway

aldosterone deficiency (non salt-losers) form, salt loss is mild and adrenal insufficiency may not occur except in stressful circumstances. The salt loser form (absolute aldosterone deficiency) manifests as adrenal crisis in the neonatal period.

11-hydroxylase deficiency accounts for 5-8% of CAH and is also inherited as an autosomal recessive trait. Salt retention, volume expansion, hypertension and hypokalemia (due to excess mineralocorticoid activity of 11-deoxycorticosterone) are the primary clinical manifestations that distinguish 11-hydroxylase deficiency from 21-hydroxylase deficiency.

Deficiency of **3β-HSD** occurs in fewer than 5% of infants with CAH. Deficiency of 3β-HSD results in decreased synthesis of cortisol, aldosterone and androstenedione but increases secretion of DHEA (Figure 23.4). Infants with 3β-HSD are usually salt losers but less virilized.

DIAGNOSIS

Serum Electrolytes

Monitoring of serum chemistry is very important in infants with suspected CAH. Infants with 21-hyroxylase or 3β-HSD deficiency are typically salt losers with underproduction of mineralocorticoids. The classic serum electrolyte pattern (hyponatremia, hyerkalemia and metabolic acidosis) may not be evident during the first 3-4 days of life. High urinary sodium concentration in presence of normal or low serum sodium indicates salt wasting. Infants with mild salt wasting may have normal serum and urinary electrolytes. Infants with 11-hydroxylase deficiency have increased formation of deoxycorticosterone (DOC), which is a moderately potent mineralocorticoid. Serum sodium is normal or mildly elevated but hypokalemia is consistently present in infants with 11-hydroxylase deficiency.

Serum Adrenal Steroids

Serum 17-OHP level will be increased (100-1000 fold) in infants with 21-hydroxylase deficiency and 11-hydroxylase deficiency. The CAH panel (ACTH, cortisol, DHEA, 17-hydroxyprenenolone and 11-deoxycortisol levels) can be measured to exclude other rare enzyme deficiencies in the steroids synthesis pathways (Figure 23.4). Deoxycortisol and DOC levels are increased in infants with 11-hydroxylase deficiency. In infants with 3β-HSD deficiency, serum DHEA and 17-hydroxyprenenolone levels are markedly increased.

MANAGEMENT

Medical Management

All infants with suspected CAH require early diagnosis and

replacement therapy to prevent adrenal crisis and vascular collapse. The goals of the treatment of CAH are to normalize ACTH secretion, to lower ACTH stimulated precursors and their side products, and to provide replacement or correction of end products (cortisol, aldosterone and sex steroids).

1. *Glucocorticoid/Mineralocorticoid Therapy:* Stress doses of glucocorticoids should be initiated in all infants in whom CAH is a consideration. The stress dose of hydrocortisone is 100 mg/m^2/day divided every six hours. Once the infant is stable and the diagnosis of salt losing CAH is confirmed, the infant should receive glucocorticoid and mineralocorticoid replacement therapy. Oral hydrocortisone (10-20 mg/ m^2/day) and fludrocortisone (0.05-0.1 mg/day) can be used as replacement therapy. The doses require adjustment for growth and during the period of stress. Infants with 11-OH deficiency are treated with glucocorticoids alone. The hypertension may persist even after adequate suppression of mineralocorticoid excess; antihypertensive therapy with spironolactone, amiloride, and calcium channel blockers has proven effective and may be required.
2. *Fluid and Electrolytes:* Serum electrolyte should be monitored closely. Urgent IV fluids are required for any evidence of salt wasting. An IV bolus of 10-20 ml/kg of normal saline should be administered in infants with hypovolemia. 5% dextrose in normal saline should be used as the initial maintenance fluid. Acidosis, hyperkalemia and hypoglycemia should be corrected.

PSYCHOSOCIAL ISSUES/GENDER ASSIGNMENT/SURGERY

Discussed earlier (*vide supra*).

Prenatal Diagnosis and Treatment

Prenatal diagnosis is technically possible when a fetus is known to be at risk because of an affected sibling. The prenatal diagnosis is important for the affected female fetus as therapy is available to minimize or prevent masculinization of the external genitalia. The CAH can be diagnosed by DNA analysis and HLA genotyping of chorionic villus cells in the first trimester. Measurement of 17-OHP and androstenedione in the amniotic fluid along with DNA analysis and HLA typing of amniotic fluid cells can be performed during the second trimester. Treatment with maternal dexamethasone (20 µg/kg/day) can effectively suppress fetal ACTH and prevent or minimize virilization of female fetus.[9] The treatment of the fetus at risk is begun optimally at 5 to 6 weeks of fetal age. Once the sex of the fetus is determined, maternal steroids can be discontinued in the male fetus. In the female fetus, the mother should be treated with steroids during the whole pregnancy if diagnosis of CAH cannot be made by DNA analysis or HLA typing.

Newborn Screening

Newborn screening programs using capillary heel blood on filter paper may include the measurement of 17-OHP and allow for early identification of males and females with CAH.

REFERENCES

1. Clarkson MJ, Harley VR: Sex with two SOX on: SRY and SOX9 in testis development, Trends Endocrinol Metab 2002;13:106.
2. Lee MM, Donahoe PK, Hasegawa T, *et al.*: Mullerian inhibiting substance in humans: Normal levels from infancy to adulthood, J Clin Endocrinol Metab 1996; 81:571.
3. Lee PA, Mazur T, Danish R: Micropenis: Criteria, etiologies and classification, Johns Hopkins Med J 1980;146:156-163.
4. Callegari C, Everett S, Ross M, Brasel JA: Anogenital ratio: Measure of fetal virilization in premature and full-term newborn infants, J Pediatr 1987;111:240.
5. Grumbach MM, Auchus RJ: Estrogen: Consequences and implications of human mutations in synthesis and action, J Clin Endocrinol Metab 1999; 84:4677.
6. Forest MG: Pattern of the response of testosterone and its precursors to human chorionic gonadotropin stimulation in relation to age in infants and children, J Clin Endocrinol Metab 1979; 49:132.
7. American Academy of Pediatrics, Committee on Genetics, Evaluation of the newborn with developmental anomalies of the external genitalia, Pediatrics 2000;106:138-142.
8. Diamond M, Sigmundson HK: Management of intersexuality: Guidelines for dealing with persons with ambiguous genitalia, Arch Pediatr Adolesc Med 1997;151:1046-1050.
9. Mercado AB, Wilson RC, Cheng KC, Wei JQ, New MI: Prenatal treatment and diagnosis of congenital adrenal hyperplasia owing to steroid 21-hydroxylase deficiency, J Clin Endocrinol Metab 1995;80:2014-2020.

24 NEONATAL NECROTIZING ENTEROCOLITIS

Akhil Maheshwari and
Vineet Bhandari

INCIDENCE AND EPIDEMIOLOGY

Necrotizing enterocolitis (NEC) is the most common gastrointestinal emergency occurring in the neonatal period. The incidence of NEC varies between centers; overall estimates are 0.5-2/1000 live births, 1-3% of neonatal intensive care unit (NICU) admissions, or 4-11% of very low birth weight (VLBW) neonates.[1]

ETIOPATHOGENESIS

Although the etiopathogenesis of NEC is not fully understood, existing evidence points towards an interaction of mucosal injury, luminal bacteria, feedings, and an immature host response.

Mucosal Injury May be An Early Event in NEC

NEC is characterized by leukocyte infiltration, mucosal edema, ulceration and coagulative necrosis. The presence of coagulative necrosis suggests that gut ischemia may be involved, although it is unclear whether ischemia is a primary initiator or the end result of intestinal injury.[2-4] NEC has been associated with perinatal events such as hypotension, asphyxia, polycythemia, exchange transfusion, lung disease and cyanotic congenital heart disease, factors that can reduce splanchnic blood flow/oxygen delivery. Ischemia is more likely to be only one of the many possible initial insults in NEC because:

1. Aforementioned insults are not recorded in many neonates who develop NEC and some recent studies do not confirm these associations.
2. These events are recorded most frequently in the early neonatal period and do not explain why NEC typically occurs later, beyond the late 2nd week of life.[5,6]

Bacteria Play An Important, Essential Role in the Pathogenesis of NEC

Although no specific infectious agent(s) have been identified, mucosal bacteria play an important role in the development of NEC:

1. NEC does not occur before bacterial colonization; gut injury prior to colonization may cause strictures or atresia, but not NEC.[7]
2. *Pneumatosis intestinalis*, the pathognomonic finding in NEC, results from bacterial fermentation of intraluminal contents.[1]
3. Enteral antibiotics reduce the incidence of NEC;[8] and
4. NEC-like lesions do not develop in germ-free animals.[9,10]

The precise role of bacteria in the pathogenesis of NEC remains unclear. The risk of NEC may be related to the pattern of bacterial colonization of the neonatal gut mucosa. In some reports, early duodenal colonization with *Enterobacteriaceae* and *Clostridia* is correlated with later development of NEC.[11,12]

NEC Usually Occurs in Infants Who are Receiving Enteral Feedings

Although NEC can occur in neonates who have never been fed, 90–95% of cases occur in infants with a history of recent volume advancement or re-initiation of enteral feedings.[13] The introduction of feedings into the intestinal lumen presumably causes a disruption of mucosal integrity, blood flow and motility. A substantially higher incidence of NEC has been reported in formula-fed infants compared with exclusively breast-fed infants, which has been attributed to abnormal bacterial colonization and a lack of immunoprotective factors in infant formula.[14,15]

Prematurity is the Most Important Predictor of NEC

More than 90% of all cases of NEC occur in premature infants, suggesting that host immaturity is an important factor in NEC.[16-18] The role of prematurity is underscored by the fact the mucosal injury, altered permeability and bacterial translocation are common events in critically ill intensive care admittees of all ages, but NEC occurs only in this specific patient population.[19-21]

NEC in Full-Term Infants

Although more than 90% of the patients with NEC are premature, about 10% of infants with NEC are born full term. Unlike preterm infants who develop NEC in the second-third week (median 12 days), most term cases are seen within the first week (median 2 days).[6] NEC in term infants is usually 'secondary' and is associated with birth asphyxia, **Down's syndrome, congenital heart disease**, rotavirus infections, and **Hirschsprung's disease**.[22]

PATHOLOGY

The disease is localized most often to the ileo-colic region. In some extremely low birth weight (ELBW) infants, there might be total gut necrosis ('NEC totalis'). Lesions are characterized by coagulation necrosis (Figure 24.1A), bacterial overgrowth,

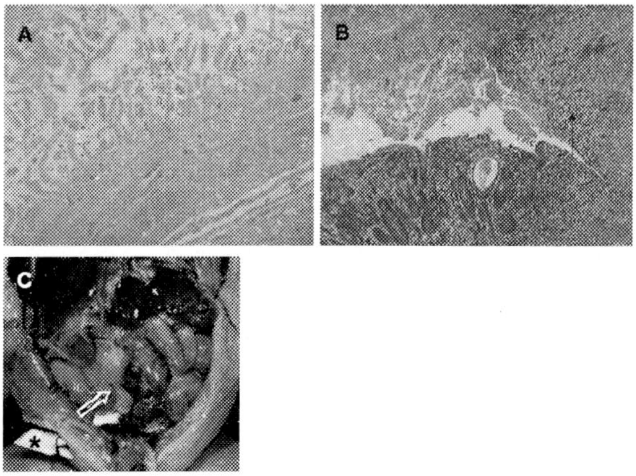

Fig. 24.1: Pathological changes in NEC. A. Classical change of NEC with coagulative necrosis—note the loss of cellular outline. B. Subacute NEC with onset of chronic inflammation (arrow) and reparative changes. C. NEC with peritonitis. Note purulent secretions (open arrow) and the peritoneal drain (*)

inflammation, and depending on the age of the lesions, reparative changes (Figure 24.1B).

CLINICAL FEATURES

Initial symptoms may be subtle and can include feeding intolerance, increased pre-feed residuals or delayed gastric emptying, abdominal distention and/or tenderness, ileus/decreased bowel sounds. In definite cases, signs of peritonitis appear, including abdominal wall erythema and tenderness. Advanced stages are associated with abdominal distension.

NEC is staged by using the **modified Bell's criteria** (Table 24.1).[23] Changes in NEC seem to follow an initial stage of systemic inflammatory response, a 'definite' stage of localized peritonitis, and an advanced stage of diffuse peritonitis (Figure 24.1C).

DIAGNOSIS

Radiographic features remain the mainstay of definitive diagnosis (Figure 24.2). Bowel loop dilation is seen in suspect NEC (as also in ileus; defined as loop diameter larger than the vertebral body

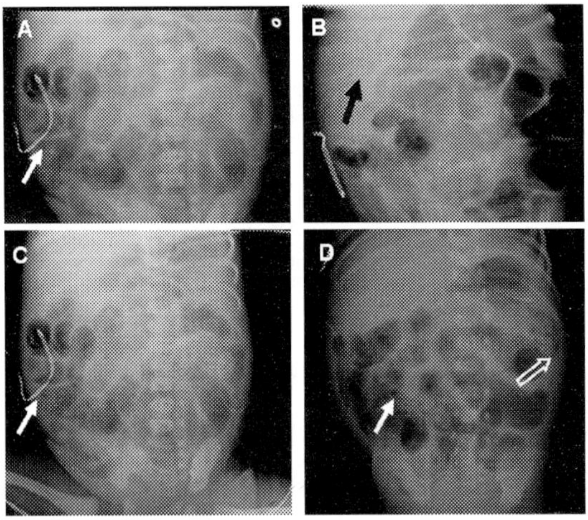

Fig. 24.2: Radiological features of NEC. Serial radiographs (A-D) from the same patient show increasingly evident pneumatosis. Solid white arrows indicate 'bubbly' submucosal pneumatosis whereas the linear subserosal pneumatosis is indicated by the open arrow. Portal venous air was seen transiently (B)

Table 24.1: Modified Bell's staging criteria for NEC [7]

Stage	*Classification*	*System signs*	*Intestinal signs*	*Radiological signs*
IA	Suspected NEC	Temperature instability, apnoea, bradycardia, lethargy	Increased pregavage residuals, mild abdominal distention, emesis, guaiac positive stool	Normal or intestinal dilation, mild ileus
IB	Suspected NEC	Same as above	Bright-red blood from rectum	Same as above
IIA	Proven NEC—mildly ill	Same as above	Same as above, plus absent bowel sounds, with or without abdominal tenderness	Intestinal dilation, ileus, pneumatosis intestinalis
IIB	Proven NEC—moderately ill	Same as above, plus mild metabolic acidosis and mild thrombocytopenia	Same as above, plus absent bowel sounds, definite abdominal tenderness, with or without abdominal cellulitis or right lower quadrant mass	Same as IIA, plus portal vein gas, with or without ascites
IIIA	Advanced NEC—severely ill, bowel intact	Same as IIB, plus hypotension bradycardia, severe apnoea, combined respiratory and metabolic acidosis, disseminated intravascular coagulation, and neutropenia	Same as above, plus signs of generalized peritonitis, marked tenderness, and distention of abdomen	Same as IIB, plus definite ascites
IIIB	Advanced NEC—severely ill, bowel perforated	Same as IIIA	Same as IIIA	Same as IIB, plus pneumoperitoneum

at the same level). The pathognomonic sign for NEC is the presence of air within the bowel wall, **'pneumatosis intestinalis'**. These radiolucent shadows appear 'bubbly' when air is sub-mucosal and become 'linear' when sub-serosal. **Portal venous gas** is associated with poor prognosis. Sonographic appearance of portal air is an early sign and although diagnostic for NEC, might not have the same prognostic significance as the presence of portal venous gas on plain radiographs.

In definite NEC, **bowel wall edema** (bowel wall thicker than the intervertebral disc at the same level) and fixed bowel loops are seen. In advanced NEC, ground glass appearance (suggestive of ascites) and later, pneumoperitoneum are seen. The ground glass appearance on X-rays is important only in association with clinical features of NEC—it is otherwise quite common in ventilated infants receiving gastric suction.

We typically use AP films to diagnose NEC and repeat films every 6-8 hours. A cross-table lateral view may be helpful in earlier detection of free air. Repeat radiographs are indicated for 48-72 hours after onset of NEC as most perforations tend to occur within this period. A good review of radiology of NEC can be found elsewhere.[24]

Leukocytosis is seen in NEC, often with neutrophilia. Platelets are low in stage II. Cultures may be positive, usually showing organisms common in the NICU as causative of late-onset sepsis. Disseminated intravascular coagulation (DIC) may be evident in advanced NEC (Figure 24.3).

Occult gastric bleeding is often seen in sick newborns and is non-specific. We do not use breath hydrogen or other testing as it was never found to have discriminant value.

TREATMENT

Medical management is designed to provide bowel rest, with decompression, antibiotics, and fluid administration. Infants stay NPO for 3-5 days in NEC stage I, and 10-14 days in stages II and III. We use antibiotics similar to our protocol for late onset sepsis, namely Vancomycin with an aminoglycoside. Anaerobic coverage is considered in infants with stage 3 NEC or with underlying Hirschsprung's disease. Ongoing nutritional support is essential

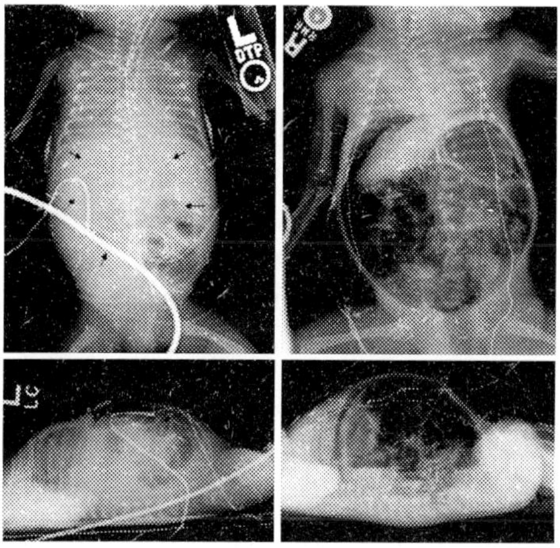

Fig. 24.3: Advanced NEC. A. Serial AP and cross-table lateral radiographs from the same patient (A, B) show the development of pneumoperitoneum. The radiographs on the left show a small non-dependent air pocket (marked by arrows) on a background of ground-glass opacity due to ascites

with total parenteral nutrition (TPN). These infants may need blood products, pressor supoort and ventilation.

Surgical management may include **peritoneal drainage or exploratory laparotomy** depending on the surgical risk of the patient.[25] In ELBW infants, both approaches might have similar results.[26] Patients who are severely affected require intestinal resection. In rare cases, the entire intestine can be involved, precluding surgical intervention. Depending on the location and extent of the bowel removed, long-term morbidities can include the need for colostomy, repeated surgical procedures, prolonged parenteral nutrition, poor nutrition, malabsorption syndromes, failure to thrive, and multiple hospitalizations.

PROGNOSIS

Mortality rates range between 20–50%. Approximately 27–63% of affected infants require surgical intervention. Upto 50% infants may die in the post-operative period.[23,24]

Subacute complications include **strictures** (often in left colon), malabsorption, bowel dysmotility, and complications of **short gut syndrome**. NEC has also been associated with poor neurodevelopmental outcome (as an independent predictor).[11]

PREVENTION

Strategies on prevention of NEC have focused on feeding practices (initiation, advancement, composition). Other measures that are being researched include amino acid supplementation, platelet activating factor (PAF) antagonists or PAF-acetylhydrolase administration, polyunsaturated fatty acid administration, epidermal growth factor administration, and the use of pre- and probiotics.[12, 13]

REFERENCES

1. Neu J, Weiss MD: Necrotizing enterocolitis: Pathophysiology and prevention, JPEN J Parenter Enteral Nutr 1999;23:S13-17.
2. Nowicki P: Intestinal ischemia and necrotizing enterocolitis, J Pediatr 1990;117:S14-19.
3. Nowicki PT: Ischemia and necrotizing enterocolitis: Where, when and how. Semin Pediatr Surg 2005;14:152-158.
4. Nowicki PT, Nankervis CA: The role of the circulation in the pathogenesis of necrotizing enterocolitis, Clin Perinatol 1994;21:219-234.
5. Neu J: Necrotizing enterocolitis: The search for a unifying pathogenic theory leading to prevention, Pediatr Clin North Am 1996;43:409-432.
6. Neu J: The 'myth' of asphyxia and hypoxia-ischemia as primary causes of necrotizing enterocolitis, Biol Neonate 2005;87:97-98.
7. Hsueh W, Caplan MS, Tan X, MacKendrick W, Gonzalez-Crussi F: Necrotizing enterocolitis of the newborn: Pathogenetic concepts in perspective, Pediatr Dev Pathol 1998;1:2-16.
8. Bury RG, Tudehope D: Enteral antibiotics for preventing necrotizing enterocolitis in low birthweight or preterm infants, Cochrane Database Syst Rev 2001:CD000405.
9. Lin PW, Stoll BJ: Necrotising enterocolitis, Lancet 2006;368:1271-1283.
10. Chan KL, Ng SP, Chan KW, Wo YH, Tam PK: Pathogenesis of neonatal necrotizing enterocolitis: A study of the role of intraluminal pressure, age and bacterial concentration, Pediatr Surg Int 2003;19:573-577.
11. Hoy CM, Wood CM, Hawkey PM, Puntis JW: Duodenal microflora in very-low-birth-weight neonates and relation to necrotizing enterocolitis, J Clin Microbiol 2000;38:4539-4547.
12. de la Cochetiere MF, Piloquet H, des Robert C, Darmaun D, Galmiche JP, Roze JC: Early intestinal bacterial colonization and necrotizing enterocolitis in premature infants: The putative role of clostridium, Pediatr Res 2004;56:366-370.
13. Stoll BJ: Epidemiology of necrotizing enterocolitis, Clin Perinatol 1994;21:205-218.
14. Lucas A, Cole TJ: Breast milk and neonatal necrotising enterocolitis, Lancet 1990;336:1519-1523.

15. Hsueh W, Caplan MS, Qu XW, Tan XD, De Plaen IG, Gonzalez-Crussi F: Neonatal necrotizing enterocolitis: Clinical considerations and pathogenetic concepts, Pediatr Dev Pathol 2003;6:6-23.
16. Chandler JC, Hebra A: Necrotizing enterocolitis in infants with very low birth weight, Semin Pediatr Surg 2000;9:63-72.
17. Snyder CL, Gittes GK, Murphy JP, Sharp RJ, Ashcraft KW, Amoury RA: Survival after necrotizing enterocolitis in infants weighing less than 1,000 g: 25 years' experience at a single institution, J Pediatr Surg 1997;32:434-437.
18. Rowe MI, Reblock KK, Kurkchubasche AG, Healey PJ: Necrotizing enterocolitis in the extremely low birth weight infant, J Pediatr Surg 1994;29:987-990; discussion 990-981.
19. Gatt M, Reddy BS, MacFie J: Review article: Bacterial translocation in the critically ill–evidence and methods of prevention, Aliment Pharmacol Ther 2007;25:741-757.
20. MacFie J, Reddy BS, Gatt M, Jain PK, Sowdi R, Mitchell CJ: Bacterial translocation studied in 927 patients over 13 years, Br J Surg 2006;93:87-93.
21. Stechmiller JK, Treloar D, Allen N: Gut dysfunction in critically ill patients: A review of the literature, Am J Crit Care 1997;6:204-209.
22. Maayan-Metzger A, Itzchak A, Mazkereth R, Kuint J. Necrotizing enterocolitis in full-term infants: Case-control study and review of the literature, J Perinatol 2004;24:494-499.
23. Walsh MC, Kliegman RM: Necrotizing enterocolitis: Treatment based on staging criteria, Pediatr Clin North Am 1986;33:179-201.
24. Buonomo C: The radiology of necrotizing enterocolitis, Radiol Clin North Am 1999;37:1187-1198, vii.
25. Pierro A: The surgical management of necrotising enterocolitis, Early Hum Dev 2005;81:79-85.
26. Moss RL, Dimmitt RA, Henry MC, Geraghty N, Efron B: A meta-analysis of peritoneal drainage versus laparotomy for perforated necrotizing enterocolitis, J Pediatr Surg 2001;36:1210-1213.

25

NEONATAL SEPSIS

Gautham Suresh and
Wendy McKenney

DEFINITIONS

Neonatal bacterial sepsis is a clinical syndrome characterized by systemic signs of infection and accompanied by bacteremia in the first month of life.[1,2] Although microbiologic confirmation of the bacteremia is necessary to rigorously define bacterial sepsis, in settings where microbiologic confirmation is difficult, sepsis can also be defined clinically, based on the presence of clinical signs.[3] In the absence of a positive blood culture, a diagnosis of "presumed" or "suspected" sepsis may be made in the presence of clinical signs (for example lethargy, feeding intolerance, temperature instability, see Table 25.2) and supportive laboratory investigations (see below) that, in the clinician's judgement, warrant at least a week of antibiotic therapy.

Based on the timing of clinical presentation, neonatal sepsis is often categorized into "early-onset" and "late-onset" sepsis. "Early-onset" sepsis is usually defined as any infection presenting in the first 72 hours of life, while "late-onset" sepsis occurs after 72 hours of post-natal life.

INCIDENCE

Neonatal sepsis is a common and potentially fatal condition, with an incidence of less than 1 to 8.6 cases per 1000 live births in developed countries,[1,2] and upto 38 cases per 1000 live births in developing countries.[3] World-wide, neonatal sepsis is responsible for the death of 1.6 million neonates each year.[2]

ETIOLOGY

The common organisms that cause neonatal sepsis are **Gram negative bacteria** (*Escherichia Coli, Klebsiella* species, *Enterobacter* species, *Pseudomonas* species, *Serratia marscescens,* and *Citrobacter* species), and **Gram positive bacteria** (*Staphylococcus aureus,* coagulase-negative staphylococcus - also known as *Staphylococcal epidermidis* - and *Streptococcal* species, especially Group B streptococcus). Rarely, *Listeria monocytogenes* and anaerobic bacteria cause neonatal sepsis. Viruses (especially herpes simplex and enterovirus) and **fungi** (especially *Candida albicans and Malassezia furfur*) are important causes of neonatal infection and should be considered in the differential diagnosis when a neonate presents with clinical features of neonatal sepsis.

PATHOGENESIS

A neonate can get infected with one of the organisms above in several ways:

1. Surface colonization of the fetus by organisms from the mother's genital tract after rupture of the membranes during labor or the process of vaginal birth. The colonization can then turn into infection when the bacteria invade the bloodstream or specific organs.
2. Fetal aspiration of infected amniotic fluid, which in turn, is the result of vaginal bacteria ascending the birth canal after rupture of membranes and causing infection of the fetal membranes, umbilical cord and placenta.[1]
3. Surface colonization by organisms after birth from the nursery environment, that subsequently turns into infection when the bacteria enter the bloodstream through skin punctures or indwelling invasive devices.
4. Transmission from persons—health-care professionals or the parents or siblings—coming in contact with the infant. This is the usual mechanism involved when infectious organisms spread from patient to patient in a neonatal unit and in nursery epidemics.

The latter two categories include **nosocomial** (hospital-acquired) **infection**, which is an important preventable category of neonatal infection and includes vascular catheter-related blood stream infection.

5. Rarely a neonate can acquire infection by hematogenous spread *in utero* from the mother across the placenta, by direct inoculation of bacteria into the skin and soft tissues by obstetric instruments during labor, or by bacteremia resulting from mucous membrane trauma following endotracheal suction, umbilical stump infection (omphalitis), or an infected circumcision site.[1]

Infection can be disseminated, with bacteremia, or can be localized to a specific body site (for example pneumonia, meningitis or osteomyelitis).

Risk Factors for Neonatal Sepsis

The risk of neonatal sepsis is increased in the presence of several antenatal (maternal), intrapartum and postnatal factors (listed in Table 25.1). Asymptomatic neonates with one or more of these risk factors should be closely observed for clinical signs of sepsis, and may require treatment with antibiotics until the possibility of sepsis is ruled out.

Table 25.1: Risk factors for neonatal sepsis
Maternal Group B *Streptococcal* colonization
Maternal infection (including chorioamnionitis and bacteremia)
Premature rupture of membranes (i.e. prior to the onset of labor)
Prolonged rupture of membranes (greater than 18 hours prior to delivery)
Traumatic delivery,
Resuscitation at birth
Low birth weight
Prematurity
Male gender
Presence of invasive devices such as vascular catheters and endotracheal tubes
Use of parenteral nutrition
Specific risk factors for fungal sepsis: Extreme prematurity, prolonged broad-spectrum antibacterial therapy, glucocorticoid therapy, hyperglycemia, neutropenia, necrotizing enterocolitis, spontaneous intestinal perforation, abdominal surgery, prolonged hospitalization.

CLINICAL FEATURES

Neonatal sepsis can present in a wide variety of ways. Presentation can be acute or indolent and may consist of a variety of clinical features, which are listed in Table 25.2.

Early-onset sepsis, of which Group B streptococcal infection is a well-recognized sub-category, is usually acquired from the maternal genital tract, and usually presents in a fulminant manner, with respiratory distress from pneumonia being a prominent feature.

Late-onset sepsis may be acquired from the maternal genital tract or from the neonate's environment after birth, present fulminantly or indolently, and often presents with focal clinical signs, which can include meningitis.

DIAGNOSIS

In the presence of clinical symptoms and signs (as outlined above), a "sepsis work up" should be done, which consists of laboratory tests to identify the organisms causing infection, assessment of antibiotic sensitivity and adjunctive tests.

Table 25.2: Clinical presentation of neonatal sepsis
General: Decreased activity and responsiveness, lethargy, excessive sleepiness. Concern on the part of the nurse or mother that the infant is 'not right'.
Thermoregulatory: Hypothermia or hyperthermia.
Respiratory: Respiratory distress or apnea.
Cardiovascular: Tachycardia, bradycardia, hypotension, shock, poor peripheral perfusion.
Gastrointestinal: Paralytic ileus, feeding intolerance, vomiting, hepatomegaly, splenomegaly, jaundice (conjugated hyperbilirubinemia), signs of necrotizing enterocolitis. Diarrhea is uncommon.
Neurologic: Lethargy, seizures, decreased muscle tone, movement and reflexes. A bulging fontanel, neck retraction, shrill cry and seizures can be signs of meningitis.
Cutaneous: Skin rash (vesicular with herpes infection), mottling, burn-like dermatitis with disseminated *Candidiasis*, ecthyma gangrenosum with pseudomonas infection, and sclerema.
Focal signs of infection: Abscess, omphalitis, arthritis, osteomyelitis, ophthalmitis, mastoiditis or mastitis.

Blood Culture

A positive **blood culture** is the gold standard test to establish the diagnosis of neonatal sepsis. Occasionally, blood culture may not grow an organism even in the presence of proven sepsis (false negative result). Two blood culture samples are preferred (each from a different site). At least one ml of blood should be instilled into each blood culture bottle. Smaller volumes (e.g., 0.5 ml) may detect heavy bacteremia but may miss light bacteremia with a low number of colony-forming units per ml of blood. The antibiotic sensitivities of organisms grown on the blood culture provide valuable information to guide antibiotic therapy. Cultures of coagulase negative *Staphylococcus* strains are usually not tested for antibiotic susceptibility.

Cerebrospinal Fluid Analysis and Culture

Infants with the onset of signs suggestive of sepsis after 72 hours of life should, undergo a lumbar puncture and **cerebrospinal fluid (CSF) analysis** to diagnose meningitis. A positive CSF culture or identification of pathogenic organisms on a CSF Gram stain confirms the diagnosis of meningitis. Other CSF parameters that are generally considered abnormal and indicative of meningitis are noted in Table 25.3. However, neonatal meningitis can occur without any abnormality in cerebrospinal fluid parameters and no single CSF value can reliably confirm or rule out meningitis.[4]

Urine Culture

A urine sample, preferably obtained by suprapubic aspiration, should be cultured in infants with suspected late-onset sepsis.

Culture of Other Material

Culture of material (e.g. pus) from sites of focal infection can also help identify the organisms. Tracheal aspirate cultures in intubated neonates are generally not useful since they most often represent colonization of the indwelling endotracheal tube and not actual infection of the lungs. Routine surveillance cultures of skin, umbilicus or other body areas are also not useful.

Buffy Coat Smear

Sometimes Gram stain of the buffy coat smear can indicate the

Table 25.3: Adjunctive laboratory test abnormalities associated with neonatal sepsis

Laboratory test	*Result suggestive (but not diagnostic) of sepsis*
Total white cell count	Less than 5000/ microliter. Elevated counts (e.g. greater than 20,000/ microliter) are less useful
Cytoplasmic changes	Presence of toxic granulation, Dohle bodies
Absolute neutrophil count	Less than 1500 - 1800 /microliter Exact values for age can be obtained from original articles[15,16]
Immature to total neutrophil ratio (ratio of promyelocytes, metamyelocytes, band cells and other early neutrophil precursors to total neutrophils)	> 0.16 in the first 24 hours > 0.12 after 60 hours of age. (Some studies report the upper limit of normal as 0.2 at all ages)
CRP	>1mg/dl (result is laboratory specific). Reaches peak elevation at approximately 50 hours. Does not begin to rise for several hours after infection sets in. Serial CRP estimation may be useful in excluding infection
CSF	>10-20 WBC/microliter Protein level > 100 - 200 mg /dl (preterm infants can have high protein levels without meningitis) Decreased glucose level (< 20-30 mg/dl)

presence of organisms and provide information about whether they are Gram-positive or negative.

Hematologic Abnormalities

Several **hematologic abnormalities** may be associated with sepsis[5]: an elevated total white cell count, neutropenia, an elevated ratio of immature to total neutrophils, an increase in the band cell count, morphologic changes in neutrophils such as toxic granulations and Dohle bodies, and thrombocytopenia. These abnormalities are listed in Table 25.3.

Acute Phase Reactants

Sepsis may be accompanied by an increase in the levels of **acute phase reactants** such as the C-Reactive Protein (CRP), and in the micro-ESR (Table 25.3). The utility of a variety of new tests, such as estimation of procalcitonin levels, interleukin 8 levels and the neutrophil CD64 index, is also being investigated.[6-8]

It is important to realize that the sensitivity of leukocyte abnormalities in sepsis varies widely across different studies, ranging from 1 to 90% and the specificity similarly ranges from 44 to 98%.[5] The sensitivity of the CRP level ranges from 60-82% and the specificity ranges from 93-96%.[7] Studies reporting the test characteristics of these, and other 'rapid diagnostic tests' are often methodologically flawed.[5] Also, the criteria for categorizing the results of these tests as abnormal vary across different studies and often depend on the age of the neonate and the time elapsed since the onset of infection. Tests that depend on the morphology of leukocytes, such as the immature: total neutrophil (IT) ratio, are subject to significant inter-observer variation. Therefore none of these tests can conclusively confirm the presence or absence of sepsis and excessive reliance should not be placed on such tests.[9,10] Positive results on these tests are suggestive, but not diagnostic for neonatal sepsis. Negative results do not conclusively rule out neonatal sepsis.

Metabolic Derangements

Hypoglycemia and hyperglycemia are both common accompaniments of neonatal infection and blood glucose levels should be closely monitored. Metabolic acidosis may be present as well.

Imaging

Chest radiographs are useful when neonatal pneumonia is suspected. Other imaging tests should be obtained only if specific clinical indications arise.

MANAGEMENT

Supportive Treatment

Neonates with infection should undergo close monitoring of their respiratory, cardiovascular and metabolic status and appropriate support should be provided as required. This may involve, as necessary, mechanical ventilation, volume expansion, use of pressors, glucose infusions and correction of electrolyte abnormalities. Transfusion of packed red blood cells may be required if the hemoglobin level is low and to increase the oxygen carrying capacity of the blood. Unstable neonates should not be fed enterally and they should receive parenteral nutrition until they are stable enough to tolerate enteral feeds. Close attention should be paid to thermoregulation. In severe cases unresponsive to antibiotic therapy and usual supportive treatment, exchange transfusion is sometimes tried, but the efficacy of this intervention is unproven. There is no role for intravenous immunoglobulin therapy in the prevention or treatment of sepsis.

Indwelling central vascular catheters (such as umbilical venous catheters or percutaneously inserted central venous catheters) should be removed if blood cultures are positive for any organism except for coagulase-negative *Staphylococcus*. Some cases of coagulase-negative *Staphylococcal* sepsis can be treated by administering antibiotics through the central venous catheter.

Specific Treatment

Empiric antimicrobial therapy should be commenced without delay in neonates with clinical features that are suggestive of sepsis and in those who are asymptomatic but are at high risk for developing sepsis (such as those with multiple perinatal risk factors). Each unit should develop policies for the empiric antibiotic combinations to be used for early-onset and late-onset sepsis, based on the local pattern of the results of cultures of blood and other specimens. If the culture results are positive, antibiotic therapy should be modified based on the organism identified and its antibiotic sensitivities. If culture results are negative, the likelihood that the result is falsely negative should be assessed. False negative cultures occur when the neonate has received antibiotic therapy prior to obtaining samples for blood culture, when an inadequate volume of blood has been inoculated into the specimen bottle, and when bacteremia is intermittent or low-level.

Duration of Antibiotics

The recommended duration of treatment for neonates with proven (positive blood cultures) *Streptococcal* or *Staphylococcal* sepsis and for uncomplicated Gram-negative sepsis is 10-14 days.[11]

Infants with clinical signs of sepsis who have negative results on blood and other cultures are generally treated for seven days or longer, based on clinical judgment, rapidity of clinical response, persistence of clinical signs, and the results of adjunctive tests such as white blood cell counts or CRP.

The recommended duration of treatment for uncomplicated meningitis is 14 days for meningitis caused by Gram-positive organisms, and 21 days for that caused by Gram-negative organisms.[11]

Infants who develop complications of meningitis such as ventriculitis, and those with a brain abscess require a prolonged duration of antibiotic therapy, for example, 6-12 weeks or longer. They may also require neurosurgical intervention, such as drainage of the abscess or placement of an external ventricular drain.

Recommended durations of treatment for other infections are as follows: neonatal pneumonia, 10 days; urinary tract infection, 7-10 days; osteomyelitis, 14-21 days; septic arthritis, 2-3 weeks.[11] Short-term antibiotic therapy (1-3 days) for urinary tract infection is not recommended because of a lack of evidence to support it.[12]

Amphotericin and/or fluconazole are the drugs of choice for neonatal *Candidiasis*.[11] Duration of therapy varies. Infection limited to an indwelling catheter without positive blood culture can be treated by removing the catheter and treating for 7-10 days. Infants with positive cultures should be treated for 2-3 weeks beyond the time when there has been resolution of signs of infection and a negative blood culture.[11] Disseminated infection requires longer treatment and is dependent on the involvement of organ systems. It may take weeks to months to resolve renal or hepatosplenic disease. All symptoms must be resolved, including neutropenia, before discontinuing drug therapy.[11] *Malassezia furfur* infection is treated with cessation of intravenous lipid infusions and removal of the indwelling catheter as well as anti-fungal drug therapy.[13]

Acyclovir is the treatment of choice for neonatal herpes

infection. Recommended treatment duration is 14 days for infection of skin, eyes or mouth. Treatment for disseminated disease or disease involving the central nervous system is 21 days. Ocular involvement should be treated with a topical ophthalmic drug in addition to acyclovir.[11]

PROGNOSIS

The mortality rate from neonatal sepsis ranges from 4-20%, but can be as high as 70% with fulminant sepsis.[1, 3, 10] The mortality is higher in preterm infants than with term infants, and with Gram-negative organisms. Survivors of neonatal sepsis are at risk of long-term neurodevelopmental sequelae, even in the absence of meningitis, but especially if meningitis accompanies the sepsis.[14]

PREVENTION

The key steps in the **prevention of nosocomial infection** are:

- Hand hygiene.
- Full barrier precautions when inserting central venous catheters.
- Adequate skin preparation with povidone-iodine prior to insertion of vascular catheters and other indwelling devices.
- Early removal of vascular catheters.
- Proper environmental hygiene.
- Use of breast milk for enteral feeds.

Early onset Group B *Streptococcal* infection can be prevented (though not completely) by using intrapartum penicillin prophylaxis for mothers who are Group B *Streptococcus* carriers.

REFERENCES

1. Palazzi DL, Klein JO, Baker CJ; Chapter 6: Bacterial sepsis and meningitis, In: Infectious diseases of the fetus and newborn infant, sixth edition, Eds: Remington JS, Klein JO, Wilson CB, Baker CJ, Philadelphia, Elsevier Saunders; 2006.
2. Haque KN: Definitions of bloodstream infection in the newborn, Pediatr Crit Care Med 2005;6:S45-49.
3. Vergnano S, Sharland M, Kazembe P, Mwansambo C, Heath PT: Neonatal sepsis: An international perspective, Arch Dis Child Fetal Neonatal Ed 2005;90:F220-224.
4. Garges HP, Moody MA, Cotten CM, Smith PB, Tiffany KF, Lenfestey R,

Li JS, Fowler VG Jr, Benjamin DK Jr: Neonatal meningitis: What is the correlation among cerebrospinal fluid cultures, blood cultures, and cerebrospinal fluid parameters? Pediatrics 2006;117:1094-1100.

5. Fowlie PW, Schmidt B: Diagnostic tests for bacterial infection from birth to 90 days—A systematic review, Arch Dis Child Fetal Neonatal Ed 1998;78:F92-98.
6. Malik A, Hui CPS, Pennie RA, Kirpalani H: Beyond the complete blood cell count and C-reactive protein. A systematic review of modern diagnostic tests for neonatal sepsis, Arch Pediatr Adolesc Med 2003;157:511-516.
7. Mishra UK, Jacobs SE, Doyle LW, Garland SM: Newer approaches to the diagnosis of early onset neonatal sepsis, Arch Dis Child Fetal Neonatal Ed 2006;91:F208-212.
8. Bhandari V, Wang C, Rinder C, Rinder H: Hematologic profile of sepsis in neonates: Neutrophil CD_{64} as a diagnostic marker, Pediatrics 2008;121:129-134.
9. Ng PC, Lam HS: Diagnostic markers for neonatal sepsis, Curr Opin Pediatr 2006;18:125-131.
10. Gerdes JS: Diagnosis and management of bacterial infections in the neonate. Pediatr Clin North Am 2004;51:939-959, viii-ix.
11. American Academy of Pediatrics. Summaries of infectious diseases, In Pickering, LK; Baker, CJ; Long, S.; McMillan, JA (Eds.) Red Book: 2006 report of the committee on infectious diseases, 27th edition, Elk Grove Village, IL: American Academy of Pediatrics 2006: 201-734.
12. Kennedy, T. UTI's. In Rudolph, C; Rudolph, A; Hostetter, M; Lister, G; Siegal, N (Eds.), Rudolph's Pediatrics, 21st edition, McGraw-Hill Medical Publishers Division, Dubuque, IL 2003: 1667-1673.
13. Devlin, R: Invasive fungal infections caused by candida and malassezia species in the neonatal intensive care unit, Adv Neonatal Care 2006;6:68-77.
14. Adams-Chapman I, Stoll BJ: Neonatal infection and long-term neurodevelopmental outcome in the preterm infant, Curr Opin Infect Dis 2006;19:290-297.
15. Manroe BL, Weinberg AG, Rosenfeld CR, *et al.:* The neonatal blood count in health and disease I, Reference values for neutrophilic cells, J Pediatr 1979;95: 89-98.
16. Mouzinho A, Rosenfeld CR, Sanches PJ, Risser R: Revised reference ranges for circulating neutrophils in very-low-birth-weight neonates, Pediatrics 1994;94: 76-82.

26 ACUTE RENAL FAILURE IN THE NEWBORN

Subrata Sarkar

Acute renal failure in the newborn is characterized by the inability of the kidneys to adequately regulate salt and water balance and/or eliminate waste products. It is usually accompanied by a sudden decrease in the **glomerular filtration rate (GFR)** and an elevated **serum creatinine**.

FUNCTIONAL DEVELOPMENT OF THE KIDNEYS [1]

The principal and unique function of the fetal kidney is the continuous provision of fluid and solutes into the amniotic cavity for maintenance of amniotic fluid volume. After birth, the kidneys are responsible for maintenance of fluid and electrolyte balance and excretion of waste products. This transition in kidney function occurs as a result of three changes viz. renal blood flow, GFR, and tubular functions.

RENAL BLOOD FLOW

The renal blood flow in the fetus accounts for only 2-3% of the cardiac output. At birth, the renal blood flow rapidly increases to 15-18% of the cardiac output.

GLOMERULAR FILTRATION

The pelvicalyceal system is well delineated in the 13th or 14th week of gestation. The nephrons continue to form through 34 weeks' gestation upto the total number of one million nephrons per kidney. Since nephrogenesis proceeds through 34 weeks' gestation, any insult to the developing kidney in a premature infant cannot not only result in acute renal failure but may potentially lead to long-term complications of interrupted nephrogenesis. Before 34 weeks' gestation there is a gradual increase in glomerular filtration rate (GFR) through the period of nephrogenesis and then the GFR remains stable between 34 weeks and term gestation. The GFR increases dramatically after birth resulting in a progressive decline in the serum creatinine to about 0.4 to 0.6 mg/dL by 2 weeks of age. This increase in GFR occurs more gradually and the decline in serum creatinine is much slower in preterm infants born before 34 weeks' gestation.

Serum creatinine may be high in the newborn shortly after birth but it may be a reflection of maternal renal function and can not be used to assess the renal function in the newborns. Thus, the gestational age at birth, the postnatal age, and the maternal serum creatinine should be taken into account when serum creatinine is used to assess the renal function in the newborns.

TUBULAR FUNCTION

Preterm infants conserve sodium less effectively because of decreased proximal tubular reabsorption, and decreased response to aldosterone. Tubular reabsorption of sodium remains low until 34 weeks' gestation with fractional excretion of sodium (FE_{Na}) ranging from 5-10%. After 34 weeks' gestation, 99% of filtered sodium is reabsorbed, resulting in FE_{Na} of less than 1%.

Preterm infants also have difficulty in excreting a potassium load because of decreased distal tubular secretion of potassium from immaturity of Sodium-Potassium-ATPase, reduced permeability of peritubular cells, and diminished GFR.

Similarly, the hydrogen ion excretion is also decreased in preterm infants. Both term and preterm infants waste bicarbonate because of altered threshold for bicarbonate reabsorption. In term infants the bicarbonate wastage resolves by 1-2 weeks of age, but in preterm infants it may be persistent.

Although the capacity to dilute urine is normal, the newborn infant has a limited ability to concentrate urine because of decreased response to arginine vasopressin and lower tonicity of renal medullary interstitium.

ETIOLOGIES [2,3]

Acute renal failure may be secondary to renal hypoperfusion without intrinsic damage (prerenal), or from intrinsic renal disease, vascular insult, and congenital anomaly (intrarenal), or due to obstructive uropathy (postrenal) (Table 26.1).

Table 26.1: Causes of acute renal failure

A. **Prerenal Failure**
   1. Hypovolemic: Hemorrhage, Dehydration (Gastrointestinal losses, Diabetes insipidus), Necrotizing enterocolitis and Sepsis (third space losses).
   2. Normovolemic: Asphyxia, Congestive heart failure, Patent ductus arteriosus, Polycythemia, Drugs (non-steroidal anti-inflammatory drugs (NSAIDs), Tolazoline).

B. **Intrarenal (Intrinsic) Renal Failure**
   1. Uncorrected prerenal failure (Acute tubular, medullary or cortical necrosis).
   2. Congenital renal anomalies: Renal agenesis, Renal hypoplasia or dysplasia, Polycystic kidneys.
   3. Vascular lesions: Renal arterial or venous thrombosis.
   4. Nephrotoxins: Aminoglycosides, NSAIDs, Angiotensin-converting enzyme (ACE) inhibitors, Radiographic contrast media.

C. **Postrenal (Obstructive)**
   1. Posterior urethral valves (most common), Urethral strictures, Ureteropelvic or ureterovesical obstructions, Megacystitis-megaureter syndrome.
   2. Functional urinary tract obstruction e.g. neurogenic bladder.

Prerenal failure is the most common cause of renal failure but if not corrected promptly it may lead to **acute tubular necrosis (ATN)** or intrinsic renal failure. However, the progression of prerenal failure to intrinsic renal failure is not sudden and several compensatory mechanisms (such as relaxation of afferent arteriole, increased catecholamine secretion, and generation of vasodilatory prostaglandins) work together to maintain renal perfusion when it is otherwise compromised. Administration of NSAIDs, e.g. indomethacin for closure of the patent ductus arteriosus can inhibit these compensatory mechanisms and can precipitate acute renal failure during renal hypoperfusion. Similarly, in presence of low renal perfusion pressure as in renal artery stenosis, the intraglomerular pressure necessary to drive filtration is partly mediated by increased generation of angiotensin II, and administration of ACE inhibitors in such conditions may precipitate acute renal failure by eliminating the pressure gradient needed for filtration.

The prognosis of ATN in newborns is good except in cases when the insult is of sufficient severity to lead to development of cortical necrosis because of microthrombi formation and vasculature injury. The chances of recovery of renal function in ATN depend on the underlying events that precipitated the hypoxic ischemic insult or toxic injury, and is much worse in neonates with multiorgan failure. Return in renal function in ATN is usually accompanied by a diuretic phase with excessive urine output at a time when the tubules have begun to recover from the insult but have not recovered sufficiently to appropriately reabsorb solute and water. Close attention to fluid and electrolyte balance is paramount during diuretic phase to ensure adequate fluid management to facilitate recovery from ATN and prevent additional renal injury.

Intrarenal failure may be prenatal in onset due to congenital abnormalities such as renal agenesis or dysplasia with or without obstructive uropathy and from genetic conditions such as autosomal recessive polycystic kidney disease, or may be acquired postnatally due to hypoxic ischemic insult or toxic injury. Prenatal onset of renal failure may be associated with maternal oligohydramnios and development of Potter's syndrome and oligohydramnios sequence in the newborns which is characterized by pulmonary hypoplasia manifested as severe pulmonary hypertension after birth, flat facies, low-set ears, and joint contractures.

Nephrotoxic acute renal failure in newborns is commonly associated with aminoglycoside antibiotics and NSAIDs for closure of the patent ductus arteriosus. Nephrotoxicity from both the medications is usually reversible once these medications have been discontinued. However, after the aminoglycosides are discontinued, the serum creatinine may continue to rise for several days because of ongoing tubular injury from continued high parenchymal level of the aminoglycosides.

Acute renal failure due to **renal artery or renal vein thrombosis** usually occurs with bilateral involvement and may present with gross or microscopic hematuria, hypertension and abdominal mass, in addition to oliguria. Renal artery thrombosis is usually associated with polycythemia, presence of umbilical arterial catheter, or patent ductus arteriosus. Renal scan typically shows enlarged kidneys with no or little blood flow and function.

DIAGNOSIS [2,3]

Diagnosis of acute renal failure is made in presence of the following suggestive history viz. maternal oligohydramnios, perinatal asphyxia, hemorrhage, umbilical arterial catheter, congenital heart disease, nephrotoxic medications, and physical examination viz. Potter facies, preauricular skin tag or pit, two-vessel umbilical cord, edema vs. volume depletion, abdominal mass (palpable bladder or kidneys), in addition to oligo-anuria. Newborns with prerenal failure, and intrinsic renal failure due to hypoxic ischemic insult, acute tubular, or cortical necrosis usually present with **oliguria** (<0.5 mL/kg/h) or **anuria** whereas newborns with intrinsic renal failure from aminiglycoside or radiograph contrast nephropathy usually have normal urine output. **Polyuria** (>4 mL/kg/h) is more common with renal dysplasia or obstructive uropathy.

The diagnosis is confirmed by serum/urine laboratory studies (serum electrolytes, BUN, creatinine, calcium, phosphorus, magnesium, albumin, and urine sodium if oliguric and not on diuretics), renal ultrasound, renal radionuclide scan (uncommonly used), and renal biopsy (rarely used). Increased BUN and creatinine are diagnostic of all forms of renal failure, but a markedly increased BUN: creatinine ratio is suggestive of prerenal acute renal failure. Serum sodium is usually decreased; and serum potassium may be normal in the beginning, but increases subsequently with severe renal failure. Serum calcium is decreased and serum phosphorus is increased frequently, especially if renal failure progresses to subacute or chronic stage. Serum bicarbonate is usually decreased as a part of an increased anion gap metabolic acidosis.

Abnormal urinary indices are used to differentiate prerenal failure from intrinsic failure/ATN. This differentiation is based on the premise that the tubules are working properly in prerenal failure and are therefore able to conserve salt and water appropriately while in ATN the tubules have irreversible injury and are unable to appropriately conserve sodium. Renal indices to differentiate prerenal and intrinsic renal failure are summarized in the Table 26.2. The use of these indices for differentiation requires that the patient has normal tubular function initially and has not had diuretics. For this reason premature infants with tubular immaturity may have prerenal failure with urinary indices suggestive of ATN.

Table 26.2: Renal indices to differentiate prerenal and intrinsic renal failure

Indices	*Prerenal*	*Intrinsic*
Urine osmolality (mOsm/L)	>400	<400
Urine sodium (mEq/L)	<20	>20
Urine/Plasma creatinine	>20	<10
Fractional excretion of sodium (FE_{Na})	<1%	>2%
Urinalysis	Normal	Hematuria, proteinuria, or casts

MANAGEMENT [2,3]

Diagnosis and management of acute renal failure should proceed simultaneously to correct the underlying cause as quickly as possible. Management of acute renal failure involves appropriate management of fluid balance, electrolyte status, acid-base balance, nutrition, and initiation of renal replacement therapy. Placement of a Foley catheter to monitor urine output greatly enhances the management. **Hypovolemia** should be corrected aggressively by replacing blood or fluid losses.

FLUID AND DIURETIC CHALLENGE TEST

Fluid challenge followed by diuretics should be considered if intravascular volume depletion is suspected. In newborns suspected to have acute renal failure, normal saline 10-20 ml/kg can be given over 1 hour if there is no evidence of fluid overload followed by 1mg/kg of furosemide over 30 min. No response suggests intrinsic or postrenal failure.

Once the diagnosis of intrinsic renal failure is established, conversion of oliguric to nonoliguric failure by stimulating urine output using diuretics does not significantly alter the course of acute renal failure but it makes the management of acute renal failure easier. Furosemide (1-5 mg/kg/dose) increases urine flow rate, decreases intratubular obstruction, and minimizes oxygen consumption by the damaged tubules by inhibiting Sodium-Potassium-ATPase. If the neonate does not respond to diuretic therapy, continued high doses of diuretics is not justified and may put the neonate at risk for ototoxicity. In neonates unresponsive to diuretics, continuous infusions may be more effective, and may cause less toxicity than the bolus administration.

Infusion of low dose **dopamine** (0.5 to 5 mcg/kg/min) to improve renal perfusion and urine output after a hypoxic ischemic insult or toxic injury is a common practice but there are no definitive studies that "renal" dose of dopamine is effective in decreasing the mortality or the need for dialysis.

For persistent **hypotension** (e.g. septic shock, congestive heart failure) consider vasopressor (dopamine and/or dobutamine) treatment and echocardiogram to assess cardiac function. Serum potassium should be monitored closely and to be treated aggressively, if present. **Metabolic acidosis** is corrected using NaHCO3, 1-3 mEq/kg/d IV or PO divided three times a day.

Fluid management in newborns with acute renal failure includes meticulous monitoring of all fluids and **electrolytes**, and renal and nonrenal output. Once intrinsic renal failure has become established and the infant is normovolemic, restrict fluid intake to insensible losses plus urine output (Insensible water loss: Term infant on days 1-3: 0.7-1.0 mL/kg/h, Preterm infant: 2.0-2.5 mL/kg/h). Urine output needs to be replaced milliliter for milliliter with electrolytes matched to urinary electrolytes, usually with 0.2-0.45% NaCl. All other output is also replaced milliliter for milliliter based on fluid composition. Strict intake and output measurements, daily weights, frequent monitoring of electrolytes especially for potential hyperkalemia or hyponatremia are essential for appropriate fluid management. Use of radiant warmer should be considered to augment insensible water loss in presence of fluid overload. Drug doses should be adjusted for the degree of renal failure, and should be dosed only by trough levels where possible. Adequate nutrition (at least 100 kcal/kg/d) should be provided and hypertension if present also should be treated.

RENAL REPLACEMENT THERAPY OPTIONS

Peritoneal Dialysis

It is one of the most commonly used options for renal replacement therapy and is indicated when conservative treatment has been unsuccessful in correcting the complications of acute renal failure i.e. refractory hyperkalemia, severe fluid overload, refractory metabolic acidosis, and refractory severe or symptomatic uremia. Peritoneum is semipermeable to proteins but freely permeable to electrolytes, glucose and urea. Peritoneal dialysis is unlikely to cause disequilibrium syndrome as it corrects electrolyte disturbances relatively slowly. It is relatively easy to perform, does not require heparinization, and the neonate does not need to be hemodynamically stable to undergo peritoneal dialysis. One should consult nephrology if peritoneal dialysis is indicated.

Continuous Renal Replacement Therapy (CRRT)

Continuous arteriovenous or venovenous hemofiltration, and continuous arteriovenous or venovenous hemodialysis: provides precise control of fluid removal and better tolerated by hemodynamically unstable patients. Less commonly used.

Hemodialysis

Fastest way to correct metabolic abnormalities and fluid overload but the disadvantages include need for heparinization, vascular access, and skilled personnel. Hemodialysis is employed more often to treat metabolic disorders associated with hyperammonemia because it is more effective to clear solute from the body than either peritoneal dialysis or any type of CRRT.

Prognosis

Outcome of the newborns with acute renal failure is dependent on the underlying cause of the renal failure. Most of the neonates who receive the appropriate treatment for renal failure have an excellent prognosis. Newborn infants with nonoliguric acute renal failure have better outcome compared to infants with oliguric renal failure. Infants with intrinsic renal failure have a poorer prognosis than other groups and for infants with congenital urinary tract obstruction the outcome depends on the degree of renal dysplasia.

REFERENCES

1. Vogt BA, Davis ID, Avner ED: The kidney, In Klaus MH, Fanaroff AA (eds): Care of the High Risk Neonate, 5th ed, Philadelphia, W.B. Saunders 2001, pp 425-446.
2. Andreoli SP: Acute Renal Failure, Current Opinion in Pediatrics 2002;17:713-717.
3. Karlowicz MG, Adelman RD: Acute renal failure in the neonate, Clin Perinatol 1992; 19:139-158.

27 RETINOPATHY OF PREMATURITY

Amuchou Singh Soraisham

DEFINITION

Retinopathy of prematurity (ROP) is a vasoproliferative disorder of the eye affecting premature infants. It is an important cause of visual impairment and blindness in children in the world. ROP accounts for between 5-40% of childhood blindness.[1,2] Retinopathy of prematurity, formerly known as **retrolental fibroplasia**, was originally described in 1942 by Terry who first suggested the association with premature birth.[3] In 1952, Campbell, a pediatrician in Melbourne, Australia, provided the first link between the use of oxygen and ROP.[4] She suggested that the toxic effects of uncontrolled supplemental **oxygen** to newborns were responsible for the epidemic of ROP.

INCIDENCE

The incidence of ROP is inversely proportional to the gestational age and birth weight. The overall incidence of ROP in infants < 1251 gm in **CRYO-ROP** study was 65% and for infants with <1000 gm, the incidence was about 80%.[5] The incidence of ROP decreases to about 10% in infants with birth weight >1500 gm. The incidence of ROP in survivors at 23 completed weeks was 71.4%; at 24 weeks was 70.7%; at 25 weeks was 45.5%, at 26 weeks was 44.6%; at 27 weeks was 35.4%; and at 28 weeks was 18.6%.[6] Severe forms of ROP have been reported in bigger and more mature infants in developing countries.[7,8] Threshold or worse ROP was reported in

124/275 eyes (45.1%) in infants >1250 gm in a recent report from India.[8]

ETIOLOGY

The exact cause of developing ROP is not known. The occurrence of ROP is linked strongly to the degree of prematurity, low birth weight, and exposure to supplemental oxygen.[9,10] In general, ROP occurs more in the white race than in black and more in male than in females.[11,12] Caucasian and Hispanic children developed a more aggressive ROP that tend to progress to retinal detachment.

A number of risk factors have been suggested as contributors to ROP although it is unclear whether these are truly independent risk factors or simply indicators of the compromised health of the neonate. These factors include respiratory distress, prolonged mechanical ventilation, bronchopulmonary dysplasia, number of blood transfusions, exchange transfusion, hypotension, hypercapnia, acidosis, patent ductus arteriosus, necrotizing enterocolitis, intraventricular hemorrhage and candida sepsis.[13-16] Recent reports suggest elevated glucose may also play a role in developing ROP.[17,18] No relation exists between ROP and maternal smoking, maternal alcohol intake[16] or exposure of the retina to light.[19] Maternal pre-eclampsia is associated with a favorable outcome for premature infants, perhaps because hypertension causes intrauterine stress and subsequent maturation of the eyes.[13] A recent study has estimated that **genetic factors** accounted for 70.1% of the variance in liability for ROP.[20]

PATHOGENESIS

During retinal development, retinal vascularisation originates from centre of optic disc and progresses radially outwards towards the ora serrata. In the human, retinal blood vessel development is initiated during the 4th month of gestation and reaches the retinal periphery just before birth. Mature vessels extend to the nasal ora serrata by 36 weeks of gestation and to the temporal ora serrata by 39-41 weeks.

The fundamental process underlying the development of ROP is **incomplete vascularisation** of the retina and the ophthalmoscopic findings stem from this arrested development. ROP is a biphasic disease consisting of an initial phase of vessel loss followed by a second phase of vessel proliferation.[21] The first phase of ROP develops at 30-32 weeks post conceptional age, regardless of the gestational age at delivery. ROP is initiated with delayed retinal vascular growth after premature birth. Insufficient vascularisation of the developing retina creates hypoxia, which causes the release of growth factors stimulating new and abnormal blood vessel growth. Second phase of ROP is characterized by hypoxia induced retinal neovascularisation and begins around 32-34 weeks post-menstrual age. New vessels form at the junction between the vascularised retina and avascular zone of retina. Over time, pathological growth of vessels produces a fibrous scar extending from the retina to the vitreous gel and lens. Retraction of this scar separates the retina from the retinal pigment epithelium, resulting in retinal detachment and blindness.

The current thought of pathogenesis of ROP is the two-phase mechanism regulated by certain growth factors. ROP develops because of abnormalities in both oxygen-regulated and non-oxygen-regulated factors, which affect both phases of the disease. **Vascular endothelial growth factor (VEGF)** is an important oxygen-regulated factor that, if suppressed, inhibits normal vessel growth, but in excess, precipitates retinal neovascularisation. A critical non-oxygen-regulated growth factor is **insulin-like growth factor (IGF-1)**. Similar to VEGF, low levels of IGF-1 prevent normal vessel growth (phase I), and higher levels allow neovascularization.[22]

Genetics may play a role in the development of ROP.[20, 23] But studies so far have found only associations, rather than casual relationships. Vannay *et al.*[24] conclude that VEGF -460TT/+405CC haplotype was more prevalent in the treated patients than in the untreated patients (13 of 86 versus 1 of 115; $p < 0.001$), and the association remained significant even after the adjustment for risk factors of ROP (gestational age, supplemental oxygen therapy and gender). Hutcheson *et al.*[25] studied Norrie disease gene sequence variants in an ethnically diverse population with ROP in the U.S., and found a weak association.

CLINICAL FEATURES

Staging of ROP

The original international classification of retinopathy of

prematurity (ICROP) was described first in 1984 and later expanded in 1987.[26,27] The original ICROP dealt with the early phases of the disorder and was based on several key observations essential in describing the retinopathy. These include: (a) the location of retinal involvement by zone, (b) the extent of retinal involvement by clock hour, (c) the stage or severity of retinopathy at the junction of the vascularized and avascular retina, (d) the presence or absence of dilated and tortuous posterior pole vessels (plus disease). ICROP was revised in 2005 and the aspects that differ from the original classification include introduction of, (e) the concept of a more virulent form of retinopathy observed in the tiniest babies (aggressive, posterior ROP), (f) a description of an intermediate level of plus disease (pre-plus) between normal posterior pole vessels and frank plus disease, and (g) a practical clinical tool for estimating the extent of zone I.[28]

a. *Location of Disease*

The retina is divided into three zones, centered on the optic disc.

Zone I: (the innermost zone) the posterior most region around the optic disc and macula, consists of a circle (Figure 27.1),

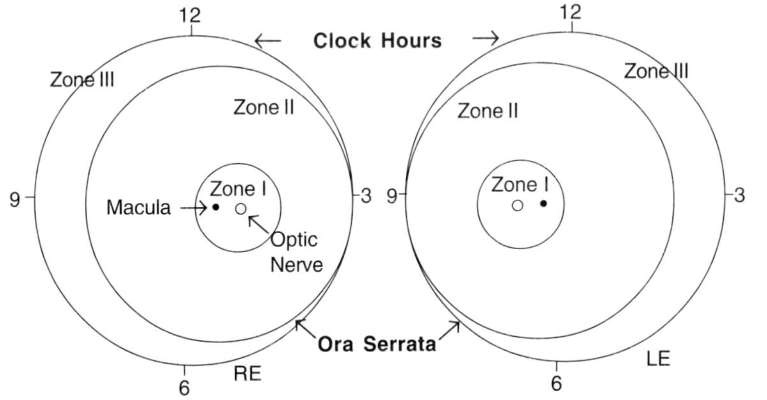

Fig. 27.1: Scheme of retina of right eye (RE) and left eye (LE) showing zone borders and clock hours used to describe the location and extent of retinopathy of prematurity (adapted the Committee for the Classification of Retinopathy of Prematurity)

with a radius of twice the distance from the macula to the optic disc, and is the most critical region for development of visual acuity.

Zone II: extends centrifugally from the edge of zone I to the nasal ora serrata (at the 3 O'clock position in the right eye and the 9 O'clock position in the left eye) and to approximately the equator on the temporal side.

Zone III: extends from the outer edge of zone II in a crescentic fashion to the ora serrata.

b. Extent of Disease

This is recorded as hours of the clock or as 30° sectors along the junction of the avascular and vascular portions of the retina.

c. Staging of the Disease

In a normal preterm infant, vascularisation of the retina is incomplete or "immature". On the basis of indirect ophthalmoscopy findings, ROP is classified into 5 stages:

Stage 1: Presence of clear demarcation line between the vascular and avascular portions of the retina.

Stage 2: Formation of a pink, ridge-like structure between the two regions.

Stage 3: Extra-retinal fibrovascular, fine vessels are seen growing from the ridge-like structure into the vitreous.

Stage 4: Partial detachment of the retina, which could be extra-foveal (4a) or foveal (4b); and

Stage 5: Total retinal detachment.

d. Plus Disease

Plus disease is defined as presence of dilated and tortuous retinal blood vessels in the posterior pole of the eye in at least 2 quadrants of the eye.

In the revised ICROP 2005, the following has been added.

e. Aggressive Posterior ROP

Previously known as "rush disease", it is a rapidly progressive severe form of ROP. The fundus appearance is characterized by prominent plus disease and flat neovascularisation. This ROP bypasses the Stage 1, 2 and proceeds from immature retina directly to neovascular (Stage 3) disease. Without treatment, it may rapidly progress to partial retinal detachment (Stage 4) and complete retinal detachment (Stage 5).

f. Pre-plus Disease

Pre-plus disease is any vascular abnormalities of the posterior pole that are insufficient for the diagnosis of plus disease but that demonstrate more arterial tortuosity and more venous dilatation than normal.

SCREENING AND DIAGNOSIS

ROP is a preventable cause of blindness. It is important that ophthalmologists before discharge should examine all high-risk preterm infants. The American screening guidelines[29] for ROP are described below in Table 27.1. In developing countries "larger" and "older" preterm infants are now more likely to develop ROP, than in developed countries. Developing countries may require modification of this screening guideline. There is no consensus guideline for screening ROP in developing countries. Every unit uses their own modification depending on the incidence on ROP in their own neonatal units.

Routinely, examination of retina is performed using the binocular indirect ophthalmoscope (a head mounted scope with light source) and a lens for focusing. Recently, another method of screening ROP is by using **RetCam**, a camera used to photograph the retina of infants. This camera is being tested as a method for screening for ROP.[30]

Preparation Prior to ROP Screening

Pupils should be dilated at least 30 minutes before the examination to allow a view of the retina. The dilating eye drops most commonly used is Phenylephrine 1% and Cyclopentolate 0.2%, a combination of dilute Phenylephrine and Cyclopentolate. Topical Proparacaine (0.5%) or other anesthetic eye drops are applied immediately before the examination. Indirect ophthalmoscopy and/or direct ophthalmoscopy through an infant gonioscopy lens of the entire retina are performed.

Table 27.1: Screening guidelines for retinopathy of prematurity

Event	*Criteria*
• Screening	
	– All infants with a birth weight ≤1500 gram.
	– All infants with gestational age ≤30 weeks.
	– Infants with birth weight between 1500 gm and 2000 gm or gestation > 30 weeks with an unstable clinical course and who are thought to be high risk.
	– Initial examination: 4-6 weeks postmenstrual age (initial exam by 31 weeks postmenstrual age or 4 weeks chronological age, whatever is later).
• Follow-up examination	
	– As recommended by examining ophthalmologist on the basis of retinal finding. Suggested follow-up include:
	– ≤1 week follow up: For zone I; stage 1 or 2 ROP and Zone II stage 3 ROP.
	– 1-2 weeks follow up: Zone I; no ROP or regressing ROP and zone II stage 2 ROP.
	– 2 weeks follow up: Zone II; stage 1 and regressing ROP.
	– 2-3 weeks follow-up: Zone II; no ROP or Zone III; stage 1 or 2 or regressing ROP.
• Conclusion of screening	
	– Based on age and retinal opthalmoscopic findings.
	– Attainment of 45 weeks postmenstrual age without prethreshold ROP or worse.
	– Progression of retinal vascularisation in zone III without previous zone I or II ROP.
	– Full retinal vascularisation.
	– Regression of ROP.

TREATMENT

Treatment of ROP consists of destroying the portion of the retina that is unvascularised in order to preserve the rest of it. The rationale for why this works is thought to be that the avascular retina is a source of growth factors that promote abnormal neovascularisation. When the avascular retina is destroyed, the release of growth factors ceases, and neovascularisation involutes and regresses.[31]

a. Laser Photocoagulation and Cryotherapy

Laser photocoagulation and cryotherapy are used in the treatment of severe ROP. However, laser photocoagulation is preferred over the cryotherapy. Long-term structural and functional outcomes suggest that laser photocoagulation is superior to cryotherapy. The difference is most dramatic in eyes with posterior ROP; favourable anatomic results have been reported in 83% of eyes treated with laser, whereas cryotherapy provided favourable outcomes in only 25% of eyes with zone 1 disease.[32-34] The clinical indication where cryotherapy is preferred instead of laser in the management of ROP includes poor fundus visibility (vitreous hemorrhage or anterior segment problems) and lack of availability of laser.[35] Cryotherapy is a painful and inflammatory procedure. Adverse effects include conjunctivitis, eyelid swelling, hypotony, infection, glaucoma and retinal detachment. The most common complication of laser is undertreatment, or 'skip areas' leading to continued abnormal vascularity with progression to retinal detachment. Although laser is less inflammatory than cryotherapy, adverse effects include anterior segment ischemia, hyphema, cataract, uveitis and burns in cornea, iris or tunica vasculosa lentis. Following the above procedures, topical cyclopegics, antibiotics and steroid drops are recommended for about 1 week.

Indication for Treatment

Early treatment of ROP **(ETROP)** before **threshold ROP** improves the outcome.[36] Treatment of ROP is indicated for the following retinal findings:

1. Zone I ROP: Any stage with plus disease.
2. Zone I ROP: Stage 3 – no plus disease.

3. Zone II ROP: Stage 2 or 3 with plus disease.

Using this criteria in ETROP trial,[36] treatment of high risk prethreshold ROP showed a benefit of earlier treatment compared to conventional management in the primary outcome measures of grading visual acuity at 9 months corrected age (14.3% vs 19.8%, p <0.005) and a much greater benefit for structural outcome at 6 and 9 months corrected age (9% versus 15.6%, p<0.001).

b. Scleral Buckling and Vitrectomy

Scleral buckling and vitrectomy (with or without scleral buckling) are indicated for treatment of retinal detachment associated with ROP stages 4 and 5. Scleral buckling performed at an earlier stage of retinal detachment (i.e. peripheral detachment) could prevent progression of retinal detachment or lead to reattachment.[37] Lens sparing vitrectomy allows primary retinal reattachment in at least 90% of eyes with stage 4A ROP.[38]

Surgery for stage 5 ROP remains controversial.[39] The natural history of stage 5 ROP is progression to no light perception vision. Some recent reports have shown that form vision can be obtained by vitrectomy for stage 5 ROP.[40] The use of intravitreal triamcinolone in vascularly active stage 5 ROP has been reported to increase success rate to 60%.[41]

PROGNOSIS

Most stage 1 and 2 ROP regresses. ROP in zone III usually have a good prognosis. The most serious long-term sequela of ROP is blindness. Infants treated for ROP may have some peripheral vision loss because of the destruction of peripheral retina. Despite early treatment for prethreshold ROP, 12% of eyes in ETROP study progressed to retinal detachment. Follow-up of infants treated with laser for ROP at 5.5 years found that 26% had required vitrectomy surgery, 18% had required cataract surgery, 20% had amblyopia and 10% required strabismus surgery for misaligned eyes.[42] Similarly, at the 15 years and final follow-up of the original CRYO ROP cohort, about 45% of cryo treated eyes and 64% of untreated control eyes were legally blind (visual acuity 20/200 or worse).[43] Therefore, it is recommended a close ophthalmologic follow-up be done regularly during the first several years of life for all preterm infants who had ROP during childhood.

PREVENTION

Prevention of ROP depends on the prevention of preterm delivery and its associated illnesses. Oxygen alone is neither sufficient nor necessary for development of ROP. However, restricted oxygen therapy may reduce serious ROP. Supplemental vitamin E for its antioxidant properties has been tried but do not reduce ROP.

REFERENCES

1. Gilbert C, Rahi J, Eckstein M, O'Sullivan J, Foster A: Retinopathy of prematurity in middle-income countries, Lancet 1997 Jul 5; 350:12-14.
2. Steinkuller PG, Du L, Gilbert C, Foster A, Collins ML, Coats DK: Childhood blindness, J AAPOS 1999; 3:26-32.
3. Terry TL: Extreme prematurity and fibroplastic overgrowth of persistent vascular sheath behind each crystalline lens: I preliminary report, Am J Ophthalmol 1942; 25: 203-204.
4. Campbell K: Intensive oxygen therapy as a possible cause of retrolental fibroplasia: A clinical approach, Med J Aust 1951; 2:48-50.
5. Palmer EA, Flynn JT, Hardy RJ, *et al.*: Incidence and early course of retinopathy of prematurity. The Cryotherapy for Retinopathy of Prematurity Cooperative Group, Ophthalmology 1991; 98:1628-40.
6. Hussain N, Clive J, Bhandari V: Current incidence of retinopathy of prematurity, 1989-1997, Pediatrics 1999; 104:e26.
7. Chen Y, Li X: Characteristics of severe retinopathy of prematurity patients in China: A repeat of the first epidemic? Br J Ophthalmol 2006; 90:268-71.
8. Vinekar A, Dogra MR, Sangtam T, Narang A, Gupta A: Retinopathy of prematurity in Asian Indian babies weighing greater than 1250 grams at birth: Ten-year data from a tertiary care center in a developing country, Indian J Ophthalmol 2007; 55:331-6.
9. Lutty GA, Chan-Ling T, Phelps DL *et al.*: Third International Symposium on Retinopathy of Prematurity: An update on ROP from the lab to the nursery, Mol Vis 2006; 12:532-80.
10. Chiang MF, Arons RR, Flynn JT, Starren JB: Incidence of retinopathy of prematurity from 1996 to 2000: Analysis of a comprehensive New York state patient database, Ophthalmology 2004; 111:1317-25.
11. Tadesse M, Dhanireddy R, Mittal M, Higgins RD: Race, Candida sepsis, and retinopathy of prematurity, Biol Neonate 2002; 81:86-90.
12. Yang MB, Donovan EF, Wagge JR: Race, gender, and clinical risk index for babies (CRIB) score as predictors of severe retinopathy of prematurity, J AAPOS 2006; 10:253-61.
13. Seiberth V, Linderkamp O: Risk factors in retinopathy of prematurity: A multivariate statistical analysis, Ophthalmologica 2000; 214:131-35.
14. Dutta S, Narang S, Narang A, Dogra M, Gupta A: Risk factors of threshold retinopathy of prematurity, Indian Pediatr 2004; 41:665-71.
15. Shah VA, Yeo CL, Ling YL, Ho LY: Incidence, risk factors of retinopathy

of prematurity among very low birth weight infants in Singapore, Ann Acad Med Singapore 2005; 34:169-78.

16. Arroe M, Peitersen B: Retinopathy of prematurity: Review of a seven-year period in a Danish neonatal intensive care unit, Acta Paediatr 1994; 83:501-05.
17. Ertl T, Gyarmati J, Gaál V, Szabó I: Relationship between hyperglycemia and retinopathy of prematurity in very low birth weight infants, Biol Neonate 2006;89:56-59.
18. Blanco CL, Baillargeon JG, Morrison RL, Gong AK: Hyperglycemia in extremely low birth weight infants in a predominantly Hispanic population and related morbidities, J Perinatol 2006; 26:737-41.
19. Phelps DL, Watts JL: Early light reduction for preventing retinopathy of prematurity in very low birth weight infants, Cochrane Database Syst Rev 2001; (1):CD000122.
20. Bizzarro MJ, Hussain N, Jonsson B, *et al.*: Genetic susceptibility to retinopathy of prematurity, Pediatrics 2006; 118: 1858-63.
21. Chen J, Smith LE: Retinopathy of prematurity, Angiogenesis 2007; 10:133-40.
22. Smith LE: Pathogenesis of retinopathy of prematurity, Growth Horm IGF Res 2004; 14 Suppl A: S140-4.
23. Csak K, Szabo V, Szabo A, Vannay A: Pathogenesis and genetic basis for retinopathy of prematurity, Front Biosci 2006;11:908-20.
24. Vannay A, Dunai G, Bányász I *et al.*: Association of genetic polymorphisms of vascular endothelial growth factor and risk for proliferative retinopathy of prematurity, Pediatr Res 2005;57:396-98.
25. Hutcheson KA, Paluru PC, Bernstein SL, *et al.*: Norrie disease gene sequence variants in an ethnically diverse population with retinopathy of prematurity, Mol Vis 2005; 11:501-08.
26. An international classification of retinopathy of prematurity. The Committee for the Classification of Retinopathy of Prematurity, Arch Ophthalmol 1984; 102:1130-34.
27. An international classification of retinopathy of prematurity. II. The classification of retinal detachment. The International Committee for the Classification of the Late Stages of Retinopathy of Prematurity. *Arch Ophthalmol* 1987;105:906-912.
28. An International Committee for the Classification of Retinopathy of Prematurity. The International Classification of Retinopathy of Prematurity revisited, Arch Ophthalmol 2005 Jul;123(7): 991-99.
29. Sections on Ophthalmology, American Academy of Pediatrics, American Academy of Ophthalmology and American Association of Pediatric Ophthalmology and Strabismus. Screening examination of premature infants for retinopathy of prematurity, Pediatrics 2006; 117:572-6. Erratum in: Pediatrics 2006; 118(3):1324.
30. Wu C, Petersen RA, VanderVeen DK: RetCam imaging for retinopathy of prematurity screening J AAPOS 2006; 10:107-11.
31. Drack A: Retinopathy of prematurity, Adv Pediatr 2006; 53:211-26.
32. Ng EY, Connolly BP, McNamara JA, Regillo CD, Vander JF, Tasman W: A

comparison of laser photocoagulation with cryotherapy for threshold retinopathy of prematurity at 10 years: Part 1. Visual function and structural outcome, Ophthalmology 2002; 109(5):928-34.
33. Connolly BP, Ng EY, McNamara JA, Regillo CD, Vander JF, Tasman W: A comparison of laser photocoagulation with cryotherapy for threshold retinopathy of prematurity at 10 years: Part 2. Refractive outcome, Ophthalmology 2002; 109:936-41.
34. Pearce IA, Pennie FC, Gannon LM, Weindling AM, Clark DI: Three-year visual outcome for treated stage 3 retinopathy of prematurity: Cryotherapy versus laser, Br J Ophthalmol 1998; 82:1254-59.
35. Quiram PA, Capone A Jr: Current understanding and management of retinopathy of prematurity, Curr Opin Ophthalmol 2007; 18:228-34.
36. Good WV: Early Treatment for Retinopathy of Prematurity Cooperative Group. Final results of the Early Treatment for Retinopathy of Prematurity (ETROP) randomized trial, Trans Am Ophthalmol Soc 2004; 102:233-48.
37. Hinz BJ, de Juan E Jr, Repka MX: Scleral buckling surgery for active stage 4A retinopathy of prematurity, Ophthalmology 1998; 105:1827-30.
38. Capone A Jr, Trese MT: Lens-sparing vitreous surgery for tractional stage 4A retinopathy of prematurity retinal detachments, Ophthalmology 2001; 108:2068-70.
39. Capone A Jr, Trese MT: Stage 5 retinopathy of prematurity: Then and now, Retina 2006; 26:721-23.
40. Mintz-Hittner HA, O'Malley RE, Kretzer FL: Long-term form identification vision after early, closed, lensectomy-vitrectomy for stage 5 retinopathy of prematurity, Ophthalmology 1997; 104:454-59.
41. Lakhanpal RR, Fortun JA, Chan-Kai B, Holz ER: Lensectomy and vitrectomy with and without intravitreal triamcinolone acetonide for vascularly active stage 5 retinal detachments in retinopathy of prematurity, Retina 2006; 26:736-40.
42. Repka MX, Summers CG, Palmer EA, Dobson V, Tung B, Davis B: The incidence of ophthalmologic interventions in children with birth weights less than 1251 grams. Results through 5-1/2 years. Cryotherapy for Retinopathy of Prematurity Cooperative Group, Ophthalmology 1998; 105:1621-27.
43. Palmer EA, Hardy RJ, Dobson V, *et al.*: Cryotherapy for Retinopathy of Prematurity Cooperative Group. 15-year outcomes following threshold retinopathy of prematurity: Final results from the multicenter trial of cryotherapy for retinopathy of prematurity, Arch Ophthalmol 2005; 123:311-18.

28 SURGICAL CONDITIONS IN THE NEWBORN

Manoj Biniwale

INTRODUCTION

Newborns may be born with congenital anomalies that need urgent surgical evaluation and intervention. Some of these anomalies can be detected prenatally and thus management of these fetuses should be started during pregnancy. Common surgical problems in the newborn are described in this chapter.

I. GASTROINTESTINAL TRACT

1. Esophageal Atresia/Tracheoesophageal (TE) Fistula

Incidence

It occurs in 1 to 2 per 5000 live births, although usually sporadic. Upto 70% have at least one other anomaly. It is most likely seen with **VACTERL** association – vertebral, anorectal, cardiac, tracheoesophageal, renal/genitourinary and limb structures.

Etiology

Abnormal infolding of foregut at four weeks of gestation leads to failure of separation of trachea from esophagus.

Clinical Features

Prenatal: Most cases are not diagnosed prenatally. Combination of maternal polyhydramnios and a small or absent stomach can lead to the diagnosis.[1] High resolution ultrasound or MRI of dilated upper pouch in the neck can be diagnostic.

Postnatal: Infant usually has symptoms depending on the type of TE fistula (Table 28.1).

Diagnosis

In most of the infants diagnosis is made in the immediate postnatal period. Inability to pass nasogastric tube distally is diagnostic. Chest radiograph demonstrates coiling of radio-opaque catheter in the upper pouch. Presence of luminal gas below the diaphragm establishes diagnosis of distal fistula. H-type fistula is diagnosed much later while investigating for aspiration pneumonias. It can be diagnosed either by contrast injected through a tube positioned in the thoracic esophagus with the infant prone and in

Table 28.1: Types of esophageal atresia /TE fistula and the presentations

Type	*Percentage of cases*	*Presentation*
Esophageal atresia with distal TE fistula above carina	85%	Distended abdomen Excessive drooling Risk of reflux of gastric secretions into lung
Isolated esophageal atresia with no tracheal communication	8 - 10%	Scaphoid abdomen Excessive drooling
Isolated TE fistula – H type	4 - 5%	Often asymptomatic Coughing during feeding Aspiration pneumonia
Double TE fistula with separate attachments with upper and lower esophagus	1-2%	Distended abdomen
Upper pouch fistula	1-2%	Excessive drooling Risk of reflux of gastric secretions into lung Scaphoid abdomen Excessive drooling Salivary aspiration

Trendelenberg position or by rigid bronchoscopy. All infants with TE fistula need further work up including echocardiogram and renal ultrasound to rule out VACTERL association.

Management

Medications are administered for gastric acid blockade while infant is maintained in head up position. A small catheter is placed in the pouch for intermittent suction. Broad spectrum antibiotics are administered preoperatively. Spontaneous ventilation is preferred. Use of continuous positive airway pressure (CPAP) is contraindicated. For infants needing positive pressure ventilation, mean airway pressure should be kept as low as possible.

Surgical: Three types of repairs are performed depending on specific anatomic variant. Rigid bronchoscopy is performed prior to surgery to confirm diagnosis, location of fistula, number of fistulas, and assess structural status of trachea.

- *Primary:* Immediate single layer end to end anastomosis between proximal esophageal pouch and distal esophageal segment is done in majority of patients with small gaps. Laparoscopic repair can be done in selective cases.
- *Delayed primary:* Repair is delayed in these infants who have underlying complications.
- *Staged:* Infants with pure esophageal atresias and TE fistulas with long gaps are managed with this technique. Initial gastrostomy performed with ligation of fistula. Serial esophageal dilations are done followed by subsequent repair at 2 to 3 months of age. Infants with persistent long gaps defined by gap of greater than four vertebral bodies with segments in neutral position or two vertebral bodies with segments stretched toward each other are unsuitable for successful anastomosis. These infants require stomach, small intestine or colon for lengthening esophagus.

Complications

Anastomotic ischemia followed by fibrosis and stricture, anastomotic leak, recurrent fistula, aspiration pneumonias, and gastro-esophageal (GE) reflux are some of the known problems after surgery. Strictures are managed by periodic dilations; anastomotic leak, if persistent and severe, may necessitate second surgery.

Prognosis[2]

The prognosis depends on birth weight and presence of congenital heart disease (CHD) (Table 28.2). Larger infants without presence of CHD have better chances of survival. Prognosis is also poor in infants with chromosomal anomalies such as trisomy 21.

Table 28.2: Survival rates of infants with esophageal atresia/TE fistula based on birth weight and presence of CHD

Group	*Characteristics*	*Survival*
I	Birthweight>1500 g without major CHD	97%
II	Birthweight<1500 g or CHD	59%
III	Birthweight<1500 g and CHD	22%

2. Hypertrophic Pyloric Stenosis

Acquired condition in which circumferential muscle layer of pyloric sphincter becomes thickened, resulting in narrowing and elongation of the pyloric channel.

Incidence

It ranges between 0.1 to 1% in the population with male predominance of 4:1.

Multifactorial inheritance is described with risk of 19% in boys and 7% in girls if mother has pyloric stenosis and 5% in boys and 2.5% in girls if father has the disease.[3]

Etiology

It is largely unknown for this condition. It may develop from discoordination between gastric peristalsis and pyloric relaxation resulting in work hypertrophy of pylorus. Maternal and infant exposure to erythromycin has been identified.[4] Possible delay of pyloric sphincter development and primary abnormality of enteric nervous system have also been postulated as other theories.

Clinical Features

Typical presentation is at 3 to 6 weeks of age with progressive nonbilious projectile vomiting. Infants appear significantly dehydrated. Blood chemistry reveals hypochloremic, hypokalemic contraction **metabolic alkalosis** with paradoxical aciduria. Hypoglycemia can lead to seizures. Unconjugated hyperbilirubinemia may be present with normal liver function tests.

Diagnosis

Small mobile ovoid mass in epigastrium on physical exam can be diagnostic. Ultrasound of the abdomen in pyloric area showing overall diameter of 17 mm or more, muscular wall thickness of 4 mm or more, and channel length of 17 mm or higher strongly suggest the diagnosis. Narrow pyloric canal (**string sign**) can be demonstrated on upper gastrointestinal (GI) study in equivocal cases.

Differential Diagnosis

Viral gastroenteritis, gastroesophageal reflux, pylorospasm, congenital adrenal hyperplasia, metabolic disorders.

Management

Medical management includes fluid support with correction of electrolyte imbalance.

Surgical: Treatment of choice is **pyloromyotomy**. Minimally invasive laparoscopic approach is preferred. Feeding is started within 4 to 8 hours of surgery. Most infants are discharged within 24 to 48 hours after surgery. Complications, though rare, include gastric perforation, incomplete myotomy causing persistent vomiting, or complete obstruction.

Prognosis

Prognosis is excellent for short- and long-term outcomes.

3. Duodenal Atresia

Incidence

Its occurrence is 1 in 7000 live births.

Etiology

It is related to failure of recanalization of embryonic duodenum. It can be present as a luminal web or membrane, fibrous cord, or complete discontinuity between the segments. Incidence of associated congenital anomalies is 50 to 80%. Congenital heart disease and **trisomy 21** are most commonly associated conditions (30% each).[5] Other common associations include intestinal malrotation (20%), esophageal atresias and imperforate anus (10 to 20%) and genitourinary anomalies (11%).

Clinical Features

Prenatal: Majority of mothers present with polyhydramnios in pregnancy. Demonstration of two dilated fluid filled structures consistent with double bubble on ultrasound is diagnostic.

Postnatal: Infants present with bilious vomiting within first 24 hours. These infants typically have distention of only the upper abdomen.

Diagnosis

Plain radiograph of abdomen shows classic double bubble sign resulting from dilated stomach and duodenum. Distal intestinal tract is gasless.

Differential Diagnosis

Extrinsic obstruction due to malrotation with Ladd's bands, preduodenal portal vein, gastroduodenal duplications, cysts or pseudocysts of pancreas and biliary tree and annular pancreas.

Management

Medical management includes nasogastric decompression, fluid and electrolyte replacement, and thorough evaluation of associated anomalies.

Surgical: Duodenal web is corrected by surgical excision and enteroplasty to widen lumen. True atresia and annular pancreas are managed by diamond duodenoduodenostomy between dilated proximal and small distal duodenum. Postoperative problems include delayed transit with dyskinetic proximal duodenum, gastroesophageal reflux and injury to biliary tree.

Prognosis

Survival rates are 95%. Morbidity and mortality are related to the associated anomalies.

4. Malrotation and Midgut Volvulus

Incidence

It is about 1 in 6000 infants.

Etiology

It is due to abnormal rotation and fixation of the bowel. It can be isolated or associated with other conditions such as congenital diaphragmatic hernia, intestinal atresia, gastroschisis and Beckwith-Weidemann syndrome.

Clinical Features

Half of the patients present within first month of life with bilious emesis. Infants who also have volvulus present with rectal bleeding and shock.

Diagnosis

Plain radiograph of abdomen showing dilated stomach with obstruction in sick appearing infant is diagnostic of volvulus. Upper GI series demonstrates the site of obstruction in second or third portion of duodenum appearing as bird's beak. Partial obstruction gives corkscrew appearance to the proximal jejunum. Malrotated duodenojejunal junction appears anterior, low, and midline or right of midline. Contrast enema should be done when results of upper GI are unclear.

Management

Volvulus presenting as an acute episode requires urgent surgical intervention. Time is critical to avoid bowel ischemia. Surgery includes evisceration of the bowel, detorsion of the volvulus, division of **Ladd's bands**, widening mesenteric base, relieving duodenal obstruction, appendectomy and nonrotational return of bowel to abdomen.

Prognosis

Mortality of operative correction is 3 to 9%. Prognosis worsens with volvulus, intestinal necrosis, prematurity and other anomalies. Recurrent volvulus occurs in less than 10% cases. Midgut volvulus accounts for 20% of cases of short gut syndrome.

5. Meconium Peritonitis

Etiology

It occurs from *in utero* bowel necrosis and intestinal perforation with meconium spillage into the peritoneal cavity. This could be secondary to meconium ileus, volvulus, atresia, peritoneal bands, gastroschisis or internal hernia. It is often associated with intestinal obstruction or mesenteric vascular occlusion. Tests for **cystic fibrosis** should be considered for infants with meconium ileus.

Clinical Features and Types

- **Fibroadhesive meconium peritonitis:** Meconium in the peritoneal cavity along with intestinal necrosis can cause inflammatory reaction leading to calcification and scarring sealing off of the perforation. It is associated with intestinal obstruction. Abdominal radiograph reveals calcification in the affected area.
- **Meconium pseudocyst:** Loop of bowel and necrotic tissue can scar leading to fibrous tissue surrounding the meconium causing pseudocyst formation.
- **Meconium ascites:** If perforation occurs just prior to birth then large amount of meconium stained fluid fills the peritoneal cavity leading to ascites.
- **Infected meconium peritonitis:** Intestinal perforation may not seal and may allow seeding of microorganisms in the peritoneal cavity.

Management

If perforation is sealed and infant is asymptomatic without any signs of obstruction, no surgical intervention is required. Surgical management for bowel obstruction includes laparotomy with resection of bowel or temporary intestinal diversion or both. Volvulus can be relieved by untwisting bowel. Resection is required for necrosis, atresia or perforation of bowel. Postoperatively infants receive parenteral nutrition, electrolyte replacement, nasogastric decompression, and antibiotic therapy. Ostomy irrigation can facilitate further meconium evacuation. Bowel function usually returns in 3 to 5 days. Surgical closure with reanastomosis can be delayed upto 4 to 6 weeks in premature infants.

Prognosis

Survival rates are near 100% due to advances in surgical techniques and postoperative care. Infants in whom removal of part of bowel is necessary are at risk for short gut syndrome.

6. Hirschsprung Disease

Incidence

It is the most common cause of intestinal obstruction in the neonate. It occurs in 1 in 5000 births with male to female ratio of 3.4:1. Down syndrome is the most common associated anomaly occurring in 8 to 16% of patients. Familial Hirschsprung disease is present in 4 to 8% of cases.[6] Other associations include heterochromia, **Waardenburg syndrome**, congenital deafness, 13q deletion, pheochromocytoma, neurofibromatosis and neuroblastoma.

Etiology

Failure of complete cranial to caudal migration of neural crest cells at 8 to 10 weeks of gestation leads to an aganganglionic segment with no parasympathetic intervention to distal colon. Thus it leads to abnormal peristalsis and functional constipation in infants.

Only rectosigmoid portion is involved in 75 to 80% of cases whereas 5 to 10% of patients have complete colonic involvement. Normal intestine proximal to the **aganglionic segment** gets thickened due to excess stimulation.

Clinical Features

Infants present with abdominal distention and no passage of meconium in 24 hours. Physical examination reveals a large soft distended abdomen. Rectal examination can produce explosive stool. Some infants may present with foul smelling liquid stools or bloody diarrhea. About 10% of patients present in the post-neonatal period with Hirschsprung associated enterocolitis. These infants present with fever, abdominal distention, vomiting, explosive diarrhea and sepsis.

Differential Diagnosis

Distal ileal atresia, colonic atresia, meconium ileus.

Diagnosis

Contrast enema is diagnostic in 80% of cases. Findings include a rectum with smaller diameter than sigmoid colon, a **transition zone**, normal caliber colon and failure to completely evacuate contrast at the 24 hours delayed film. Definitive diagnosis is made by demonstrating absence of ganglionic cells on acetylcholinesterase staining along with hypertrophy of nerve trunks.

Management

Most patients undergo diverting colostomy proximal to transition zone in the neonatal period followed by definitive treatment by laparoscopy Soave pull through of colon at 6 to 12 months of age. Routine anal dilations are recommended in selective cases to avoid further narrowing. Postoperative complications include strictures, enterocolitis, retained aganglionic segment leading to constipation and anal sphincter achalasia.

Prognosis

Approximately 90% patients achieve normal or near normal bowel function.

7. Imperforate Anus

Incidence

It occurs in 1 of 5000 newborns. It could be associated with other one or more VACTERL anomalies including genitourinary (20% to 50%), gastrointestinal (13%), cardiac (10%), skeletal (5%) or central nervous system (6%). Tethered cord is associated with 25% of cases.

Etiology

Failure of normal separation and division of the cloaca into anterior urogenital sinus and posterior intestinal canal.

Types

Previous terminology included high, intermediate and low. Recent terminology divides type according to location of rectal fistula as this has both prognostic and clinical implications.

Males: More than 80% of male patients have fistulous connections between rectum and urinary tract. It can be rectovesical, rectoprostatic or rectobulbar depending on position. If fistula opens onto perineal skin it is called perineal fistula. Unusually in patients with Down syndrome, the rectum ends blindly in the pelvis.

Females: In perineal fistula, it opens on the perineal skin anterior to the anal dimple. Vestibular fistula opens in the posterior aspect of introitus outside hymen. A cloaca is a complex malformation of rectum, vagina and urethra.

Clinical Features

Diagnosis is made on the first clinical examination. Anal opening may be normal if only rectal atresia is present. Those babies present with abdominal distention and failure to pass meconium. Rocker bottom perineum suggests sacral agenesis and carries poor prognosis with fecal incontinence. In the male infant presence of a well developed midline groove between buttocks, a prominent anal dimple and meconium exiting from fistula anterior to the sphincter are indicative of perineal fistula. On the other hand infant with rectourethral fistula presents with flat buttocks with no perineal opening and passage of meconium through urine. In the female infant a single perineal opening in place of urethra indicates cloaca where as normal urethra with opening in the vestibule is seen in the infant with rectovestibular fistula.

Management

Infants can be managed by the type of fistula they have (Figures 28.1 and 28.2). Two important decisions are made within first 24 hours of life. First is whether the infant needs colostomy versus definitive repair and other is to determine whether associated urogenital anomalies need more urgent attention. It takes upto 24 hours for enough pressure to build up in the colon to push meconium out of perineal fistula. Cross table lateral film is obtained for infants when diagnosis is in doubt. Distance is measured from anal dimple marked by lead marker and end of dilated bowel loop. Primary repair is attempted if distance is less than 1 cm. Main purpose of colostomy in patients who do not qualify for definitive repair is to provide immediate relief of bowel obstruction. Postoperatively feeding is begun once colostomy is functioning. Anal dilations are performed after 2 to 3 weeks of surgery in patients who have anorectoplasty and continued upto 6 to 12 months.

Prognosis

These patients need life-long follow-up. Common post-operative

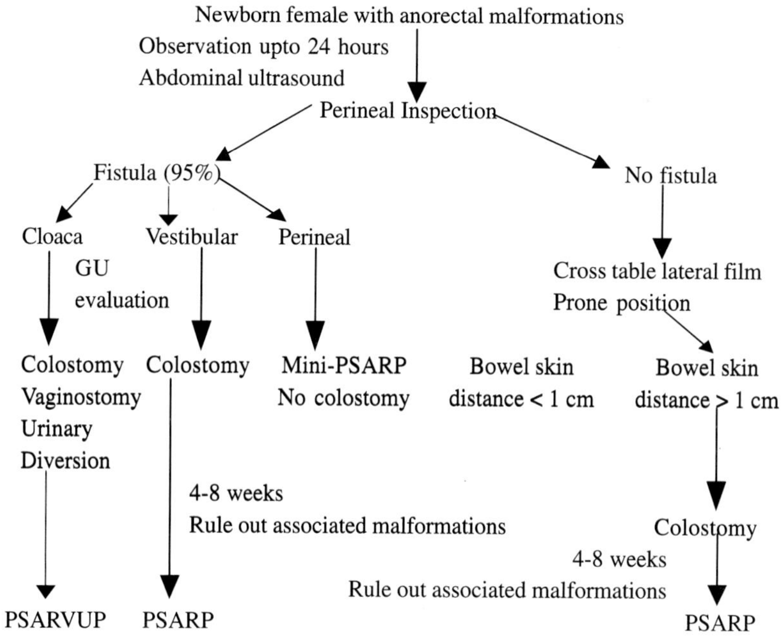

Fig. 28.1: Management of anorectal malformations in female neonates (Modified from[7])

PSARP–Posterior sagittal anorectoplasty, PSARVUP—Posterior sagittal anorectal vaginourethroplasty.

problems include perianal excoriation, constipation and fecal incontinence (25%). In female patients who have cloacae, the presence of urinary incontinence frequently requires diversion (20%) or intermittent catheterization (20 to 30%).

8. Abdominal Wall Defects [7]

Most common abdominal wall defects seen in newborns are omphalocele and gastroschisis. Comparison of these two conditions is shown in Table 28.3.

A. Omphalocele

Etiology

Omphalocele results from a failure of umbilical ring to contract leaving a round defect of variable size. Failure of closure is related to the aberrant development and migration of abdominal wall

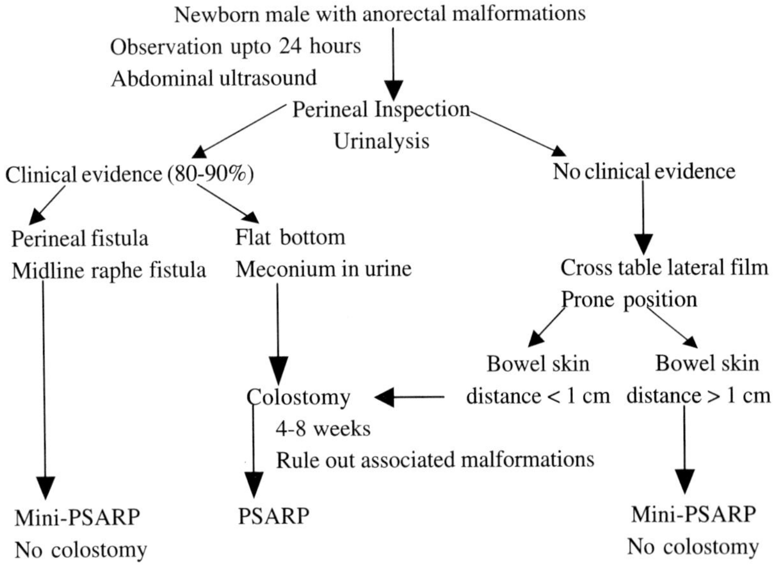

Fig. 28.2: Management of anorectal malformations in male neonates (Modified from[7])
PSARP – Posterior sagittal anorectoplasty.

muscular components by 18 weeks of gestation or to a failure of the developing midgut to return to the abdominal cavity by 11 weeks of gestation. Amnion covered sac contains intestines along with parts of liver. Rarely the defect extends to produce a complex deformity called as **Pentalogy of Cantrell**: Sternal, diaphragmatic and pericardial defects, upper abdominal omphalocele and ectopia cordis. Other syndromes associated with omphalocele include VACTERL association, **Beckwith-Weidemann syndrome** (macrosomia, macroglosia, visceromegaly, hemihypertrophy, hypoglycemia, renal defects) and **OEIS complex** (omphalocele, exstrophy, imperforate anus and spinal defects).[8]

Clinical Features

It can be diagnosed accurately by prenatal ultrasound in second trimester. Careful examination is recommended because of the risk of having other anomalies. Amniocentesis is performed to rule out chromosomal abnormalities.

Postnatally defect can be small (<5 cm) or large. Large omphaloceles frequently contain liver in addition to bowel.

Table 28.3: Comparison of gastroschisis and omphalocele (Modified from[9])

Characteristic	*Gastroschisis*	*Omphalocele*
Incidence	1 in 4,000 to 20,000	1 in 3,000 to 10,000
Maternal age	Younger	Older
Male to female ratio	1:1	3:1
Location of defect	Right of umbilical cord	Within umbilical cord
Umbilical cord	Intact and normal	Within covering sac
Size of defect	<4 cm	>4 cm
Organs in defect along with intestines	Stomach	Liver, spleen, bladder, uterus, ovaries
Covering sac	Absent	Present
Appearance of bowel	Matted, foreshortened, edematous	Normal
Additional anomalies	10 to 20%	45 to 80%
- GI	Intestinal atresia, midgut volvulus, intestinal stenosis	Rare
- Non GI	Rare	Cardiac (25%), GU (20%), Craniofacial (20%), diaphragmatic hernia (12%)
- Chromosomes	Normal	Trisomies common
- Syndromes	None	Beckwith-Wiedemann syndrome, Pentalogy of Cantrell
Surgery	Primary closure in 80%	Primary closure for defects <5 cm otherwise multistaged repair
Bowel function after surgery	Slow	Normal to slow
Survival	>90%	90% in absence of anomalies, 60 to 70% with other anomalies

Management

Small lesions may be delivered vaginally. Larger defects warrant C-section for delivering these infants without risk of rupturing the sac. A careful assessment of physiologic status is necessary to guide anesthetic management and identify prognostic factors. Abdominal wall closure can be done in a primary or staged repair.

Prognosis

Mortality can be as high as 30 to 40% mainly related to underlying complications. Factors affecting survival include large defect, ruptured sac, low birth weight, presence of additional congenital anomalies and early respiratory failure. Complications include gastrointestinal dysmotility, bowel obstruction, perforation of viscus, GE reflux and sepsis.

B. Gastroschisis [9]

Etiology

Exact mechanism is unknown but it is thought be due to a defect in abdominal wall related to vascular injury. Involution of the right umbilical vein creates a potential weak spot at the junction of the right aspect of umbilical ring and abdominal wall. Teratogenic exposures such as solvents, aspirin, ibuprofen, pseudoephedrine and cocaine can cause increased risk of developing gastroschisis in the fetus.[10] Partial closure of the defect can cause constriction around intestinal mesentery leading to luminal lymphatic and venous flow obstruction. It can further cause impaired absorption, reduced brush border enzyme synthesis and motility disorder related to rigidity of the bowel wall.

Clinical Features

Prenatal ultrasound can accurately detect the defect at second trimester screening. Amniocentesis is not necessary as there are no associated anomalies. Amniotic alpha fetoprotein is elevated in these fetuses.

Postnatally defects are visualized at right side of umbilicus with eviscerated intestinal loops prolapsing without a covering sac. The umbilical cord is intact. Intestinal loops may be thickened, foreshortened or covered with a fibrous peel.

Management

Early delivery after lung maturation followed by repair may improve intestinal function and help reduce morbidity. Almost all the infants are delivered vaginally without any problems. Emergent closure or coverage of the defect is the highest priority to limit intestinal injury. Transparent surgical bowel bag is placed around the infant immediately after delivery. A gastric decompression tube is placed to prevent intestinal dilation. The defect can be repaired by primary or staged closure depending on size discrepancy and the infant's physiologic status. Placement of temporary prosthetic silo allows for more gradual reduction of intestine into abdominal cavity.

Prognosis

More than 90% survive with good long-term health. Factors associated with a prolonged hospital stay include prematurity, low birth weight, staged silo repair and presence of intestinal atresia. Long-term problems include nonspecific abdominal pain, strictures and repeated abdominal surgery.

9. Necrotizing Enterocolitis

Necrotizing enterocolitis can lead to bowel ischemia and perforations needing surgical intervention in severe cases. Please see chapter on necrotizing enterocolitis for details.

10. Inguinal Hernia

Incidence

It is about 10 to 20 per 1000 live births. Incidence in extremely low birth weight premature infants is almost upto 30%. It is much more common in males and can be associated with undescended testes.

Etiology

In premature infants the inguinal canal is extremely short and has not developed an oblique direction through the abdominal wall. The external ring is situated almost directly over the internal ring. Testes usually descend into scrotum by 32 weeks of gestation. Contraction of the female inguinal canal and narrowing of the canal of Nuck occurs at a similar gestational age. Increase in intra-abdominal pressure in the preterm infants prior to contraction of the inguinal canal predisposes them to have the hernia. Some of the other associations include exstrophy of the bladder, Ehlers-Danlos syndrome, prune belly syndrome, and ventriculo-peritoneal shunts.

Clinical Features

Premature infants who have received positive pressure ventilatory support are at risk for developing inguinal hernia during their second month of stay in the neonatal intensive care unit (NICU). There is usually a history of an intermittent bulge appearing in the groin, scrotum, or labia, especially noted at times of increased intra-abdominal pressure, such as crying or straining. If a loop of bowel becomes entrapped in a hernia, the infant becomes extremely irritable and develops intense pain, followed by signs of intestinal obstruction. If the hernia is not reduced, the blood supply may be compromised (strangulated hernia), leading to perforation and peritonitis.

Differential Diagnosis

A hydrocele is differentiated from a hernia by the ability to palpate above the mass and not feel continuity between the scrotal hydrocele and the inguinal canal at the level of the internal ring. Occasionally an acute hydrocele of the cord cannot be differentiated clinically from an incarcerated inguinal hernia, and surgery is required. A transilluminant mass does not rule out an incarcerated hernia. Torsion of the testicle may also be misdiagnosed as an inguinal hernia. There is acute, severe pain with vomiting. Examination reveals an exquisitely tender mass in the inguinoscrotal region that does not extend through the internal ring into the inguinal canal.[11]

Management

All infants with inguinal hernia require referral to a pediatric surgeon because of the high incidence of complications. Unlike umbilical hernias, inguinal hernias do not spontaneously resolve and all must be repaired. These infants can be monitored in the NICU as long as the hernia remains reducible. Repair of the hernia is performed just prior to discharge or when the infant reaches

1800 to 2000 grams. Decision of contralateral exploration in infants with unilateral hernia is made by surgeons individually for each clinical situation.

Postoperative complications are almost always related to general anesthesia causing apnea, respiratory distress and failure of extubation requiring assisted ventilation. For selected premature infants caudal block can be used, instead of general anesthesia.

Prognosis

The prognosis is excellent, once repair is done. The risk of recurrence is rare.

II. RESPIRATORY SYSTEM

1. Choanal Atresia

Incidence

Its incidence is about 1 in 5000 live births. About two third of cases are unilateral. It is more common in girls and right side is affected more frequently than left side. About half of the patients have associated syndromes–**Apert**, **Treacher Collins**, **Down**, orofacial-digital, **Crouzon** and **CHARGE** (**C**oloboma, **H**eart Disease, Choanal **A**tresia, Mental **R**etardation, **G**enital Hypoplasia and **E**ar Anomalies).

Etiology

Obstruction can be secondary to membranous (10%) covering or dense cartilage (90%). Abnormal embryogenesis of neuro-ectodermal cell lines can lead to anomalies in CHARGE association.

Clinical Features

Classic presentation is cyanotic infant who gets better when cries. As the infants are predominant nose breathers they are at risk for respiratory failure if oral breathing is not established in a timely manner. Failure to pass a 6 Fr catheter through the nares into the nasopharynx is a simple diagnostic measure. CT scan or MRI is obtained to differentiate it from stenosis and to determine if atresia is bony or membranous.

Unilateral choanal atresia is usually asymptomatic and diagnosed in neonatal period only when the other nare is obstructed by catheter or feeding tube. These patients may remain asymptomatic for years and may present with respiratory distress associated with upper respiratory tract infections.

Management

Urgent establishment of oral airway or intubation is necessary for these infants to avoid hypoxia. It depends on severity of obstruction and presentation. Usually unilateral atresia is corrected at 4 to 5 years. In patients with bilateral atresia if oral airway is tolerated the repair is done at 4 to 6 weeks. If infant needs intubation then immediate repair is preferred. Tracheostomy is preferred in CHARGE patients. Repeated dilations may be necessary in infancy to maintain patency of nares.

Prognosis

Overall prognosis is good except in the patients with multiple anomalies.[12]

2. Congenital Diaphragmatic Hernia (CDH)

Incidence

It occurs in approximately 1 in 2500 to 5000 live births. Associated anomalies are seen in about 30 to 50% and chromosomal anomalies occur in 10 to 20% of infants. Eighty-five percent of defects occur due to a posterolateral defect on left side involving the **foramen of Bochdalek.**

Etiology

Failure of closure of embryonic pleuroperitoneal canal leading to a herniation of intestines at 8 weeks of gestation. The ipsilateral lung can be hypoplastic and shows decreased airway and alveolar numbers. Pulmonary artery is also smaller on affected side. Contralateral lung can also be abnormal with decrease in alveolar numbers.

Clinical Features

Prenatally it can be asymptomatic or can present as polyhydramnios. Prenatal ultrasound shows presence of abdominal viscera in left or right hemithorax above the level of inferior margin of scapula or at the level of four chamber view of heart. **Lung to head circumference ratio (LHR)** is used to predict severity of the condition. Newborns usually present with scaphoid abdomen, mediastinal displacement and varying degrees of respiratory distress depending on severity of pulmonary hypoplasia. Cardiac sounds are heard on the right and decreased breath sounds on the left. Infants may need mechanical ventilation. Pneumothoraces can occur due to the hypoplastic lung.

Diagnosis

Plain radiograph demonstrates presence of bowel loops in the hemithorax and the heart deviated to other side.

Management

Prenatal: Figure 28.3 show the algorithm for decisions in prenatal management of these infants. Fetoscopic balloon tracheal occlusion is being investigated for the most severe cases.[13] Another approach is the **exutero intrapartum treatment (EXIT)**-to-extracorporeal membrane oxygenation (ECMO) strategy reserved for high risk cases to avoid hypoxia, hypotension and acidosis.

Postnatal: Infants should be delivered at the tertiary care centers so that optimum ventilatory care and surgical expertise are available. One strategy is to have delayed repair to maximize infant's cardiovascular condition and decrease reactive pulmonary hypertension. ECMO has been used pre, intra and postoperatively to increase poor survival rate secondary to persistent pulmonary hypertension in the newborn (PPHN). Current management strategy is shown in Figure 28.4.

Prognosis

Survival has increased from 50 to 79% with advancement of perioperative care. Late complications include recurrence of hernia, pulmonary insufficiency, small bowel obstruction, GE reflux and thoracolumbar scoliosis. Infants are also at risk for cerebral injury leading to the developmental delay.

3. Congenital Malformations of the Lung

During the development of lungs a variety of bronchopulmonary

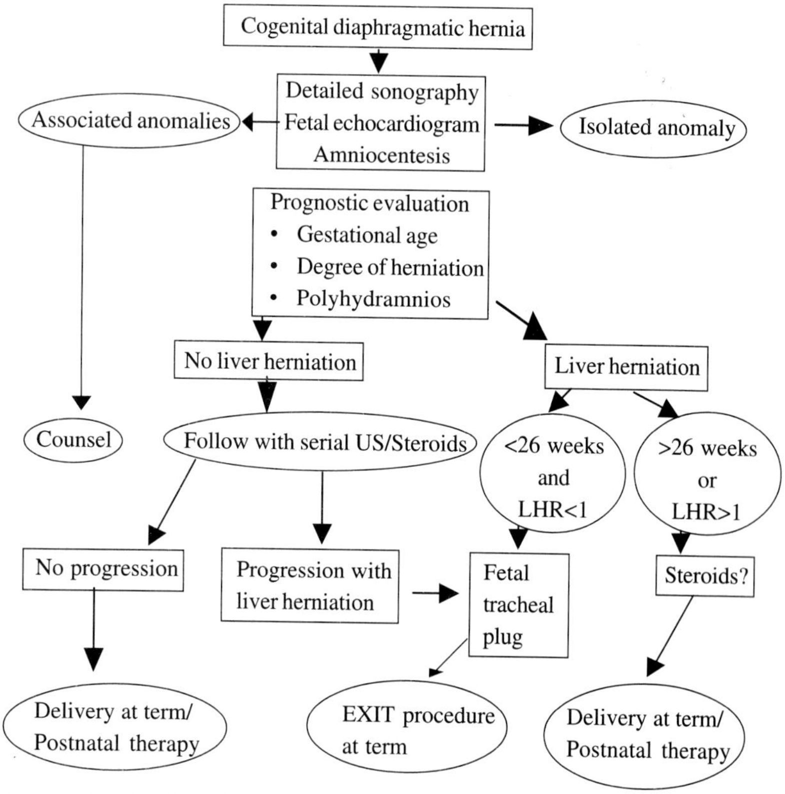

Fig. 28.3: Algorithm for prenatal management of congenital diaphragmatic hernia (Modified from[13])
EXIT: Exutero intrapartum treatment; LHR: Lung to head circumference ratio; US: Ultrasound.

malformations can occur from mesodermal and endodermal lung components.

A. Congenital Lobar Emphysema

It is the most common cystic malformation resulting from air trapping in one of the lobes of lung. Left upper lobe is most commonly involved followed by right middle or upper lobe. Deficiency of cartilage within large airway leads to overdistention of the affected lobe. Bronchial compression can also be caused by an external compression due to blood vessels or mediastinal masses. Infants can be asymptomatic or may have mild respiratory distress. Physical exam reveals decreased breath sounds in the

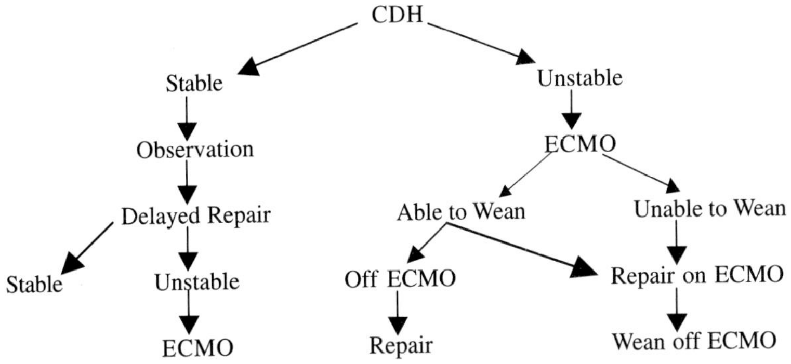

Fig. 28.4: Current algorithm for postnatal management of congenital diaphragmatic hernia (CDH)
ECMO: Extra corporeal membrane oxygenation.

affected area. Chest radiograph demonstrates a hyperinflated lobe causing mediastinal shift and compression of other areas of the lung. CT scan or MRI of the lungs along with angiography may be indicated to demonstrate vascularity of adjacent structures. Asymptomatic infants are monitored conservatively. Lobectomy is reserved for persistent symptomatic or severely affected infants.[14]

B. Congenital Cystic Adenomatoid Malformation (CCAM)

It presents as numerous cystic lesions composed of the lung tissue confined to a single lobe. It is caused by failure of mesenchyme to progress to normal bronchopulmonary development. It can be associated with polyhydramnios, hydrops and pulmonary hypoplasia. It manifests with respiratory distress at birth in about half of cases and worsens as cysts fill with air causing mediastinal shift. Majority of infants present by one year of age. Three types of CCAM are described based on size of the cysts—type I (2-10 cm), type II (0.5 to 2 cm) and type III (<0.5 cm). Prenatal treatment is offered for fetuses developing hydrops. Aspiration is performed for large cysts. Thoracoamniotic shunting is performed for recurrence. Solid type III CCAM can be resected by fetal surgery.[15] Infants are monitored closely for respiratory distress. Selective intubation is considered for unilateral CCAM to ventilate contralateral bronchus. Complete resection is recommended for the risk of complications. Resection can be delayed with close monitoring in asymptomatic neonates. Prognosis is excellent for type I (90% survival). Types II and III are associated with other anomalies and have 60% survival.

C. Bronchogenic Cyst

These cysts can be air filled or solid. The cysts can change in size depending on degree of obstruction. Majority are asymptomatic. Infants having multiple cysts usually present with some respiratory distress. Complications include stridor if pressing on the airway, pneumothorax or infection. Asymptomatic infants are managed conservatively while infants having symptoms due to pressure effects require resection.

D. Bronchopulmonary Sequestration

It occurs due to presence of non-functioning lung tissue lacking connection with bronchus and receiving blood supply from systemic vessels. Almost three-quarters of the lesions are intralobar (abnormal tissue within normal lung) and remaining lesions are extralobar (outside visceral pleura). These infants are often asymptomatic but occasionally cause respiratory distress and mediastinal shift. Over time, the sequestrations do not grow and eventually become smaller. Large or symptomatic lesions require resection.

III. CENTRAL NERVOUS SYSTEM

1. Myelomeningocele

Incidence

It affects 1 in 2000 live births. Supplementation of folic acid by the mother soon after conception decreases risk by 70%. Maternal diabetes and medication use (e.g. valproate and carbamazepine) may increase risk.

Etiology

Initial defective spinal cord development is caused by a mesodermal migration defect. Neurologic insult may also result from an abrasion of exposed spinal cord by the uterine wall or by constituents of amniotic fluid.

Classification

A. ***Meningocele:*** Meninges herniated through the defect form cystic structure filled with spinal fluid.
B. ***Myelomeningocele:*** Spinal cord along with meninges herniates through the defect.
C. ***Spina bifida oculta:*** Posterior arches of spines fail to fuse. It can be associated with tethering of the cord.

Clinical Features

Severity of the defect depends on extent of neural tissue involvement and level of the defect. Infants with defects in the cervical and thoracic region are not able to ambulate compared to those with defects involving lumbosacral and sacral region who can ambulate with or without short braces. Defects involving lumbar area require full braces and crutches. These infants are prone for hip dislocation, bladder and bowel problems and sensory deficits.

Diagnosis

Prenatal: Maternal serum alpha-fetoprotein (AFP) is diagnostic in 75% of cases. Elevation of the amniotic fluid AFP and acetylcholinesterase is indicative of a neural tube defect. Second trimester screening ultrasound identifies the structural defect. Lemon sign can be visualized on ultrasound in which frontal bones are scalloped inwards. Leg and foot movement should be assessed and full skeletal survey should be performed to rule out associated malformations. Fetal MRI can provide additional anatomic details of the defect.[16]

Postnatal: Clinical exam reveals the defect. CT scan or MRI should be done to rule out hydrocephalus and other associated anomalies.

Management

Prenatal: Surgical resection and covering of the defect are still experimental procedures with variable success rates.

Postnatal: The defect is covered with warm normal saline and a sterile dressing. Decision to perform surgical repair is based on a number of factors including size and location of lesion, technical feasibility of surgical closure, prognosis for ambulation, presence or absence of associated anomalies, availability of personnel and a facility to provide adequate care for the infant, infant's family structure, and attitude of the family toward the defect and its consequences. Usual decision is early closure within 72 hours. Ventriculoperitoneal shunt is placed at later stage for infants developing hydrocephalus. Long-term follow-up is arranged with neurosurgery, orthopedics and urology.

Prognosis

It depends on the level and extent of the defect and associated anomalies. These infants are at increased risk for developmental delay and learning disability.

2. Hydrocephalus

Hyrdocephalus develops when there is imbalance between the rate of cerebrospinal fluid (CSF) formation and absorption. It most commonly develops secondary to impaired absorption. Choroid plexus papilloma is the only exception where hydrocephalus is secondary to increased production of CSF. It is classified into obstructive and ex vacuo. Ex vacuo hydrocephalus is due to decrease in cerebral tissue volume and is not associated with macrocephaly (e.g. lissencephaly).

Etiology

Causes of **obstructive hydrocephalus** are enumerated in Table 28.4.

Clinical Features

Most infants present with rapid head growth, full and enlarged anterior fontanelles, and split cranial sutures. Advanced cases reveal prominent forehead, sparse hair and thin skull. Cracked pot sound appears on percussion of the head (Macewan sign). In infants with thin cortex transillumination may reveal accumulation of CSF. Paresis of abducens nerve can occur. These infants may also demonstrate "setting sun" sign with conjugate downward deviation of eyes.[17]

Diagnosis

Cranial ultrasound is the initial investigation of choice. CT scan or MRI is obtained to visualize the anatomic details.

Table 28.4: Types and etiology of obstructive hydrocephalus

Non-communicating
- Aqueductal stenosis
  - Aqueductal gliosis secondary to perinatal infection or bleeding
  - Viral infections (mumps, rubella, parainfluenza)
  - X-linked hydrocephalus (Bickers-Adams syndrome)
  - Autosomal recessive with VACTERL
- Atresia of foramen of Monro
- Dandy-Walker malformation (cystic transformation of fourth ventricle, agenesis of cerebellar vermis and enlarged posterior fossa)
- Arnold Chiari II malformation (caudal displacement of cerebellar tonsils, fourth ventricle, choroid plexus and medulla into cervical spinal canal)
- Agenesis of corpus callosum
- Posthemorrhagic hydrocephalus
- Intrauterine infection – toxoplasmosis, cytomegalovirus (CMV)
- Vein of Galen malformation
- Radiation exposure
- Maternal malnutrition
- Intraventricular neoplasm

Communicating
- Congenital absence of arachnoid granulation
- Leptomeningeal inflammation
- Group B streptococci ventriculitis
- Subarachnoid hemorrhage

Management

It depends on the cause of hydrocephalus. Most of the patients with hydrocephalus need extracranial shunting procedure. Ventriculoperitoneal shunt is usually the treatment of choice. Ventriculostomy is reserved for premature sick infants as a temporizing measure. These infants are followed by neurosurgery to monitor complications related to shunting procedures. Main complications include shunt infection and obstruction. Shunt infection usually occurs within months after placement of shunt. It is caused by skin microorganisms such as *Staphylococcus epidermidis* and is treated with vancomycin. As the child grows, these shunts also require periodic revisions.

Prognosis

These infants are at risk for neurodevelopmental disabilities. Visual problems, decrease in IQ, memory problems and behavioral problems are seen in these children.

3. Intracranial Hemorrhage

A. Subdural Hemorrhage

It is most often related to birth trauma. Related mechanisms include tear in dura due to precipitous delivery or instrumentation, breech delivery causing extension of neck leading to occipital diastasis, or rupture of bridging veins. Infants are born at term and present with lethargy, apneas, bradycardia, seizures, full fontanelle, unequal pupils or irritability. Diagnosis is confirmed by CT scan.

Management involves close monitoring, providing necessary respiratory support and surgical intervention for infants demonstrating significant neurological signs. Severe bleeding is associated with a poor outcome. Less severe cases which are recognized early have normal outcome (80% to 90%). About 10% to 15% have hydrocephalus requiring shunt placement.

B. Subarachnoid Hemorrhage

Small subarachnoid bleeds most frequently occur in premature infants (7%). It can be secondary from leaking of blood after intraventricular hemorrhage. Infants are often asymptomatic but rarely present with seizures.[18] Diagnosis is by CT scan and management is supportive. These infants carry a good prognosis.

C. Cerebellar Hemorrhage

It is more common in very premature infants.[19] Infants may have symptoms related to brainstem compression and present with apneas, bradycardia and lateral deviation of eyes. Diagnosis is made by posterior fontanelle ultrasound. Management is usually supportive. Follow-up MRI may show cerebellar atrophy. Infants may have long-term neurodevelopmental problems.

D. Intraventricular Hemorrhage

It is common in premature infants and is discussed in a separate chapter.

IV. GENITOURINARY SYSTEM

1. Posterior Urethral Valves (PUV)

Incidence

It is the leading cause of prenatally diagnosed urinary tract obstruction with an incidence of 1 in 5000 births.

Etiology

It is caused by a thin membrane of tissue in the posterior urethra that further causes an obstruction to urinary flow out of the bladder. Some authors postulate that these valves result from anomalous development of the mesonephric duct, while others believe that they originate from the urogenital sinus.

Clinical Features

Usually these patients are admitted to the NICU after prenatal diagnosis of suspected PUV. Postnatally these infants may present with poor urinary stream, urinary tract infection (UTI), an enlarged bladder, or failure to thrive. Severely affected infants present with sepsis, renal failure, respiratory distress, and electrolyte disturbances including hyponatremia and hyperkalemic metabolic acidosis.

Diagnosis

Urinary abnormalities are detected on prenatal ultrasound as early as 12 weeks of gestation. The findings supporting diagnosis of PUV include enlarged bladder, thickened bladder walls, posterior urethral dilation, bilateral hydronephrosis, and hydroureters. After birth evaluation should include renal ultrasound (including images of the ureters and bladder), **voiding cystourethrogram (VCUG)**, urinalysis, urine culture, and serum electrolytes, creatinine and blood urea nitrogen. Renal ultrasound is done to assess the degree of hydronephrosis, bladder wall thickening, and posterior urethral dilatation. Renal ultrasound can also provide evidence of renal dysplasia. VCUG is the gold standard for the diagnosis of PUV; a diagnostic linear filling defect is seen in a markedly dilated posterior urethra. VCUG also confirms presence of vesicoureteral reflux (VUR) that occurs in 25-50% of patients with PUV.

Management

Prenatal: Percutaneous vesicoamniotic shunting is offered prenatally in fetuses with no evidence of pulmonary hypoplasia. Alternatively, vesicostomy can be done in fetuses in which vesicoamniotic shunting has failed to resolve urinary obstruction.

Postnatal: After delivery, the treatment of infant should start promptly to provide respiratory support, fluid resuscitation if the patient is volume depleted, correction of electrolyte abnormalities, and initiation of antibiotics, if clinically indicated. Insertion of a urinary catheter usually relieves acute obstruction. When the infant is stable, primary valve ablation with endoscopic incision of the PUV is the procedure of choice. Premature or small infants may not have a large enough urethra to insert an 8F resectoscope. These infants often require urinary diversion with a cutaneous vesicostomy. Urinary diversion is also done for persistent urethral dilatation after valve resection. Treatment should also include prophylactic antibiotics if associated with VUR.[20]

Prognosis

The prenatal detection of PUV before 24 weeks gestation results in a poorer prognosis with upto 50% chance of death secondary to pulmonary hypoplasia or long-term morbidity secondary to chronic renal failure. Other poor prognostic indicators include moderate or severe hydronephrosis and increased echogenicity or cystic changes indicating renal dysplasia. Although prenatal diagnosis allows for prompt intervention of the infant before septic and metabolic complications occur, the overall outcome of PUV may not improve significantly with prenatal treatment.

V. SOLID TUMORS

1. Neuroblastoma

It constitutes more than 50% of tumors in newborns.[21] These tumors originate in neural crest cells. Most common primary site is adrenal gland. These infants present with abdominal mass, hypertension, heterochromia iridis, opsoclonus or subcutaneous nodules. It can be detected during a prenatal ultrasound. Urine homovanillic acid and vanillylmandelic acid levels are diagnostic as these tumors secrete catecholamines. Surgery, chemotherapy and radiation are offered depending on site and stage of tumors. Infants have better prognosis than older children with disease free survival of 75%.

2. Teratoma

These are the most common neonatal germ cell tumors. These tumors constitutes intermix of tissues belonging to more than one germ layer that originate from pluripotent stem cells. The most common tumors are sacrococcygeal teratomas. It presents as a mass in the region of buttocks. Infants may present with rectal or urinary obstruction and associated vertebral anomalies. Treatment is by surgical resection and outcome is excellent.

3. Wilm's Tumor

It usually manifests between ages 1 to 5 years but rarely can be diagnosed in the neonatal period.[22] Congenital anomalies are present in 15% of cases. Associations include congenital aniridia, hemihypertrophy, genitourinary anomalies, male pseudohermaphroditism and Beckwith-Weidemann syndrome. Treatment depends on the stage and the extent of the tumor. The prognosis is good in most of the cases when tumor is not aggressive.

4. Retinoblastoma

It is the most malignant tumor affecting eyes in neonates. About 50% of cases are diagnosed by leukokoria. Infants can also present with strabismus, decreased vision, secondary glaucoma, or spontaneous hyphema. Ultrasound, CT scan and MRI are done to identify calcification and extent of the tumor. Treatment depends on size and location. It includes combination of chemotherapy, surgery, radiation, thermotherapy, photocoagulation and cryotherapy. Limitation of tumor to the eye carries a good prognosis.[23]

REFERENCES

1. Stringer MD, McKenna KM, Goldstein RB, Filly RA *et al.*: Prenatal diagnosis of esophageal atresia J Pediatr Surg 1995;30:1258-1263.
2. Spitz L, Kiely EM, Morecroft JA, Drake DP: Esophageal atresia: At-risk groups for the 1990s J Pediatr Surg 1994; 29:723-725.
3. Mitchell LE, Risch N: The genetics of infantile hypertrophic pyloric stenosis: A reanalysis, Am J Dis Child 1993;147:1203-1211.

4. Mahon BE, Rosenman MB, Kleiman MB: Maternal and infant use of erythromycin and other macrolide antibiotics as risk factors for infantile hypertrophic pyloric stenosis, J Pediatr 2001;139:380-384.
5. Grosfeld JL, Rescorla FJ: Duodenal atresia and stenosis: Reassessment of treatment and outcome based on antenatal diagnosis, pathologic variance, and long-term follow-up. World J Surg 1993;17:301-309.
6. Holschneider A, Ure BM: Hýrschsprung's disease, In: Ashcraft KW, Murphy JP, Sharp RJ, Sigalet DL, Snyder CL (eds) Pediatric Surgery 3rd ed, WB Saunders Company, Philadelphia, PA 2000, pp 453-472.
7. Magnuson DK, Parry RL, Chwals WJ: Selected Abdominal Gastrointestinal Anomalies in Martin RJ, Fanaroff AA, Walsh MC Eds; Neonatal Perinatal Medicine: Diseases of the fetus and infant 8th ed, Elsevier Mosby, Philadelphia, PA 2006, pp 1381-1403.
8. Gilbert WM, Nicolaides KH: Fetal omphalocele: Associated malformations and chromosomal defects, Obstet Gynecol 1987;70:633-35.
9. Martin, C and Fishman S: Gastroschisis, In: Manual of Neonatal Surgical Intensive Care (Hansen A and Puder M), B.C. Decker, Inc Hamilton, ON 2003, pp 203-212.
10. Torfs CP, Katz EA, Bateson TF, Lam PK, Curry CJ: Maternal medications and environmental exposures as risk factors for gastroschisis, Teratology 1996;54:84-92.
11. Kapur P, Caty MG, Glick PL: Pediatric hernias and hydroceles, Pediatr Clin North Am 1998;45:773-789.
12. Hall BD: Choanal atresia and associated multiple anomalies, J Pediatr 1979;95:395-398.
13. Crombleholme TM: Selected Surgical treatment of the fetus in Martin RJ, Fanaroff AA, Walsh MC Eds; Neonatal Perinatal Medicine: Diseases of the fetus and infant 8th ed, Elsevier Mosby, Philadelphia, PA 2006, pp 231-254.
14. Bailey PV, Tracy T Jr, Connors RH, deMello D, Lewis JE, Weber TR: Congenital bronchopulmonary malformations, Diagnostic and therapeutic considerations, J Thorac Cardiovasc Surg 1990;99:597-602.
15. Duncombe GJ, Dickinson JE, Kikiros CS: Prenatal diagnosis and management of congenital cystic adenomatoid malformation of the lung, Am J Obstet Gynecol 2002;187:950-954.
16. Adzick NS, Walsh DS: Myelomeningocele: Prenatal diagnosis, pathophysiology and management, Semin Pediatr Surg 2003;12:168-74.
17. Kirkpatrick M, Engleman H, Minns RA: Symptoms and signs of progressive hydrocephalus, Arch Dis Child 1989;64:124-28.
18. Paneth N, Rudelli R, Kazam E, Monte W: Brain Damage in the Preterm Infant: Subarachnoid hemorrhage, Clin Dev Med 1994:131;138-162.
19. Merrill JD, Piecuch RE, Fell SC, Barkovich AJ, Goldstein RB: A new pattern of cerebellar hemorrhages in preterm infants, Pediatrics 1998;102:E62.
20. Becker A, Baum M: Obstructive uropathy, Early Hum Dev 2006;82:15-22.

21. Büyükpamukçu M, Varan A, Tanyel C, Senocak ME, *et al.*: Solid tumors in the neonatal period, Clin Pediatr (Phila) 2003;42:29-34.
22. Hrabovsky EE, Othersen HB Jr, deLorimier A, Kelalis P, Beckwith JB, Takashima J: Wilms' tumor in the neonate: A report from the National Wilms' Tumor Study, J Pediatr Surg 1986;21:385-387.
23. Chantada G, Fandiño A, Dávila MT, Manzitti J, *et al.*: Results of a prospective study for the treatment of retinoblastoma, Cancer 2004;100:834-842.

29

FOLLOW-UP OF HIGH RISK NEONATES

Abhay Lodha,
Heather Christianson
and Reg Sauvé

INTRODUCTION

Advancements in technology and improved obstetrics and neonatal care have made survival of extremely premature infants progressively more likely. Increasingly, these infants are thought to benefit from close longitudinal multidisciplinary follow-up to monitor their growth and development and to facilitate intervention when it is needed.

Neonatal care is based on a continuum, which extends from the antenatal period to the Neonatal Intensive Care Unit (NICU) and continues to the Follow-Up Clinic. Members of **Neonatal Follow-up Programs** typically provide detailed assessments of each infant's functioning in a variety of areas. A **multidisciplinary team** approach allows for comprehensive assessment and initiation of interventions if needed. Neonatologists, pediatricians, ophthalmologists, nurse specialists, speech/language pathologists, audiologists, orthoptists, psychologists, occupational therapists, physiotherapists, social workers and dietitians may staff the clinics. Volunteers can also play an integral role in optimal running of follow-up clinics.

The information obtained by each follow-up program is very useful to those providing care to neonates in the NICU and assists in joint decision-making with parents about ongoing care.[1-4]

GOALS [5]

Follow-up of high-risk infants in a follow-up clinic is an important component of NICU care. The mandates of neonatal follow-up programs vary, but they may include education, research and clinical goals. In many follow-up programs, data are routinely collected on an "audit" population of very low birth weight babies to monitor outcomes of babies born in specified regions. Some babies may be referred to follow-up clinics because of specific clinical risk factors by community physicians or others. A third group enrolled may be those participating in externally funded research projects or registries. All three groups are managed with specific assessment protocols, with additional appointments as clinically indicated.

Overall, neonatal follow-up programs are often comprehensive in their goals, which may be studied, in three broad categories.

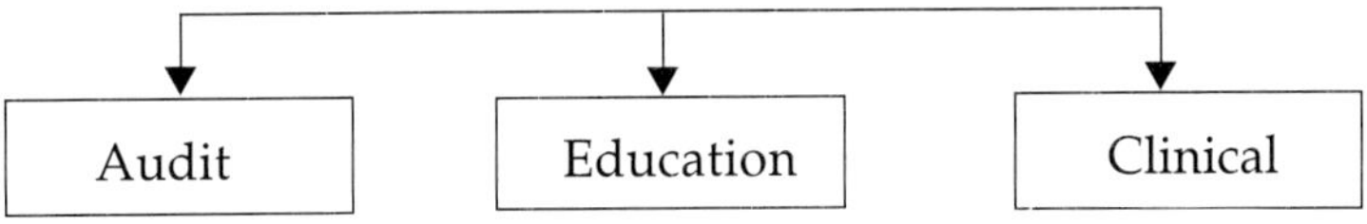

Examples of goals could be:

1. Ensure appropriate ongoing specialized care for high risk neonates discharged from the NICU
2. Identify neurodevelopemental and neurosensory problems and facilitate further follow-up and early intervention to optimize the future potential of these infants.
3. Audit the care provided in the NICU with a view to both future research potential and direction of neonatal care.
4. Educate health care professionals and the general public and create awareness of the association between perinatal problems and pediatric outcomes.

Criteria for Follow-up [5, 6]

Every institution must identify groups of high-risk infants who need follow-up, for example.

1. **Low birth weight and gestational age**, which may vary from institute to institute but are generally ≤1250 grams or ≤28 weeks.
2. **Other conditions:**
   - Perinatal asphyxia.

- Hypoxic ischemic encephalopathy.
- Ventriculomegaly with or without intraventricular hemorrhage.
- Post hemorrhagic hydrocephalus with/without shunt.
- Seizure disorders.
- Meningitis.
- Long-term ventilatory assistance.
- Congenital diaphragmatic hernia.

3. **Infants receiving experimental or newer therapy:**
   - Inhaled nitric oxide, high frequency ventilation, extracorporeal membrane oxygenation (ECMO), total body/ selective head cooling for hypoxic ischemic encephalopathy.
4. **Multiple births.**
5. **Infants with ongoing complications beyond the neonatal period:**
   - Bronchopulmonary dysplasia (whether or not they remain oxygen dependent).
   - Infants with tracheostomies.
6. **Infants with neonatal complications:**
   - Septicemia.
   - Hypoglycemia.
   - Hyperbilirubinemia.
   - Complex congenital heart disease.
   - Solid organ transplants.
   - Feeding difficulties with or without gastrostomy tubes.
7. **Fetal interventions in the antenatal period:**
   - Twin to twin transfusion with laser therapy.
   - Fetal surgery for hydrocephalous, neural tube defects.
   - *In utero* blood transfusion/blood exchange transfusion.

Outcomes

Consistency of outcome measures is important particularly in the audit and research roles. We recommend the model proposed by the NCMRR (National Centre for Medical Rehabilitation Research, National Institute of Health, 1993). This model is also recognized by the American Academy for Cerebral Palsy and Developmental Medicine.[7]

Grades	*Functional Dimension*	*NCMRR Dimension*
I	Cell/Tissue	Pathophysiology
II	Body	Impairment
III	Individual (Person)	Functional limitations
IV	Social (Life situations)	Disabilities
V	Environment	Societal limitation

Outcomes of Importance in Follow-up

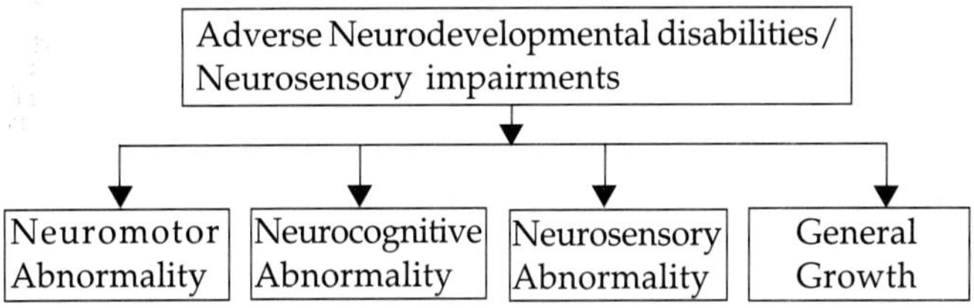

Neuromotor Abnormality

The most common condition in this category is cerebral palsy. This is a non-progressive neuromotor impairment syndrome secondary to lesions in the brain. Major neurologic disability is usually classified as moderate to severe cerebral palsy (spastic diplegia, spastic quadriplegia, or spastic hemiplegia or paresis), hydrocephalus (with or without associated cerebral palsy or sensory deficits). Neuromotor impairment includes ambulatory or non-ambulatory impairment.

Neurocognitive Abnormality

This is identified by standardized psychological assessment. A significant neurocognitive abnormality is defined as a score more than 2 standard deviations below the mean on standardized testing. The intellectual outcome of children with neuromotor abnormality may differ greatly according to the neurologic diagnosis.

Neurosensory Abnormality

This category broadly involves hearing and vision. Severe visual impairment is defined when any infant's vision is below 20/200 or who is considered completely or legally blind. Severe hearing impairment is defined as the presence in any infant of a sensorineural hearing loss of > 70 db with voice range (250-4000 Hz) or requiring amplification (e.g., hearing aids, cochlear implant).

General Growth

High-risk infants are prone to have growth delay. This could be due to poor nutritional intake, malabsorptive function of the gut, post surgical gut impairment, short bowel syndrome, feeding technique issues and GI motility abnormalities. These problems all demand optimal nutrition. Proper monitoring of growth and community support focused on infant growth and feeding is mandatory for early recognition of problems and their management.

Identification of Functional Difficulties [8-10]

Functional status of high risk populations is generally determined in several domains in the follow-up clinics:

- Fine and gross motor skills.
- Cognitive skills.
- Language skills.
- Social/adaptive skills.
- Learning skills.

Methods of Identification

Three levels of identification can be considered in different situations:

Surveillance

In populations at risk of neurodevelopmental problems.

Screening

Using cost effective instruments/tools with known specificity, sensitivity, reliability and validity to identify those infants/children with an increased likelihood of having an adverse finding.

Formal Testing

Using standardized measures to confirm the presence and severity of adverse findings.

One important convention is to use corrected gestational age for the follow-up visits. Prematurity is corrected by subtracting the number of weeks of prematurity from the chronological age of the child to give an adjusted or corrected age until the second birthday.[11]

PRACTICAL POINTS

Timing of Assessments

The timing of visits is usually determined by several factors:

Staff resources, nature of the high-risk population, the type of surveillance used and the purpose of the visits.

Frequency of Visits

Ideally, the frequency of visits is usually linked to key developmental milestones or achievements. An example of "core" assessments based on corrected age is:

4 Months:

Nursing review, general physical exam, Amiel-Tison longitudinal neurological examination, physiotherapy assessment, ophthalmology exam, social work assessment, and audiology screening, if not previously done.

8 Months:

Nursing review, general physical exam, Amiel-Tison exam, audiology, and nutrition.

21 Months:

Nursing review, physiotherapy, psychology, speech/language pathology and social work.

36 Months:

Nursing review, general physical and neurologic exam, psychology, speech/language pathology, orthoptics and social work.

5 Years:

Nursing review, general physical and neurological exam, ophthalmology, psychology, speech/language pathology, and social work. This visit may be offered only to children at greatest risk of difficulties, which become evident only near school age (e.g. birth weights of 1000 grams or less).

Common tools have included:

- Alberta Infant Motor Scale.[12, 13]
- Movement Assessment of infants (MAI).[14-16]
- Ages and Stages Questionnaires (ASQ).[17, 18]
- **Bayley Scales of Infant and Toddler Development (BSID-III).[19]**
- Gross Motor Function Classification System (GMFCS).[20-22]
- Vineland Adaptive Behavior Scales.[23]
- Amiel-Tison exam.[24]

Children with birth weight less than 750 gm have higher rates of functional limitations, greater compensatory dependence, and an increased need for services compared with those with birth weights higher than 750 gm.[25] Overall the incidence of health problems and neurodevelopmental sequelae increase with decreasing birth weight (Tables 29.1 to 29.5).

School-Age Outcome of Infants with Very Low Birth Weight (VLBW)

VLBW infant who survive at age 5 to 8 years revealed significantly more major as well as subtle neurological dysfunction and lower intelligence, performed less well on tests of language and academic achievement and had more behavioral problem than control groups.[26] Extremely low birth weight (ELBW) adolescents scored

Chapter 29

Table 29.1: Birth weight-specific neurodevelopmental outcomes[26]

Variables		*Birth weight (kg)*			
		<1	*1-1.49*	*1.5-2.49*	*≥2.5*
Neurologic abnormality (%)		20	15	8	<5
Cerebral palsy (%)		>5	4	2	<0.4
Intelligence					
	Mean IQ	88	96	96	103
	IQ<70 (%)	13	5	5	0-3
Behavioral problems (%)		29	28	29	21

Table 29.2: 20 months neurosensory outcomes of children with birth weight of <1000 g [25]

Outcomes	*Percent of children*
Major neurologic abnormality	20
Cerebral palsy	15
Diplegia	7
Dihemiplegia	1
Hemiplegia	3
Quadriplegia	4
Hypertonia	2
Hypotonia	2
Shunt dependent hydrocephalous	1
Blindness (unilateral or bilateral)	1
Deafness (unilateral or bilateral)	9

Table 29.3: 20 months developmental outcomes of children with birth weight of <1000g [25]

Bayley Scales of Infant Development	*Total*
Mental Developmental Index (MDI)	
Mean ± SD score	75 ± 17
<70	42%
70-84	26%
≥85	32%
Psychomotor Developmental Index	
Mean ± SD score	73 ± 17
<70	40%
70-84	31%
≥85	29%
Neurodevelopmental impairment MDI <70 and/or neurosensory abnormality.	48%

lower on all measures, especially mathematics. A high proportion of VLBW adolescents (15-20%) and even higher proportion of ELBW adolescents (30-50%) were receiving remedial assistance.[1] Some reports suggest that there is an increased number of behavioral problems in VLBW adolescents.[1]

Table 29.4: Health outcomes by birth weight at eight years [26]

Variables	*Birth weight (kg)*			
	<1	*1-1.49*	*1.5-2.49*	*≥2.5*
Asthma (%)	20	15	8	<5
Rehospitalization previous year (%)	7	7	5	2
Limitation of >1 activity of daily living because of health (%)	46	34	27	17

Table 29.5: Outcome variables [25]

	Birth weight 501-800 g	*Gestational Age (Weeks)*		
		23	24	25
Total followed (N)	1000	77	323	554
Severe disability	9-37%	34%	22-45%	12-35%
Cerebral palsy	5-37%		11-15%	3-20%
Subnormal cognitive (MDI <70)	13-47%		14-39%	10-30%
Blindness	2-25%		0-9%	3-10%
Deafness	0-7%			

Outcome of Infants with Extremely Low Birth Weight

Neonatology, the medical subspecialty devoted to the medical care of the newborn infant, has made remarkable advances in diagnostic and therapeutic techniques during the past 30 years. Survival at a birth weight less than 750 gm increased from 32% to 46% in the early 1990s to 57% to 67% in more recent years.[27-29] The major morbidities influencing later development include severe brain injury, occurring in 12% to 19%; chronic lung disease, occurring in 39% to 61%; necrotizing enterocolitis, occurring in 30% to 50%; and retinopathy of prematurity, occurring in 12% to 33% of survivors.[2, 30] Other factors reported to correlate with later outcome include maternal chorioamnionitis and transient hypothyroxinemia. A review of literature on survivors of a birth weight less than 750 gm reveals that during early childhood, the rates of severe neurosensory disability range from 9% to 37%, with cerebral palsy occurring in 5 to 37%, blindness in 2% to 25%, and deafness in 0% to 7%. Cognitive function is subnormal in 15 to 47% of survivors in this group.[31-33]

Early Intervention

The role of a comprehensive early intervention program was studied in a clinical trial. The program, which provided intensive educational enrichment to preterm infants with low birth weight, improved the IQ scores of the children at 3 years of age, however, the extremely low birth weight infant group were less responsive to the intervention.[34] Subsequent follow-up of the cohort at 8 years demonstrated only minimal effects of the intervention on cognitive status, school achievement, or behavior.[35] Early intervention programs can provide educational support to parents and considered to be beneficial for children from deprived families.

Detailed information on functional difficulties is best obtained after the age of 2 years. With growth and maturity, learning, motor, language and behavior skills are more clearly defined. If Neonatal Follow-up Programs choose to continue following children beyond the age of 2 years, they will require more detailed screening, standardized assessments tools and expertise of multidisciplinary team members.

REFERENCES

1. Barrington K, Saigal S: Long-term caring for neonates, *Paediatr Child Health* 2006;11(5):265-266.
2. Hack M, Fanaroff AA: Outcomes of children of extremely low birth weight and gestational age in the 1990's, *Early Hum Dev.* Jan 1999;53(3):193-218.
3. Hack M, Friedman H, Fanaroff AA: Outcomes of extremely low birth weight infants, *Pediatrics,* Nov 1996;98(5):931-937.
4. Sauve R, Lee K: Neonatal follow-up programs and follow-up studies: Historical and current perspectives, *Paedaitr Child Health* 2006;11(5):267-270.
5. Bernbam J, Gerdes M, Spitzer A: Follow-up of the high-risk neonate, In: Spitzer A, ed. *Intensive care of the fetus and neonate,* St. Louis: Mosby 1996:729-741.
6. McCormick MC: The outcomes of very low birth weight infants: Are we asking the right questions? *Pediatrics,* Jun 1997;99(6):869-876.
7. *National Institute of Health, Research Plan for the National Center for Medical Rehabilitation Research, Washington DC: US Department of Health and Human Services,* 1993.

8. Astbury J, Orgill AA, Bajuk B, Yu VY: Sequelae of growth failure in appropriate for gestational age, very low birth weight infants, *Dev Med Child Neurol,* Aug 1986;28(4):472-479.
9. Asztalos E: Follow-up of the high-risk neonate, In: Kirpalani H, Moore A, Perlman M, eds, *Resident Handbook of Neonatology,* Hamilton,Canada: B.C. Decker Inc 2007:496-502.
10. Aylward GP, Pfeiffer SI, Wright A, Verhulst SJ: Outcome studies of low birth weight infants published in the last decade: A metaanalysis, *J Pediatr* Oct 1989;115(4):515-520.
11. Ross G, Lawson K: Using the Bayley-II: Unresolved issues in assessing the development of prematurely born children, *J Dev Behav Pediatr,* Apr 1997;18(2):109-111; discussion 112-103.
12. Campbell SK, Kolobe TH, Wright BD, Linacre JM: Validity of the Test of Infant Motor Performance for prediction of 6-, 9- and 12-month scores on the Alberta Infant Motor Scale, *Dev Med Child Neurol,* Apr 2002;44(4):263-272.
13. Darrah J, Piper M, Watt MJ: Assessment of gross motor skills of at-risk infants: Predictive validity of the Alberta Infant Motor Scale, *Dev Med Child Neurol,* Jul 1998;40(7):485-491.
14. Harris SR, Haley SM, Tada WL, Swanson MW: Reliability of observational measures of the Movement Assessment of Infants, *Phys Ther,* Apr 1984;64(4):471-477.
15. Harris SR, Swanson MW, Andrews MS, *et al.*: Predictive validity of the "Movement Assessment of Infants", *J Dev Behav Pediatr,* Dec 1984;5(6):336-342.
16. Swanson MW, Bennett FC, Shy KK, Whitfield MF, Identification of neurodevelopmental abnormality at four and eight months by the movement assessment of infants, *Dev Med Child Neurol,* Apr 1992;34(4):321-337.
17. Squires J, Bricker D, Potter L: Revision of a parent-completed development screening tool: Ages and Stages Questionnaires, *J Pediatr Psychol,* Jun 1997;22(3):313-328.
18. Squires J, Potter L, Bricker D: *The ASQ user's guide for the ages and stages questioners: A parent-completed, child-monitoring system,* 2nd Edition ed. Baltimore: Paul H. Brookes Publishing; 1995.
19. Bayley N: *Manual for the Bayley Scales of Infant and Toddler Development,* Third edition ed, San Antonio (TX): The Psychological Corporation; 2006.
20. Palisano R, Rosenbaum P, Walter S, Russell D, Wood E, Galuppi B: Development and reliability of a system to classify gross motor function in children with cerebral palsy, *Dev Med Child Neurol,* Apr 1997;39(4):214-223.
21. Palisano RJ, Hanna SE, Rosenbaum PL, *et al.*: Validation of a model of gross motor function for children with cerebral palsy, *Phys Ther,* Oct 2000;80(10):974-985.
22. Wood E, Rosenbaum P: The gross motor function classification system for cerebral palsy: A study of reliability and stability over time, *Dev Med Child Neurol,* May 2000;42(5):292-296.

23. Sparrow S, Ball D, Cicchetti D: *Vineland adaptive behavior scales,* Circle Pines: American Guidance Service; 1984.
24. Amiel-Tison C: *How to follow through childhood, the neurological trace of a cerebral disorder of perinatal origin, Canadian Paediatric Society Update*: Multimed Inc.; 1991.
25. Hack M, Taylor HG, Klein N, Mercuri-Minich N: Functional limitations and special health care needs of 10- to 14-year-old children weighing less than 750 grams at birth, *Pediatrics,* Sep 2000;106(3):554-560.
26. Hack M, Klein NK, Taylor HG: Long-term developmental outcomes of low birth weight infants, *Future Child,* Spring 1995;5(1):176-196.
27. Fanaroff AA, Wright LL, Stevenson DK, *et al.*: Very low birth weight outcomes of the National Institute of Child Health and Human Development Neonatal Research Network, May 1991 through December 1992, *Am J Obstet Gynecol* Nov 1995;173(5):1423-1431.
28. Horbar JD, Onstad L, Wright E. Predicting mortality risk for infants weighing 501 to 1500 grams at birth: A National Institute of Health Neonatal Research Network report, *Crit Care Med,* Jan 1993;21(1):12-18.
29. Stevenson DK, Wright LL, Lemons JA, *et al.*: Very low birth weight outcomes of the National Institute of Child Health and Human Development Neonatal Research Network, January 1993 through December 1994, *Am J Obstet Gynecol,* Dec 1998;179(6 Pt 1):1632-1639.
30. Taylor HG, Klein N, Schatschneider C, Hack M: Predictors of early school age outcomes in very low birth weight children, *J Dev Behav Pediatr,* Aug 1998;19(4):235-243.
31. Lucas A, Morley R, Cole TJ, Gore SM: A randomised multicentre study of human milk versus formula and later development in preterm infants, *Arch Dis Child Fetal Neonatal Ed,* Mar 1994;70(2):F141-146.
32. O'Shea TM, Klinepeter KL, Meis PJ, Dillard RG: Intrauterine infection and the risk of cerebral palsy in very low birth weight infants. *Paediatr Perinat Epidemiol,* Jan 1998;12(1):72-83.
33. Reuss ML, Paneth N, Pinto-Martin JA, Lorenz JM, Susser M: The relation of transient hypothyroxinemia in preterm infants to neurologic development at two years of age, *N Engl J Med,* Mar 28 1996;334(13):821-827.
34. Enhancing the outcomes of low birth weight, premature infants. A multisite, randomized trial. The Infant Health and Development Program, *Jama,* Jun 13 1990;263(22):3035-3042.
35. McCarton CM, Brooks-Gunn J, Wallace IF, *et al.*: Results at age 8 years of early intervention for low birth weight premature infants. The Infant Health and Development Program, *Jama,* Jan 8 1997;277(2):126-132.

APPENDIX A

COMMON NEONATAL PROCEDURES

Rhishikesh Thakre

GENERAL PRINCIPLES

Basic Essentials

- Attending physician will counsel parents as to the need for and details of this procedure.
- Ensure that parental consent form has been signed.
- Adequate light should be available.
- Ensure warmth during the procedure.
- Fluid balance must be maintained during the procedure.
- An assistant should be designated for monitoring purpose.
- Multi channel monitor – heart rate, oxygen saturation and blood pressure should preferably be used.
- Oxygen and suction provision should be made.
- Resuscitation equipment and drugs should be in functional order.
- The infant should be well restrained during the procedure. Improper position and restraint are the common sources of failure in procedures.

Asepsis Basics

- Use universal precautions, always.
- All traces of antiseptics should be removed after the procedure. Antiseptic should not be allowed to pool under the baby.
- The rationale for cleaning, disinfecting, or sterilizing patient-care equipment can be understood more readily if medical devices, equipment, and surgical materials are divided into three general categories (critical items, semi-critical items, and non-critical items) based on the potential risk of infection involved in their use.

- All items that will touch normally sterile tissues are sterilized (Critical items). Items that touch mucous membranes but do not breach the continuity (semi- critical) e.g., bronchoscope, endotracheal tube, respiratory tubes, requires a disinfection process. For many non-critical items, such as blood pressure cuffs or crutches, cleaning can consist only of:
  1. Washing with a detergent or a disinfectant-detergent;
  2. Rinsing; and
  3. Thorough drying. In general, items that touch only intact skin need only be clean.

Making Use of Monitors

- Be sure that monitor alarms are functioning and are in the "ON" position.
- Alarms should never be left in the "OFF" position when the infant is unattended.
- Document and report significant changes in heart rate and/or respiratory rate.
- Leads may be used until they are no longer adhering to the skin or not conducting a good tracing. Leads may be moved to different areas on the skin for cleansing skin surfaces.
- Assess skin integrity with each lead change.

Sedatives and Analgesics

Whilst it is difficult to distinguish pain from other constructs such as fear or hunger, pain perception should be presumed in neonates in situations where a cause of pain is present and where typical pain behavior is present (e.g. grimacing).

Following are examples of painful procedures which warrant analgesic agent:

Arterial puncture	Ventilation
Heel lance	Chest / wound drain insertion / removal
Venipuncture	ICD insertion
IV access / infiltrates / phlebitis	Gastric tube insertion
Central line insertion / removal	Lumbar puncture
Removal of adhesive tape	Suprapubic urine collection
ETT intubation / extubation	ROP examination
Dressings / removal of sutures	IM injections
Birth trauma	Drugs–amphotericin B, erythropoietin etc.

Practical Strategies to Reduce Stress and Pain

- Minimize handling.

- Maintain as quiet an environment as possible.
- Assess pain using the pain assessment scale.
- Assess for, and report the following signs of pain and anxiety.
  - Restlessness, "fighting the ventilator", crying.
  - Poor tolerance of handling.
  - Changes in vital signs: Tachycardia, hypertension, tachypnea.
  - Decreased oxygenation.
- Document sedation scores at least every 4 hours during initiation and maintenance infusions.

Sedation Scale	*Description*
Awake (4)	Awake, alert
Minimal (3)	Ptosis
Moderate (2)	Spontaneous eye closure, delayed response to verbal stimulation, appropriate response to verbal/tactile stimulation
Deep (1)	Responds only to repeated or painful stimulation
Unresponsive sedation (0)	No response to painful stimulation.

- Report increased tolerance to narcotic analgesia.
- Keep naloxone and resuscitation equipment available at bedside when narcotics are continuously infusing.
- Using 24% sucrose solution for minor procedures:
  - For maximal effect, 24% sucrose in water solution, given 1ml (<34w) to 2 ml (>34w), should be administered approximately 2 minutes prior to the painful procedure.
  - Pacifier use should continue between dips of sucrose as the pacifier also provides calming, comforting and analgesic effect.
  - Oral sucrose should not be given to unstable infants. Infants with difficulty in coordinating sucking and swallowing may need to have the sucrose administered by dipping the pacifier into sucrose.
  - Administer sucrose (syringe method) by applying sucrose drop directly.
  - It is expected that the infant will become calm and quiet after 1 or 2 pacifier dips or several drops of sucrose solution.
  - Provide additional supportive measures during the procedure such as pacifier, talking to the infant and touch.

Choice of Sedative

Agent	*Bolus dose*	*Frequency*	*Infusion*
Midazolam	0.1mg/kg	2- 4 hours	10-60 mg/kg/hour
Lorazepam	0.1mg/kg	4-12 hours	NR

Appendix A

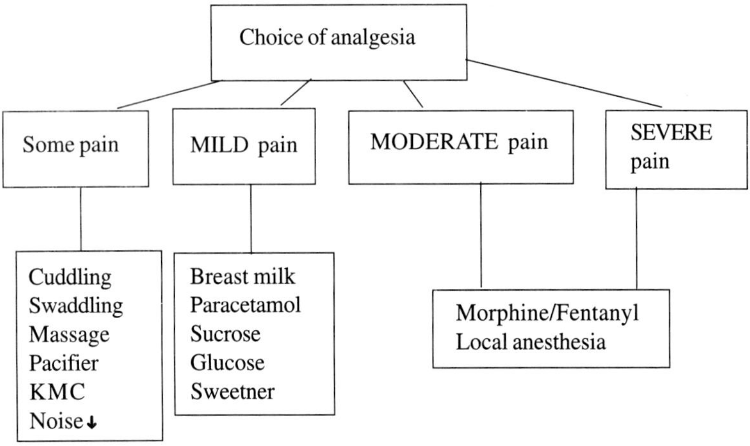

Neonatal Procedures

1. Abdominal tap
2. Assisting during X-Ray, CT scan, USG and MRI
3. Assisted ventilation
4. Bladder tap
5. Blood culture
6. Blood sampling – Capillary, arterial, venous and cord blood
7. Breast milk expression, storage and handling
8. Care of infant in radiant warmer and incubator
9. Care of jaundice in the newborn
10. Central vascular access
11. Chest physiotherapy
12. Care during non-invasive ventilation and CPAP
13. Developmentally supportive care
14. Endotracheal tube insertion, fixation and removal
15. Endotracheal suction
16. Exchange transfusion
17. Giving injections – IM, IV, ID
18. Hand washing
19. Insertion of gastric tube
20. Intercostal catheter insertion
21. Intraosseous access
22. Inverted nipple

23. Kangaroo care
24. Laryngeal mask airway
25. Lumbar puncture
26. Measuring blood glucose
27. Measuring blood pressure
28. Measuring temperature
29. Metabolic screening tests
30. Nasopharyngeal airway
31. Needle aspiration for pneumothorax
32. Nitrogen washout test
33. Oxygen therapy
34. Peripheral vascular catheters – vein and artery
35. Pericardial tap
36. Stool heme occult test
37. Surfactant administration
38. Transillumination
39. Umbilical vessel cannulation
40. Urine collection
41. Gastric aspirate shake test

1. ABDOMINAL TAP

Indications

1. Massive ascites causing respiratory distress.
2. Hydrops fetalis.
3. Nectrotizing enterocolitis.
4. Suspected peritonitis.

Supplies

- 23 G needle of 1- ½ inch length.
- Three-way stopcock, 10 cc syringe.
- Alcohol and betadine, cotton balls.
- Sterile gloves, towel.

Procedure

- Clean the abdomen with alcohol and betadine.
- Insert the needle attached to a 10 ml syringe via a 3-way stopcock through

the iliac fossa at the junction of medial 2/3 with lateral 1/3, between the anterior superior iliac spine and pubic symphysis.

- Enter perpendicularly piercing the skin, subcutaneous tissue and changing the direction towards the midline.
- Once you feel the "giving way" sensation, do not advance the needle further. Try to aspirate.

Complications

- Infection.
- Hemorrhage.
- Bowel or bladder perforation.

REFERENCE

1. Manual of neonatal nursing, Ed. Lalitha Krishnan, Published by National Neonatology Forum, 1993.

2A. ASSISTANCE DURING X-RAY

- Cover film with cloth diaper.
- Position baby properly and hold baby in place during exposure.
- A lead apron should be worn.
- Remove all metal objects (e.g. lead wires, heat probes) as well as clothing and diapers from area that will be exposed on film. Remove any objects that may interfere with ability of X-rays to penetrate.
- Clear the immediate area of all extra personnel once X-ray technician announces that X-ray will be taken.
- Staff, parents and other infants should be at least 6 feet from the X-ray machine to avoid significant exposure to X-rays.

2B. ASSISTANCE DURING COMPUTED TOMOGRAPHY (CT) SCAN/MAGNETIC RESONANCE IMAGING (MRI) /ULTRASONOGRAPHY (USG)

Preparation

- Explain to the family the reason for transfer of the baby to the radiology unit.
- Obtain informed consent for any anticipated procedures, if applicable.
- Prepare the baby for transfer:
  - Ensure that the baby's condition is stable before transfer.
  - If the baby is able to feed but the mother is unable to accompany and breastfeed the baby or the baby must be fed using an alternative feeding method, insert a naso- or oro-gastric tube.
  - Ensure that the IV line, if present, is in place and secured.
  - Gather essential equipment, supplies, drugs and fluids.

- Have a health care provider (with experience in establishing and maintaining IV lines, resuscitating a baby, and giving drugs) accompany the baby.
- Ensure that the transport vehicle has adequate lighting and insulation to keep the baby warm or to prevent overheating.
- Ask a relative to accompany the baby and mother, if possible.
  - Give sedation depending upon the needs e.g. chloral hydrate, midazolam.

Communication

- Contact the radiology unit in advance about the procedure so they can be prepared.
- Confirm that the facility is able to accommodate the baby on the scheduled time.
- Give an estimated time of arrival.
- Fill out the referral form and send it with the baby.

Care During Transfer

- Keep the baby in skin-to-skin contact with the mother or a relative. If skin-to-skin contact is not possible, keep the baby dressed and covered. Check the temperature setting and measure the baby's temperature every hour.
  - If a warming device is not available, place the baby in a box with warm water bottles. Cover the bottles with a cloth and ensure that they are secured so that they do not directly touch the baby's skin. Confirm that the surface of the covered warm water bottle is not too hot by touching it with the dorsal aspect of your hand. When the water becomes cold, refill the bottles with warm water or remove them from the box.
- Ensure that the baby receives feeds or fluid:
  - Allow the baby to breastfeed. If the baby cannot be breastfed, give expressed breast milk by naso- or oro-gastric tube.
  - If the baby is receiving IV fluids, carefully monitor the rate to ensure that the baby receives the correct volume of fluid.
  - Inspect the infusion site every hour.
  - Check the volume of fluid infused and compare to the prescribed volume.
  - Record all findings.
- If the baby is receiving oxygen, check the oxygen flow and tubing every 15 minutes.
  - Assess the baby's vital signs frequently.

Care During the Procedure

- Ensure the temperature of the environment is warm before admitting the baby in the procedure room.
- Keep the baby with the mother or guardian to assist and restrain.
- Monitor respiration, colour, activity and heart rate periodically.

- Wash hands before handling the baby.
- Assistant or guardian can stay with the infant during the USG and CT scan procedure.
- Wipe the ultrasound jelly with gauze following USG procedure.

Care During MRI Procedure

1. Before and after most MRI procedures no special preparation, diet, reduced activity, or extra medication is necessary.
2. The MRI procedure can easily be performed through clothing, but attention must be paid to ferromagnetic items, such as zippers or clasps because metal will interfere with the test. For the assistant or parent ensure they do not wear jewellery, a hearing aid, or any removable dental work.
3. Items that need to be removed by patients before entering the MR system room include:
   - Purse, wallet, money clip, credit cards, cards with magnetic strips.
   - Electronic devices such as beepers or cell phones.
   - Hearing aids.
   - Metal jewellery, watches.
   - Pens, paper clips, keys, coins.
   - Hair barrettes, hairpins.
   - Any article of clothing that has a metal zipper, buttons, snaps, hooks, under wires, or metal threads.
   - Shoes, belt buckles, safety pins.

   Examples of items or things that may create a health hazard or other problem during an MRI exam include:
   - Pacemaker.
   - Implantable cardioverter defibrillator (ICD).
   - Neurostimulator.
   - Metal implant.
   - Implanted drug infusion device.
   - Foreign metal objects, especially if in or near the eye.
   - Permanent cosmetics or tattoos.
   - Other implants that involve magnets.
4. Most MRI exams take between 15 to 45 minutes to complete depending on the body part imaged and how many images are needed, although some may take as long as 60 minutes or longer. Hence appropriate sedation should be given.
5. Cover the ears with earplugs to reduce noise.
6. Unlike contrast agents used in X-ray studies, MRI contrast agents do not contain iodine and, therefore, rarely cause allergic reactions or other problems.
7. Pillows and straps may be used to prevent movement during the procedure.

8. During the procedure the support staff cannot stay with the patient. Monitoring therefore has to be very reliable. MRI compatible monitoring devices should be used and data continuously displayed in the control room.
9. The majority of babies need to have sedation/anesthesia during the procedure.
10. MRI suite has air/oxygen/electrical outlets. A ventilator may be used alongside.
11. There is no patient heater in the MRI room, although the "tunnel" can reach 80°F during a longer scan. The baby needs to be dressed. Bundle the baby in warm blankets.
12. The MRI nurse will remove the monitor leads from the baby and replace with special leads, which are available in the MRI suite.
13. **Baby with An Intravenous (IV) Line**
    - If the baby is stable and can manage without IV fluids for one to one and a half hours, the peripheral IV is to be heparin-locked. IVs may be an intracath (i.e. Jelco or Insyte). Steel butterflies are not acceptable in the MRI suite.
    - After obtaining a physician's order, a **CVC** may be heparin-locked as per protocol.
    - **If the Baby Needs His/Her IV Fluids Maintained**
        - Only one infusing IV line is acceptable in the MRI.
        - Change IV to run via a syringe pump (volumetric pumps with metallic parts cannot be used in the MRI room).
        - Ensure 3 long extension tubes are attached to the IV/CVC prior to transporting the baby to MRI.
        - MRI has its own syringe pump bolted to the anesthetic machine – this is the only pump allowed into the room. Take along a bag of D10W (since it is not usually in stock in the MRI suite).
        - Take extra syringes if the baby is receiving large volumes of fluid.

REFERENCE

1. Sawyer-Glover AM, Shellock FG: Pre-MRI Procedure Screening: Recommendations and Safety Considerations for Biomedical Implants and Devices, J Magn Reson Imaging 2000;12:92-106.

3. ASSISTED VENTILATION

Facts

- Neonatal ventilation is teamwork.
- Neonatal ventilation is more of an art than science.
- As one learns to drive a car with supervision and gets certified, so also one must undergo specialized training for neonatal ventilation, preferable for at least 1 year under qualified supervision, before one can start on his/her own.

- Ventilation is a labor-intensive job and requires qualified nursing and trained personnel round the clock by the bedside.
- Not more than 1% of neonatal intensive care unit (NICU) admissions require ventilation.
- Neonatal illnesses are rarely limited to one system. Multi organ system involvement is the rule rather than the exception. Ventilation is providing support to one major system i.e. lungs. The prognosis is based on outcome of all the organs affected. Hence, ventilation is not a panacea in neonatology.
- Gestational age and birth weight are two major independent factors influencing outcome of ventilation. Onset of illness, timing of ventilation, evidence of multi organ involvement and presence of complications are other factors influencing the neonatal outcome.
- Ventilation in newborn is most commonly pressure limited and time cycled.
- *It is not the machine but the person behind the machine, which will determine the outcome of ventilated newborns.*

Clinical Criterion for Respiratory Distress

Downes' score	*0*	*1*	*2*
Respiratory Rate	< 60/minute	60-80/minute	> 80/minute or apnea
Retractions	None	Mild	Moderate - Severe
Cyanosis	None	In $FiO_2 < 0.4$	In $FiO_2 > 0.4$
Air Entry	Clear and equal	Decreased	Barely audible
Grunting	Absent	Audible with stethoscope	Audible without stethoscope

If the Downes' score is ≥4: This signifies clinical respiratory distress, monitor arterial blood gases (ABG). If the score is ≥ 8, this signifies impending respiratory failure.

ABG Score

	Points			
	0	*1*	*2*	*3*
PaO_2 mmHg	>60	50-60	<50	<50
pH	>7.3	7.20-7.29	7.1-7.19	<7.1
$PaCO_2$ mmHg	<50	50-60	61-70	>70

If the ABG score is 3 or more, this indicates the need for CPAP or mechanical ventilation.

Types of Ventilator

1. Pressure limited

These are simple in design, easy to operate and relatively inexpensive. They provide a fixed predetermined pressure irrespective of the tidal volume. The compliance of lungs and airway resistance affect the tidal volume.

2. Volume limited

A preset tidal volume can be delivered. They are complicated in design and costly.

Indications

1. Respiratory arrest.
2. Respiratory failure.
3. Impending respiratory failure.
4. Cardiopulmonary failure.
5. Shock.
6. Recurrent apnea non responsive to medical management.
7. Failure of continuous positive airway pressure (CPAP).
8. Post operatively for support–e.g, tracheo-esophageal fistula, diaphragmatic hernia.
9. Neurologic depression with impaired respiration – e.g, drug-induced.

Goals of Ventilation

1. To achieve and maintain adequate pulmonary gas exchange.
2. To minimize risk of lung injury.
3. To reduce the work of breathing.
4. To optimize patient comfort.

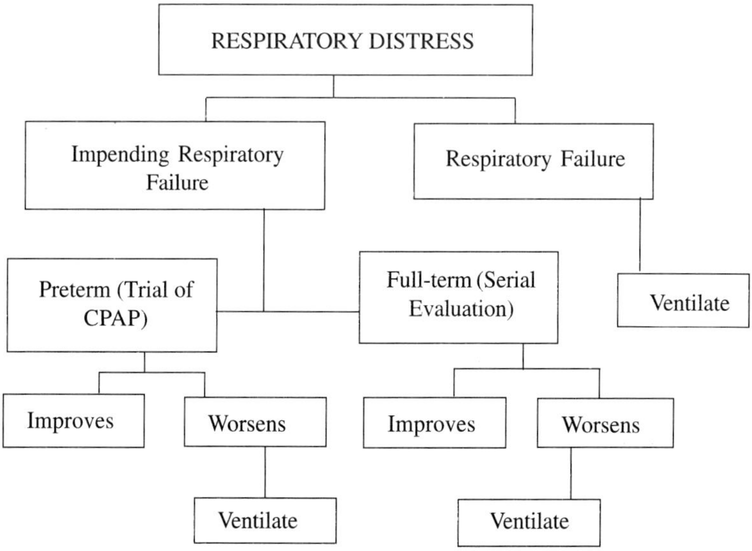

Supplies

- Ventilator circuits.
- Humidifier.
- Test lung.
- T-piece.
- Ventilator.
- Compressed air and oxygen source and tubings.
- Electric outlets.

Prerequisite

- Round the clock bedside monitoring.
- Round the clock availability of team of trained nursing staff and personnel.
- Minimum equipment support in the form of - pulse oximeter, non-invasive blood pressure monitor, ABG analysis machine and portable X-ray.
- Central oxygen support of 40 PSI.
- Battery backup for ventilator and monitors.
- Earthing and voltage stabilization with spike guard for the ventilator.
- Strict asepsis practices and infection control measures.
- Good backup services in case of ventilation malfunctioning.
- Technical know-how about the probable errors of ventilator malfunctioning.

Procedure

1. Perform endotracheal intubation of the patient.
2. Ensure standby bag, mask, intubation and suction apparatus in functional order.
3. Attach the patient to vital sign and pulse oximeter.
4. **Setting the patient circuit:** Secure the patient circuit to the ventilator with the inspiratory limb attached to the input of the humidifier, tubing from the humidifier to the T-piece with test lung, from the T-piece the expiratory limb to the expiratory outlet of the ventilator. The pressure sensor is an optional attachment from the T-piece to the pressure inlet. Heated wire from the T-piece to the humidifier is another optional attachment. Fill the humidifier jar with sterile water up to the level mark.
5. **Ventilator setting:** Secure oxygen and compressed air supplies (45 PSI). Turn on the electrical connections. Set the ventilator on the selected mode. Set the pre-decided settings on the ventilator based on clinical assessment. Check the ventilator with no alarms is delivering the desired parameters.

Choosing Ventilator Settings

1. *Flow* – Flow rate is an important determinant of the ability of the ventilator to deliver the needed peak inspiratory pressure (PIP). Usually the flow is set at 8-10 L/minute and left unchanged unless the PIP requirement rises above 30 or high rates are used.

2. *FiO_2* – All ventilators have the capability to provide a FiO_2 of 0.21 to 1.00 (or 100%). The FiO_2 is usually set 10% more than what the infant was receiving prior to ventilation. It is necessary to titrate the appropriate concentration of oxygen since both hyperoxia and hypoxemia can cause harm.
3. *PIP* – PIP is the primary factor determining the tidal volume and can affect PaO_2 and $PaCO_2$. The lowest PIP that adequately ventilates the infant is appropriate. PIP can be judged by hand ventilation using a manometer or by observing for minimal pressure required to have chest rise. High PIP (> 30 cm H_2O) is avoided because of the risk of air leaks and barotrauma. PIP of < 30 cm H_2O is usually sufficient for most respiratory disorders.
4. *PEEP* – It is routine to keep at least a positive end-expiratory pressure (PEEP) of 4 cm H_2O to keep the alveoli open. In case of RDS, a PEEP of 4-6 cm H_2O is set. However in case of meconium aspiration syndrome (MAS) a low PEEP of 3-4 cm H_2O is sufficient since the pathology is of air trapping and a high PEEP may lead to airleaks. A PEEP < 3 is not recommended for any illness in neonates.
5. *Ti* – Inspiratory time (Ti) is set depending on the requirement of the mean airway pressure (MAP) and the inspiratory to expiratory time ratio (I:E ratio). A Ti of 0.3-0.5 sec. is sufficient for most disorders. In low compliance conditions like respiratory distress syndrome (RDS), a longer Ti of 0.5 sec is used. In conditions with increased airway resistance like MAS, shorter Ti of 0.3-0.4 may be used. Ti is one parameter that is not touched unless there is persistent hypoxemia unresponsive to changes in PIP, PEEP and FiO_2. Increasing the Ti will proportionally shorten the expiratory time and increase the I:E ratio. The normal I:E ratio is 1:1- 1:3. An I:E ratio <1:1 causes air trapping and inadvertent PEEP.
6. *Te* – Expiratory time (Te) works on the same principles as Ti. The Te can be gradually prolonged as the baby gets weaned off. One must remember that expiration is passive and hence a prolonged Te does not mean the baby cannot spontaneously breathe during that time.
7. *Respiratory Rate* – Respiratory rate is the primary determinant of minute ventilation and hence CO_2 elimination. Generally rates are set at a rate the baby is breathing prior to ventilation. In majority the rates are set around 40/minute and adjusted if necessary. Higher rates may be necessary in MAS if CO_2 retention is a problem. It must be recognized that increasing the RR while keeping the Ti the same, shortens the Te, which can cause inadequate emptying of lungs. This leads to air trapping and so to inadvertent PEEP i.e. the PEEP the baby receives is higher than the set PEEP. This can cause problems with oxygenation and carbon dioxide retention.
8. *Assist Modes* – Some ventilators have various assist modes like CPAP, intermittent mandatory ventilation (IMV), assist control (AC), synchronized IMV (SIMV), pressure-regulated volume control (PRVC), pressure support ventilation (PSV) and it is up to the user to decide the right mode that is to be used. It is probably best to begin with IMV or SIMV mode and then to shift to other modes, as needed.

9. *Sensitivity or Trigger* – When weaning, sensitivity trigger to pressure, volume or flow is used to trigger ventilation. Initially a low trigger is kept which is gradually increased to train the baby in adapting to the work of breathing.

Suggested initial settings for common conditions

Ventilator parameter	*Normal lung*	*RDS*	*MAS*
PIP	**13-15**	**20-25**	**20-25**
PEEP	3	5-7	3-5
FiO_2	10% higher than on CPAP or headbox		
Rates	30-40	40-60	40-60
Flow (L/min)	8-10	8-10	8-10
Ti (sec)	0.4	0.4	0.4

Connecting the Ventilator

1. Remove the T-piece.
2. Attach the endotracheal tube (ETT) connector from the patient to the ventilator circuit.
3. Adequacy of ventilation is clinically judged by:
   - Colour
   - Chest expansion
   - Absence of chest retractions
   - Air entry
   - Improvement in oxygen saturations.
4. After 15-20 minutes of stabilization, do a blood gas.
5. Ensure minimal handling of babies.
6. Ensure strict asepsis during suction and intubation.
7. Avoid routine paralyzing, suctioning and chest physiotherapy.
8. Following the acute phase, ensure change of postures every 4-6 hours.
9. Change one setting on the ventilator at a time. Make small changes in settings rather than allowing big swings.
10. Following change of settings, blood gas analysis is done not early than 20 minutes.
11. Use heparin 5U / 10 U for flushing the syringe for ABG. ABG should be analysed within 30 minutes of drawing the sample.
12. Ensure daily weight and urine output is monitored for the ventilated babies. Ensure adequate nutritional intake – enteral and/or parenteral.
13. Anticipate sudden deterioration and check for DOPE i.e. - ETT **D**isplacement, **O**bstruction, **P**neumothroax and **E**quipment failure.
14. Ensure hematocrit is kept above 35%.

Patient Positioning During Ventilation

- Regular change of posture once acute phase of ventilation has stabilized helps aeration of lungs, and mobilises secretions. Patients with resistant hypoxaemia may benefit from being turned prone. The improved oxygenation probably results from normalisation of pleural pressure gradients within the lung.

- Supine positioning is not optimal in terms of oxygenation and energy expenditure, for which the prone position is better.

Target ABG

- There is no agreement regarding "safe" arterial oxygen concentrations in newborns. It is therefore impossible to set absolute limits for blood gases.
- Permissive hypercarbia is suggested.
- The frequent monitoring of blood gases is clearly essential during the acute stages of illness to assess the need for or effect of respiratory support.
- Acceptable blood gases: pH 7.25-7.35, $PaCO_2$ 45-55 (early phase), $PaCO_2$ 50-70 (later stage), PO_2 40-60 (early phase), 50-70 (later stage).

Effect of changing ventilator settings on pCO_2 and pO_2

Increase in:	*pCO_2*	*pO_2*	*MAP*
FiO_2	No change	Increase	No change
Rate	Decrease	Usually no change	Increase
PIP/Tidal Volume (TV)	Decrease	Increase	Increase
Ti	Usually no change	Increase	Increase
PEEP	Usually no change	Increase	Increase

Prerequisites for Weaning are:

1. The infant has been stable clinically stable for at least 24 hours.
2. Blood gases suggest improvement in gas exchange.
3. Chest radiograph shows adequate improvement in basic pathology.
4. Biochemical parameters—Electrolytes, calcium, glucose, hematocrit and blood counts are stable.
5. Respiratory drive of baby is adequate.

Comprehensive ventilation care

Monitoring	*Medications*	*Ventilator aspects*
• Clinical	• Analgesia	• Compressor
• Biochemical	• Sedation	• Humidifier
• Radiological	• Paralysing agent	• Circuit
• Microbiologic	• Nutrition	• Filters
• Lung function		• Settings
		• Airway access

Signs of Deterioration on Ventilation

1. Respiratory

- Color change: Cyanotic, grey, mottled, pallid.
- Apnea associated with color change and/or bradycardia.
- Arterial: $PaO_2 < 40$; $PaCO_2 > 60$ (early phase), > 70 (late stage), pH < 7.25 or > 7.5.
- Sustained respiratory rates > 60 or < 25.
- Diminished breath sounds.
- Increased crackles or wheezing.
- Pulmonary hemorrhage

2. Cardiovascular

- Systolic blood pressure < the 10th or > 90th percentile for gestational age and postnatal age.
- New onset heart murmur.
- Diminished heart sounds.
- Sudden drop in hematocrit.
- Continued oozing from blood sampling sites.

3. Neurologic

- Full and/or tense fontanelles.
- Activity: Seizures, jitteriness, flaccidity, hypertonia, opisthotonus posturing.

4. Excretory

- Urine output < 1-2 ml/kg/hour.
- Glycosuria > 2+
- Proteinuria > 2+
- Large gastric residues.
- Abdominal distention.
- Prominently visible bowel loops.
- Discoloration of abdomen.
- Occult or frank blood in stools.

5. Miscellaneous

- Excessive weight gain (>10% of body weight/day).
- Excessive total blood loss (>10% of estimated blood volume).
- Blood glucose < 40 mg/dl or > 125 mg/dl.

Deterioration of Infant on ETT Mechanical Ventilation

1. Respond to the infant and not to the monitor.

2. Assess for breathing.
3. If breathing is inadequate, check the ETT lip mark. If the tube is above or below the fixed lip mark, it suggests tube dislodgement. Reposition the ETT.
4. If there are any visible secretions in the oropharynx or ETT, do a quick suction. Reassess.
5. If there is increased work of breathing, sudden collapse, diminished air entry and shift of mediastinum, suspect pneumothorax. Perform an intercostal needle insertion to confirm/treat the diagnosis.
6. Check the equipment is functioning properly.

Bedside ETT Suction Card

Front Side

Babies Name:

Weight (gm):

Date tube inserted: cm:

Tube position: cm above carina:

ET size: Catheter depth:

Back Side

Tube Size	*CUT cm*	*Catheter depth cm*
2.5 mm	11	14.5 cm
3.0	13	17 cm
3.5	13	17 cm
4.0	14	18 cm

1. Rapid Sequence Intubation

- *Check equipment:* Appropriate and functioning ETT, laryngoscope blade, stylet, suction catheter, suction machine (pressure set to 100 cm of H_2O), medications (atropine, midazolam, vecuronium), oxygen, ambu bag, oxygen reservoir, face mask, fixing tape, scissors, tincture benzoin, and shoulder pads.
- Use universal precautions.
- *Apply monitors:* Pulse oximeter, cardioscope.
- Provide 100 % oxygen and bag the baby for 2-3 minutes.
- Designate assistant and check heart rate every 30 seconds.
- Injection Atropine, 0.01 mg/kg IV, followed 2 minutes later by midozolam, 0.1mg/kg, IV (In emergent situations, this step may be omitted).
- Ask assistant to apply cricoid pressure if required.

- Injection Vecuronium, 0.1 mg/kg IV bolus (optional).
- Under vision intubate the trachea. Introduce the ETT till the vocal cord guideline lies across the vocal cords or predetermined distance (wt + 6 cm at the lip). If using stylet, remove it keeping the ETT in place.
- Do not spend more than 20 seconds to intubate. If unable to intubate or heart rate drops below 100/minute, abandon procedure and continue oxygen and bag/mask ventilation.
- Confirm placement of ETT in trachea by checking for equal bilateral chest expansion, equal air entry in both axillae, improvement in colour, absence of sounds over abdomen.
- Assess and re-assess adequacy of ventilation and heart rate.
- Fix the ETT. Clean the area with tincture benzoin to prevent peeling or excoriation of skin. Apply cotton tape and with adhesive tape fix the ETT.
- Connect to the ventilator.
- Get a chest X-ray to confirm proper ETT placement.

2. Daily Care of the Ventilator

- Attach the ventilator to electrical source. Use voltage stabilizer with spike guard and UPS / generator backup.
- Connect the ventilator to oxygen and compressed air source. If no compressed air line, compressor should be turned on to generate 50 PSI pressure.
- Fix the patient circuit – inspiratory limb, expiratory limb, humidifier bottle and air traps.
- Ensure the bacterial filter is in the inspiratory limb and the expiratory limb ends at the exhalation valve.
- Clean the compressor filter with tap water and allow it to dry at room temperature every day.
- Change patient circuit every 3 days. Sterilize with gas sterilization or with use of 2% glutardehyde. For disinfection – clean tubings, humidifier jar, with soap and water, remove visible stains, allow it to immerse in freshly prepared 2% glutardehyde (efficacy for 14 days) for 8 hours, immerse the tubings in sterile water and allow the tubings to air dry.

3. Humidification

- Piped medical oxygen and air are completely dry. Warming and humidification of inspired gases can help reduce the problem of tube blockage.
- The upper airway may not be able to supply enough heat and moisture to fully saturate them. Inadequate humidification of inspired gases destroys the ciliated epithelium lining the upper airway. This stops secretions from being cleared from the lungs and increases the risk of infection.
- Set humidifier temperature at 37°C and humidity at 70%.

- Use deionised or sterile water in the humidifer jar upto the watermark. Check periodically. Use sterile filter paper in the humidifier. Change filter paper every 24 hours.
- The adequacy of humidification is judged by miminal water condensation in the ventilatory circuit.

4. Choosing Mode of Ventilation

There is no consensus on the choice of mode for initiation or weaning. Use assist control (AC) or IMV mode during initiation and stabilization and SIMV (also known as patient triggered ventilation or PTV) during weaning. When using CPAP on ventilator, only the "PEEP" and FiO_2 needs to be set.

	IMV
Adv	Fixed ventilator breaths are delivered at regular interval irrespective of patient's respiratory rate.
Disadv	1. Patient breathes spontaneously which causes ineffective gas exchange depending upon whether the baby breathes with or against the ventilator. 2. Asynchrony has the potential to lead to gas trapping and air leaks. 3. Asynchrony is associated with irregularities in arterial blood pressure, cerebral blood flow velocity, and intraventricular hemorrhage in preterm infants.
	SIMV
Adv	Mechanical breath is timed to the onset of a spontaneous breath if it occurs within a "timing window".
Disadv	1. Expiratory asynchrony may occur if the baby's inspiratory time is less than the clinician's set time. 2. Baby may breathe spontaneously between mechanical breaths but the only additional support is provided by PEEP. 3. Spontaneous breaths in excess of the preset number are not supported, resulting in uneven tidal volumes (V_T) and potentially a high work of breathing, especially during weaning.
	AC
Adv	All spontaneous breaths that exceed the trigger threshold result in delivery of mechanical breaths at the onset of inspiration.
Disadv	If AC breaths are cycled strictly by time, expiratory asynchrony can still occur if the machine Ti exceeds the baby's spontaneous Ti.
	Pressure Support
Adv	Provides an inspiratory pressure assist to spontaneous breaths during mechanical ventilation. A spontaneous breath that meets

	the trigger threshold causes delivery of a mechanical breath that is pressure-limited and flow-cycled (with a Ti limit). The patient controls its onset, duration and frequency.
Disadv	Not many studies in neonatal period.

TROUBLE SHOOTING

Apnea Alarm Ventilator Troubleshooting

Responding to Alarms and Abnormal Waveforms

If alarm situation or abnormal waveform is present, do the following in all situations:

1. Look at the patient to evaluate distress.
2. Assess patient to be sure of ventilation and oxygenation.
3. If necessary, disconnect patient from ventilator and manually ventilate, increasing FiO_2.
4. Check the alarm parameters are set appropriately.
5. Once the cause of problem has been determined, resolve the cause.
6. If the problem cannot be resolved, change the ventilator.

COMMON ALARM SITUATIONS

Low Pressure Alarm

1. Check for patient disconnection.
2. Check for leaks in the patient circuit, related to the artificial airway, and through chest tubes.
3. Check the proximal airway pressure sensor (Paw) line to be sure it is connected and not obstructed.
4. This alarm may be accompanied by a low tidal volume (TV) alarm.

High Pressure Alarm

1. If patient is coughing, be sure that secretions have not built up in the airway and that patient is not biting on the tube.
2. Check for kinking, and/or malpositioning of the ETT.
3. Check to see if the patient's airway resistance has increased or if compliance has decreased.
4. Be sure that the main inspiratory or expiratory lines are not kinked or obstructed.
5. Check that patient is breathing synchronously with ventilator.
6. Determine if auto-PEEP has developed.
7. Be sure that expiratory valve is functioning.

Low PEEP/CPAP Alarms

1. Check the low PEEP alarm setting to be sure it is below the PEEP level.
2. See if the patient is actively inspiring below baseline.
3. Determine if a leak is present.
4. Check to be sure that the patient is not disconnected.
5. Assess the proximal Paw to be sure it is not occluded.

Apnea Alarm

1. Determine if the patient is apneic.
2. Check for the presence of leak.
3. Check the sensitivity setting to be sure the ventilator can detect patient effort.
4. Check the alarm time interval and the volume setting is appropriate.

Low Source Gas Pressure or Power Input Alarm

1. Check 50 PSI gas source (e.g. wall connection or air compressor).
2. Check high pressure nose connections to the ventilator.
3. Check electrical power supply, and reconnect if necessary.
4. Check line fuse or circuit breaker.
5. Try the reset button.
6. If alarms continue, replace the ventilator.

Ventilator Inoperative Alarm and/or Technical Error Message

1. Internal malfunction present; try turning ventilator off and restarting it.
2. If alarm continues, replace the ventilator.

Operative Settings are Incompatible with Machine Parameters

1. Error message usually indicates that a parameter must be reset (e.g. flow is not high enough to deliver TV within an acceptable Ti to keep I:E ratio below 1:1.
2. Readjust the appropriate controls.

I:E Ratio Indicator and Alarm Activated

1. Usually indicates an I:E ratio of greater than 1:1.
2. If inverse I:E ratio is a goal, disable the I:E ratio limit.
3. If normal I:E ratio is a goal, check alarm causes:
   - Has increased airway resistance or decreased compliance resulted in a lower flow? Treat the cause.
   - Is the flow setting too low for the desired TV delivery? Increase flow or change flow waveform.

Other Possible Alarms

1. High PEEP / CPAP alarms*.
   Similar to causes of high pressure alarms.
   - In flow-cycled modes, check for system leaks.
2. Low TV and/or low flow alarms.
   - Similar to situations that cause low pressure alarms.
   - The patient's spontaneous ventilation has decreased for some reason.
   - The alarm may be set inappropriately.
   - Flow sensor disconnection or malfunction.
3. High TV and/or high flow alarm.
   - Check machine sensitivity for auto-triggering.
   - Be sure alarms are set appropriately.
   - If external nebulizer is in use, reset the alarm setting until the treatment is finished.
   - Check flow sensor for miscalibration, contamination or malfunction.
4. Low FiO_2 and high FiO_2 alarm.
   - Check gas source.
   - Check built in oxygen analyzer for proper functioning.

Common Causes of High Pressure Alarm Situations

- Circuit leaks
  - Patient coughing
  - Secretions or mucus in the airway
  - Patients biting on tube (oral intubation)
- Airway problems
  - Kinking of tube inside the mouth in the back of the throat
  - Impinging of the tube on the carina
  - Change in the tube position
- Patient-related conditions
  - Reduced compliance (e.g. secretions, mucosal edema, or bronchospasm)
  - Patient fighting the ventilator (e.g. dyssynchrony with ventilator settings)
- Ventilator circuit
  - Accumulation of water in the patient circuit
  - Kinking in the circuit
  - Ventilator's inspiratory or expiratory valves malfunction

Common Causes of Low Pressure Alarm Situations

- Patient's disconnection from ventilator
- Circuit leaks
  - Mainline connections to

- Humidifiers
- Filters
- Water traps
- In-line metered dose inhalers
- In-line nebulizers
- Proximal pressure monitors
- Flow monitoring lines
- Exhaled gas monitoring devices
- In-line closed suction catheters
- Temperature monitors
- Exhalation valve leaks: Cracked or leaking valves
- Unseated valves, improperly connected valves

• Airway leaks
  - Use of minimum leak technique
• Chest tube leaks

REFERENCES

1. Hermansen CL, Lorah KN: Respiratory distress in the newborn, Am Fam Physician 2007;76:987-94.
2. Owen LS, Morley CJ, Davis PG: Neonatal nasal intermittent positive pressure ventilation: What do we know in 2007? Arch Dis Child Fetal Neonatal Ed 2007;92:F414-18.
3. Massimo Bellettato, Wally Carlo: Assisted Ventilation of the Newborn, Accessed on www.emedicine.com. Updated June 2006.
4. Mammel MC, Bing DR: Mechanical ventilation of the newborn: An overview, Clin Chest Med 1996; 17: 603-13.
5. Bancalari E, Sinclair JC: Mechanical ventilation, In: Sinclair JC, Bracken ME, eds. Effective Care of the Newborn Infant, New York: Oxford University Press; 1992.
6. Boynton BR, Hammond MD: Pulmonary gas exchange: Basic principles and the effects of mechanical ventilation, In: Boynton BR, Carlo WA, eds.: New Therapies for Neonatal Respiratory Failure, New York: Cambridge University Press; 1994.
7. Greenough A, Milner AD, Dimitriou G: Synchronized mechanical ventilation for respiratory support in newborn infants, Neonatal Collaborative Review Group, NICHD Cochrane Neonatal Reviews.

4. BLADDER TAP

Indication

• Sample for urine culture.

Supplies

- 23 G needle.
- 5-10 cc syringe.
- Alcohol and betadine swabs, cotton balls.
- Sterile gloves, towel, gauze pads.

Prerequisite

- Ensure the infant has not passed urine in the last 1 hour.

Procedure

- An assistant holds the legs of the patient in the frog-leg position.
- Locate the site of puncture, which is 0.5 – 1 cm above the pubic symphysis in the midline.
- Use universal precautions.
- Clean prepubic region with alcohol and betadine.
- Introduce a 23 G needle attached to a 5 or 10 cc syringes in the midline just above the pubis symphysis with the needle held perpendicular.
- Advance the needle while aspirating at the same time. Do not advance once urine is aspirated in the syringe.
- Aspiration usually takes place by a distance of 2-3 cm.
- Withdraw the needle and maintain pressure over the site of puncture.
- Label and transfer the urine specimen to the lab.
- If no urine is aspirated, re-attempt 3-4 hours later.

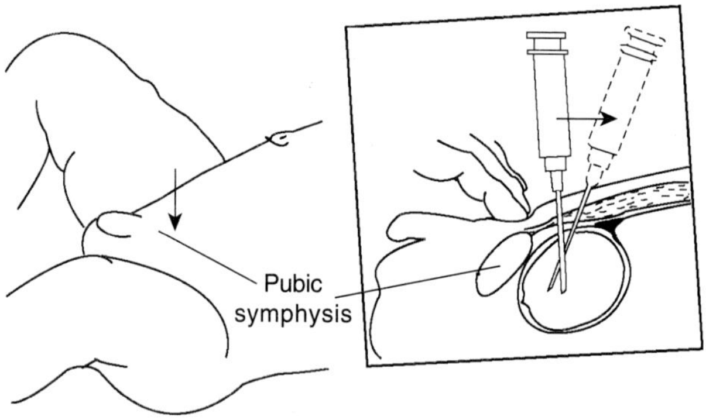

Complications

- Infection.
- Transient hematuria.
- Perforation of bowel.
- Osteomyelitis of suprapubic bone.

REFERENCE

1. Manual of neonatal nursing, Ed, Lalitha Krishnan, Published by National Neonatology Forum, 1993.

5. BLOOD CULTURE

Blood cultures aid in identifying the specific type of organism causing a blood stream infection, and when combined with antibiotic sensitivity tests, can provide information to the physician about therapeutic interventions.

Indications

- Prior to initiation of antibiotics.
- Part of sepsis screen.
- Clinical suspicion of sepsis.

Supplies

- Alcohol and iodine prep pads.
- Sterile 2 × 2 or 4 × 4 gauze.
- Syringe(s).
- Appropriate blood culture specimen bottle(s) obtained from Microbiology.

Procedure

- Drawing blood from a small infant is usually a 2-person procedure.
- Immobilization of the extremity is mandatory.
- Cleanse the skin with alcohol swabs 3 times, or until the swabs appear entirely free of surface dirt after application.
- Allow to dry.
- Apply 10% povidone-iodine, or (preferably) 2% iodine solution, or (ideally) 2% tincture of iodine in 70% alcohol, 3 times, in centrifugal circles from the anticipated site of arterial or vene-puncture.
- After 3rd swab, allow to dry at least 60 seconds.
- During this period, prepare lids (tops) of blood culture bottles with iodine and/or alcohol; lay out sterile gloves, and use paper wrapper as a sterile field for the needle and syringe (not necessary if using a Vacutainer system).
- Wipe off dry iodine at puncture site with alcohol.
- Anchor the artery or vein and smoothly insert the needle, bevel up. Attach syringe to hub of butterfly tubing. Obtain blood; place upto 0.5 ml. in each bottle (these bottles constitute 1 blood culture *set*).
- Attach syringe to blood culture dome. Inoculate bottles without changing needles. While firmly holding syringe and dome with one hand and the blood culture bottle with the other, push needle into the bottle. Blood will flow freely into the bottle.
- Repeat at different sites for requisite number of blood culture *sets*.

PRACTICE POINTERS

1. Timing of Specimen

The yield is higher prior to initiation of antibiotic therapy. Contrary to proper belief yield is not higher at the spike of fever. In cases of bacteremia or in septicemia with spiking fever, the best time to draw blood cultures is just before or at the rise in temperature.

2. The Number of Samples

At least one set of blood cultures is indicated in the diagnosis of most infants and more than one set usually is neither necessary nor valuable. If administration of antibiotics is clinically indicated, 2 sets of cultures separated by 20 to 30 minutes should be obtained prior to initiation of antibiotic therapy. Multiple sets of cultures obtained at one time would heighten the risk of missing the period of bacteremia, which is usually intermittent.

3. Volume of Blood Samples

Approximately 1 mL per 2.5 kg (4 mL per 10 kg of body mass). A single *set* of blood cultures is the total volume of blood obtained from a single site that is inoculated into media.

4. Growth Characteristics of the Medium

Bottles to be Obtained
Aerobic bottles only unless patient has peritonitis or fasciitis (in which case draw standard aerobic and anaerobic cultures).
If anaerobic infection is unlikely, use aerobic bottles only unless the patient is immunocompromised.
In the immunocompromised, consider a bottle for fungal culture (usually effective in aerobic bottles, but consult the microbiology laboratory).
If anaerobic infection is suspected, each set consists of 1 aerobic and 1 anaerobic bottle.

Collection of blood samples from the indwelling catheters for the cultures may be used in cases of suspected line infection; this should always be combined with cultures obtained from peripheral sites.

5. Method Used for Detection of Growth in Cultures

Certain antibiotic removal devices are commercially available that can be of considerable help in patients who are already on antibiotics. It is essential that the culture request contain the information that antibiotics have been given, unless they have been stopped for more than 1 week. Media containing resins are often used to adsorb antibiotics that may be present in a patient's blood and to improve microbial detection.

6. False Positive Culture Report

Features of false-positive blood cultures are as follows:

1. Coagulase-negative staphylococci (*S. epidermidis*) and *S. viridans* in a single bottle in patients not suspected of infectious endocarditis and without chronic indwelling IV access catheters are usually contaminants.
2. Corynebacteria (previously known as "diphtheroids"), *Propionibacterium acne*, and *Bacillus* spp. are usually contaminants, but they can be pathogenic in immunocompromised patients.
3. Multiple organisms in a series suggest contamination.
4. Late-appearing growth: Species that grow out after prolonged culture have a higher likelihood of being contaminants.
5. The patient's symptoms have resolved or are inconsistent with sepsis (beware of infectious endocarditis, which can have an indolent course).
6. A primary infected source (e.g., sputum or urine) yields a different pathogenic isolate.

Documentation

Document on lab requisition form:

- Location of culture site.
- Date and time of specimen collection.
- Name of nurse obtaining specimen.
- Date, time and location of blood culture.
- Patient response to procedure.

REFERENCES

1. Gerdes JS: Diagnosis and management of bacterial infections in the neonate, Pediatr Clin North Am 2004; 51: 939-59.
2. Roberts, GC, Goodman, NL, Land, GA, Larsh, HW, McGinnis, MR: Manual of Clinical Microbiology, 4th Edn, Lennette, EH, Balows, A, Hausler, WJ, Shadomy, HJ (eds), Washington, DC, AMS, pp. 500-513, 1985.
3. Isaacman, D. J., R. B. Karasic, E. A. Reynolds and S. I. Kost: Effect of number of blood cultures and volume of blood on detection of bacteremia in children, J. Pediatr 1996;128: 190-195.

6. BLOOD SAMPLING

Most laboratory tests are performed on whole blood (collected in tubes containing anticoagulants), plasma or serum.

The Steps of Blood Collection

- Properly identifying the patient by name and date of birth, or medical record number.
- Assessing the patient and environment before proceeding.

- Properly completing the lab requisition slip and labels.
- Verifying order, and deciding on appropriate collection method.
- Assembling proper (safety) equipment.
- Selecting an appropriate site (palpate the site).
- Using universal precautions.
- Properly preparing the site (cleanse the site.)
- Performing the venepuncture.
- Recognizing and appropriately intervening when complications occur.
- Controlling of bleeding.
- Recording the procedure—Properly obtaining, handling, and labelling specimens: Patient's first and last name, Unique patient ID number, Date and time specimen was collected, Identity of the phlebotomist who collected the specimen, Properly charting procedure into patient record.
- Practising infection control.
- Maintaining specimen integrity during transit.

CAPILLARY SAMPLING

Supplies

- Sterile 2 mm lancet.
- Sterile alcohol swab.
- Sterile gauze pads.
- Soft cloth.
- Blood collection form.
- Blood collection tube or dry blood spot paper.
- Gloves.

Indications

- pH determination.
- Hematocrit.
- Complete blood count (CBC), micro erythrocyte sedimentation rate (ESR).
- Biochemical estimations.

Procedure

- Ensure the infant is kept in the normal range of temperature during the procedure.
- *Preparing the site:*

  Warm the heel for 3 minutes prior to puncture by using "heel warmers" or if not available, by wrapping a moist warm wash cloth upto 41°C. Moist heat helps to increase blood flow to the area to be punctured. The increase in blood flow has been found to be as much as sevenfold. The blood specimen must be collected immediately after the 3 minutes warming, because the wash cloth will rapidly cool the heel as it cools and this will actually slow the blood flow.

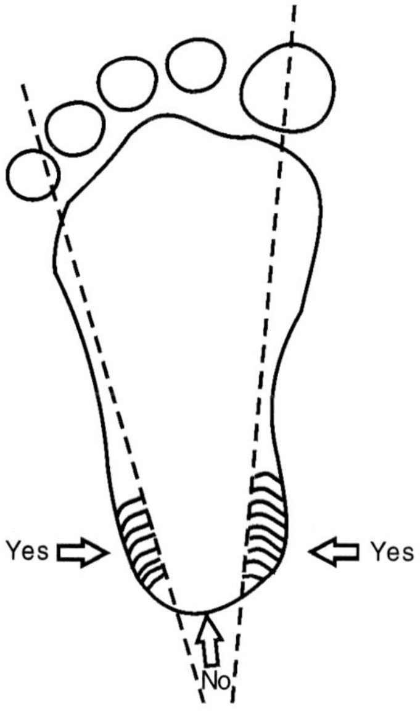

- *Cleansing the site*

  As with venepunctures, it is important to cleanse the puncture site. The antiseptic – povidone iodine, should remain in contact with the skin for at least 1 minute and should be rubbed off with a dry, sterile swab. If the site is not dried well, the antiseptic can mix with the specimen and the blood will not "bead up" well at the puncture site. Rather, the blood will spread over the moist area, making it difficult to collect.
- Thoroughly scrub your hands and arms to the elbow with soap and water, and put on disposable gloves. *Positively identify the patient.*
- Place neonate on stomach if possible and place his/her limb lower than the level of the heart to increase blood flow to the foot.
- Keep a gauze piece below the site of collection. Do not spill blood.
- Perform a swift, clean puncture on the plantar surface of the heel at a 45-60 degree angle.

  Note: The "crown" portion of the heel should not be used. It is too close to the calcaneus.
- Wipe away the first drop of blood. Gently and progressively squeeze the lower leg and ankle using a "tennis racket" grip. A large drop of blood should form on the skin. Touch the drop of blood with a heparinised glass capillary tube and the blood will run into the tube if it is held horizontally or slightly downwards. Close one end of the capillary tube with plasticine.

- Stop the bleeding by applying pressure with a dry swab for a few minutes. Do not apply adhesive over site of puncture.
- Watch for any signs of distress from the patient that are unusual or appear to impair cardiopulmonary function. Be careful not to displace any lines or monitoring devices attached to the patient.
- Discard contaminated materials properly.
- Label specimen cards or tubes correctly.

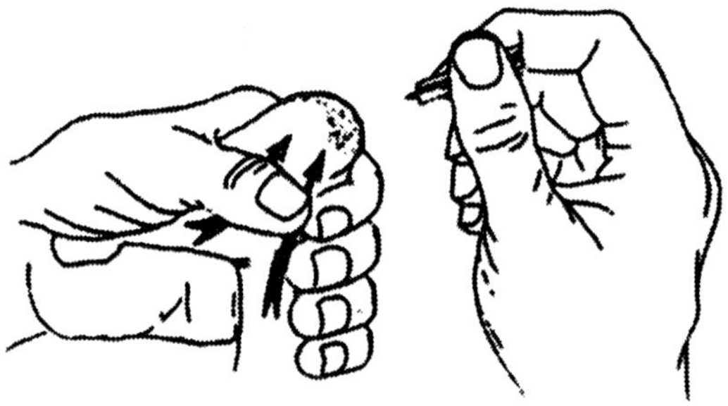

- *Watch for:*
  a. Prolonged bleed from puncture site.
  b. Local hematoma.
  c. Bluish / reddish discoloration at local site.
  d. Swelling of the limb.

Complications

- Neonatal osteomyelitis.
- Maceration.
- Infection.

Artefacts in arterial blood gas

	pH	*pCO_2*	*HCO_3*	*pO_2*
Excess heparin	Low	Low	Low	-
Delayed analysis	Low	High	-	Low
Air bubble	-	Low	-	High

USING A MICROCENTRIFUGE

The sample of blood in the capillary tube must be spun down in a microcentrifuge for 2 minutes. All level 2 and 3 nurseries should have a microcentrifuge.

A microcentrifuge should be used as follows:

1. The power lead can be left plugged in and switched on all the time.

2. Open the lid of the microcentrifuge and unscrew the cover.
3. Place the capillary tube in one of the radiating grooves in the centrifuge plate so that the end of the tube, which is blocked with plasticine, is right up against the outside edge of the plate. Many capillary tubes can be centrifuged (spun) at the same time if needed. The capillary tube must be balanced by another tube (filled with water if necessary) placed in the groove opposite it.
4. Replace the cover and screw it tightly closed.
5. Close the lid.
6. Set the timer for 2 minutes.
7. Switch the microcentrifuge on.
8. After 2 minutes the microcentrifuge will automatically switch off. Allow it to stop. Some microcentrifuges can be manually slowed down with a brake.
9. When the microcentrifuge has stopped completely, open the lid, unscrew the cover and remove the spun capillary tube.

You will notice that the red cells have all been spun to one end of the tube. The rest of the tube is filled with serum. Where the red cells and the serum meet, you will see a 1 mm white band. This is formed by the white blood cells.

DETERMINING THE PACKED CELL VOLUME (PCV)

A special instrument called a packed cell volume reader (or a micro-haematocrit reader) is used to measure the packed cell volume. Two different types of PCV reader are available. One type measures the PCV while the capillary tubes are still in the microcentrifuge while the other type is completely separate from the microcentrifuge.

MEASURING THE PACKED CELL VOLUME ON THE MICROCENTRIFUGE

1. Centrifuge (spin) the capillary tube as described above.
2. Place the perspex reader over the plate holding the capillary tubes.
3. While holding the plate still with one hand so that it does not turn, twist the knob on the reader with the other hand until the baseline (i.e. 0) crosses the capillary tube at the point where the red cells meet the plasticine.
4. Now hold the knob still with one hand and rotate the perspex reader with the other hand until the top line (i.e. 100%) crosses the capillary tube at the top of the serum (not the top of the tube).
5. Determine which line crosses the capillary tube at the point where the red cells meet the serum. Follow that line along to either the left or the right and read the PCV.

MEASURING THE PACKED CELL VOLUME OFF THE MICROCENTRIFUGE

1. Remove the capillary tube from the microcentrifuge and place it in the vertical groove of the reader so that the junction of the plasticine and the red cells lies on the bottom line.

2. Slide the capillary tube holder to the left or the right until the top of the serum (not the top of the tube) falls on the top line.
3. Move the perspex arm up so that the line falls on the junction of the red cells and the serum.
4. Read the PCV.

VENOUS BLOOD SAMPLING

Indications

- Blood chemistry studies.
- Blood culture.

Site

Veins on dorsum of hand, foot, scalp, antecubital vein, saphenous vein.

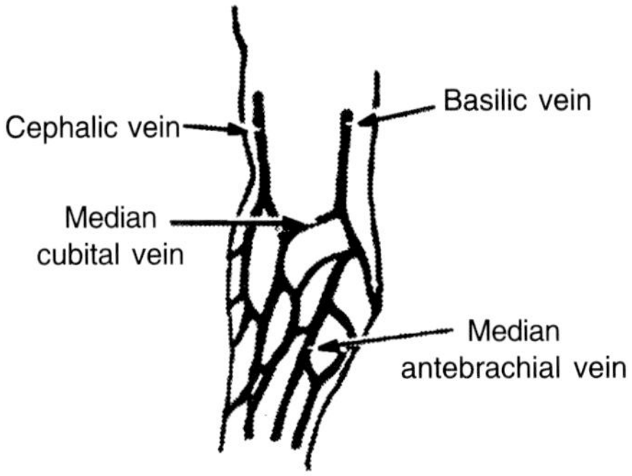

Antecubital veins

Supplies

- Sterile 22 / 23 G needle.
- Sterile alcohol swab.
- Sterile gauze pads.
- Soft cloth.
- Blood collection form.
- Blood collection tube / bulbs.
- Gloves.

Procedure

- Ensure the infant is kept in the normal range of temperature during the procedure.
- Cleanse the puncture site with povidone iodine. Let it remain in contact with the skin for at least 1 minute. Wipe with alcohol. Allow it to room dry.

- Thoroughly scrub your hands and arms to the elbow with soap and water, and put on disposable gloves.
- Keep a gauze piece below the site of collection. Do not spill blood.
- Keep the extremity firm and fixed. Manipulate the limb to visualize the vein and to make it prominent.
- The bevel of the needle should be directed up while entering the skin and lying parallel to and above the vein and after entering for about 3-4 mm the vein should be pierced so that the needle remains securely in place. Allow the blood to flow by gravity. At times you may have to alternately squeeze and release the extremity to pump out the blood. Other alternative is to break the needle hub before piercing the skin and allow blood to flow directly into a bulb or tube.
- Collect the necessary amount of blood in the collection tube/bulb.
- After collection remove the needle and press the puncture site with a sterile gauze for 1-2 minutes or till bleeding stops.

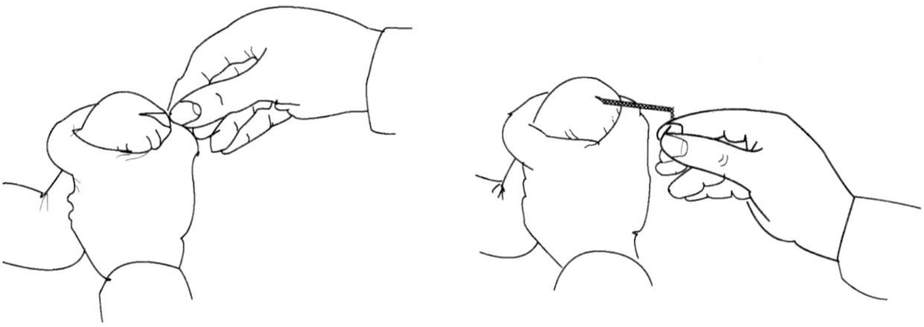

Broken needle technique for venous blood collection

Complications

- Hematoma.
- Infection.
- Extravasation.

ARTERIAL BLOOD SAMPLING

Indications

- Arterial blood gas estimation.
- Blood culture.
- Biochemical estimations (usually if larger volumes are needed, compared to those that can be obtained by heel or venepuncture).

Sites

Radial artery, Temporal artery, Posterial tibial artery and Dorsalis pedis artery. Avoid femoral and brachial arteries.

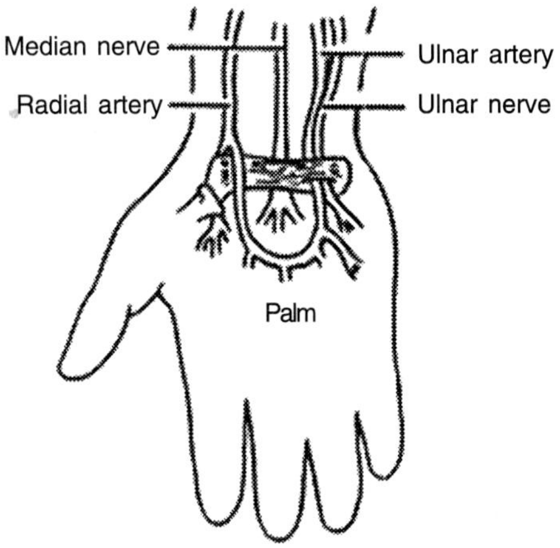

Supplies

- Alcohol wipes.
- Povidone iodine wipes.
- Sterile gauze.
- Butterfly needle (#23 or #25) or 22-gauge, 1-inch needle.
- 2 ml heparinised syringe.
- Adhesive bandage and adhesive tape.
- Blood collection form.
- Gloves.

Procedure

- Ensure the infant is kept in the normal range of temperature during the procedure.
- Thoroughly scrub your hands and arms to the elbow with soap and water, and put on disposable gloves.
- Keep a gauze piece below the site of collection. Do not spill blood.
- Heparinise the syringe and butterfly set to prevent clotting of blood. Flush the syringe and butterfly with 10U/ml of heparin. Ensure no heparin is left in the circuit, as it will alter blood gas values.
- Radial artery is the preferred site, but dorsalis pedis, posterior tibial, and physicians may use ulnar arteries with documented ability.

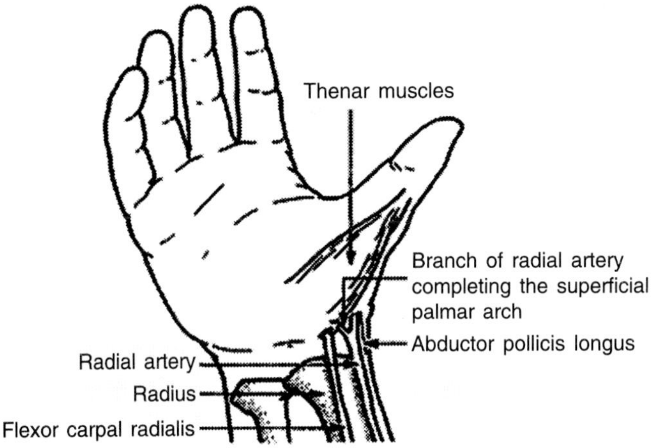

Anatomy of radial artery

- Perform Allen's test if radial artery is punctured to check for collateral circulation (See below). If collateral circulation is not adequate **DO NOT PERFORM** arterial puncture.
- ***Allen's Test:*** Elevate patient's hand. Make a fist of patient's hand and apply pressure over the radial and ulnar artery. Open the hand of the patient and release pressure from the ulnar artery. Return of color to the palm within 6 seconds indicates adequate collateral circulation by way of the ulnar artery. This represents a negative Allen's test.
- ***Modified Allen's Test:*** Elevate patient's feet. Occlude dorsalis pedis artery; then blanch the great toe by compressing the toenail for several seconds. Release pressure on the nail and observe for flushing (rapid return of color indicates adequate collateral flow).

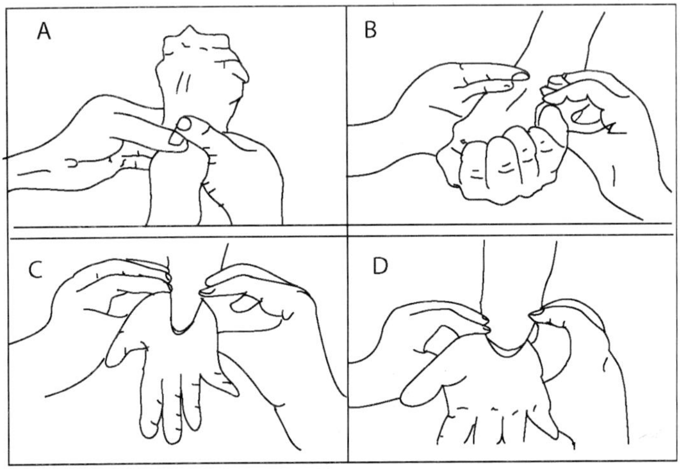

Appendix A

- Keep the extremity firm and fixed. Arteries that are difficult to visualize or palpate in the neonate may be outlined by diffusing light through the extremity from a transilluminator placed under the limb.
- Palpate artery with index and middle finger of the non-dominant hand. Check for a strong, steady pulse and good skin color around hand.

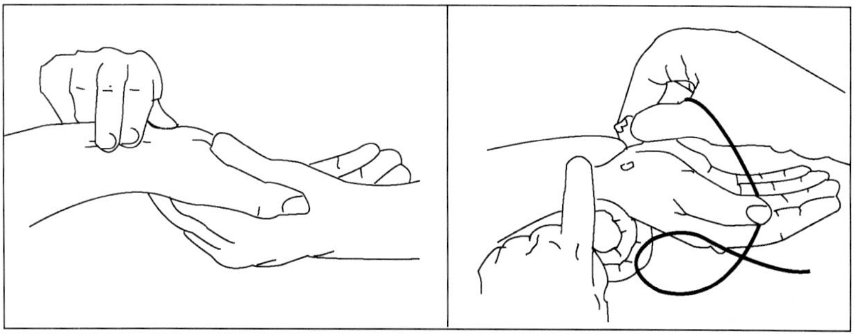

- Separate fingers on non-dominant hand over the artery continuing to feel the pulse under each finger. The site between the nurse's separated fingers is the puncture site.
- Cleanse area with antiseptic solution going in a circular motion moving from inward to outward. Allow to dry for at least 30 seconds prior to puncture. Continue to palpate artery with separated index and middle fingers. **Do not touch** prepped insertion site with fingers.
- Infiltrate the skin if local anesthetic is to be used or apply EMLA cream (1 hour prior). Insert needle at a 5-15 degree angle with the bevel directed upward such that it only extends into the epidermis. The entire bevel should be covered and lay just under the skin.
- Continue to palpate artery with separated fingers. With bevel of needle up, gently and slowly insert butterfly or needle of heparinized syringe into artery using a 30°-45° angle. A pulsatile backflow of blood into the tubing of the butterfly or the hub of the syringe indicates the artery has been punctured.
- Stabilize needle and obtain sample: 0.3 – 0.6 ml for ABG, more for blood culture or biochemical estimations (as needed). Remove needle and place in jelly cube located in ABG syringe package or engage protective sheath over butterfly needle. Apply firm pressure over puncture site with sterile 3x3 gauze. Hold pressure for 5 minutes or longer until bleeding has stopped.
- Discard needle appropriately in needle box. Place tip of syringe in dead ender cap.
- Observe frequently for hematoma or bleeding.
- Remove any air bubbles from syringe if present. To remove air, gently tap side of the syringe or roll the barrel of syringe in palm of the hand. Rotate syringe gently back and forth for 20 seconds to mix heparin and blood.

- Label specimen patient's ID. Record on the label the initials of the one who obtained the sample, the date and the time.
- If sample is hand delivered to lab, place syringe on ice to prevent alteration in values.

CORD BLOOD SAMPLING

Indications

- Babies born to Rh-negative mother.
- Suspected intrauterine infection.
- Ante partum hemorrhage.
- Metabolic screen.
- Intrapartum fetal distress.

Procedure

Blood can be obtained by puncturing the umbilical vein or by releasing the cord clamp (maternal) while the placenta is till in the uterus or after delivery the blood can be obtained by puncturing the veins on the fetal side of the placenta.

Note: Direct Coombs' test may be falsely negative if the cord blood is contaminated by Wharton's jelly.

SAMPLING FROM INDWELLING ARTERIAL LINE

Indications

- Blood gas estimation.
- Biochemical estimations (usually if larger volumes are needed, compared to those that can be obtained by heel or venepuncture).

Supplies

- Preheparinised 1 ml (1) and 2 ml syringe (2).
- Sterile gauze.
- Gloves.

Procedure

- Undo and remove the cap from the T limb of the 3-way stopcock.
- Switch off the tap to the infusion pump and on to the cannulated artery.
- Swith off the infusion pump.
- Take 2 ml preheparinised syringe and draw 1.5-2 ml of dead space and blood in it.

- Partially rotate the tap control to occlude the catheter and prevent blood loss.
- Remove syringe 1. Cap it with sterile needle and keep aside after expelling bubbles of air.
- Insert preheparinised 1 ml syringe into the port. Turn tap to on position for catheter and withdrawal blood sample. Turn 3-way to occlude blood loss.
- Replace the initial blood withdrawn in syringe 1 back into the patient by turning the tap position on for the catheter and syringe. Ensure it is free of air bubbles.
- Switch on the infusion pump.
- Attach the syringe 3 (2 ml syringe with 1 ml heparinised saline) to the port and inject 0.5 cc of heparinised saline.
- Turn the tap to off position for syringe and on position for catheter and infusion pump.
- Withdraw syringe from the 3-way stopcock.
- Close the port with cap.
- Document the blood drawn.

REFERENCES

1. Manual of neonatal nursing, Ed, Lalitha Krishnan, Published by National Neonatology Forum, 1993.
2. Essential Newborn Nursing for Small Hospitals. In resource restricted countries, Learners Guide, Published by Division of Neonatology, Department of Pediatrics, AIIMS, New Delhi 2004.

7. BREAST MILK EXPRESSION

All women who choose to breastfeed or provide breast milk to their baby need to be supported in initiating and maintaining lactation unless it is medically contraindicated. This support should be provided by staff (lactation consultants, if available) throughout the infant's hospitalization.

Clinical Assessment and Care

Assess the following parameters:

1. Maternal comfort and readiness for pumping (consider effects from narcotic and/or magnesium sulfate administration, C-section, etc.).
2. Infant's medical condition as it affects the ability to breastfeed.
3. Contraindications for breastfeeding.
4. Medications taken on a regular basis should be evaluated for safety with breastfeeding.

Breast Pumping– Manual

- Obtain a clean cup or container to collect and store the milk.

- Wash hands thoroughly.
- Ask the mother to sit or stand comfortably and hold the container underneath her breast.
- Support the breast with four fingers and place the thumb above the areola. Squeeze the areola between the thumb and fingers while pressing backwards against the chest.
- Express each breast for at least 4-5 minutes alternating breasts until the flow of milk stops.
- If the milk does not flow well:
  a. Ensure the mother is using the correct technique.
  b. Have the mother apply warm compresses to her breasts.
  c. Have someone massage mother's back and neck.

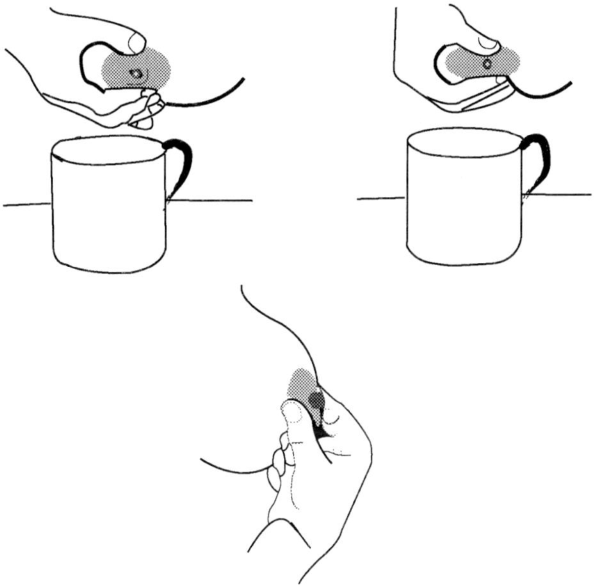

Method of expression of breast milk

Breast Pumping–Mechanical

Supplies

- Breast pump.
- Breast pump kit.
- Milk storage containers.
- Labels preprinted with baby's identification number.

- Dishwashing soap.
- Sanitizing cleaning wipes.
- Hand hygiene products.
- Paper towels.
- Clock.
- Sink.

Procedure

Preparation of Mother

- Pump kits are available for hand (manual), single pumping, or double pumping (electric). Select desired breast pumping kit.
- Demonstrate for mother the procedure of wiping clean the hospital breast pump before each use using an approved sanitizing agent.
- Using instructions located in package, attach parts to pump.
- Wash hands thoroughly prior to pumping.
- Apply warm, wet washcloths to breasts for 1 to 2 minutes before pumping, or take a warm shower. This promotes let down to get milk flowing. Mothers do not need to clean the breasts before pumping.
- Hand massages nipple/areola area for 1 to 2 minutes.
- Select a comfortable chair and/or area for pumping. Use pillows for good body posture.

Pumping Instructions

- Make sure suction lever is on minimum setting prior to turning machine on.
- Place appropriate sized flange on one or both breasts, making sure flange opening is centered over nipple. Improper positioning of flange can lead to nipple trauma.
- Turn machine on after flange/ flanges are in place. If using double pumping kit, you may place second flange on breast after machine is turned on. Remove flange only after machine has been turned off.
- Position upper body slightly forward to facilitate milk flow into receptacle. Improper posture will allow milk to flow back into flange causing moisture to form on flange resulting in decreased suction.
- Instruct mother to express milk every 2 to 3 hours during the day and night or at least 8 times in 24 hours, which approximates the feeding pattern of a newborn. Frequent breast stimulation and milk removal stimulate milk production.

Timing of Pumping

- If single pumping, pump one side then the other for approximately 10 minutes each side. The duration of pumping is not as critical as assessment of milk transfer. More or less pumping time may be needed.

- If double pumping, pump both breasts simultaneously for about 10 minutes during the first few days of lactation.
- When milk has transitioned, pump until the milk flow stops. Instruct mother to pump for an additional 2 minutes after cessation of milk flow to ensure that the breasts have fully emptied. The degree of breast emptying stimulates the breast to make more milk.

Equipment Care

- Always wash breast pump parts that come in contact with milk in hot, soapy water after each use. Allow to air dry on a clean towel after washing.
- Wipe the pump itself with the sanitizing wipes that are available on the unit.

Breast Milk Storage and Handling

Human milk must be kept in a separate refrigerator/freezer or container designated only for human milk.

Supplies

- Designated refrigerator or freezer.
- Appropriate container (bottle or bags).
- Patient labels.

Procedure

- Label individual containers of human milk with infant's name, medical record number and date pumped.
- Store pumped milk in "feeding-sized" volumes as soon as possible after receiving from infant's mother. Keep all containers of pumped milk for each infant together in a plastic bag or box.
- Verify infant's name and medical record number at the time a container of milk is removed from the refrigerator/freezer.
- Refrigerate or freeze milk immediately after pumping.
- Fresh milk, if available, should be used prior to frozen milk
- Fresh milk may be used for upto 4 hours at room temperature after pumping.
- Freshly refrigerated milk must be used within 24 hours while baby is in the nursery.
- Frozen milk may be kept in a standard home freezer (attached to refrigerator) at 0ºC, or an upright chest or freezer for 6 months
- Thaw frozen milk in a labelled cup: inside the refrigerator over several hours or place the cup inside a glove and allow to sit in standing warm water on a covered surface. After defrosting, the milk should be labelled with the date and time it is completely thawed.
- Keep thawed milk refrigerated until used or discarded.
- Frozen milk should be used within 24 hours of thawing.

- Label continuous or intermittent feeding with the infant's name, date and the time the feeding was begun. No more than 4 hours of feeding should be hung or drawn up at one time
- Replace syringe of milk every 4 hours (every 2 hours with the addition of Human Milk Fortifier).
- Refrigerator temperature should be kept between 0°C and 7°C. Freezer temperature should be kept at -20°C or lower.

Transporting Breast Milk

- Transport frozen breast milk to the hospital in a tightly packed cooler without ice. A clean towel, newspaper, or freezer gel pack may be used to fill dead air space. Ice is warmer than frozen milk and may actually contribute to thawing.
- Transport non-frozen breast milk in a chilled state.
- If partial thawing of less than 50% of the milk volume occurs during transport, the milk can be refrozen.

Thawing Breast Milk

- Wash hands before handling breast milk.
- Thaw frozen milk in the refrigerator or under cool running water. Do not submerge the cap in water.
- Label thawed milk with date and time thawed and expiration date (24 hours).
- Do not refreeze breast milk that has been thawed.

Warming Breast Milk for Feeding

- Wash hands before handling breast milk.
- Place milk container into warm water or under warm running water until warm. Do not place in hot or boiling water. Do not heat in microwave. Do not submerge the cap in water. Overheating may cause considerable loss of nutrients and may adversely affect anti-infective factors.
- Use warmed milk within the hour of starting to feed the infant.

Fortification of Breast Milk

- Use human milk fortifier (HMF) packets as ordered to provide optimal nutrition for premature or compromised infants.
- After the fortifier is added, gently swirl the milk – do not shake vigorously.
- Gentle mixing is needed to avoid breaking of the fat globules. This can cause fat to stick to the sides of the container, which can decrease the calories in the milk.

Strategies to Overcome Lactational Insufficiency

1. Encourage increased duration or frequency of pumping, if appropriate. Increasing frequency will have a better effect on supply as long as she is emptying her breasts.

2. Increase fluids—suggest that mother make more effort to drink fluids. Six to eight glasses of water per day are recommended; more, if the mother is thirsty.
3. Encourage "time out" for themselves—activities, which may be helpful to promote relaxation and decrease stress. Most mothers note an increase in milk supply when they are feeling better and starting to do more activity. Regular naps may increase the milk supply.
4. Suggest double pump set-up if mother is using a single set-up or electric pump if mother is using a manual pump.
5. Suggest skin-to-skin contact with baby, followed by pumping, if possible. Pumping at the bedside may facilitate relaxation as well.
6. Suggest that the mother keep a record of her pumping schedule and milk volumes. This may be helpful in figuring out her milk supply problems.
7. If, after a few days of the above interventions are in place, and the milk supply is still low, you may recommend metaclopromide (Reglan). It should not be used if the mother has a history of depression.
8. Getting the baby to breast will usually improve the milk supply also.
9. Communicate about the progress of the baby and involve mother in day-to-day care.
10. Ask the mother to contact mother support groups, lactational consultant or other mothers in nursery. Sharing problems relieves stress.

8. CARE OF BABY IN A WARMER / INCUBATOR

Indications

1. Acutely ill infants.
2. Any infant with temperature instability in an isolette.
3. Any infant on an open warmer which is turned on.

Supplies

- Thermometer.
- Radiant warmer.
- Incubator.

Purpose of Thermal Care

The purpose is thermal protection which is series of measures taken at birth and during the first few days ensure that the baby:

- Maintains a normal body temperature (36.5°C - 37.5°C).
- Does not become too cold (<36.5°C =hypothermia).
- Does not become too hot (>37.5°C = hyperthermia).

Choice of Heating Equipment

The thermal care equipment available is radiant warmer, incubator, warm room, local heating devices and skin-to-skin contact. Warming devices should only be used in institutions that have a reliable electricity supply, skilled personnel to care for babies in warming devices, staff skilled in maintaining, cleaning and repair of the warming device, and availability of spare parts.

The decision of using incubator or radiant warmer in hospital care is based upon:

1. Familiarity and ease of use.
2. Experience of the staff.
3. Quality of infection control measures.

- There are no contraindications for a baby to be cared for in incubators. All interventions including ventilation, central lines etc. can be safely carried out in incubators. The only disadvantage of incubators is risk of infection, and cleaning requires lot of maintenance and time.
- **Type of incubator:** The concept of an incubator with additional insulation, namely a double wall of plexiglass, is appealing as it may help very low birth weight (VLBW) infants maintain this appropriate temperature environment. Studies have assessed the effects of double-walled incubators compared to single-walled incubators on the energy needs and water balance of VLBW infants. The double-walled incubators have advantages as far as decreasing heat loss and decreasing heat production. The infants cared for in these incubators seemed to be in the best temperature range, as their need to burn energy was less. However, these effects were small and did not provide any evidence of any long-term improvement regarding duration of hospitalization or survival. Although it appears that caring for extremely small infants in double-walled incubators may result in certain metabolic advantages, the Cochrane review was unable to find any data in the literature to support or refute this theory. Available data is insufficient to directly guide clinical practice.
- Radiant warmers result in increased insensible water loss (IWL) compared to incubators. This needs to be taken into account when calculating daily fluid requirements. There is insufficient evidence about choice of equipment on important outcomes to guide clinical practice.
- Therefore primarily the choice of equipment for thermoregulation would be defined by the familiarity, ease and experience.

Following babies may be candidates for incubator care:

a. Care of extremely LBW (ELBW) babies for humidification.
b. For isolating an infected baby to achieve barrier nursing.
c. For use at low ambient temperature or when there is lot of convective currents where a radiant warmer fails to work.
d. For transporting babies.

- All staff using the equipment must have received the appropriate on-the-job training in its use. An instruction manual must always be available for reference purposes. A specific procedure for cleaning and maintenance of equipment must be specified and adhered to.

USING A RADIANT WARMER

- Turn on the warmer and set the temperature usually between 36°C and 37.5°C in skin mode for LBW babies during the first week of life.
- When it is known beforehand that a baby is to arrive in the newborn unit, turn on the warmer to pre-warm the linen and mattress so that the baby does not initially lie on a cold surface.
- Ensure that the baby's head is covered and the baby is clothed or covered unless it is necessary for the baby to be naked or partially undressed for observation or a procedure.
- Ensure the baby is placed at the centre of warmer.
- Ensure that the probe is firmly fixed at the abdomen with transparent tape.
- Turn the baby frequently while under the warmer, if possible.
- Increase the volume of fluid by 10% of the total daily volume per day
- Check the temperature of the warmer and of the room every hour, and adjust the temperature setting accordingly.
- Wash hands and check the axillary temperature as per protocol.
- Wash hands and change the diaper or sheet on passing urine or stool.
- Do not forget to turn on the heater if it has been shut for hyperthermia or X-ray.
- Shut the system prior to moving the upper unit of the warmer out for X-ray.
- Do not leave the side panels down at any time.
- If alarm occurs for high temperature, check probe site, take axillary temperature, shift to manual mode and recheck the baby temperature after 10 minutes.
- If alarm occurs for low temperature, check probe site, take axillary temperature, shut off the fan and recheck temperature after 10 minutes
- Inform if:
  a. System failure alarm occurs.
  b. Baby develops hypothermia (< 36.5°C) / hyperthermia (>37.5°C).
  c. Overheating of coil occurs.
- Document infant's temperature and nursing actions taken on record.

Using An Incubator

- Determine the appropriate temperature for the incubator based on the baby's weight and age as shown below.
- Warm the incubator to the desired temperature before placing the baby inside.
- Clean the mattress and cover it with a clean linen sheet.
- Ensure that the incubator's water reservoir is empty; microrganisms may grow in the water and infect the baby. Leaving the reservoir dry will not affect the function of the incubator.

- Ensure that the baby's head is covered and the baby is clothed or covered unless it is necessary for the baby to be naked or partially undressed for observation or a procedure.
- Ensure the baby is placed at the centre of warmer.
- Ensure that the probe is firmly fixed at the abdomen with transparent tape.
- Close the hood as quickly as possible after placing the baby inside, and keep the portholes of the incubator closed at all times to keep the incubator warm.
- Check the temperature of the incubator every hour for the first eight hours, and then every three hours.
- Wash hands and change the diaper or sheet on passing urine or stool.
- If the temperature of the incubator does not match the set temperature, the incubator may not be functioning properly; adjust the temperature setting until the desired temperature is reached inside the incubator, or use another method to warm the baby.
- Measure the baby's temperature every hour for the first eight hours, and then every three hours: If the baby's temperature is less than 36.5°C or more than 37.5 °C, adjust the temperature of the incubator accordingly. If the baby's temperature remains less than 36.5°C or more than 37.5°C in spite of the incubator being kept at the recommended setting, manage for abnormal body temperature.

Weight of baby	*Incubator temperature by Age*			
	35°C	*34°C*	*33°C*	*32°C*
< 1500 grams	1-10 days old	11 days to 3 weeks old	3-5 weeks old	> 5 weeks old
1500 to 2000 grams		1 to 10 days old	11 days to 4 weeks old	> 4 weeks old
2100 to 2500 grams		1 to 2 days old	3 days to 3 weeks old	> 3 weeks old
> 2500 grams			1 to 2 days old	> 2 days old

If the incubator is single-walled, increase the incubator temperature 1°C for every 7°C difference in temperature between the room and the incubator.

Clinical Assessment For Thermal Well Being

Signs of hypothermia

- Cool skin temperature
- Pallor
- Mottling of extremities
- Decreased pulses
- Prolonged capillary refill time

Signs of hyperthermia

- Increased heart rate
- Increased respiratory rate
- Flushed appearance
- Extended posture
- Skin warm to touch

- Apnea
- Heart rate changes
- Decreased activity
- Brisk capillary refill
- Apnea

MODE OF THERMAL CONTROL—SKIN VERSUS AIR MODE

Each method has its pros and cons.

Skin Mode

The heater output is controlled by the baby's skin temperature, which is set at a desired level. The heater cycles to keep the skin temperature at that constant.

Advantages

1. Useful in re-warming of hypothermic babies in a graded manner.
2. A set skin temp of 36°C would suffice for all LBW babies.
3. Reduced need for close monitoring of infant temperature.

Disadvantages

1. Marked fluctuations in air temperature.
2. If the skin probe gets partially dislodged or displaced, overheating occurs.
3. Inappropriately low ambient temperature if the infant is febrile.
4. Fever is likely to be missed unless infant temperature is checked frequently.
5. Masking of hypo- and hyper-thermia in baby.

Air Mode

The air temperature is set to a desired level and a thermostat in the airflow maintains this temperature.

Advantages

1. Proportionate heat control.
2. Fluctuations in air temperature minimal.

Disadvantages

1. If the air probe is placed away from the body it will cause variable heating.
2. If the air probe is covered it will cause variable temperature changes.

Site of Temperature Probe

- The thermal sensor in skin mode needs to be fixed over abdomen firmly if the baby is in supine position.
- In prone position, the flank may be used.
- Areas with high metabolic rate as the right hypochondrium (due to underlying liver) need to be avoided.
- Probe should not be applied over bruised or broken skin.

Setting the Temperature

- During at least the first week after birth, LBW babies should be provided with a carefully regulated thermal environment that is near the thermoneutral point.
- For LBW babies in incubators, this can be achieved by adjusting incubator temperature to maintain an anterior abdominal skin temperature of at least 36°C, using either servo-control or frequent manual adjustment of incubator air temperature.

Managing a Cold Baby

1. Active intervention must be done if the baby temp is < 36.5°C (axillary).
2. The method, or combination of methods selected will depend on the severity of the hypothermia and the availability of staff and equipment.
3. The re-warming process should be continued until the baby's temperature reaches the normal range.
4. Ensure feeding and euglycemia if baby is active or start IV fluids and check sugar.
5. Every hypothermic newborn should be assessed for infection.

Moderate Hypothermia (32 to 36.4°C)

- Remove cold or wet clothing, if present.
- Ensure skin-to-skin contact with mother, if the baby does not have other problems.
- If the baby is unstable, dress the baby in warm clothes, cap and cover with a warm blanket.
- Warm the baby using a radiant warmer.
- Encourage the mother to breastfeed more frequently. If the baby cannot be breastfed, give expressed breast milk using an alternative feeding method.
- Measure blood glucose. If the blood glucose is less than 45 mg/dl (2.6 mmol/l), treat for hypoglycemia.
- Measure the baby's temperature every hour for three hours.
- If the baby's temperature is increasing at least 0.5°C per hour over the last three hours, re-warming is successful; continue measuring the baby's temperature every two hours.
- If the baby's temperature does not rise or is rising more slowly than 0.5°C per hour, look for signs of sepsis (e.g. poor feeding, vomiting, breathing difficulty).
- Once the baby's temperature is normal, measure the baby's temperature every three hours for 12 hours.
- If the baby's temperature remains within the normal range, discontinue measurements.
- If the baby is feeding well and there are no other problems requiring hospitalization, discharge the baby.

- Advise the mother how to keep the baby warm at home.

Severe Hypothermia (< 32°C)

- Warm the baby immediately using a pre-warmed radiant warmer.
- Remove cold or wet clothing, if present. Dress the baby in warm clothes and a hat, and cover with a warm blanket.
- Evaluate and treat for sepsis, if appropriate.
- Secure IV line and start maintenance I.V. fluids.
- Measure blood glucose. If the blood glucose is less than 45 mg/dl (2.6 mmol/l), treat for hypoglycemia.
- Assess the baby periodically.
- Look for signs of clinical deterioration (i.e. respiratory rate less than 20 breaths per minute, gasping, not breathing, or shock) every hour.
- Measure the baby's temperature every hour.
- If the baby's temperature is increasing at least 0.5°C per hour over the last three hours, re-warming is successful; continue measuring the baby's temperature every two hours.
- If the baby's temperature does not rise or is rising more slowly than 0.5°C per hour, ensure that the temperature of the warming device is set correctly.
- Assess readiness to feed every four hours until the baby's temperature is within the normal range.
- If the baby shows signs of readiness to suckle, allow the baby to begin breastfeeding. If the baby cannot be breastfed, give expressed breast milk using an alternative feeding method.

Managing Hyperthermia (>37.5°C)

Hyperthermia as a result of overheating or underlying infection can be ruled out by following bedside clues:

Overheated infant	*Febrile infant*
1. Extended posture.	1. Flexed posture.
2. Healthy appearance.	2. Looks unwell.
3. Pink skin color.	3. Pale skin.
4. Warm hands and feet.	4. Cool hands and feet.
5. High rectal temperature.	5. High rectal temperature.
6. Abdominal – skin temperature difference of <2°C.	6. Abdominal – skin temperature difference of >3°C.

1. Put off the heat source.
2. Do not give antipyretic drugs to reduce the baby's temperature.
3. If hyperthermia is due to overheating, reduce the temperature setting on the warming device.

   a. Undress the baby partially or fully for 10 minutes and then clothe the baby.
   b. Observe for signs of sepsis (e.g. poor feeding, vomiting, breathing difficulty) and repeat when the baby's temperature is within the normal range.
   c. Measure the baby's temperature every hour until it is within the normal range.
   d. Review nursing care practices to ensure that the problem does not happen again.
4. If the hyperthermia is due to exposure to a high ambient temperature or sun exposure:
   a. Place the baby in a normal temperature environment (25°C to 28°C).
   b. Undress the baby partially or fully for 10 minutes, then dress and cover the baby.
   c. If the baby's temperature is more than 39°C: Sponge the baby or give the baby a bath for 10 to 15 minutes in water that is about 4°C lower than the baby's current temperature. Do not use cold water or water that is more than 4°C lower than the baby's temperature.
   d. Measure the baby's temperature every hour.
   e. If the baby's temperature is still abnormal after two hours, evaluate and treat for sepsis, if appropriate.
5. Allow the baby to begin breastfeeding at the earliest. If the baby cannot be breastfed, give expressed breast milk using an alternative feeding method.
6. If there are signs of dehydration (sunken eyes or fontanelle, loss of skin elasticity, or dry tongue or mucous membranes):
   a. Establish an IV line and give IV fluids at maintenance volume according to the baby's age. Increase the volume of fluid by 10% of the baby's body weight on the first day that the dehydration is noted.
   b. Measure blood glucose. If the blood glucose is less than 45 mg/dl (2.6 mmol/l), treat for hypoglycemia.
   c. Once the baby's temperature is within the normal range, measure the baby's temperature every three hours for 12 hours. If the baby's temperature remains within the normal range, discontinue measurements.
   d. If the baby is feeding well and there are no other problems requiring hospitalization, discharge the baby.
7. Advise the mother how to keep the baby warm at home and protect from overheating.

PRACTICE POINTERS

1. The method used to keep the baby warm will depend on its weight, gestational age, and health as well as on the availability of staff and equipment.

2. No heating device can function efficiently in a cold room.
3. The head has the greatest potential for heat loss due to its surface area, therefore, cover the head to minimize heat losses in smaller babies.

Best Preventive Practices in Delivery Room for Thermal Control

- Warm delivery room.
- Pre-warming surface.
- Drying the newborn immediately, especially the head.
- Wrapping in pre-warmed dry blankets that cover the head.
- Eliminating drafts.
- Promoting early skin-to-skin contact with mother.
- Use of special plastic wraps especially in VLBW babies.
- Delay bathing and weighing.
- Promote early breastfeeding.

Best Preventive Practices in Nursery for Thermal Control

- Cover items that come in contact with infant (scale, X-ray plates) and do not place on cold surface.
- Warm caregiver's hands and equipment, such as stethoscope.
- Ensure equipments are in draft free area.
- Ensure room temperature of 22°-24°C.
- Administer warmed, humidified gases with ETT, CPAP, or supplemental oxygen.
- Maintain dry linens.
- Keep diapers dry, especially while on radiant warmer.
- Use a warmed, humidified environment for infants at risk for increased insensible water loss.
- Delay bathing until infant's temperature is stable and cardiorespiratory stability is assured.
- Use heat shields on radiant warmers or double walled incubators: with birth weights of 1.0 kg or less.

Key Points

1. The newborn cannot regulate its temperature as well as an adult and therefore needs to be protected from cold and heat.
2. Hypothermia of the newborn is due more to lack of knowledge than to lack of equipment.
3. Heat loss is mainly due to ***evaporation*** from the baby's body. But loss of body heat also occurs by ***conduction*** if the baby is placed naked on a cold surface (e.g. a table, weighing scale or cold mattress); by ***convection*** if the naked newborn is exposed to cooler surrounding air; and by ***radiation***

from the baby to cooler objects in the vicinity (e.g. a cold wall or a window) even if the baby is not actually touching them.

4. In trying to keep babies warm, it is important to make sure they do not become overheated. Hyperthermia is as dangerous as hypothermia.
5. There is no single environmental temperature that is appropriate for all sizes, gestational ages and conditions of newborn babies.
6. Every hypothermic newborn should be assessed for infection.

REFERENCES

1. VJ Flenady, PG Woodgate: Radiant warmers versus incubators for regulating body temperature in newborn infants, Cochrane Database of Systematic Reviews 2007 Issue 4.
2. N Laroia, DL Phelps, J Roy: Double wall versus single wall incubator for reducing heat loss in very low birth weight infants in incubators, Cochrane Database of Systematic Reviews 2007 Issue 4.
3. JC Sinclair: Servo-control for maintaining abdominal skin temperature at 36°C in low birth weight infants, Cochrane Database of Systematic Reviews 2007 Issue 4.
4. EM McCall, FA Alderdice, HL Halliday, JG Jenkins, S Vohra: Interventions to prevent hypothermia at birth in preterm and/or low birth weight babies, Cochrane Database of Systematic Reviews 2007 Issue 4.
5. Thermal protection of the newborn: A practical guide. Department of Reproductive Health and Research (RHR), World Health Organization, 1997.

9. CARE OF JAUNDICE IN THE NEWBORN

Management Strategy

1. To prevent total serum bilirubin (TSB) from rising.
2. To reduce TSB level.
3. To prevent neurotoxicity.

Principles of Treatment in Jaundiced Infants

1. Treatment decisions are based on TSB.
2. Gestation is more important than birth weight of the baby. A higher cut-off can be used for a small for gestational age baby.
3. Postnatal age in hours should be considered when deciding treatment.
4. Sick baby refers to presence of asphyxia, hypothermia, sepsis, acidosis, hypoxia, hypercapnia and evidence of hemolysis.

COMPONENTS OF A PHOTOTHERAPY UNIT

A number of commercial or hospital-made phototherapy units are available. Their main components are:

1. The Light Tubes

Most phototherapy units contain 4 or more blue fluorescent tubes with 2 white tubes. Increasing the number of fluorescent tubes improves the efficiency of the phototherapy. Ultraviolet tubes are NEVER used, as they will burn the infant very seriously. Fluorescent tubes have a limited life span and, therefore, must be replaced every 1000 hours (or 6 months if the hours in service are not recorded). A special photometer can be used to measure the light output of a phototherapy unit. This helps in deciding when to replace the tubes.

2. The Light Box

The fluorescent tubes are fixed into a special light box, which usually has a fan to keep the tubes cool. Otherwise the tubes and the infant will overheat. Most light boxes have a time counter, which indicates how many hours the tubes have been used.

A thick sheet (1 cm) of clear perspex (plastic) must be placed under the tubes to protect the infant from falling glass if a tube explodes. The perspex does not lessen the effect of the phototherapy but it does reduce the amount of heat reaching the infant.

3. The Stand

All phototherapy units have some form of stand to support the lighting box. Usually the stand allows the height of the light box to be raised or lowered. The tubes usually are placed 40 cm above the infant. The closer the tubes are to the infant the more effective is the treatment as more light is provided. Therefore the tubes are often moved closer if the infant is severely jaundiced. However, the infant may overheat if the tubes are brought too close. Sometimes more than one phototherapy unit is used for an infant with a high TSB.

PHOTOTHERAPY (PT) LIGHTS

a. Halogen Spotlights

These appear white and deliver an irradiance of 20 - 25 mW/cm^2/nm. Positioning of the light is critically important to the spotlight's effectiveness. They are most effective when delivered from directly above the infant at a distance of 52 cm. This should be measured in a vertical distance from the infant with a tape measure. Directing the light from the side of the crib or allowing the circle of light to move off the infant's largest surface area e.g. abdomen, significantly reduces the dose delivered. Choose the number 4 setting and the widest aperture.

b. 4 Special Blue + 2 White Fluorescent Lights

This combination should deliver 12 μW/cm^2/nm. They degenerate with time, so replacement of tubes should be done if more than 6 months old, more than 1000 hours of usage or when blackening is observed at the ends of PT tubes, even though they still appear to be working.

c. Biliblanket

This is a halogen light source directed into a fiberoptic mat. The three settings deliver: low = 7 $\mu W/cm^2/nm$; medium = 12 $\mu W/cm^2/nm$; high = 15 $\mu W/cm^2/nm$. The blanket must be positioned directly next to the infant's skin to be effective. It can be used as the sole source of phototherapy or as an adjunct to conventional treatment by laying the infant on the blanket to give "double" phototherapy i.e. increasing the surface area exposed. Biliblankets are not to be used on infants less than 28 weeks gestation or infants with broken/reduced skin integrity. Biliblanket alone does not require eye pads.

d. Light Emitting Diode (LED) Phototherapy

Recently, high intensity gallium nitride light emitting diodes (LEDs) have been developed which generate significantly higher light irradiance levels compared to all currently available conventional phototherapy units. Blue LEDs emit a high intensity narrow band of blue light overlapping the peak spectrum of bilirubin breakdown, resulting in potentially shorter treatment times. The incidence of rebound hyperbilirubinemia with LED phototherapy seems to be less than conventional phototherapy.

e. Compact Fluorescent Lamp (CFL) Phototherapy

A set of 4-6 CFL are used. The flux emitted is > 20 $\mu w/cm^2/nm$.

CARE OF BABY UNDER PHOTOTHERAPY

1. Keep the infant at the centre of phototherapy.
2. Ensure eyes are always covered.
3. Adjust distance of PT unit to keep babies skin temp at 36.5°C. If the temperature of baby is >36.5°C increase the baby – PT distance, if the temperature of baby is <36.5°C decrease the baby – PT distance.
4. Change baby position every 4 hourly.
5. Turn off the light during feeding and while performing any procedure on infant.
6. Breastfeeding on demand is continued. More frequent breast feeds are encouraged and if hydration is not maintained or infant cannot be fed orally, 10-20% extra IV fluids in addition to maintenance fluids are provided.
7. Serum bilirubin is measured every 12 hours or 4-6 hourly, if severely jaundiced.
8. In most circumstances, it is not necessary to remove the infant's diaper, but when bilirubin levels approach the exchange transfusion range, the diaper should be removed until there is clear evidence of a significant decline in the bilirubin level.

9. *Inform if:*
   A. Temperature > 37.5°C
   B. Baby develops diarrhea.
   C. If baby passes dark yellow urine.
   D. If baby passes white stool.
   E. If baby does not accept feeds.
10. *Assess and Document:*
    - Temperature, pulse and respiration rate 4 hourly.
    - Posture of the baby.
    - Oral intake.
    - Urine passed.
    - Stools.
    - Skin turgor and mucous membranes.
    - Rash.

PARENT/CAREGIVER INSTRUCTIONS

- Reinforce importance of treatment, length of treatment, laboratory tests and sufficient fluid intake.
- Instruct parents to keep infant's eyes covered if bili-lights are used.
- Emphasize length of time infant may be in mother's room/out from under bili-lights.
- Instruct parents/caregiver to inform nurse of intake and output while infant is in mother's room.
- Instruct parents/caregiver to notify infant's nurse if infant refuses feeding or displays change in activity level, e.g. twitching, tremors and lethargy.

Contraindications

1. Cholestatic jaundice.
2. Porphyria.

Strategies to Increase the Effectiveness of Phototherapy

i. As much of the skin as possible should be exposed to the bili-lights.
ii. Phototherapy unit should be as close to the baby as permissible.
iii. Use double surface phototherapy / biliblanket, if possible.
iv. Surround the adjoining area of the baby with a reflector surfaces such as silver foil or white cloth.
v. Measure the flux of phototherapy unit by fluxmeter periodically.
vi. Ensure good air circulation to the phototherapy unit to prevent overheating of light because irradiance declines with rising temperature.
vii. Use 20W, 2 ft, and blue fluorescent tubes TL-52 for phototherapy unit.
viii. Presence of darkening of tube ends by rings, if present, need immediate tube replacement.

Phototherapy should be interrupted in a newborn only during breastfeeding and diaper changes.

PRACTICAL TIPS

Clinical assessment is unreliable if a newborn has been receiving phototherapy and if the baby has dark skin.

Phototherapy Issues

a. *Light source:* The most effective light sources currently commercially available are those that use special blue fluorescent tubes or a specially designed light-emitting diode light. The special blue fluorescent tubes are labelled F20T12/BB or TL52/20W.

b. *Distance from the light:* The phototherapy unit should be as close to the baby as possible ensuring normothermia. Hyperthermia makes the phototherpy less effective. Halogen lamp PT however needs specific distances and manufacturer's instructions should be followed.

c. *Surface area:* In most circumstances, it is not necessary to remove the infant's diaper, but when bilirubin levels approach the exchange transfusion range, the diaper should be removed until there is clear evidence of a significant decline in the bilirubin level.

d. *Intermittent versus continuous phototherapy:* In most circumstances, phototherapy does not need to be continuous. Phototherapy may be interrupted during feeding or brief parental visits. Individual judgment should be exercised. If the infant's bilirubin level is approaching the exchange transfusion zone, phototherapy should be administered continuously until a satisfactory decline in the serum bilirubin level occurs or exchange transfusion is initiated.

e. *Intensive phototherapy* is recommended for those with "higher risk" based on age specific nomograms. It implies the use of high levels of irradiance in the 430- to 490-nm band (usually 30 $\mu W/cm^2$ per nm or higher) delivered to as much of the infant's surface area as possible. If TSB levels approach or exceed the exchange transfusion line, the sides of the bassinet, incubator, or warmer should be lined with aluminum foil or white material to increase the performance of phototherapy. If the TSB does not decrease or continues to rise in an infant who is receiving intensive phototherapy, this strongly suggests the presence of hemolysis.

f. *When should PT be stopped:* There is no standard for discontinuing phototherapy. The TSB level for discontinuing phototherapy depends on the age at which phototherapy is initiated and the cause of the hyperbilirubinemia. If phototherapy is used for infants with hemolytic diseases or is initiated early and discontinued before the infant is 3 to 4 days old, a follow-up bilirubin measurement within 24 hours after discharge is recommended.

Side Effects of Phototherapy

1. Dehydration.
2. Temperature fluctuations.
3. Loose stools.
4. Rash.
5. Hypocalcemia.
6. Bronze baby syndrome.

Failure of Phototherapy

Inability to document a decline in bilirubin of 1-2 mg/dl after 4-6 hours and/ or to keep the bilirubin below the exchange transfusion level.

Causes of Inadequate Response to Phototherapy

1. Occult sepsis.
2. Urinary tract infection
3. Inadequate hydration / nutrition.
4. Ongoing hemolysis, e.g., minor blood group incompatibility, G6PD deficiency.
5. Drugs: Sulfisoxazole, benzyl alcohol etc.
6. Concealed hemorrhage.
7. Inadequate dose of phototherapy.

Contraindications to PT

Congenital porphyria or a family history of porphyria is an absolute contraindication to the use of phototherapy, as is the concomitant use of drugs or agents that are photosensitizers.

USING A BILIRUBINOMETER

Before the TSB can be measured with a bilirubinometer, a sample of blood has to be collected into a capillary tube and spun down as described above. A number of different types of bilirubinometers are available. Bilirubinometer are electrically powered, expensive and have to be carefully standardized at least once a week. The care and use of a bilirubinometer, therefore, should be the responsibility of a trained medical technologist.

USING A BILIRUBIN FLUX METER

- Place the phototherapy light(s) over the infant.
- Turn the radiometer on. It should read between 003 - 025 $\mu W/cm^2$ under normal fluorescent ceiling lights.
- Hold the radiometer near the infant's skin, at the abdomen or back. The reading will stabilise after a few seconds.

- The radiometer measures irradiance in mW/cm^2. To convert: divide the reading on the radiometer by 80 (the effective bandwidth).
- Document the dosage. Keep a record of the readings.

Assessing Jaundice

- Assessment for jaundice is not by visual impression. Assessment is by inspection after blanching the skin for yellowish discoloration.
- Always assess jaundice in bright natural light.
- Do not rely on clinical assessment if baby is receiving phototherapy.
- Recognize that visual estimation of the degree of jaundice can lead to errors, particularly in darkly pigmented infants.
- If there is any doubt about the degree of jaundice, estimate serum bilirubin.
- Degree of jaundice can be assessed by Kramers criterion.

Kramer's Criterion

Head and neck	4-8 mg/dl
Upper trunk	5-12 mg/dl
Lower trunk and thighs	8-16 mg/dl
Arms and lower legs	11-18 mg/dl
Palms and soles	>15 mg/dl

Not applicable for preterm and for babies receiving phototherapy

- When in doubt about extent of jaundice, do serum bilirubin.

Criterion for Physiologic Jaundice

Type of bilirubin	Indirect bilirubin. Direct bilirubin never more than 2 mg/dl or less than 15% of total bilirubin.
Appearance	After 36 hours of age.
Rate of rise of bilirubin	Less than 5 mg/dl per day.
Severity of jaundice	Usually does not exceed 15 mg/dl.
Natural course	Peak TSB levels are seen between 3rd-5th days of life in term and 3rd-7th day in preterm and disappears by 2 weeks.
Clinical condition	Healthy newborn.

Note: All the features must be present to label as physiologic jaundice. Physiological jaundice is a *diagnosis of exclusion* based on history, clinical and lab findings.

Criterion for Pathological Jaundice

a. Clinical jaundice in the first 36 hours of life.
b. TSB > 15 mg/dl.

c. Rate of TSB increase > 0.2 mg/dl/hour or 5 mg/dl/day.
d. Direct serum bilirubin > 2 mg/dl or > 15% of total bilirubin.
e. Clinical jaundice persisting for > 2 weeks.

Approach to a Jaundiced Newborn

- Identify "high risk" newborns at delivery likely to develop jaundice.
- Ensure appropriate follow up for jaundice.
- Emphasize need for early, exclusive breast-feeds and ensure adequacy of breast-feeding.
- Assess clinical condition (well or ill).
- Ascertain birth weight and gestation.
- Evaluate jaundice with post-natal age in hours.
- Perform systematic evaluation – history and physical examination.
- Decide whether jaundice is physiological or pathological.
- If physiological and baby well, only observation is required.
- If deeply jaundiced, look for signs of bilirubin encephalopathy (lethargy, poor feeding, shrill cry, assymetric Moro reflex, hypertonia, opisthotonus or convulsions).
- If jaundice is pathological perform laboratory tests.
- Initiate appropriate measures to reduce elevated bilirubin.
- Counsel parents.

Which Jaundiced Newborns are Investigated?

1. Jaundice in preterm.
2. Jaundice in sick infant.
3. Jaundice appearing in first 36 hours.
4. Jaundice persisting beyond 14 days.
5. Jaundice with high coloured urine or clay stools.
6. Jaundice with anemia or hepatosplenomegaly.
7. Jaundice requiring phototherapy.

Management of hyperbilirubinemia in the healthy term newborn
TSB (mg/dl)

Age (hours)	*Consider phototherapy*	*Phototherapy*	*Exchange transfusions if intense phototherapy fails*	*Exchange transfusion and intense phototherapy*
< 24	-	-	-	-
25 – 48	≥ 12	≥ 15	≥ 20	≥ 25
49 – 72	≥ 15	≥ 18	≥ 25	≥ 30
> 72	≥ 17	≥ 20	≥ 25	≥30

American Academy of Pediatrics, Practice parameter: Management of hyperbilirubi-nemia in the healthy term newborn, Pediatrics 1994; 94:558-567.

Management of neonatal hyperbilirubinemia in low birth weight babies based on bilirubin levels (mg/dl)

Weight (gm)	*Phototherapy*	*Consider exchange transfusion*
500-750	5-8	12-15
750-1000	6-10	>15
1000-1250	8-10	15-18
1250-1500	10-12	17-20
1500-2500	15-18	20-25

a. These are guidelines; each baby should be individualized.

b. As a rough guide, start phototherapy in a well VLBW baby if the bilirubin levels are about one per cent of birth weight and exchange blood transfusion at a value of above plus additional 5 g/dl.

c. A sick VLBW baby requires intervention earlier.

Cashore WJ: Bilirubin and jaundice in the micropremie, Clin Perinatol 2000; 27: 171-179.

Ineffective and Potentially Dangerous Practices in Jaundice Management

- Sunlight exposure.
- Routine use of phenobarbitone.
- Supplemental feeds for baby receiving phototherapy.
- Stopping breastfeeding.
- Using plain blue or white tubes for phototherapy.

A. Early Exchange Blood Transfusion

- Cord bilirubin ≥5 mg/dl.
- Cord Hemoglobin ≤10 mg/dl.
- In case of severe sensitization to remove antibodies in baby (suggestive history of severe affection, raised indirect Coombs' titre in mother, positive direct Coombs' test in baby).

B. Subsequent Exchange Transfusion

Age (hr)	*TSB (mg/dl)*
< 24	≥ 10
25-48	≥ 15
> 48	≥ 20

When rate of rise of serum bilirubin 0.5 mg/dl per hour

C. Intensive Phototherapy

Indicated at a bilirubin level, which is 5 mg/dl less than that for exchange blood transfusion.

D. Preterm/LBW Babies

Correspondingly lower values should be used. A level equal or greater to 0.5 and 1 per cent of birth weight in grams can be used as a rough guide for phototherapy and exchange blood transfusion, respectively.

Maisels MJ: Jaundice, *In:* Neonatology: Pathophysiology and Management of the Newborn, 4th edn. Eds, Avery GB, Fletcher MA, McDonald MG, Philadelphia, J.B. Lippincott, 1994; p 765.

Best Preventive Practices for Hhyperbilirubinemia

1. Promotion and practice early, exclusive and frequent breastfeeding.
2. Ensure adequacy of hydration by noting the weight, urine frequency and colour.
3. Discourage use of prelacteals to the newborn.
4. Ensure administration of Anti-D injection to Rh-negative mother with Rh +ve newborn, if not sensitized.
5. Ensure all infants are routinely monitored for the development of jaundice
6. Identify "high risk" newborns for jaundice. Assess for jaundice twice daily in these high-risk babies. Ensure follow-up at 72-96 hours of age.
7. Respond appropriately to parental concerns about jaundice, poor feeding and changes in newborn behavior.
8. Clinical judgment should be used in determining follow-up. Earlier or more frequent follow-up should be provided for those who have risk factors for hyperbilirubinemia.
9. Educate parents and health care providers about the potential risks of jaundice during the newborn period.
10. Perform periodic checks of phototherapy units to make sure that an adequate irradiance is being delivered.

REFERENCES

1. American Academy of Pediatrics Subcommittee on Hyperbilirubinemia. Management of hyperbilirubinemia in the newborn infant 35 or more weeks of gestation, Pediatrics 2004 Jul;114(1):297-316.
2. Alkalay AL, Simmons CF: Hyperbilirubinemia guidelines in newborn infants, Pediatrics 2005;115:824-825.
3. Bhutani VK, Johnson LH, Schwoebel A, Gennaro S: A systems approach for neonatal hyperbilirubinemia in term and near-term newborns, J Obstet Gynecol Neonatal Nurs 2006;35:444-455.

4. Agrawal R, Aggarwal R, Deorari AK, Paul VK: Jaundice in the newborn. Indian J Pediatr 2001;68:977-980.
5. Tan KL: Phototherapy for neonatal jaundice, Acta Paediatr 1996;85:277-279.

10. CENTRAL VASCULAR ACCESS

Basic Principles for Central Venous Catheter

- Use an aseptic technique when inserting the catheter and any subsequent injections or changing fluid lines.
- Keep the entry site covered with a dry sterile dressing.
- Ensure the line is well secured to prevent movement (this can increase risks of infection and clot formation).
- Change the catheter if there are signs of infection at the site.
- Remember to remove the catheter as soon as it is no longer needed. The longer the catheter is left in, the greater the risks of sepsis and thrombosis.
- Some people suggest changing a catheter every 7 days to reduce the risks of catheter related sepsis and thrombosis. However, provided that the catheter is kept clean (sterile injections and connections) and there are no signs of systemic sepsis, routine replacement may not be necessary. Repeated cannulation to change lines on a routine basis, rather than based on clinical need, can increase the risks to the patient.
- Always clamp the line before the line is opened. Keep the line clamped until continuity of the system or system closure is reestablished. Under no circumstances should central lines be opened to air.
- Platelet transfusions should not be infused into central catheters.
- Central line dressings must be occlusive. A dressing is no longer occlusive if an edge of the dressing is "rolling up" and not adherent to the skin. There should be no pockets of air under the dressing. The edges of a central line dressing should not be reinforced with tape. Dressings must be changed if one observes that the dressing is no longer occlusive.
- Dressing changes are to be a two-person procedure in order to ensure asepsis and to prevent dislodging the catheter.

Types of Central Venous Catheters

- A peripherally inserted central catheter (PICC) line is a central venous catheter inserted into a vein in the arm rather than a vein in the neck or chest.
- A tunneled catheter (for e.g. Broviac®) is surgically inserted into a vein in the neck or chest and passed under the skin. Only the end of the catheter is brought through the skin through which medications can be given.

Single and multilumen catheters

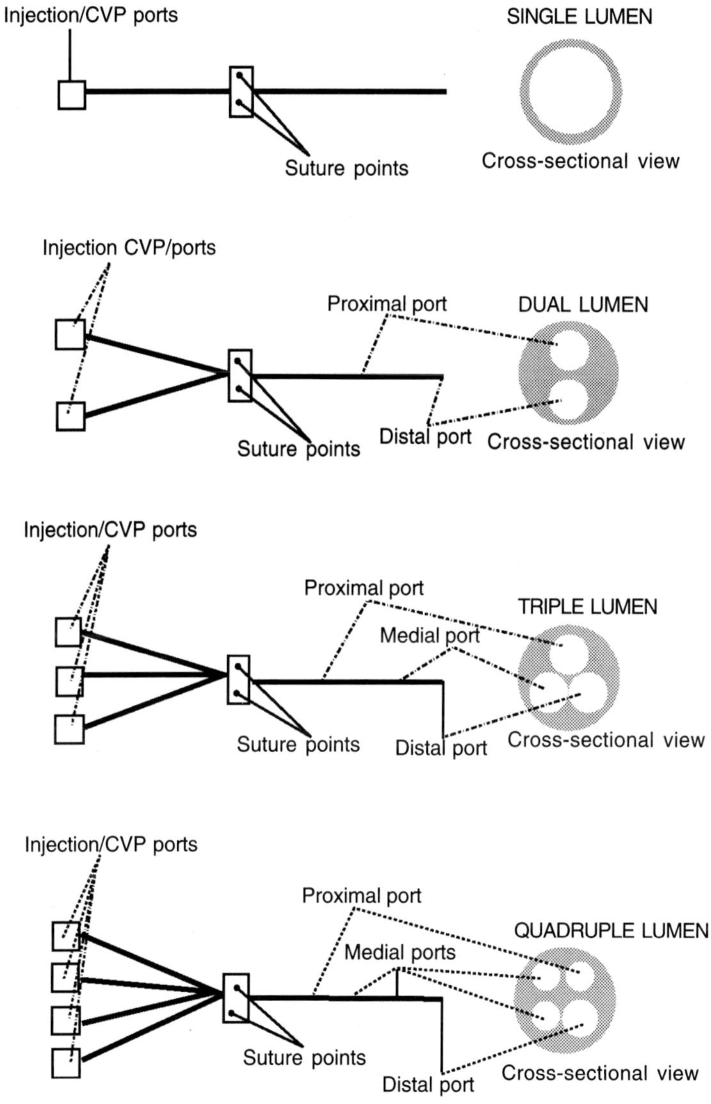

Placement of Central Venous Catheters

- The insertion of a long line should not be considered a routine. However, infants who are VLBW, likely to be slow to reach full enteral feeds, have IV access problems or long-term **IV nutrition needs** (NEC, major surgical problems etc.) may require line placement.

- In babies <1000 g insertion of an **umbilical venous catheter** (UVC) on admission is the preferred option. In those who are very small, sick or have respiratory distress an **umbilical artery catheter** (UAC) should be considered at the same time. In sick term babies a double lumen UVC should be used as they may require several infusions.

Indications

- Placement of venous access line when other peripheral sites are unavailable.
- Prolonged hyperalimentation.
- Monitoring central venous pressure.

Contraindications

- Infection over the insertion site.
- Coagulopathies.

Sites

- External jugular vein.
- Subclavian vein.
- Basilic vein.
- Saphenous vein.
- Internal jugular vein.

Subclavian catheter

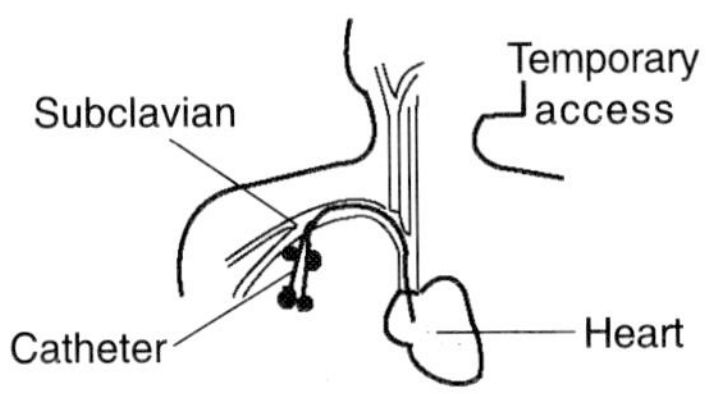

Internal jugular catheter

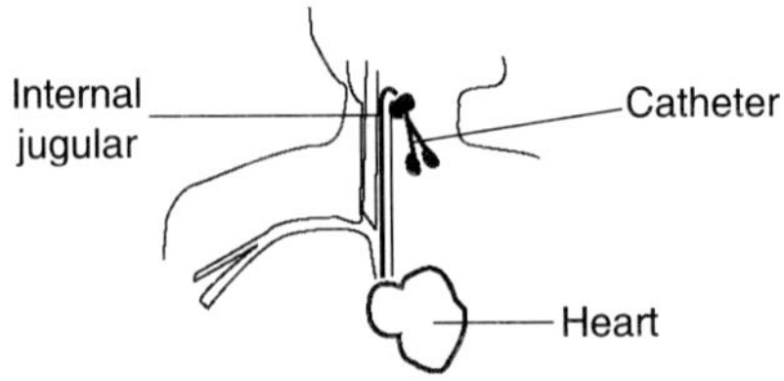

The vessels with the highest success rate of catheterization are those, which have not been previously used for peripheral IV's.

	Advantages	*Disadvantages*
Arm veins (cephalic, basilic)	Simple to access, veins visible and palpable No vital organs close Patient comfort	Failure to achieve central position High incidence of thrombosis Low maximum infusion rates
Internal jugular	Simple to insert Direct route to central veins High flow rate, low risk of thrombosis Lower risk of pneumothorax	Patient discomfort Higher rate of late complications, especially infection Tunnelling more difficult to chest wall
Subclavian/axillary	Less patient discomfort Lower risk of long-term complications	Curved insertion route Difficult to access Acute complications– pneumothorax, haemothorax, nerve damage
Femoral	High flow Easy insertion	Higher rate of infection/ /thrombosis More discomfort

Supplies

- Cap, mask, sterile gloves and sterile gown.

Basic Methods of Inserting the Central Venous Catheter

- ***Catheter over the needle:*** This is a longer version of a conventional intravenous cannula and may be quickly inserted with a minimum of additional equipment. The catheter is larger than the needle, which reduces the leakage of blood from the insertion site, but using a larger needle to find the vein makes the consequences of accidental arterial puncture more serious. In addition, it is easy to over-insert the needle.
- ***Catheter over guide wire (Seldinger technique):*** This is the preferred method of insertion. A small diameter needle (18 or 20 gauge) is used to find the vein. A guide wire is passed down the needle into the vein and the needle removed. The guide wire commonly has a flexible J-shaped tip to reduce the risk of vessel perforation and to help negotiate valves in the vein e.g the external jugular vein (EJV). Once the wire is placed in the vein, the catheter is passed over it until positioned in the vein. The wire should not be over-inserted as it may kink, perforate the vessel wall or cause cardiac arrhythmias. This technique allows larger catheters to be placed in the vein after the

passage of appropriate dilators along the wire and a small incision in the skin at the point of entry.

- ***Catheter through the needle or catheter through cannula:*** The catheter is passed through a cannula or needle placed in the vein. The technique is becoming less popular as the hole made in the vein by the needle is larger than the catheter that is passed leading to some degree of blood leakage around the site. If a problem is encountered during threading the catheter, withdrawal of it through the needle risks shearing part of the catheter off with catheter embolisation into the circulation. This technique is mainly reserved for the antecubital route.

Procedure

- Flush the long line with 0.9% NaCl leaving syringe attached.
- Cut round the IV cannula at the hub leaving cannula on the introducer.
- Position the infant maximising access i.e. open the incubator door, slide tray out and use overhead heater. Secure limbs if necessary.
- If an assistant is required, he/she must wear a gown and sterile gloves.
- Clean the skin with the chlorhexidine solution appropriate for the infant's gestation. Wait about 1 minute until it dries otherwise it will not be an effective skin prep.
- Create a sterile field with sterile guards.
- Apply tourniquet above site.
- Position line, syringe and forceps on sterile field.
- Insert cannula, advance cannula off the introducer and withdraw introducer.
- Insert long line with forceps and feed to pre-measured distance releasing tourniquet when catheter is through the cannula.
- Withdraw cannula over the long line ensuring the long line is stable by using pressure on the limb above the cannula.
- Detach long line at blue connection, remove cannula and reattach connection, ensuring air is not introduced. The black marker that lies over the metal insert must not be visible.
- Flush long line with 0.5ml of heparinised saline (10U/ml).

SUBCLAVIAN VEIN (SCV) CANNULATION

Preparation and Positioning

- The patient should be supine, both arms by the sides, with the table tilted head down to distend the central veins and prevent air embolism.
- Turn the head away from the side to be cannulated unless there is cervical spine injury.
- Normally the right SCV is cannulated since the thoracic duct is on the left and may occasionally be damaged during SCV cannulation.

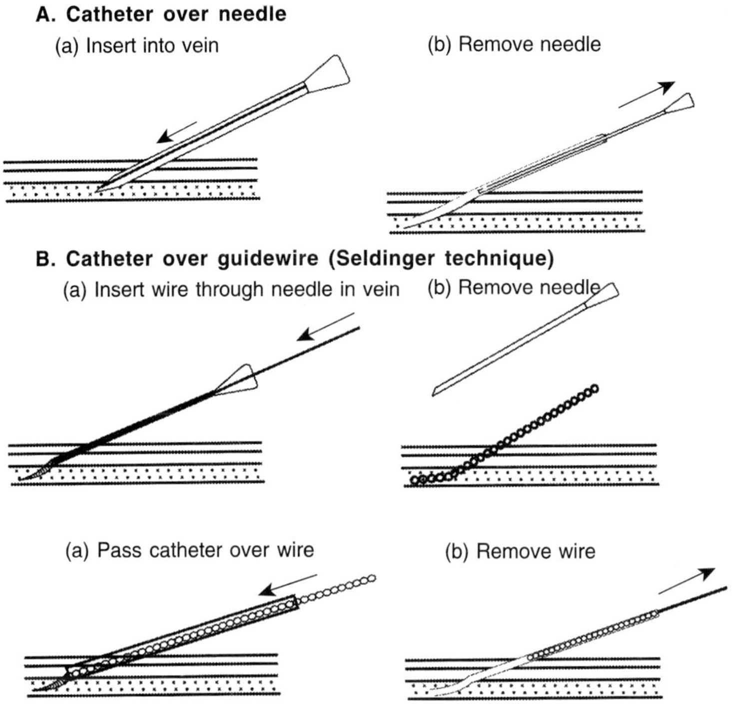

Technique

- Infraclavicular route is preferred.
- Keep the infant supine in Trendelenburg position at 20–30 degrees with a roll between scapula and head turned away from the side to be punctured. Site of insertion is the junction of middle and medial thirds of the clavicle. Prepare the site with aseptic precautions and infiltrate local anaesthetic.
- Introduce the needle attached to a syringe just under the clavicle puncturing the skin.
- Direct the needle towards a finger tip placed in the suprasternal notch.
- The syringe and the needle should be parallel to the frontal plane directed medially and slightly cephalad, behind the clavicle towards the posterior superior aspect of the sternal end of the clavicle.
- Advance needle applying gentle suction with syringe.
- On free flow of blood rotate the level of needle caudally clockwise 90 degrees to facilitate placement of the catheter.
- Disconnect the syringe and occlude the hub of the needle with a finger to prevent the aspiration of air. Remove syringe during exhalation. Remove syringe during inhalation if the infant is on respiratory support.

- Insert guide wire and pass it, now place the catheter over the guide wire and remove the wire.
- Catheter tip should be at the level of the junction of SVC and right atrium and should be confirmed by radiography.

Practical Problems Specific to the Subclavian Route

- *Keep hitting the clavicle:* Check that you are starting from the correct position. Redirect the needle slightly more posterior whilst being careful not to enter the chest. Try bending the needle slightly to encourage it to pass beneath the clavicle. Try placing a pillow under the shoulders or getting someone to pull gently down on the arms.
- *Cannot find the vein:* Direct the needle a little more cephalad.
- *Fail after repeated attempts:* DO NOT PERSIST since the likelihood of complications increase. Try an alternative route ON THE SAME SIDE unless chest radiography is available to exclude any possible pneumothorax.
- *The catheter tip is not in the chest:* Usually detected on chest X-ray, or if the fluid level in the central venous pressure (CVP) manometer does not rise and fall with breathing.

INTERNAL JUGULAR VENOUS CANNULATION

- The right side of the neck is preferred in infants as risk of damage to thoracic duct is less, path of the right atrium is more direct and the dome of the right lung and pleura is lower than the left.
- Approach can be by the anterior, posterior or central route.

Preparation and Positioning

- The patient should be supine, both arms by the sides, with the table tilted head down to distend the central veins and prevent air embolism.
- Slightly turn the head away from the side to be cannulated for better access (turning it too far increases the risk of arterial puncture).

Technique

- Stand at the head of the patient.
- Locate the cricoid cartilage and palpate the carotid artery lateral to it at this level.
- Keeping a finger gently over the artery, insert the needle at an angle of 30-40° to the skin and advance it downward towards the nipple on the same side. Always direct the needle away from the artery under your finger.
- The vein is usually within 2-3 cm of the skin. If the vein is not found, redirect the needle more laterally.

Practical Problems

- *Cannot feel the artery:* Check the patient. Try the carotid on the other side. It

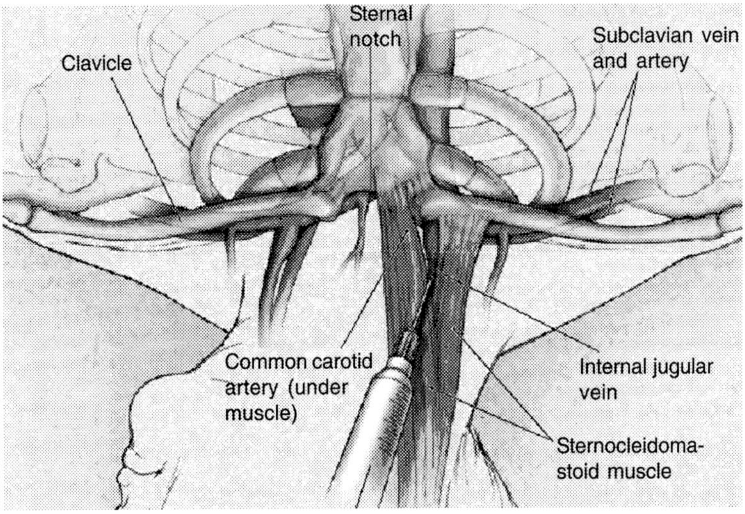

is safer to consider a different approach rather than 'blindly' try to find the jugular.

- *Arterial puncture:* Remove needle and apply firm pressure over the puncture site for 10 minutes.
- *Cannot find the vein:* Recheck your position. Ensure that you are not pressing firmly on the artery as this can compress the vein next to it. Try tipping the patient further head down if possible. If the patient is hypovolemic, and central venous access is not immediately required to correct it, give intravenous fluids and wait until the veins are fuller. Try inserting the needle a little closer to the artery but beware of puncture.

EXTERNAL JUGULAR VEIN (EJV) CANNULATION

Preparation and Positioning

- The patient should be supine, both arms by the sides, with the table tilted head down to distend the central veins and prevent air embolism.
- Turn the head away from the side to be cannulated for better access.

Technique

- Stand at the head of the patient and identify the EJV as it crosses the sternocleidomastoid muscle.
- If it is not palpable or visible then choose an alternative vein for catheter placement.
- Insert the needle in line with the vein where it is most easily seen or palpated.
- Thread the guide wire and then the catheter.

Practical Problems

- *Cannot see the vein:* If mechanically ventilated, briefly hold the lungs in inspiration. Press on the skin above the midpoint of the clavicle where the vein enters the chest. If none of these make the EJV visible, then use a different vein.
- *Catheter will not pass into chest:* Press on the skin where the vein enters the chest. Try rotating the catheter or flushing it with saline as you insert it. If using a guide wire, rotate the wire when it reaches the bottom of the vein. Try slowly turning the head in either direction. It may be useful to insert a normal plastic cannula into the vein first, and then thread the guide wire down this. By doing this, the wire can be pushed, pulled and rotated without the risk of it being cut which could occur if the wire is manipulated through a needle.

FEMORAL VEIN (FV) CANNULATION

Preparation and Positioning

Abduct and externally rotate the thigh slightly.

Technique

- Identify the pulsation of the femoral artery 1-2 cm below the inguinal ligament.
- Insert the needle about 1cm medial to the pulsation and aim it towards the head and medially at an angle of 20-30° to the skin.

Practical Problems

- *Cannot feel the artery:* Try the other side. Check the blood pressure. Treat any hypotension and retry. If there is no other venous access then it may be acceptable to try to locate the FV with a small needle starting medially to avoid the femoral nerve. Once found, change to the normal needle and continue the procedure. If the artery is accidentally punctured, apply direct pressure with your fingers and insert the normal needle medial to the puncture site.
- *Cannot locate the vein:* Recheck the anatomical landmarks. It is possible for the FV to be compressed by the fingers on the artery. Release pressure but leave the fingers resting on the skin over the artery and retry. Cautiously redirect the needle closer to the artery and in a more lateral direction.

ANTECUBITAL VEINS

Preparation and Positioning

Apply a tourniquet to the upper arm to distend the veins and select the best one. The order of preference for veins are:

- A vein on the medial side of the antecubital fossa—the basilic or median cubital vein. Even when not visible, these veins are often easily palpable when engorged.

- A vein on the postero-medial aspect of the forearm—a tributary of the basilic vein. Rotation of the arm may be required.
- The cephalic vein.

Lie the patient supine with the arm supported at 45° to the body and the head turned towards you (helps prevent the catheter passing into the IJV on that side).

Technique

- Stand on the same side of the patient.
- Estimate the length of catheter needed to reach the superior vena cava (SVC).
- Puncture the chosen vein with the needle and cannula and remove the needle.
- Insert the catheter through the cannula and advance it a short distance (1-2 cm), then release the tourniquet.
- Steadily advance the catheter along the vein until it is estimated to be in the correct position.

Practical Problems

- *Cannot thread the catheter along the vein*

Do not use force to pass it. If using a catheter-through-needle technique and you are sure that the catheter is in the vein, remove the needle from the vein and slide it to the end of the catheter. This will allow you to advance and withdraw the catheter without risk of cutting it on the needle. Try flushing the catheter with saline whilst advancing. Try the arm in different positions. Rotate the catheter whilst insertion.

Care of Percutaneously Inserted Central Catheters

- The dressing is not routinely changed.
- Blood samples should not be drawn through the catheter.
- To confirm the site of catheter tip, a post-insertion single AP X-ray view of the lower chest and upper abdomen is taken.
- IV fluids need not contain heparin if the flow rate is 5 ml/hr or greater; if flow rate is < 5 ml/hr, fluid should contain heparin, usually at a concentration of 0.25 - 0.5 unit/ml, but at a rate not to exceed 100 U/kg day; (50 U/kg/day in infants <1000 g).
- IV rates should be kept at 3 ml/hr or greater, and less than that recommended by the catheter manufacturer (generally <20 ml/hr for a 27 or 28-gauge catheter).
- At the time of its removal, the length of the catheter from its tip to entry point into the plastic hub should be measured and recorded on the special form in the patient's chart.
- Weigh infant prior to central venous line placement to decrease later need for manipulation. Use bed scales, if possible.

- Be aware of tenuous nature of catheter when positioning. Gather and secure tubings in such a way to avoid tension on the site. Consider use of Velcro wrap around tubings to achieve this.
- Kangaroo care should be avoided for the first week after surgical placement of a central venous line.

Securing Long Line

- Coil long line next to site without crossing long line.
- *Apply dressing:* Do not use antibacterial ointment. Do not use benzoin for adherence. If the catheter length is sufficient, the catheter may be looped under the dressing to reduce the risk of catheter dislodgement.
- *For gauze dressing*: Place a sterile folded 2 × 2 over the site. Tape the gauze dressings on all sides with a non-porous tape or cover with a transparent dressing to create a occlusive dressing.
- *For transparent dressing*: Apply transparent dressing smoothly over the catheter, avoiding wrinkling and air pockets under the dressing.

Confirm Position

- Wrap syringe in sterile guard until position confirmed by X-ray.
- X-ray with *contrast medium* prior to connecting fluids. This must be done using sterile technique.
- Record in the clinical notes the date, insertion site and length of catheter. Enter the procedure in the neonatal database.
- It is also important that we note the catheter tip position in the clinical record.
- If the long line is clearly *well into the heart* (particularly if it is **curled**) and needs to be withdrawn, another radiograph must be taken after manipulation to ensure that it has been withdrawn far enough and is in an acceptable position.

Dual Lumen Central Venous Catheter

- Each lumen is separate all the way to the end, so separate infusions can run in each lumen and *do not* need to be compatible.
- It is generally best to infuse fluids through both lumens. However, if one lumen is not used, it should be flushed every 12 hours with 1 cc of Heplock solution.
- Blood may be drawn from either lumen. Once a lumen is chosen to be the blood drawing lumen, every effort should be made to draw blood from the same lumen. The blood drawing lumen should be labelled at the stopcock end and identified.
- When drawing blood samples from one port, turn off infusate on the other port(s) until blood draw is complete (to avoid contamination of blood samples with IV solutions).

Problems During Central Venous Cannulation

Arterial puncture Usually obvious but may be missed in a patient who is hypoxic or hypotensive. If unsure, connect a length of manometer tubing to the needle / catheter and look for blood flow which goes higher than 30 cm vertically or is strongly pulsatile. Withdraw the needle and apply firm direct pressure to the site for at least 10 minutes or longer if there is continuing bleeding. If there is minimal swelling then retry or change to a different route.

Suspected pneumothorax If air is easily aspirated into the syringe (note that this may also occur if the needle is not firmly attached to the syringe) or the patient starts to become breathless. Abandon the procedure at that site. Obtain a chest radiograph and insert an intercostal drain if confirmed. If central access is absolutely necessary then try another route ON THE SAME SIDE or either femoral vein. DO NOT attempt either the subclavian or jugular on the other side in case bilateral pneumothoraces are produced.

Arrhythmias during the procedure Usually from the catheter or wire being inserted too far (into the right ventricle). Withdraw the wire or catheter if further than this.

Air embolus This can occur, especially in the hypovolemic patient, if the needle or cannula is left in the vein whilst open to the air. It is easily prevented by ensuring that the patient is positioned head down (for jugular and subclavian routes) and that the guide wire or catheter is passed down the needle promptly.

The wire will not thread down the needle Check that the needle is still in the vein. Flush it with saline. Try angling the needle so the end of it lies more along the plane of the vessel. Carefully rotate the needle in case the end lies against the vessel wall. Reattach the syringe and aspirate to check that you are still in the vein. If the wire has gone through the needle but will not pass down the vein it should be very gently pulled back. If any resistance is felt then the needle should be pulled out with the wire still inside, and the procedure repeated. This reduces the risk of the end of the wire being cut off by the needle tip.

Persistent bleeding at the entry Apply firm direct pressure with a sterile dressing. Bleeding should usually stop unless there is a coagulation abnormality. Persistent severe bleeding may require surgical exploration if there is an arterial or venous tear.

REFERENCES

1. Hermansen MC, Hermansen MG: Intravascular catheter complications in the neonatal intensive care unit, Clin Perinatol 2005;32:141-156.
2. Statter MB: Peripheral and central venous access, Semin Pediatr Surg 1992;1:181-187.
3. Shah P, Shah V: Continuous heparin infusion to prevent thrombosis and catheter occlusion in neonates with peripherally placed percutaneous central venous catheters, Cochrane Database Syst Rev 2005;(3):CD002772.
4. Pettit J: Assessment of infants with peripherally inserted central catheters: Part 1. Detecting the most frequently occurring complications, Adv Neonatal Care 2002; 2:304-315.

11. CHEST PHYSIOTHERAPY

To assist with clearance of secretions in specific pulmonary conditions.

Indications

- Consolidation.
- Lung collapse or aspiration on chest X-ray.
- Excessive or tenacious secretions.

Contraindications

- Unstable infant, low blood pressure, apneas, bradycardias or severe desaturation on handling.
- Recent intraventricular hemorrhage.
- Hypothermia.
- Recent pneumothorax and risk of reoccurrence.
- Pulmonary hemorrhage.
- Thrombocytopenia.
- Evidence of osteopenia on X-ray.

Procedure

- Observe heart rate and oxygen saturation.
- Observe ventilator settings and modality: If on SIMV/PSV reduce the sensitivity of trigger from 1.0 to 1.6 to avoid triggering due to artefacts like manual vibration.
- Auscultate: Perform suction as necessary.

Postural Drainage

- Position infant according to affected lung segments to be treated under direction from the physiotherapist.
- Use gravity to facilitate mobilisation of secretions towards the trachea.
- Can be used when secretions are thin and easily removed.

- No head down position to be used as this raises intracranial pressure and augments gastro-oesophageal reflux.

Vibration

- Infant in a postural drainage position.
- Fingers cupped around the chest, contralateral support of thumb, apply gentle vibration with minimal compression in time with the ventilator expiratory phase or expiration. Other hand is cupped and supports the infant's head.
- Vigorous vibration can cause rib fractures.

Percussion

- Used to loosen tenacious secretions.
- Place infant in postural drainage position tapping with fingers or face mask over the area of the lung to drain followed by vibration.
- Hold infant's head to prevent shaking. Do not use percussion on infants 1200 grams or less, and/or with a gestational age <33 weeks at the time of intervention.

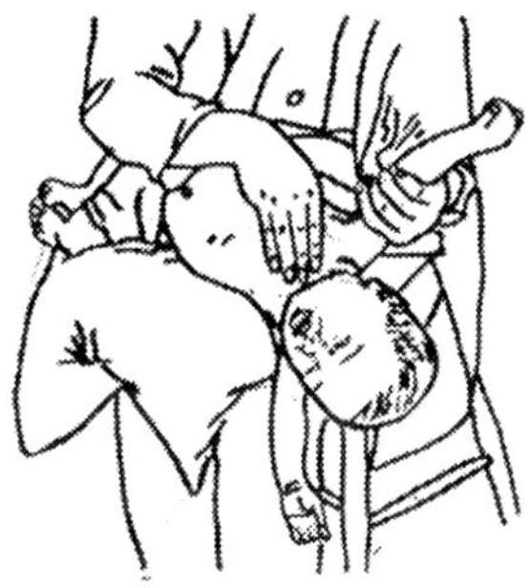

Right middle lobe

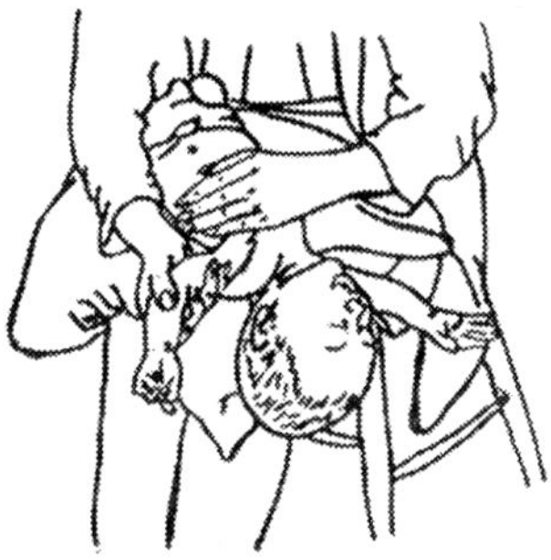

Lingular segment of left upper lobe

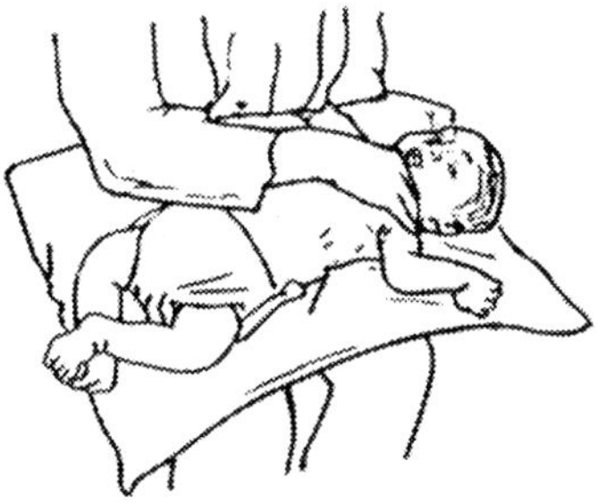

Anterior segment of left upper lobe

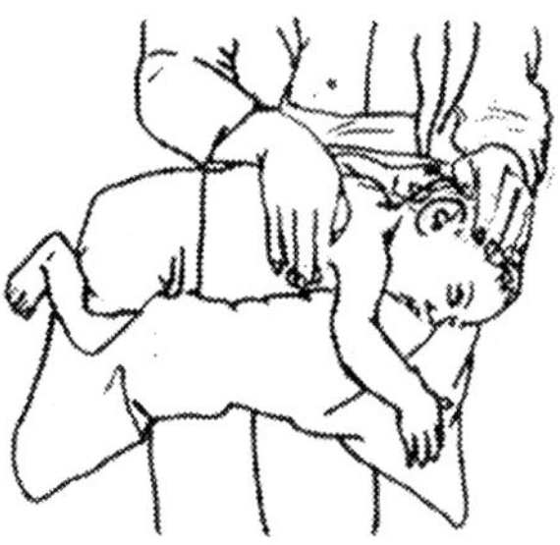

Superior segment of right lower lobe

12. CARE DURING NON-INVASIVE VENTILATION

- Non-invasive ventilation (NIV) refers to the use of nasal continuous positive airway pressure (NCPAP) and/or nasal intermittent positive pressure ventilation (NIPPV) as a means of providing respiratory support to the sick neonate.
- NIPPV is a form of non-invasive ventilatory assistance combining NCPAP and IPPV.
- NIPPV may be synchronized (SNIPPV) or non-synchronized. The *primary mode* of either form of respiratory support refers to its use soon after birth. The *secondary mode* refers to its use following a period of IPPV, usually for respiratory distress syndrome (RDS).
- CPAP is a non-invasive modality for respiratory support in a *spontaneously breathing* newborn.

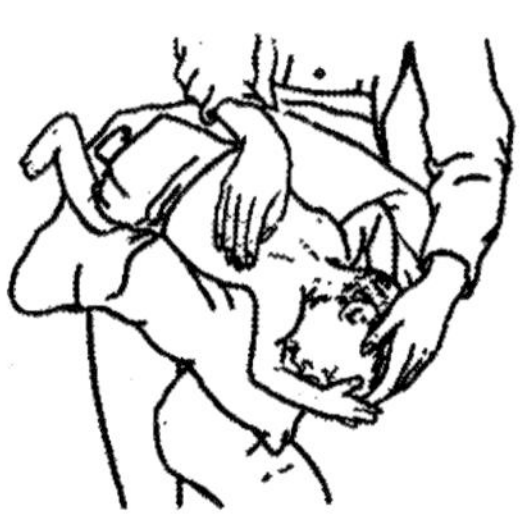

Posterior segment of right lower lobe

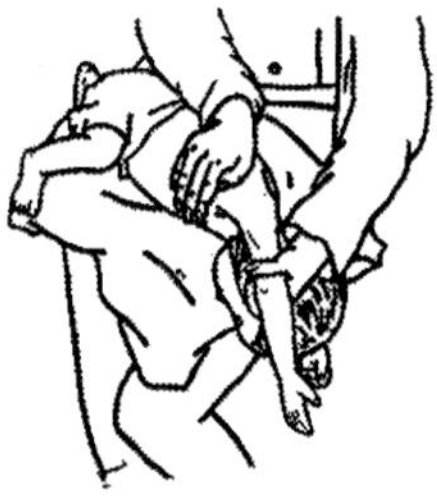

Lateral segment of right lower lobe

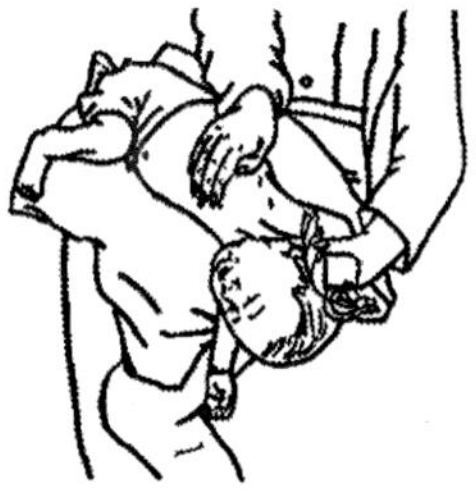

Anterior basal segment of right lower lobe

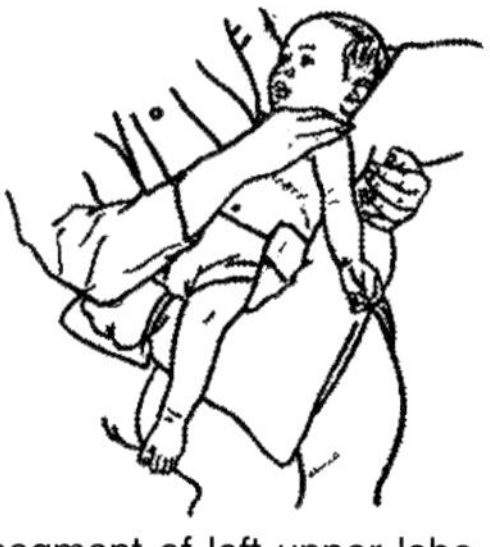

Apical segment of left upper lobe

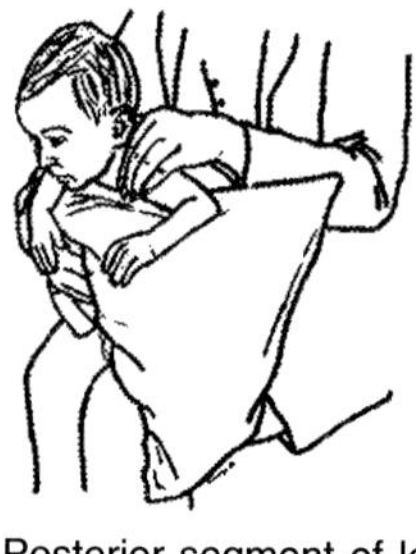

Posterior segment of left upper lobe

Indications for CPAP

a. Post-extubation support of preterm infants.
b. Primary treatment for RDS.
c. Apnea of prematurity.

Prerequisite

- Assess airway, breathing and circulation.
- Decompress the stomach and decrease diaphragmatic pressure, by placing

a 6.5 Fr naso- or oro-gastric (NG/OG) tubes in patients < 1 kg and an 8 Fr NG/OG for patients >1 kg. Use OG tube because NG tube will increase airway resistance.

The Basic Components of CPAP are:

1. Continuous gas flow.
2. Humidifier.
3. Reservoir bag.
4. One-way check valve.
5. Under water tube/valve to produce expiratory pressure.

CPAP—Types

- Head Box (not recommended for long-term use).
- Face Chamber (not recommended for long-term use).
- Face mask (not recommended for long-term use).
- Endotracheal (not recommended for long-term use).
- Nasal mask
- Nasopharyngeal—Uninasal/Binasal.
- Nasal Uninasal/Binasal.

Supplies

A. Infant Star 500/950™ time cycled pressure limited infant ventilator (other time-cycled, pressure-limited ventilators can be used for NIPPV).
B. Star Sync™ with abdominal probe (for SNIPPV).
C. V-SIL™ binasal airway
   1. 2.5 mm (4.0 cm length).
   2. 3.0 mm (4.0 cm length).

   Or

D. Argyle™ CPAP nasal cannula kit
   1. X-small.
   2. Small.
E. Neobar™ endotracheal tube holder
   1. Ultra.
   2. Micro.
   3. Small.
F. Tape.
G. Surgical lube.
H. Orogastric tube.
I. Suction catheter.

Setting up Nasal CPAP

1. *Select the correct size prong* based on the infant's weight. If no weight is available, there is a ring that contains sample prongs, which can be used to estimate proper size. Select the correct size prong (small, medium or large) by measuring the prong diameter against the infant's nares. Use the largest prong size that will fit the infant's nares. If the prongs are too small, you will have a poor seal and loss of CPAP. Prongs that are too large will distort the nose. Prongs are set inside the nares and there is some space between the prong set and the infant's nose. Properly placed prongs should only have 1/3 to 1/2 of the prongs in the nares. Prongs fit snuggly in the nares.
2. *Select the appropriate sized bonnet:* The bonnet should fit snuggly on the infant's head. If the bonnet that is supplied with the prongs is too large or too small for the infant's head, the proper bonnet must be obtained. Bonnet size will need to be reassessed with head growth or with changes after birth as edema and molding subside. If the bonnet is too large, it can slip over the eyes and cause the prongs to be released from the nose. If the bonnet is too small, it will ride up on the head, put excess tension on the prongs and distort the nose.
3. *Secure the Stay:* Flex tubing to the bonnet with the Velcro tab.
   a. Place the bonnet well down over the infant's head ensuring that the ears are well covered and flat against the head.
      1. The string ties should be in the midline facing to the front.
      2. The front edge of the bonnet should be at the eyebrow line.
      3. The back of the bonnet should cover the entire skull.
   b. Secure the fixation straps by placing them in between the Velcro tabs located on the sides of the cap.
   c. Tie the inspiratory and pressure lines to the bonnet with the string ties.
4. Assess the following to ascertain correct placement of the prongs.
   a. Eyes clearly visible.
   b. Nose in "normal position" and not pushed upward.
   c. Stay-Flex tubing is positioned just above the ears and away from the eyes.
5. Attach the prongs to the generator; ensure that the prongs are correctly situated.
6. Place on ventilator.

Monitoring

1. Work of breathing
   - Atelectasis with decreased breath sounds on auscultation and decreased chest excursion.
   - Tachypnea with rapid respiratory rate, or very shallow respirations with poor air movement.
   - Nasal flaring with chest wall retractions.
   - Apnea, bradycardia and cyanosis.

2. CPAP apparatus
   - Assure proper positioning of the CPAP apparatus and head straps when nasal prongs are used to prevent skin breakdown.
   - Follow prescribed nasal CPAP apparatus instructions for proper hat and nasal prong sizing.
   - Maintain spacing between apparatus and end of nose per package instructions.
   - Inspect the condition of the septal skin area under the apparatus every 3-6 hours noting pressure-related injury.
   - Inspect pinna for pressure-related injuries every shift.

Ongoing Care

- Maintain neck in a neutral position.
- Maintain neutral thermal environment.
- Maintain minimal stimulation, i.e., suction only when necessary, decrease light, noise, and touch by clustering care.
- Utilize non-invasive methods to assess gas exchange, i.e., pulse oximeter and transcutaneous blood gas measurements.
- Change infant's position every 3-6 hours as tolerated.
- Adjust oxygen percent and flow rate to keep saturation within ordered parameters.
- Maintain patent airway by suctioning the nares as required.
- Maintain airway pressure by keeping patient calm, with nursing measures, and follow with sedation.
- Assess integrity of skin and mucous membranes at least every 4 hours.
- Assess that CPAP bonnet and prongs are correct and properly positioned at least every hour.
- Assess internal nares, using a laryngoscope or pen light, at least every 24 hours.
- Assess trends in oximetry every hour.
- Assess abdominal girth at least every 8 hours – more frequently if distended.
- Assess and record settings hourly (PEEP, FiO_2, mean airway pressure, humidity). Maintain settings as ordered, checking level of CPAP after suctioning or manipulating of the prongs.

Troubleshooting

a. *To keep prongs securely in the nose:*
   1. Verify that prongs are correctly placed on the generator.
   2. Check the size and position of the bonnet and fixation straps and that the exhalation line is free.
   3. Try the next larger sized prongs.

b. *If unable to maintain the desired level of CPAP:*
   1. Check if the mouth is open and creating a pop-off.

2. The prongs may be too small; try the next larger size.
3. Check if there is an NG tube in place, which may distort the prongs.

Prerequisites for Weaning

1. The infant has been stable clinically stable for at least 24 hours.
2. Blood gases suggest improvement in gas exchange.
3. Chest radiograph shows adequate improvement in basic pathology.
4. Biochemical parameters—Electrolytes, calcium, glucose, hematocrit and blood counts are stable.
5. Respiratory drive of baby is adequate.

"Failure" Criteria for Infants Treated with CPAP

1. Persistent apnoeic episodes.
2. $PaCO_2$ of ≥60 mm Hg.
3. FiO_2 of ≥0.6 to maintain acceptable oxygen saturation.

Indications for NIPPV

1. A method of non-invasive ventilatory assistance in the spontaneously breathing infant with impending or existing ventilatory failure due to increased work of breathing (WOB).
2. A form of weaning from invasive conventional mechanical ventilation in the spontaneously breathing patient with an increased work of breathing (WOB).

Contraindications

Upper airway abnormalities:
1. Choanal atresia.
2. Cleft palate.
3. Tracheoesophageal fistula.
4. Severe cardiovascular instability.

CLINICAL MANAGEMENT

A. (S)NIPPV (Primary Mode)

1. Settings:
    - Frequency 25-40/min.
    - PIP 4 cm H_2O > than PIP required during manual ventilation. Adjust PIP for effective aeration per auscultation.
    - PEEP 4 - 6 cm H_2O.
    - Ti 0.35-0.45 sec.
    - FiO_2 adjusted to maintain oxygen saturations (SpO_2) of 85 - 93%

- Flow 8-10 l/m.

2. Monitor SpO_2, heart rate and respirations.
3. Obtain blood gas in 15-30 minutes.
4. Adjust ventilator settings to maintain blood gas parameters within normal limits.
5. Suction mouth and pharynx and insert clean airway
6. Clean original airways with soap and water, rinse with sterile water and dry. Place in plastic bag for next changing.
7. Maximal support recommendations:
   ≤1000 gm MAP 14 cm H_2O.
   >1000 gm MAP 16 cm H_2O.

B. (S)NIPPV (Secondary Mode)

1. *Extubation criteria while on conventional ventilation:*
   - Frequency ≤15-25/min.
   - PIP ≤16 cm H_2O.
   - PEEP ≤5 cm H_2O.
   - FiO_2 ≤0.35.
   - Hematocrit ≥ 40%.
2. *Place on (S)NIPPV:*
   - Frequency 15-25/min.
   - PIP 2-4 cm H_2O higher than conventional ventilation settings.
   - PEEP ≤5 cm H_2O.
   - FiO_2 adjusted to maintain SpO_2 85 - 93%.
   - Flow 8-10 l/m.
3. Suction mouth and pharynx and insert clean airway
4. Clean original airways with soap and water, rinse with sterile water and dry. Place in plastic bag for next changing.
5. *Maximal support recommendations:*
   ≤1000 gm MAP 14 cm H_2O.
   >1000 gm MAP 16 cm H_2O.

(S)NIPPV Weaning to Oxyhood / Nasal Cannula (NC)

1. Minimal (S)NIPPV settings:
   - Frequency ≤ 20/min.
   - PIP ≤ 14 cm H_2O.
   - PEEP ≤ 4 cm H_2O.
   - FiO_2 < 0.3.
   - Flow 8-10 l/m.
   - Blood gases within normal limits.

2. Wean to:
   - Oxyhood: Adjust FiO_2 to keep SpO_2 85 - 93%.
   - NC: Adjust flow (1-2 l/m) and FiO_2 to keep SpO_2 85 - 93%.

Potential Hazards/Complications

A. Obstruction of prongs due to mucus plugging.
B. Feeding intolerance.
C. Abdominal distension.
D. Abdominal perforation.
E. Ventilator induced lung injury.
F. Hypoventilation.
G. Infection.
H. Nose bleed / nasal irritation.
I. Skin irritation and pressure necrosis.

REFERENCES

1. Bhandari V: Non-invasive ventilation of the sick neonate: Evidence-based recommendations, J Neonatol 2006;20:214-221.
2. Millar D, Kirpalani H: Benefits of non-invasive ventilation, Indian Pediatr 2004;41:1008-1017.
3. Upadhyay A, Deorari AK: Continuous positive airway pressure—a gentler approach to ventilation, Indian Pediatr 2004;41:459-469.
4. Morley C, Davis P: Continuous positive airway pressure: Current controversies, Curr Opin Pediatr 2004;16:141-145.
5. Halliday HL: What interventions facilitate weaning from the ventilator? A review of the evidence from systematic reviews. Paediatr Respir Rev 2004;5 Suppl A:S347-352.
6. De Paoli AG, Morley C, Davis PG: Nasal CPAP for neonates: What do we know in 2003? Arch Dis Child Fetal Neonatal Ed 2003;88:F168-172.

13. DEVELOPMENTALLY SUPPORTIVE CARE

The premature and at risk neonate are in a crucial stage of development in the first period of their life. The NICU environment, geared toward acute physical care, ironically can be a stressful and developmentally counterproductive environment for the infant. Studies have demonstrated potential detrimental effects of intensive care and the NICU environment. The NICU health care team can provide a supportive, nurturing environment that will improve developmental outcomes of hospitalized neonates.

The aim of developmental care is to modify the environment of the nursery utilising a broad range of strategies designed to reduce stress and prevent agitation, preserve energy and promote growth, enhance recovery, facilitate self-regulatory capabilities and promote central nervous system (CNS) organization.

Steps for Developmentally Supportive Care in Nursery

1. *Consistency of Caregiving*
   a. Within a 24-hour period after admission a primary team of caregivers on both day and night time shifts should be selected.
   b. The team includes representatives from medicine, nursing, occupational or physical therapy, social work, respiratory therapy and other persons providing direct patient care.
   c. Team members should work with the family to create a developmental care plan.
   d. Expectations should be discussed with the developmental team and families should be invoved in directing the plan according to their neonate's needs.
   e. The plan of care should be reviewed in daily rounds and discussed with the family frequently.
   f. Each member on the care giving team should be aware of the following:
2. *Assist Infants in Transition State*
   a. Gently approaching neonate in a slow, controlled manner and placing hands on the neonate to allow the neonate to adjust.
   b. Unwrapping neonate slowly, if swaddled.
   c. Allowing a lag in time, before doing a procedure, to allow the neonate time to adjust his/her state.
   d. Providing neonate with calming maneuvers if signs of stress are observed.
   e. Individual neonates should be monitored for 10 minutes after procedure, since behavioral and physiological changes may be delayed. As the neonate grows and matures he/she should be able to exhibit more self-regulatory and calming behaviors and caregivers should help the neonate to develop these behaviors.

Calming Measures

   a. Extremity containment.
   b. Hand clasping.
   c. Firm hand placement on top of head, back or cupping feet into flexion.
   d. Providing pacifier.
   e. Swaddling and/or nesting.
   f. Assisting the neonate with hand to mouth.
   g. Soft talking.
   h. Soothing music.
3. *Infant Assessment*
   a. Initial 24-hour observation period should be done as soon as the neonate is stabilized medically.
   b. Each neonate should be observed for a 24-hour period.

c. Observation should occur prior to and after feeding, and procedures.
d. Data collection from observation should include neonatal states, signs of stress, engagement and disengagement cues.
e. The assessment is important to determine what type of stress patterns the neonates are experiencing, how procedures are being tolerated and using the assessment to determine which procedures need to be modified in order to prevent further physiologic stress to the neonate.
f. Interventions that help the neonate to maintain physiologic and behavioral stability should be recorded during the observation period.

Signs of Stress Behaviour

- Colour changes: Mottled, dusky and cyanosed.
- Apnea, bradycardia, desaturation.
- Hiccoughing, sneezing, yawning, gagging, regurgitating feeds.
- Tremors, twitches, frantic activity, arching, frowning, gaze averting.
- Completely flaccid trunk, extremities and face.
- Easy fatiguability

4. *Family Involvement*
   a. The family members also should be educated regarding developmental issues such as premature development, positioning, feeding, infant stimulation, the NICU environment and its relation to development, signs of infant stress and developmental outcomes of all NICU diagnoses.
   b. Parental concerns and expectations should be discussed with the developmental team as well as parental knowledge of medical and developmental care.
   c. Assessment also needs to focus on behaviors of both parent and neonate and how they interact. Family dynamics should be assessed; stresses and coping abilities of family members should be determined.

Interventions for Developmentally Supportive Care in NICU

Assist infant to maintain organized behavior by:
a. Bringing hand to mouth.
b. Clustering and timing care to provide undisturbed rest and sleep periods.
c. Introducing cycled lights for the preterm infants.
d. Decreasing noise levels around the infant at all times.
e. Bringing infant to a more alert state prior to initiating procedures.
f. Providing "purposeful" touch.
g. Offering a swaddle bath.
h. Encouraging alert state during wakeful periods by enfacement, elevating infant's head and shading eyes - extending the time as tolerance develops.
i. Supporting infant after procedures or care to assist infant in regaining physiological stability through containment and gentle, "purposeful" touch.

j. Helping infant to console him/herself.

1. Clustering of Activities

a. Procedures should be scheduled so that the neonate has at least blocks of three-hour periods of uninterrupted sleep.
b. Vital signs should be taken from the monitors when the neonate is sleeping.
c. Neonates should be monitored for all signs of stress. If neonates show stress, calming behaviors should be administered.
d. Procedures may need to be adjusted and breaks should be taken in accordance with the signals of the individual neonate.
e. The neonate's caregiving schedules should be coordinated with the family.
f. Avoid non-emergency interventions during the night, e.g., bathing and weighing.

2. Positioning of Infant

a Neonate's position must be changed at least every three hours.
b. Prone is the preferred position. The optimal position is with the arms and legs flexed into the body. Place rolls along both sides of the body. A roll can also be put around the flexed legs for containment and flexion.
c. The side-lying and prone position should be used when possible.
d. Provide boundaries and use rolls/nesting to maintain desired posture, reduce agitation, conserve energy and create a feeling of "security" for the infant.
e. Rolls and positioners should be used to help promote the flexed position.
f. Neonates should be nested as much as possible in positions, which facilitate flexion of extremities and promote hands to mouth and midline.
g. To help avoid flattening of the head, the neonate should be rotated in quarter turns using small rolls to help support the head and promote molding.
h. Endotracheal tubes should be supported with towel rolls, wedges or other devices so that the neonate's head position can be changed every three hours.
i. Avoid moving an infant who has sought out his own boundaries (e.g. foot against a porthole door).

3. NICU Environment–Noise

Interventions to decrease environmental noise include:

a. Padding doors.
b. Rubber trash cans.
c. Eliminating radios / telephone.
d. Rounds away from the bedside.

e. Close incubator doors gently.
f. Avoid loud talking in nursery.
g. Incubator covers to help absorb noise.
h. Avoid placement of equipment on incubator.
i. Have a designated "quiet time" daily.
j. Encourage housekeeping to empty large trashcans outside of nursery.
k. Attending to alarms as soon as possible.
l. Turning down volume on monitors to as low as is safely possible.
m. Acoustical ceilings.
n. Avoid talking loudly, especially across open care beds.

4. NICU Environment– Light

Interventions to decrease bright lighting include:
a. Covering isolettes and open cribs.
b. Individual lighting at each bed with dimmer controls or incremental lighting in room.
c. Using natural light as much as possible and reducing overhead lighting.
d. Dimming lights especially when infants are out of incubators and being held.

5. Promote Oro-motor Competency

a. Offering pacifier or infant's fingers to suck on during OG or NG feedings or on a fixed schedule if receiving parenteral nutrition/continuous feeding.
b. Introducing taste and smell by placing a drop or two of formula/breast milk on lips or tongue during feedings.
c. Holding infant during feedings, when conditions permit.
d. Stroking cheeks and supporting chin.
e. Providing oral sucrose before performing painful procedures.

6. Facilitate and Promote Motor Development

a. Providing a support for legs and feet against which the infant can press.
b. Placing infant on his/her abdomen on a folded blanket, with arms and legs close to his/her body, in a manner that prevents external rotation.
c. Providing vestibular stimulation by holding and rocking.
d. Placing in sitting position a few moments each day, increasing as tolerated.
e. Performing range of motion exercises and stretching activities
f. Providing infant massage as tolerated for infants > 32 weeks gestation.

7. Facilitate and Promote Language, Vision and Hearing Development

a. Placing black/white/red, or high-contrast pictures and objects in line of vision 8-15 inches from face as long as infant remains relaxed and focused.

b. Providing auditory stimulation such as tapes of mother's and father's voices, music boxes, and classical music when infant is quiet, alert, relaxed and appears interested.
c. Talking or singing to infant when providing care or holding and touching him/her, using different pitches or volume in voice.
d. Allowing for face-to-face interaction with infant with or without talking, depending on infant's developmental level.

8. Facilitate Social and Behavioral Development

a. Encouraging parental/caregiver to participate in care when possible.
b. Encouraging parents/caregivers to participate in Kangaroo Care when possible.
c. Placing family pictures and mementos on bed.
d. Calling infant by first name.
e. Encouraging parents/caregivers to attempt to gain eye contact with infant.
f. Consoling infant with cuddling, swaddling, rocking or pacifier.
g. Encouraging parents/caregivers to participate in feeding infant.

9. Promoting Family Centered Care

a. Parent support groups.
b. Unrestricted visitation policies.
c. Teach parents infant behavioral principles and developmental interventions.
d. Teach parents to care for their neonates in a way that is appropriate for gestational age.
e. Parent education should be geared toward adult learning principles. Utilize a variety of health education models for teaching parents such as videos, pamphlets, hands-on.
f. Provide opportunities for kangaroo care.
g. Share developmental plan with parent/caregiver.
h. Allow for verbalization of anxiety by encouraging discussion of fears and concerns.
i. Encourage attendance at weekly support group meeting when these are offered.

Documentation

1. Implementation of developmental care of the preterm/ill infant.
2. Assessment findings.
3. Interventions and patient responses/outcomes.
4. Patient/caregiver teaching and level of understanding.

REFERENCES

1. Als, H., Lawhon, G., Brown, E., Gibes, R., Duffy, F.H., McAnulty, G., and Blickman, J.G.: Individualised behavioural and environmental care for the very low birth weight preterm infant at high risk of Bronchopulmonary Dysplasia: Neonatal Intensive Care Unit and developmental outcome, Pediatrics 1986;78: 1123-1132.
2. Blackburn, S.T. and VandenBerg, K.A. (1993): Assessment and management of neonatal neurobehavioral development, In: Kenner, C., Brueggemeyer, A. and Gunderson, L.P. (eds): Comprehensive Neonatal Nursing: A Physiological Perspective, Philadelphia: WB Saunders, 1094-1134.
3. Buehler, D.M., Als, H., Duffy, F.H., McAnulty, G.B. and Liederman, J: Effectiveness of individualised developmental care for low risk preterm infants: Behavioural and electrophysiologic evidence, Pediatrics 1995;96: 923-932.
4. Symington, A. and Pinelli, J. (2001): Developmental care for promoting development and preventing morbidity in preterm infant (Cochrane Review): The Cochrane Library, 2, 2001, Oxford: Update Software.
5. VandenBerg, K.A. (1995): Behaviourally Supportive Care for the Extremely Premature Infant, In: Gunderson, L.P. and Kenner, C. (eds), Care of the 24-25 Week Gestational Age Infant, 2nd Ed, Petaluma: NICU INK, 145-171.
6. Harrison, H: The principles of family centered care, Pediatrics 1993;92:643-649.
7. Rauh VA, Nurcombe B, Achenbach T, Howell C: The Mother-Infant Transaction Program. The content and implications of an intervention for the mothers of low birth weight infants, Clin Perinatol 1990;17:31-45.
8. VandenBerg, K. (1993): Basic competencies to begin developmental care in the intensive care nursery. Infants and Young Children: 6(2), Aspen Publishers, Pp 52-59.
9. Vergara, E., Cronin, A., and Walker, K. (1993): Foundations for Practice in the NICU and EI: A Self-Guided Practice Manual, Florida State Dept. of Education, Tallahassee, FL.
10. Gardner, S. L. and Goldson, E. (2002): The neonate and the environment: Impact on development, In G. B. Merenstein and S. L. Gardner (Eds.), Handbook of Neonatal Care (pp. 219-282), St. Louis, MO: Mosby.

14. ENDOTRACHEAL TUBE INSERTION

Indication

1. Ineffective bag and mask ventilation.
2. Tracheal suctioning for depressed meconium stained liquor in the newborn.
3. Suspected airleak or diaphragmatic hernia.

4. Administering drugs.
5. Impending respiratory failure.
6. Respiratory failure / arrest.
7. Shock non-responsive to volume expansion.
8. For procedures under anesthesia.
9. Frequent apneas not responding to medical management.
10. Post operative care following major surgery, e.g., tracheo-esophageal repair, correction of congenital diaphragmatic hernia etc.
11. Neurologic depression with impaired respiration, e.g., drug induced.

Routes

1. Nasotracheal.
2. Orotracheal.

Note: One route of intubation does not seem to be preferable to the other. Post extubation atelectasis may be more frequent after nasal intubation, particularly in VLBW infants.

Type

1. Emergency.
2. Elective.

Supplies

1. Laryngoscope – straight blade- no. 0 and 1 (with extra set of batteries).
2. Endotracheal tubes – 2.5 mm, 3 mm, 3.5 mm.
3. Suction apparatus – Upto 100 cm of water.
4. Suction catheter – 6 F, 8 F, 10 F.
5. Oxygen source and tubings.
6. Self inflating bag (250-750 ml).
7. Adhesive tape, scissors.
8. Stethoscope.
9. Manometer, stylet – optional.

Choosing the Appropriate Equipment

1. *Laryngoscope blade:* Size 0 for preterms, Size 1 for term infants.
2. *Endotracheal tube*
   a. Sterile and single use.
   b. Use transparent tubes rather than rubber or opaque tubes.
   c. Keep two sizes, 0.5 mm small and large to the calculated ETT size ready by the bedside.
   d. Uncuffed tubes are used.

e. Size of the ETT is selected as follows:

ETT Size	*Birth weight*	*Gestational age*
2. 5 mm	< 1000 grams	< 28 weeks
3.0 mm	1000-2000 grams	28-34 weeks
3.5 mm	2000 – 3000 grams	34-38 weeks
4.0 mm	> 3000 grams	> 38 weeks

f. Depth of insertion is upto the vocal cord guideline mark on the ETT.

Rule of Thumb for Lip to Tip Distance for ETT Insertion: 6 cm + wt (kg)

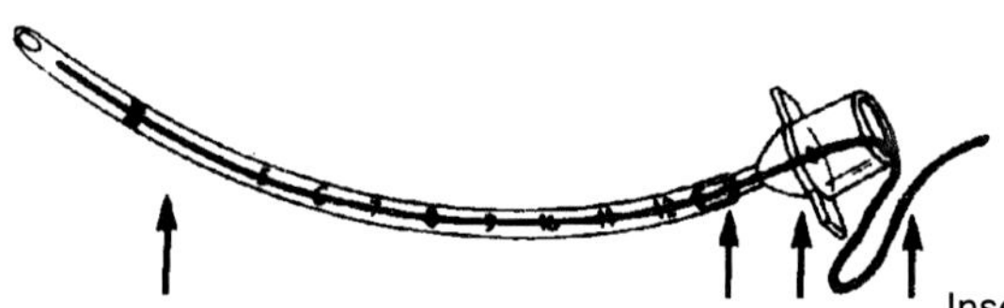

Procedure

a. Prerequisite

- Check all equipment and apparatus are in functioning order and available in different sizes.
- Ensure that the infant is kept in the normal range of temperature during the procedure.
- Always have an assistant by the side.
- Ensure the ETT tube is cut 4 cm distal to the length of insertion obliquely and adhesives have been cut appropriately.
- A pulse oximeter should be placed on the infant preferably.
- For elective intubation, rapid sequence pre-medication may be delivered as IV Morphine 0.1mg/kg, IV Atropine 20 mcg/kg and IV Suxamethonium 1-2 mg/kg.

b. Procedure: (Do not spend more than 20 seconds to intubate)

- Place the infant in "sniffing position" with the head in midline with slight extension. Stand at the head end of the patient.
- In elective intubation, pre-oxygenate the infant with 100% oxygen for 2-3 minutes.
- Hold the laryngoscope in the left hand between the thumb and forefinger

with the blade towards the baby. Turn on the light by opening the blade. If using stylet, ensures that the distal end does not protrude outside the ETT as it may cause trauma or perforation.

- An assistant directs 100% oxygen toward the neonate's nose with oxygen tubing and monitors the neonate's heart rate.
- Insert the laryngoscope blade from the right angle of the mouth and slide it over the tongue. Advance the blade further to reach beyond the base of the tongue till the tip rests in the vallecula.
- Now lift the entire blade forwards and upwards, with the movement at the shoulder (not at the wrist) to view the glottic opening. In case of difficulty in visualizing the glottic opening ask the assistant to apply pressure over the cricoid.
- If any secretions are visible, do a quick suction.
- Hold the appropriate size ETT in the right hand and introduce it from the angle of the infant's mouth and insert it through the vocal cords keeping the vocal cord guide at the level of the cords.
- Hold the tube firmly in your right hand and gently remove the laryngoscope without disturbing the tube.
- Connect the ETT to the Ambu bag and ventilate.
- Ask the assistant to confirm the tube placement by the following.

c. Confirmation of Tube Placement

Primary confirmation:

- Equal air entry bilaterally over the axilla.
- Equal chest rise bilaterally.
- Absence of air sounds over the stomach.
- Improvement in heart rate and colour.

Secondary confirmation:

- Radiology is gold standard. The confirmation of ETT on X-ray would be if the tip of the tube is 2 cm above the carina or is at T1 or T2. It is important that the chest radiograph be taken with the patient's head in neutral position. Flexion of the neck advances the tube further down the airway, and extension brings the tip up in the airway.
- Capnography.

Trouble Shooting

Problem	*Remedy*
Taking time to intubate	If unable to intubate or heart rate drops below 100 per minute, abandon procedure and continue oxygen and bag / mask ventilation.
Hypoxia	Ensure oxygenation pre and during the process of intubation by asking the assistant to provide 100% oxygen by tubing.

Fixation of Endotracheal Tube

- Cut the ETT not more than 4 cm from the lips to eliminate unnecessary dead space.
- Apply tincture benzoin over the site of fixation of the adhesive.
- Apply the first trouser leg tape to the right cheek.
- Place the upper leg across the top of the lip.
- The lower leg is placed directly on the tube and it is wrapped around the tube in a spiral fashion.
- The second trouser leg tape is applied to the left cheek, and the lower leg is placed across the lower lip.
- The upper leg is placed directly on the tube and it is wrapped around the tube in a spiral fashion.
- Secure tape high on cheekbones, NOT on fatty part of cheeks as there is too much play at this point allowing excessive in-out motion of the tube.

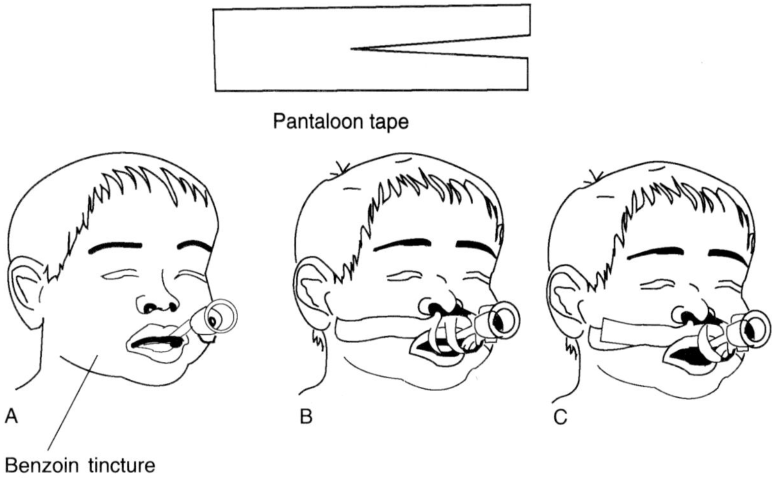

Documentation

- Size of the ETT.
- Position at the lip junction of the ETT.
- Number of attempts for intubation.
- Suction catheter size for the oral and endotracheal suction.
- Depth of insertion for the ETT suction catheter.
- Confirmation by primary and supplemented by one secondary technique.
- How ETT was secured.

MONITORING

Assessment

- Assess on insertion and every 2 hourly
  - Patency of airway by auscultation of bilateral equal breath sounds, observing for symmetrical chest expansion and effective, non-labored ventilation.
  - Secure fixation of tube.
  - Quantity and character of secretions.
  - O_2 saturations.
  - Condition of mouth/lip, nose. Observe for skin dryness, redness, irritation, and pressure areas to lip, corner of mouth or nares.
  - Assess on every shift the location of ETT by noting centimeter depth markings on emergence from mouth/gumline or nares.

Report For

- Respiratory distress.
- Extubation or malpositioned ETT.
- Absent or diminished breath sounds.
- Change in secretions.
- Difficulty in advancing suction catheter.
- Partially or totally occluded ETT.

Ongoing Care

- Monitor continuously heart rate, oxygen saturations and respiratory status.
- Provide nasal and oral hygiene every 2-4 hours.
- Administer sedation as appropriate to prevent tube dislodgement and comfort.
- Anticipate tube block, dislodgement or displacement.

Complications

- Hypoxia.
- Tachycardia and bradycardia.
- Injury to the soft tissue of the oral cavity and oropharynx.

Bedside Equipment

- Have at bedside.
- Manual ventilation bag.
- Suction equipment.
- Appropriate size face mask.

REMOVAL OF ENDOTRACHEAL TUBE

Supplies

- Bag and mask attached to oxygen source.
- Suction catheters.
- Prepared oxy-hood or nasal cannula or NCPAP or NIPPV.
- Laryngoscope and pre-cut ETT in case of need to re-intubate.

Procedure

- Assess infant's condition by observing heart rate, color, respiratory rate, respiratory effort and auscultating chest.
- Maintain on pulse oximeter.
- Suction nasopharynx at least 30 minutes prior to extubating. The nasopharynx must be patent because infants are obligatory nasal breathers. Endotracheal suction may cause atelectasis. Therefore the infant requires time to recover before the ETT is removed.
- Provide two or three breaths using the last ventilator settings delivered with a resuscitation bag just prior to withdrawing ETT. Handbagging may be used to re-expand the infant's lungs if there is not an effective cry at extubation.
- Disconnect from ventilator and gently remove/pull out ETT.
- Place infant under oxygen hood or place prongs in nares to provide NIPPV/ NCPAP.
- It is beneficial for the infant to be nursed prone following extubation. The prone position improves oxygenation due to mechanical advantages on chest wall expansion. Positioning of the infant is dependent upon their condition; surgical infants may not be able to be positioned prone.

Monitor

- Colour, cry and activity.
- Respiratory efforts, work of breathing.
- Stridor.
- Secretions.

Practice Pointers

1. The neonate's general condition should be assessed frequently.
2. Assess the heart rate periodically if interventions are done.
3. A prompt increase in heart rate is the best indicator that the tube is in the tracheobronchial tree and providing effective ventilation.
4. Two common and serious errors of endotracheal intubation are malplacement of the endotracheal tube and the use of the wrong-sized tubes.

REFERENCE

1. K Spence, P Barr: Nasal versus oral intubation for mechanical ventilation of newborn infants, Cochrane Database of Systematic Reviews 2007, Issue 4.

15. ENDOTRACHEAL SUCTION

Indications

1. Presence of visible or audible secretions in the ETT or post physiotherapy.
2. Interpretation of certain clinical changes, i.e.:
   - Decrease in SaO_2.
   - Decreased air entry / chest wall movement.
   - Decrease/increase heart rate.
   - Decreased tidal volume.
   - Deterioration in blood gas values.

Birth weight	*ETT size (mm)*	*Distance of ETT at lip(cm)*	*ETT suction catheter (Fr)*	*Depth of ETT suction catheter insertion (cm)*
< 1000 gm	2.5	7	5	7.5
1 to 2 kg	3	8	6	8.5
2- 3 kg	3.5	9	7	9.5
> 3 kg	4	9-10	8	9.5-10.5

Contraindications

1. Upto 1 hour following surfactant administration.
2. There is no role for routine suctioning of the ETT.

Procedure

- Universal precautions while handling.
- Use sterile and single use flexible PVC plastic catheters with two holes, one at the tip and the other on the side.
- Prior to suction, increase FiO_2 by 10%. Although pre-oxygenation is shown to decrease hypoxemia at the time of suctioning, other clinically important short and longer-term outcomes including adverse effects have not been assessed.
- Insert suction catheter not more than 0.5 cm distal to the ETT. The catheter should not occlude more than 2/3 of the internal diameter of the tube.
- Apply suction while withdrawing the catheter.
- Withdraw catheter by rotating or swirling movement.
- Ensure suction machine pressure has a cutoff at 100 mm of Hg.
- Instillation of normal saline for irrigation prior to suction is controversial. If thick secretions are present, instill 0.5 -1 cc normal saline, bag and then do

suction. Correct humidification settings and adequate hydration of the infant should ensure thin secretions.

- Preferably use thumb control suction catheters to control timing of suctioning.
- Use separate catheters for oral and ETT suction.
- Do not place catheters in any solution.
- Use de-ionized or sterile water for clearing the suction catheter / tubing.

Complications

- Bacteraemia.
- Hypoxaemia.
- Tachycardia and bradycardia.
- Atelectasis.
- Systemic hypertension.
- Raised intracranial pressure.

PRACTICE POINTERS

1. Based upon the results of Cochrane review, there is insufficient evidence to decide between endotracheal suctioning with or without disconnection. There is, however, evidence of some benefit from performing suctioning without disconnection for some specific short-term outcomes.

REFERENCES

1. M Pritchard, V Flenady, P Woodgate: Preoxygenation for tracheal suctioning in intubated, ventilated newborn infants, Cochrane Database of Systematic Reviews 2007, Issue 4.
2. PG Woodgate, V Flenady: Tracheal suctioning without disconnection in intubated ventilated neonates, Cochrane Database of Systematic Reviews 2007, Issue 4.

16. EXCHANGE TRANSFUSION

The nature of the exchange transfusion depends on the underlying cause for which the procedure is planned:

Double Volume

Removal of bilirubin/antibodies.

Single Volume

Correction of coagulopathies, anemia, or removal of antibodies/antigens.

Partial Volume

Polycythemia.

Indications

- Removal of antibody-coated red blood cells in hemolytic disease.
- Removal of excessive unconjugated bilirubin.
- For correction of severe anemia.
- Neutropenia associated with sepsis, or coagulation defects non-responsive to single component replacement.

Supplies

- Disposable exchange tray (contains blood filter set).
- Cut down tray with umbilical catheter.
- Sterile water.
- Sterile gloves, towel, gowns.
- Betadine solution.
- Cardiac monitor with blood pressure (BP) transducer or non-invasive BP monitor
- Pulse oximeter.
- Radiant warmer.
- Restraints.
- IV pole.
- Surgical caps and masks.

Pre-Procedure Planning

- Call blood bank to see if there is blood available and inform that exchange transfusion is needed.
- The freshest citrate–phosphate-dextrose (CPD) blood available, irradiated and less than 8 days old is desirable.
- If infant has not been type and screened on the current admission, draw specimen at this time and send to the blood bank
- Soak umbilical cord with sterile normal saline soak for 1 hour prior to exchange.
- If possible, ensure that infant is NPO × 2 hours prior to exchange.
- Agitate blood for exchange transfusion every 10-15 minutes to bring it to room temperature.
- There must be at least one doctor or one nurse exclusively involved in the monitoring of exchange throughout its progress.
- *Volume of blood needed to be exchanged:* Double volume exchange transfusion - Usually use two blood volumes (180 ml/kg). One blood volume removes 65% of baby's red cells. Two blood volumes removes 88%.
- *Partial exchange transfusion:* To correct severe anaemia without hypovolaemia; to correct for polycythaemia.

Choice of Blood for Eexchange Transfusion

Rh iso-immunization: In emergency situation use O Rh negative cells. Ideal is to use O Rh negative blood suspended in AB plasma. Cross matched baby's blood group but Rh negative can also be used.

ABO incompatibility: Blood group O types (Rh compatible) with baby. Ideal is to use blood group O (Rh compatible) suspended in AB plasma.

Other situations: Cross-matched baby's blood group.

Polycythaemia

$$\text{Volume exchanged (ml)} = \frac{\text{Blood Volume} \times (\text{PCV initial} - \text{PCV desired})}{\text{PCV initial}}$$

Anaemia

$$\text{Volume exchanged (ml)} = \frac{\text{Blood Volume (ml)} \times (\text{Hb desired} - \text{Hb initial})}{(\text{Hb Donor} - \text{Hb Initial})}$$

Procedure

- Place infant under radiant heater.
- Monitor with cardiac monitor and pulse oximeter continuously during procedure.
- Take complete set of vital signs. Knowledge of baseline vital signs facilitates decision making for interventions.
- Aspirate infant's stomach.
- Immobilize all four extremities. Restrain infant's limbs, placing arms comfortably out from his/her sides. Wrap legs together in a diaper and tape down securely.
- Make available clean surfaces for: Transfusion Pack, Exchange Transfusion Tray, Cut Down Tray.
- Connect infusion system as below. Set-ups are closed systems. Avoid breaking into the system.
- Umbilical venous catheter (UVC) is inserted by physician under strict aseptic precautions.
- Ensure sedation is prescribed and available, if necessary, for infant agitation.
- Initial blood withdrawn to be sent for lab analysis. Pre and Post exchange labs generally include: Hgb, Hematocrit, Platelets, Electrolytes, Calcium, Glucose, Bilirubin Total and Direct.
- Blood is withdrawn slowly over a minute during each draw and discarded into discard bag. Replacement blood is pushed slowly over 1 minute as tolerated.

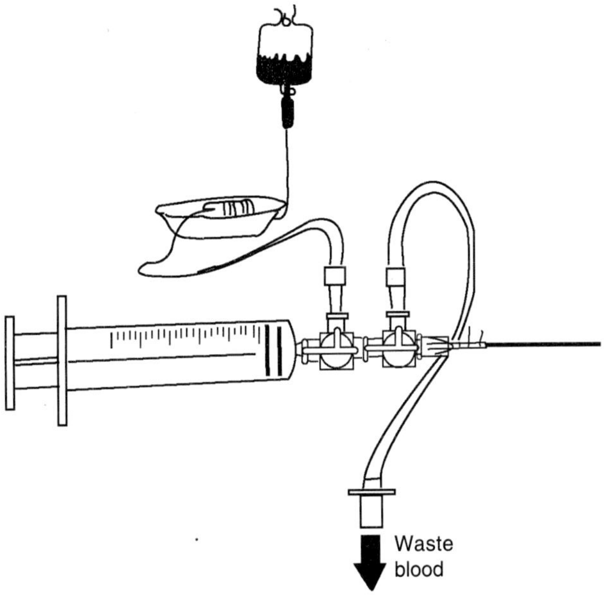

Setting the 4-way with the use of 2 stop cocks

Technique of Exchange Transfusion

a. Isovolumetric Exchange:

Remove blood from an artery while infusing through a vein at the same rate.

	IN	OUT
	Peripheral vein	Peripheral artery
or	Peripheral vein	Umbilical artery
or	Umbilical vein	Peripheral artery
or	Umbilical vein	Umbilical artery

b. Push-Pull:

This can be done through an umbilical venous catheter. Withdraw blood over 2 minutes, infuse slightly faster. Aim to exchange 180 ml/kg over 1½ -2 hours.

<1000 gms	Use 5 ml aliquots
1000-2000 gms	10 ml
>2000 gms	15 ml

- At midpoint of exchange a dose of 100 mg/kg Ca gluconate may be given.
- Ensure the infant's skin is cleansed of povidone iodine and central lines are well secured upon completion of the exchange transfusion. Remove restraints from the infant and make sure the baby is comfortable.

- Remove the umbilical venous catheter. Lines are left in place in case another exchange transfusion is required.
- Dispose of blood components and tubings according to infection control guidelines.

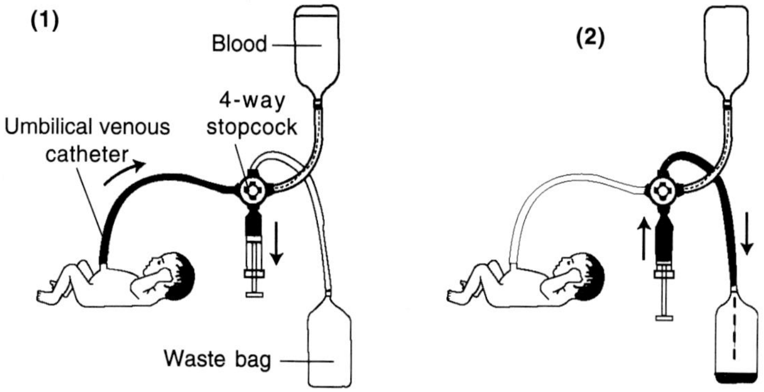

(1) Withdrawing patient blood
(2) Expelling drawn patient blood into bottle

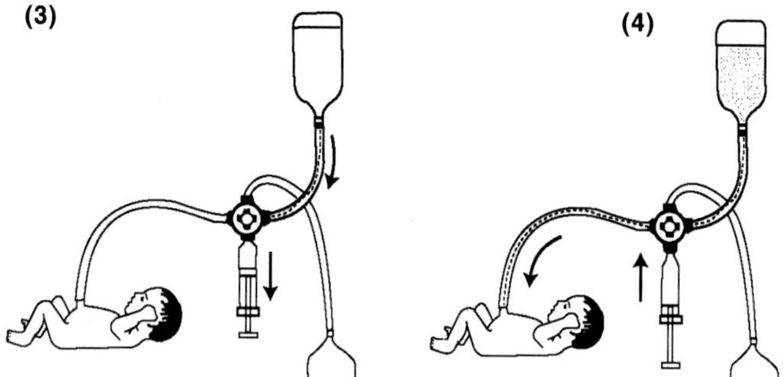

(3) Withdrawing fresh blood from the blood bag
(4) Pushing fresh blood into the patient

MONITORING

During Procedure

- Record heart rate, respiratory rate, blood pressure, perfusion, and skin temp every 15 minutes.
- Obtain axillary temp every 30 minutes.
- Monitor continuous blood volumes being removed and replaced.

Post Procedure

- Obtain vital signs:
  a. Every 30 minutes × 2, then
  b. Every 1 hour × 2, then
  c. Every 2 hours × 2, then
  d. Every 4 hours until 24 hours have elapsed since completion of exchange transfusion.
- Obtain glucose meter reading immediately after procedure, then every 1 hour × 2.

Documentation

- Record vital signs, blood in and out, blood warmer temperature on Exchange Transfusion Record.
- Blood Bank transfusion record.

Complications

During the procedure	*After the procedure*
Air embolism	Infection
Volume imbalance	Hypoglycemia
Arrythmias	Hypocalcemia
Acidosis	Hypernatremia
Respiratory distress	Thrombocytopenia
Hyperkalemia	Anemia / Polycythemia
Anemia / Polycythemia	Coagulopathy or neutropenia
	Necrotising enterocolitis
	Graft versus host disease
	Blood transmitted infections

Rh Incompatibility Jaundice

A. *Early exchange blood transfusion*

- Cord bilirubin 5 mg/dl.
- Cord Hb <10 mg/dl.

- In case of severe sensitization to remove antibodies in baby (suggestive history of severe affection, raised indirect Coombs' titre in mother, positive direct Coombs' test in baby).

B. *Subsequent exchange transfusion*

Age (hr)	*TSB (mg/dl)*
< 24	≥ 10
25-48	≥ 15
> 48	≥ 20

When rate of rise of serum bilirubin 0.5 mg/dl per hour

C. *Intensive phototherapy*

Indicated at a bilirubin level, which is 5 mg/dl less than that for exchange blood transfusion.

D. *Preterm/Low birth weight babies*

Correspondingly lower values should be used. A level equal or greater to 0.5 and 1 per cent of birth weight in grams can be used as a rough guide for phototherapy and exchange blood transfusion, respectively.

Maisels MJ, Jaundice: *In:* Neonatology: Pathophysiology and Management of the Newborn, 4th edn., Eds Avery GB, Fletcher MA, McDonald MG, Philadelphia, J.B. Lippincott, 1994; p 765.

REFERENCES

1. Okoji GO: How to do it: Neonatal exchange blood transfusion, Trop Doct 1995;25:34-35.
2. Thayyil S, Milligan DW: Single versus double volume exchange transfusion in jaundiced newborn infants, Cochrane Database Syst Rev 2006, Oct 18;(4):CD004592.
3. American Academy of Pediatrics Subcommittee on Hyperbilirubinemia: Management of hyperbilirubinemia in the newborn infant 35 or more weeks of gestation, Pediatrics 2004;114:297-316.
4. Alkalay AL, Simmons CF: Hyperbilirubinemia guidelines in newborn infants, Pediatrics 2005;115:824-825.
5. de Waal KA, Baerts W, Offringa M: Systematic review of the optimal fluid for dilutional exchange transfusion in neonatal polycythaemia, Arch Dis Child Fetal Neonatal Ed 2006;91:F7-10.
6. Dempsey EM, Barrington K: Crystalloid or colloid for partial exchange transfusion in neonatal polycythemia: A systematic review and meta-analysis, Acta Paediatr 2005;94:1650-1655.
7. Schimmel MS, Bromiker R, Soll RF: Neonatal polycythemia: Is partial exchange transfusion justified? Clin Perinatol 2004;31:545-53, ix-x.
8. Locham KK, Kaur K, Tandon R, Kaur M, Garg R: Exchange blood transfusion in neonatal hyperbilirubinemia—Role of calcium, Indian Pediatr 2002;39:657-659.
9. Jackson JC: Adverse events associated with exchange transfusion in healthy and ill newborns, Pediatrics 1999;99:e7.

10. Peripheral vessel exchange transfusion, Indian Pediatr 1999;36(9):914-917.
11. Todd NA: Isovolemic exchange transfusion of the neonate, Neonatal Netw 1995;14:75-77.
12. Todd NA: Procedural flow chart job aid for the exchange transfusion, Neonatal Netw 1993;12:63-67.
13. Sanklecha M, Khambadkone S, Irani SF: Peripheral exchange transfusions, Indian J Pediatr 1992;59:646.

17. GIVING INJECTIONS

INTRAMUSCULAR (IM) INJECTIONS

Supplies

- Sterile 1-inch needle of the smallest size that will allow fluid to flow freely (e.g. 22- to 24-gauge).
- Sterile syringe (e.g. 1- to 3-ml).
- Dry cotton-wool ball.

Sites for IM Injections

1. Quadriceps muscle group of the upper, outer thigh. This site is preferred because of the small risk of giving the injection intravenously, hitting the femur with the needle, or injuring the sciatic nerve.
2. Gluteus muscle group in the buttock. This muscle group is difficult to use for IM injection because of variable amounts of fat and subcutaneous tissue and the danger of injury to the sciatic nerve and major blood vessels in the region. If using this site, use only the upper, outer quadrant of the muscle, and always aspirate before injecting.
3. Deltoid muscle group. This site can be used for giving immunizations but should not be used for giving other injections.

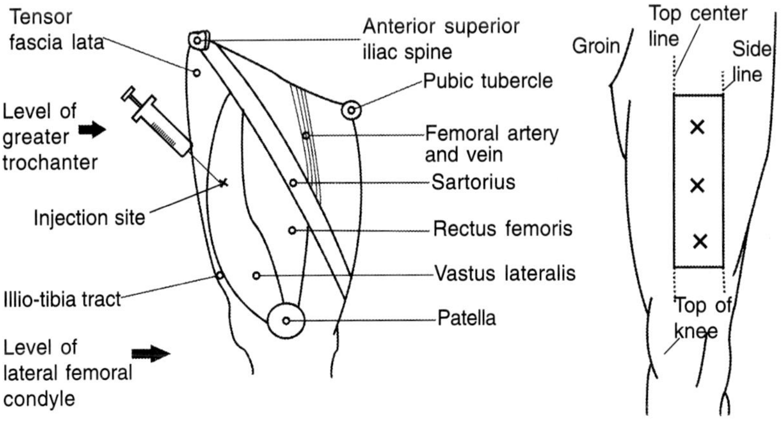

Appendix A

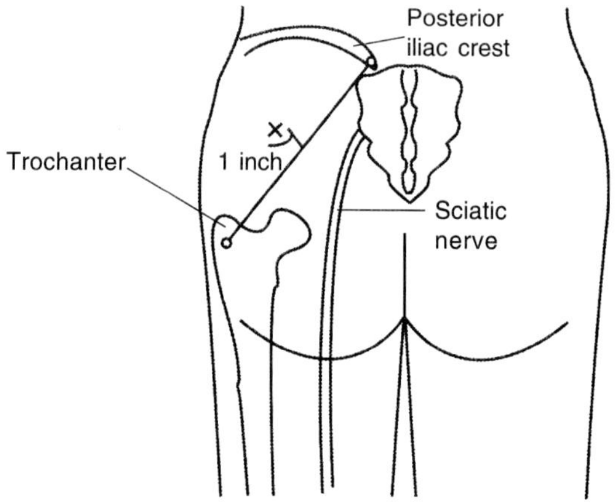

Procedure

- Gather necessary supplies.
- Wash hands.
- Select the site for injection.
- Draw the material for injection into the syringe.
- Ensure that the drug and dose are correct.
- Grasp the centre of the target muscle between the thumb and forefinger, if possible.
- Insert the needle at a 90 degree angle through the skin with a single quick motion.
- Withdraw the plunger of the syringe slightly to ensure that the tip of the needle is not in a vein (i.e. no blood should enter the needle).
- Upon completion of the injection, withdraw the needle and apply gentle pressure with a dry cotton-wool ball.
- Record the site of the injection, and rotate the site of subsequent injections.

PRACTICE POINTERS

- Use a sharp needle of the smallest diameter that will allow fluid to flow freely (e.g. 22- to 24-gauge).
- Use a minimal volume for injection (e.g. 2 ml or less at any single injection.
- Administer medication slowly.
- Establish anatomic landmarks.
- Cleanse the skin thoroughly.
- Alternate sites for subsequent injections.
- Aspirate before injection.
- Use a needle of adequate length to reach the intended injection site.

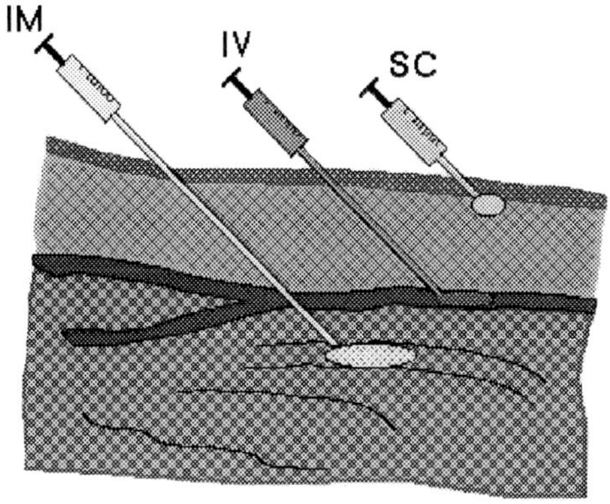

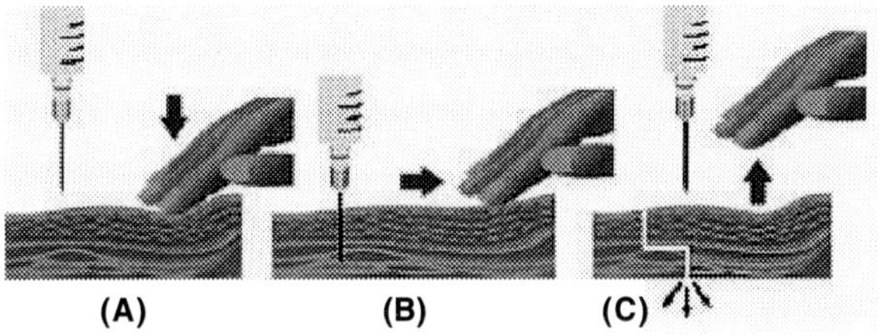

Tracking technique: An intramuscular injection is designed to deposit medications deep into muscle tissue

Complications of IM Injections

- Inadvertent intra-arterial or intravenous injection.
- Infection from contaminated injection material.
- Neural injury (typically the sciatic nerve after injections in the buttock).
- Local tissue damage due to injection of irritants.

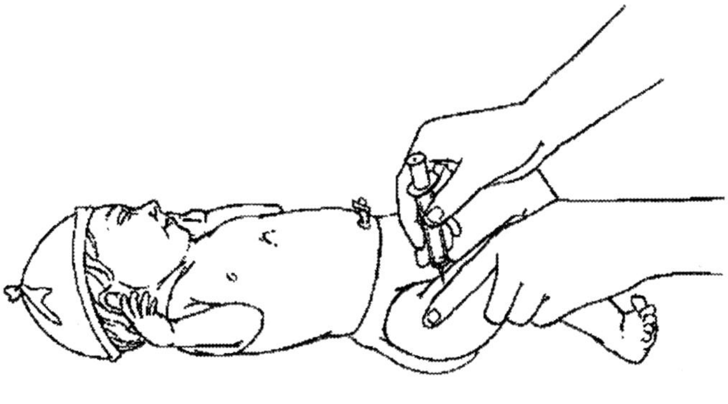

Intramuscular injection into quadriceps muscle group

Advantages:

- Larger volume can be given by IM (compared to subcutaneously).
- A depot or sustained release effect is possible with IM injections, e.g. procaine penicillin.

Disadvantages:

- Trained personnel required for injections. The site of injection will influence the absorption. Generally speaking, the deltoid muscle is the best site.
- Absorption is sometimes erratic, especially for poorly soluble drugs, e.g. diazepam, phenytoin. The solvent may be absorbed faster than the drug causing precipitation of the drug at the site of injection.

INTRAVENOUS (IV) INJECTIONS

The description is for giving an IV push injection to a baby with an IV line in place.

Supplies

- Swab or cotton wool ball soaked in antiseptic solution.
- Sterile 1-inch needles (e.g. 22- to 24-gauge).
- Sterile syringes with markings for proper dose (e.g. 1- to 3-ml).
- 2 ml IV fluid.

Procedure

- Gather necessary supplies.
- Wash hands.
- Choose the site in the IV line where an IV injection can be given nearest to the insertion site of the cannula (e.g. a valve or a soft rubber connector).
- Clean the port with the swab or cotton-wool ball soaked in antiseptic solution, and allow the area to dry.
- Draw the material for injection into the syringe.
- Ensure that the drug and dose are correct.
- If the IV fluid is infusing without problem:
  - Stop the IV infusion.
  - Insert the needle into the IV line, and inject the material slowly over two minutes, carefully observing the area around the cannula for any swelling.
- If the position of IV cannula is in doubt:
  - Stop the IV infusion.
  - Flush the IV line first with 2 ml of IV fluid, observing the area around the cannula carefully for swelling that indicates that the cannula has come out of the vein.
  - If the cannula is still in the vein, inject the material slowly over two minutes, carefully observing the area around the cannula for any swelling.

- Upon completion of the injection, withdraw the needle and restart the IV infusion.

INTRADERMAL INJECTIONS

Only use intradermal injection for the Bacille Calmette Guerin (BCG) vaccine.

Supplies

- Sterile 25- or 27-gauge needle.
- Sterile syringe (1 ml).
- Dry cotton-wool ball.

Procedure

- Gather necessary supplies.
- Select the site for injection.
- Wash hands.
- Draw the material for injection into the syringe using the 21-gauge needle.
- Ensure that the correct drug and dose are given.
- Replace the 21-gauge needle with a 25- or 27-gauge needle.
- Hold the syringe and needle almost parallel with the skin, with the bevel of the needle facing up.
- Pull the skin taut with one hand, and insert the tip of the needle barely under the skin. Advance the needle slowly until the bevel of the needle has fully entered the skin.
- Gently point the needle upward, without re-piercing the skin.
- Inject the material with steady pressure for three to five seconds (there will be significant resistance) and look for a blanching of the skin. The baby will probably cry during the injection; a true intradermal injection often burns slightly and should raise a small "bleb" under the skin that causes the skin to pucker like the skin of an orange (peau d'orange).
- Upon completion of the injection, withdraw the needle and apply gentle pressure with a dry cotton-wool ball.

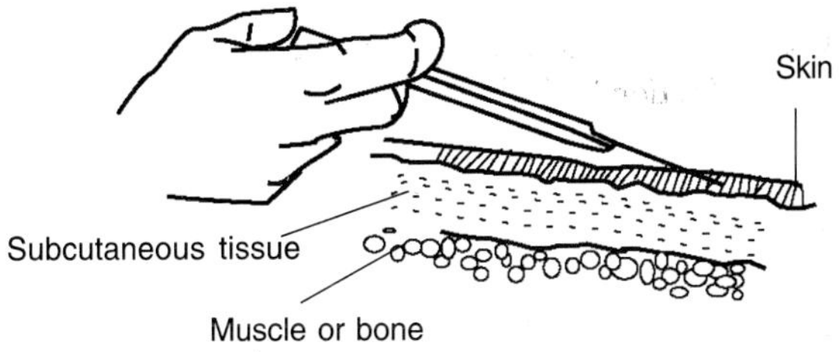

Intradermal injection

Appendix A

REFERENCES

1. Pocket book of hospital care for children, Guidelines for the management of common illnesses with limited resources, World Health Organization 2005.
2. Essential Newborn Nursing for Small Hospitals, In resource restricted countries, Learners Guide, Published by Division of Neonatology, Department of Pediatrics, AIIMS, New Delhi 2004.

18. HAND WASHING

Hand washing is vigorous, brief rubbing together of all surfaces of lathered hands, followed by rinsing under a stream of water. **Hand washing is a part of normal duty of care.**

Indications

1. Before and after touching a baby.
2. Before and after a procedure.
3. After you use the bathroom or change diapers.
4. After you blow your nose, sneeze or cough.

Purpose of Hand Washing

1. Remove all dirt and debris.
2. Reduce cross contamination.
3. Interrupt fecal oral route of infection.
4. Reduce risk of hands acting as vectors.
5. Break link in chain of infections.
6. Increase image of cleanliness of health providers and caretakers in eyes of public and patients.

Description of Procedure

1. Before entering the nurseries, all personnel are to perform an initial 3-minute scrub.
2. Remove jewellery, watch etc on hands. Roll up the sleeves above the elbow.
3. Rinse under running water. The following steps should take at least 3 minutes.
4. Lather with soap using friction both the hands (minimum 10-20 seconds). Vigorously wash hands palm-to-palm, palm over dorsum, palm-to-palm with fingers interfaced, back of fingers to opposing palms, rotating thumbs in palms followed by rotating fingers in palm.
5. Continue scrub by vigorous washing under running water of fingertips and each of the 4 planes of each finger and thumb. Follow this with vigorous washing of the back and palms of the hands. Wash the arms with firm circular motions.

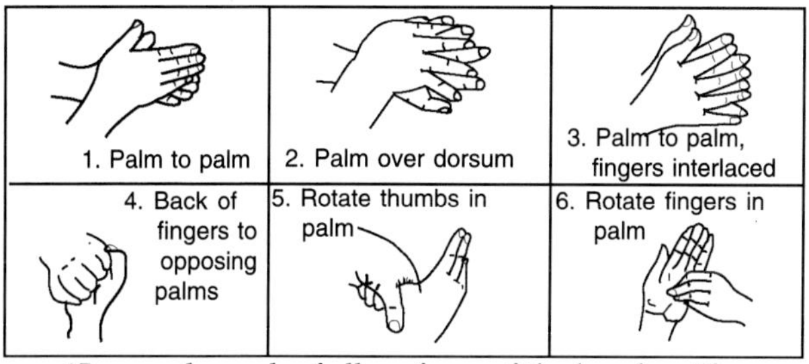

6. Vigorous 15 seconds wash of all surfaces of the hands with soap and water is required before and after each patient contact, after contact with body fluids or secretions, after contact with equipment that comes in contact with the patient, or contact with items that are potentially contaminated with microorganisms (monitors, telephones etc).
7. Rinse each arm thoroughly by allowing the water to run off the elbows.
8. Frequently missed areas are nails, nail bed, under surface of nails, thumbs, web spaces, back of fingers and hands. Turn off the water/soap by foot or elbow.

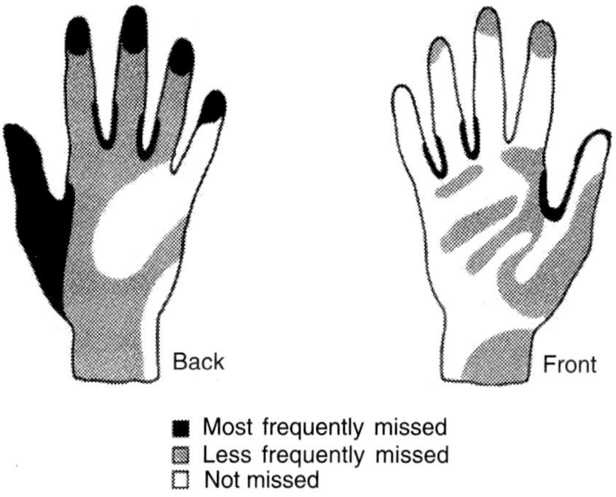

9. Dry hands thoroughly. Be sure that the hand sanitizer has completely evaporated before touching any devices, bed linens, or patients. The vapors, which have the potential to ignite in an oxygen-enriched environment, should be adequately dissipated once the hands feel dry and the cooling sensation associated with evaporation has disappeared.

DO's	*DONT's*
• Keep basins, dryers, soap at convenient sites.	• Do not use nail polish or artificial nails.
• Educate and demonstrate hand wash.	• Do not use washed hands for turning off the water source.
• Keep vigilance.	
• Use sink for hand wash only and not for any other purpose.	• Do not substitute hand washing by wearing gloves.

Types of Hand Wash

1. Mechanical - Use of soap and water.
2. Chemical - Use of antimicrobials.

Microorganism on Skin

1. *Resident:* Always present in deep layers of skin and can be cultured repeatedly. E.g.: Coagulase –ve Staphylococcus, Acinetobacter, Corynebacterium (diphtheroids or coryneforms).
2. *Transient:* Recent contamination and are the common sources of nosocomial infections. E.g.: gram-negative coliforms and Staphylococcus aureus.

Prerequisites of Hand Washing Agents

Hand washing and hand treatment scheme must:

1. Kill a broad spectrum of microorganisms (both transient and resident) especially pathogenic bacteria.
2. Maintain a residual effect where the bacterial load on the skin is controlled between applications by antimicrobial agents remaining on the skin, and
3. Be non irritating to the skin.

In any successful hand wash program, two main parameters must be considered: the immediate and persistent antimicrobial effects. The immediate antimicrobial effects depend on two attributes: the mechanical removal of contaminating microorganisms and the topical antimicrobial compounds ability to kill microorganisms upon contact. The persistent antimicrobial effects (the ability of the hand wash to keep the microbial population at a low level after washing) are dependent upon the type of anti-microbial product used.

Immediate antimicrobial effectiveness depends upon the type and amount of antimicrobial hand sanitizer used, the amount of time spent washing the hands, the mechanical pressure and friction exerted in the wash, and the temperature of the water.

Choice of Hand Washing Agent: Soap Versus Antimicrobial

The absolute indications for hand washing with plain soaps and detergents versus hand washing with antimicrobial-containing products are not known because of the lack of well-controlled studies comparing infection rates when such products are used. For most routine activities, hand washing with plain soap appears to be sufficient, since soap will allow most transient microorganisms to be washed off.

The indications for hand washing depend on:

a. The type, intensity, duration and sequence of activity;
b. The degree of contamination associated with the contact; and
c. The susceptibility to infection of the health care recipient.

Precautions in Soap Use

1. Any soap can be used such as liquid, bar, granule, or soap-impregnated tissue form.
2. If liquid soap is used, it preferably must be in disposable containers. If reusable containers are used prior to refilling, complete thorough cleaning of the container is mandatory. The dispenser should be replaced or cleaned and filled with fresh product when empty; liquids should not be added to a partially full dispenser.
3. If bar soap is used, it should be kept on racks that allow drainage of water.

Antimicrobial Hand Washing products should be used preferably in following conditions:

1. In high-risk patients—ICU, NICU, Casualty.
2. Before any invasive procedure.
3. In immunocompromised patients.
4. In barrier nursing leaving an isolation room.
5. Before contact with patients having invasive devices.

Choice of Antimicrobial Solution

Selection of an appropriate hand-washing product must be based on four criteria:

1. Efficacy.
2. Safety.
3. Cost.
4. Acceptability.

Agent	*Immediate effect*	*Residual effect*	*Remarks*
Plain Soap	Yes	No	Skin irritation, time consuming, need to be dried. Not effective if hands are soiled with dirt or heavily contaminated with blood or other organic material. Not alone for surgical scrub. Cumbersome.
Ipodophor iodine	Yes	Yes	Skin irritation.
Chlorhexidine gluconate (4%)	Yes	Yes	Skin irritation if > 4%.
> 50 % Alcohol	Yes	No	Skin irritation.
Sodium hypochlorite	Yes	No	Very irritating to hand.
Hexachlorophene	Yes	No	Only against gram positive.

The most commonly used antimicrobial hand wash in emergency care is alcohol based (70%). Following precautions must be followed for its effective use:

a. The hands must not be visibly soiled with blood or organic material.
b. The hand surface must be completely covered with antiseptic.
c. Hands must be allowed to dry.
d. Not less than 0.5 ml should be used.

Alcohol based hand washing agent

Advantage	*Disadvantage*
• Rapid reduction in microbial counts.	• May cause skin irritation.
• Easy to use.	• Sensitive to dilution with water.
• Time saving.	• Costly.
• Better compliance.	
• Eliminates use of water and drying.	
• Does not need sink, dryers.	

Hand Drying

1. Drying by means of hand dryers has had variable effects. In some studies, air dryers have been shown to reduce the number of organisms on hands after hand washing. Several studies have demonstrated that air hand dryers are unsuitable for use in critical patient care areas because of the potential for cross infection, either through airborne dissemination or contaminated personnel. Air dryers may be an impediment to hand drying because of the time taken to dry hands and the need to ensure that the equipment is functioning.
2. Drying by single use autoclaved towel is beneficial.
3. Autoclaved paper napkins are also beneficial.
4. Drying of hands by wiping to the personal wear or common towel is not advisable.

Methods to Improve Hand Washing

1. Senior staff should serve as role models.
2. Policing each other.
3. Educating the need for hand washing.
4. Demonstrating the technique.
5. Convenient placement of infrastructure like sinks, dryers etc.

KEY POINTS

1. Hand washing before and after each patient contact remains the single most important practice in the control of nosocomial infections. Hand washing

with a suitable detergent agent should be done for at least 3 minutes initially and 30 seconds in between two babies.

2. Hand washing is necessary after touching blood, body fluids, secretions, excretions, and contaminated items, whether or not gloves are worn.
3. Gloving does not replace hand washing; hand washing is imperative after removing gloves.
4. Hand washing should be encouraged whenever a health care provider is in doubt about the necessity for doing so.
5. The efficacy of a hand wash depends on the time taken and the technique.

REFERENCES

1. CDC Guideline for Hand Washing and Hospital Environmental Control, 1985 supersedes Guideline for Hospital Environmental Control. Revised by Julia S. Garner, and M S Favero, MMWR, June 24, 1988 Vol. 37 / No. 24.
2. Larson E: Current hand washing issues, Infect Control 1984;5:15-17.
3. Canada Communicable Disease Report, Infection control guidelines, Hand Washing, Cleaning, Disinfection and Sterilization in Health Care, Supplement, ISSN 1188-4169, Dec 1998, Volume 24S8.

19. INSERTION OF ORO- AND NASO-GASTRIC TUBES

Indications

1. Enteral feeding
   - Preterm (immature suck/swallow reflex).
   - Neurological disease (impaired suck reflex).
   - High respiratory rate (tachypnoea with risk of aspiration).
2. Gastric decompression
   - CPAP.
   - Necrotising enterocolitis.
   - Paralytic ileus.
   - Abdominal surgery.
3. Administration of medication.

Supplies

- Appropriate size tube
  - 5G >750 g to <1500 g feeding only.
  - 6G >1500 g feeding and/or free drainage.
  - 8G surgical cases and/or free drainage.
- Lubricant (if necessary).
- 10 ml syringe.
- Tape for securing.

- Specimen pot for free drainage.
- Sucrose if appropriate.

Prerequisite

1. The correct method of measurement for orogastric and nasogastric tube (OGT; NGT) insertion is to measure from the bridge of the nose to the ear lobe and then to the xiphoid sternum. Measurements are most accurate if taken with the infant in the supine position.
2. If there are any signs of respiratory distress or the neonate is on ventilatory support by CPAP, an OGT, not NGT, must be inserted.
3. Observe the infant for colour changes throughout the procedure. Passing an oral/nasal tube can stimulate a vagal response. Resuscitation equipment must be readily accessible.
4. If reinserting a tube that has dislodged, it is preferable to wait 1hour after a feed or ideally wait and insert prior to the next feed.

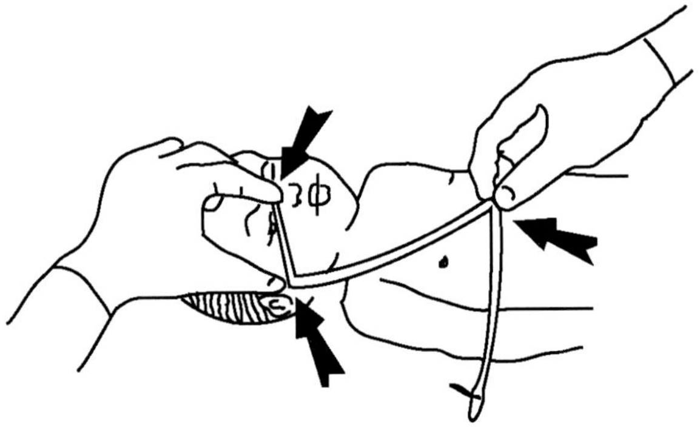

Measuring length of nasogastric tube

OROGASTRIC

Gently insert tube into mouth, aiming down and back. Flex patient's neck (unless contraindicated) when tube reaches posterior nasopharynx. Insert the tube orally and secure centrally. Tape the tube to the top lip where possible to prevent interference to the tongue. If resistance is met during insertion, stop advancement and adjust direction of tube slightly before reattempting.

NASOGASTRIC

- Insert nasally in a backward direction. If resistance persists after a reattempt then try the other nostril. Secure the tube across the cheek.
- **Gastric tubes should be changed every seven days.**

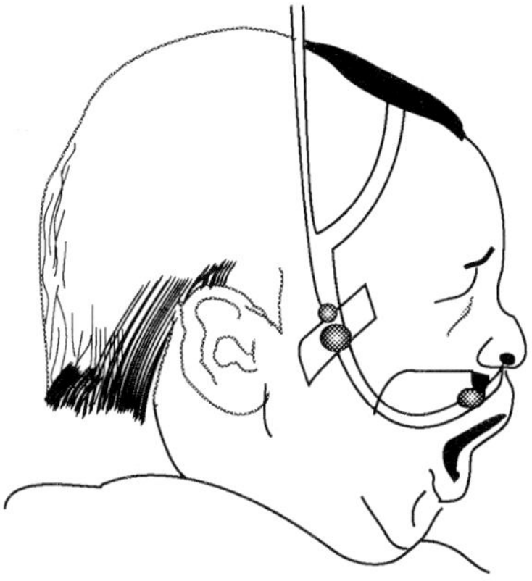

Fixation of nasogastric tube

Position Verification

Position of the tube should be verified in the following situations:

- Initial insertion.
- Prior to bolus feeds, medications.
- Following episodes of coughing, vomiting and retching.
- If displacement is suspected i.e. loose tape.

Tests Recommended for Assessing Placement

1. The 'air insertion' test (injecting air down the tube and listening) is not to be used as a primary method of testing but can be used to dislodge the exit-port of the feeding tube from the gastric mucosa. Use no more than 2 ml.
2. The presence of aspirate obtained from the gastric tube does not rule out misplacement.
3. pH indicator strip of pH 5.5 or below within 10 -15 seconds.
4. X-ray – although this is the gold standard, it is not to be used routinely due to cost and radiation exposure, but can be used if the infant is being X-rayed for other reasons.

CARE OF BABY DURING FEEDING

1. Check the amount of feed to be given in order sheet.
2. Use mother's milk for feeding whenever available.
3. Use Dexolac special care or Lactodex LBW formula for babies < 2.5 kg.
4. Use Lactodex or Lactogen I or Nan formula for babies > 2.5 kg.
5. Ensure 30 ml of boiled water with one scoop of formula and make a paste.
6. Wash hands before feeding the baby.
7. Strictly give tube feeds when ordered.

8. Keep the lid of the formula firmly covered.
9. If baby does not take complete feed orally give the remaining amount by tube and inform the doctor.
10. Burp the baby following feeds if given orally. Do not burp if given tube feeds.
11. Keep baby in right lateral position after tube feeds.
12. **Inform if:**
    A. Baby not accepting oral feeds.
    B. If aspirate is brown / red / green.
    C. If baby vomits out the feed.

CARE DURING TUBE FEEDING

1. Size of Tube:

No 6 for < 1 kg.
No 7 for 1-3 kg.
No 8 for > 3 kg.

2. Depth of Insertion:

Nasogastric – Tragus of ear to nose + Nose to lower end of sternum.
Orogastric – Lips to lower end of sternum.

3. During Feeds

- Check the amount of feed to be given.
- Use the appropriate formula.
- Confirm position of tube.
- Aspirate for contents always before feeding the baby if the abdomen appears distended.
- Keep the head end elevated by 30 degrees.
- Fill the syringe with feed and attach it to the tube.
- Allow the contents to flow by gravity.
- Do not push or flush the feeds.

4. After Feeds

- Disconnect the syringe.
- Keep baby in right lateral position.
- Do not burp the baby.

5. If Aspirate Present: Note

i. Amount: ml.
ii. Colour: Yellow / Green / Brown / Red.

6. What to do for Aspirate?

If aspirate green / red / brown: Withhold feeds. Inform doctor.

If Aspirate Yellow / White

- > 50 % of feed: Withhold feed. Inform doctor.
- < 20 % of feed: Continue feeding.
- 20 – 50 % of feed: Feed the amount tolerated.

Example:

1. Baby on 10 cc feed has 5 cc aspirate: That means 50% of feed is the aspirate: Withhold feed.
2. If the baby has 1 cc aspirate: Brown, Red, Green: Omit feed.
3. If the aspirate is 4 cc: White / Yellow: That means out of 10 cc baby is tolerating 6 cc. In the next feed give 6 cc.

Tube Removal

Perform hand hygiene and put on gloves. Flush tube with water or normal saline to remove any mucous from ports. Place the patient in upright position. Gently loosen tape or securing device from skin. Rotate tube gently, pulling slowly and steadily into towel.

REFERENCES

1. Manual of neonatal nursing: Ed, Lalitha Krishnan, Published by National Neonatology Forum, 1993.
2. Essential Newborn Nursing for Small Hospitals: In resource restricted countries, Learners Guide, Published by Division of Neonatology, Department of Pediatrics, AIIMS, New Delhi 2004.

20. INTERCOSTAL CATHETER INSERTION

Indication

- Pleural chest tubes are used to evacuate blood, pus, air and fluid, from the thoracic cavity.
- To reestablish negative pressure in the intrapleural space and thereby expand the lungs following collapse resulting from surgery or trauma.

Supplies

- Sterile surgical instrument pack.
- Size 11 scalpel blade.
- 3/0 black silk suture on a curved edge needle.
- Sterile gown, gloves and drapes.
- Skin preparation, e.g., Betadine.

- Argyle 8, 10 or 12 Fr. sterile intercostal catheter.
- Elastoplast strapping.
- 1% Lignocaine, syringe and needle.
- Underwater seal drainage system or a Heimlich valve.

Procedure

- Observe universal precautions.
- Mask, sterile gown and gloves are required as for any sterile procedure.
- Place infant under radiant heater to maintain infant's temperature, try to maintain some area of the infant visible beyond the sterile field. Place the infant with the affected side uppermost and the arm extended above the head (a nappy cloth roll may help maintain a good position). Ensure limbs are adequately restrained.
- Monitor infant's heart rate and oxygen saturation level.
- Site of insertion - The neurovascular bundle should be avoided. This can be accomplished by passing the drain through the intercostals space just above the upper border of the rib.

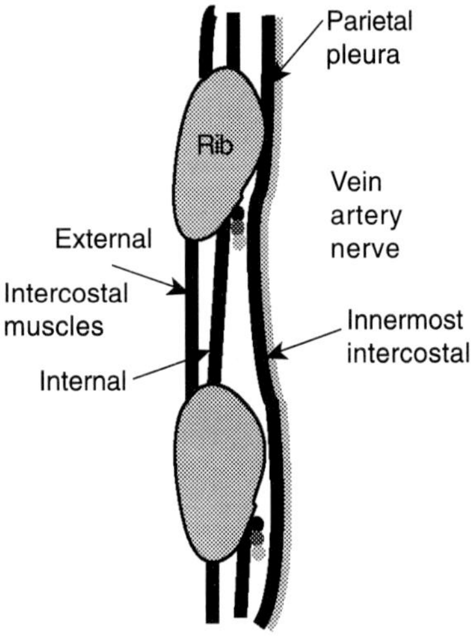

- The intercostals catheter is inserted in the 4th or 5th intercostals space in the anterior axillary's line. This corresponds to a point 4 cm lateral to and 4 cm below the nipple. The incision must be well clear of the nipple.

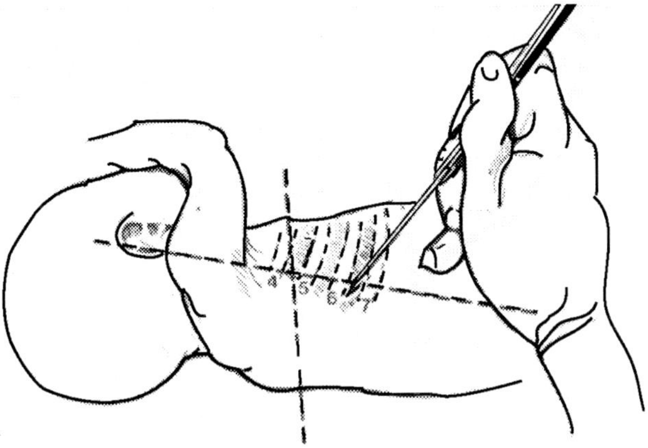

- Prepare the field with iodine solution e.g. Betadine.
- Select intercostal catheter size:

Infants	>1500 g	10 or 12 Fr
	<1500 g	8 or 10 Fr

- Water Seal Chamber must be filled first and maintained at 2 cm level to create a seal for closed drainage and keeping air from entering the cavity. This is filled regardless of whether suction is applied from the wall. After set-up routinely monitor the water level for evaporation and fill with sterile water as necessary.
- Place sterile drape in position.
- Infiltrate the insertion site with 1% Lignocaine 0.5 - 1mL (An alternate practice is to infiltrate with local anesthetic before preparing and draping the field in order to allow greater time for the anesthetic to take effect).
- Using small (number 11) scalpel blade makes a 1 cm incision through the skin and subcutaneous tissue.
- Using straight mosquito forceps to bluntly dissect away the subcutaneous tissue and intercostal muscles, the parietal pleura is reached. Aim to dissect

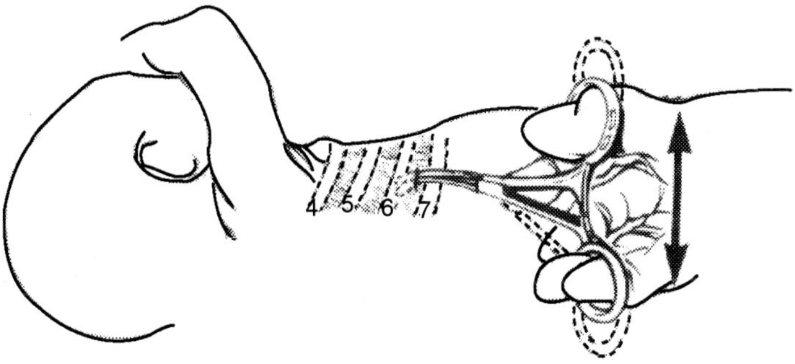

a passage just above a rib border in order to avoid the neurovascular bundles running below each rib. Open the parietal pleura by blunt dissection. At this point the hiss of air escaping the pleural space may be heard.

- Remove the trochar from the chest tube and grasp the distal end with curved artery forceps. Advance the chest tube into the pleural space 3-5 cm, i.e. at the 1-3 cm marking on the catheter directing the tip anteriorly as well as superomedially so that the tip lies beneath the anterior chest wall.
- **Drainage system:** Prepacked drainage systems are now available for drainage of pneumothoraces, haemothoraces or pleural effusions. The bottle has a screw top with two ports. One port has the underwater length of tubing attached. The second port has a shorter length of tubing attached, which acts as the venting end and is exposed to air or could be attached to a suction unit. Venting prevents the build-up of pressure in the chest drainage system, which could prevent evacuation of air or fluid.
- The underwater seal occurs when there is adequate water in the bottle. The distal end of the intrapleural drain is then attached to the underwater seal port of the chest drain bottle and immersed 2.5 cm below the level of the water. Incoming air bubbles through the water, which acts as a one-way valve and prevents the backflow of air into the intrapleural space.
- For more complicated pneumothoraces or haemothoraces, a plastic multichamber system incorporates the above one-bottle system into one unit. There are three chambers: the first is for drainage, the second chamber is the underwater seal and the third chamber is the vacuum or suction control. When this system is set up, water is placed in the water seal chamber to the indicated mark, and also placed in the suction control chamber to the

Underwater chest drainage system

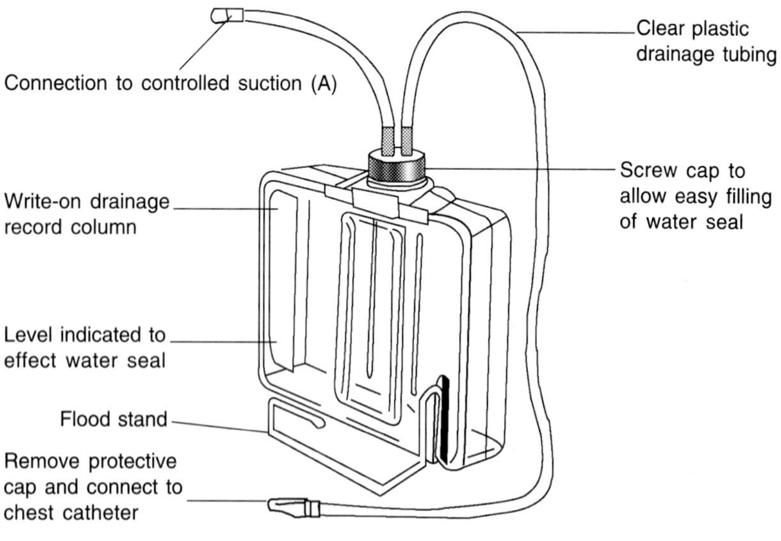

Appendix A

required level. This system is a great improvement on the previous systems and enables patient mobility.

- Connect the chest tube to a Heimlich valve or an underwater seal drainage system, and note whether the fluid is swinging and/or bubbling. Fogging within the catheter may be seen when within the pleural space.
- When there is no air leak the water level in the Water Seal Chamber should rise and fall with the patient's respirations, reflecting normal pressure changes in the pleural cavity during respiration. During spontaneous respirations, the water level should rise during inhalation and fall during exhalation. If the patient is receiving positive pressure ventilation, the oscillation will be just the opposite. Oscillations may be absent if the lung is fully expanded and suction has drawn the lung up against the holes in the chest tubes.
- Secure connection between chest tube and patient drainage connecting tubing with waterproof adhesive tape over sterile connector. Do not obliterate view of drainage.
- Place a single stitch through the wound so that the skin is drawn snugly around the chest tube. Purse string stitches are not used as they leave an unsightly scar. Wrap the ends of the suture around the chest tube several times and tie securely.
- Secure the chest tube to the chest wall. This helps to maintain the anterior position of the chest tube and minimizes trauma to intrathoracic structures due to movement of the extrathoracic portion of the chest tube.

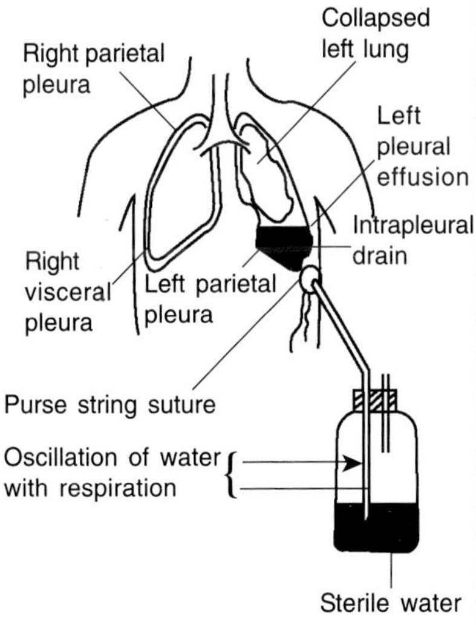

One bottle system

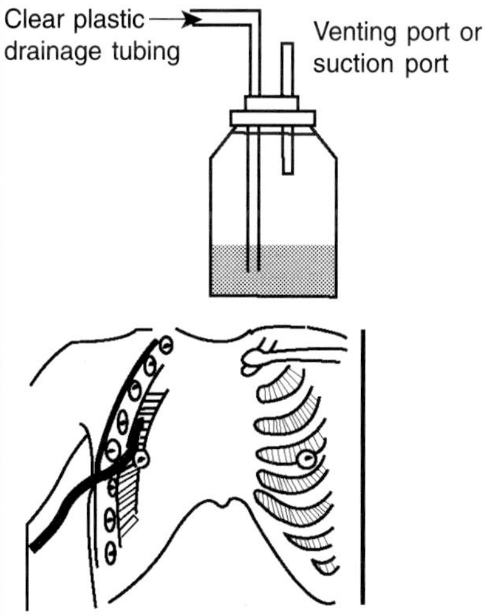

Intercostal catheter

Ongoing Care

- Check the tube position and resolution of the pneumothorax by transillumination and X-ray as soon as possible.
- The need for ongoing analgesia is based on an assessment of physiological and behavioural responses associated with pain.
- Infants requiring an intercostal catheter should be transferred to a NICU as soon as possible for ongoing care.

Suction and Its Use

The addition of suction to the drainage system increases the negative pressure, enhancing lung re-expansion. A high-volume and low-pressure suction unit should be applied. To start with 5-10 cm of H_2O suction pressure is applied. Once suction has been discontinued, the tubing to the underwater seal should be disconnected, otherwise this could cause positive pressure and may precipitate a tension pneumothorax. Wiping it with a damp cloth and a mild disinfectant solution should clean the suction unit. Most suction units are fitted with a disposable air filter capsule, between the vacuum connector and the filter capsule mount. The filter prevents cross-infection and should be changed after each patient.

Stripping/Milking of Intrapleural Drains

Milking and stripping are harmful and can result in lung damage. If the tubing becomes occluded, it should be replaced. Using the correct size of catheter should prevent tubes becoming occluded, therefore reducing the necessity of changing the drain.

Clamping of Intrapleural Drains

Clamping of drains is discouraged as this can prevent air leaving the pleural space. This in turn can cause a pneumothorax, which could progress to a life-threatening tension pneumothorax. There is also no need to clamp tubing when mobilizing or transporting patients to other departments as this may also cause a tension pneumothorax. When changing the bottle system, it may be necessary to clamp the drain and during this process the patient should be under close observation for any signs of deterioration in breathing.

Complications

- Haemorrhage.
- Lung perforation and infarction.
- Phrenic nerve damage.

Removal of Chest Drain

A chest tube is removed when it is apparent that the lung is well expanded and no air leaks from the lung or wound.

Supplies

- Sterile gloves.
- Sterile 4 × 4's.
- 2 or 4 inch adhesive tape.
- Povidone iodine.
- Vaseline gauze.
- Suture removal pack.

Procedure

- This is a two-person procedure with one sterile and one assisting.
- Dressing must be ready to apply to insertion site prior to tube removal so the vaseline gauze creates a seal to prevent air entry.
- Drape bed linen with protective pads.
- Assemble equipment at bedside.
- Perform hand hygiene and put on gloves.
- Remove the old dressing from around the chest tube.
- Clamp drainage tubing of chest tube being removed using blue slide clamp.
- Place the dressing over the insertion site immediately after the physician removes the tube.
- Cover 4 × 4 sponges completely with Tegaderm. Date and initial, leaving dressing on for 48 hours.
- Discard chest drainage system as per hospital policy.
- Anticipate follow up X-ray.
- Document events and patient's tolerance in progress notes.

REFERENCES

1. Quigley RL: Thoracentesis and chest tube drainage, Crit Care Clin 1995;11:111-26.
2. Harriss DR, Graham TR: Management of intercostal drains, Br J Hosp Med 1991 ;45:383-386.
3. Brandt ML, Luks FI, Lacroix J, Guay J, Collin PP, Dilorenzo M: The paediatric chest tube, Clin Intensive Care 1994;5:123-129.
4. Joshi JM: Intercostal tube drainage of pleura: Urosac as chest drainage bag, J Assoc Physicians India 1996;44:381-382.
5. Davies MW, Dunster KR: Insertion distance of neonatal intercostal catheters using a 10 French Argyle trocar thoracic catheter, Crit Care Resusc 2003;5:103-105.
6. Kabra NS: Use of venous catheter to drain pneumothorax, Pediatr Int 2003;45:368.

21. INTRAOSSEOUS (IO) ACCESS

The bone marrow cavity has an extensive virtually non-collapsible vascular network directly communicating with the systemic circulation. Medications or fluids given by the IO route diffuse through the medullary cavity then enter the venous circulation.

Indication

Establishing rapid venous access in an emergency.

Supplies Required

- Sterile gloves and gown.
- Dressing pack.
- Antiseptic to prepare the skin.
- Rigid needle with an inner stylet (for patients <18 months, an 18-20 lumbar puncture needle can be used).
- Syringe with 0.9% NaCl flush.
- Routine IV line tubing set-up and tape.

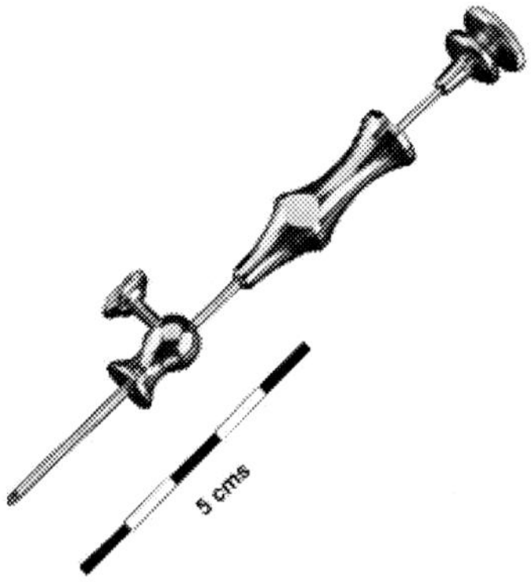

Sites of Intraosseous Puncture

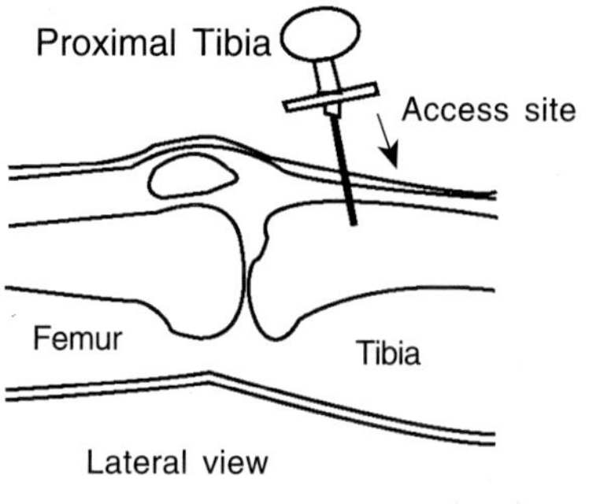

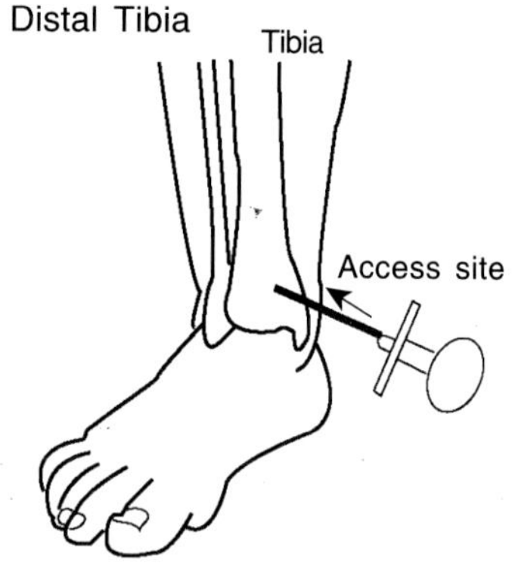

The proximal tibia is the preferred site. The entry point is a few centimetres below the tibial tuberosity at the centre of the flat antero-medial surface. The needle is directed perpendicular directed downwards, away from the upper tibial epiphysis in the line of the shaft.

The distal antero-medial surface of the tibia is an alternate site, which can be used in children of all ages.

The distal femur and sternum should ***not*** be used.

Procedure

- Observe universal precautions.
- Immobilize the extremity.
- Prepare the site with antiseptic.
- Consider use of local anaesthetic (0.5-1 mL 1% lignocaine) if time permits.
- Insert the needle. The needle handle is held in the palm of the hand while the thumb and forefinger grip the shaft about a centimeter from the point to stabilize the needle. Firm pressure is applied while using a screwing or rotary action until the bone cortex is traversed. At approximately 1 cm or less, below the skin surface, a distinct loss of resistance on entry of the bone marrow is felt.

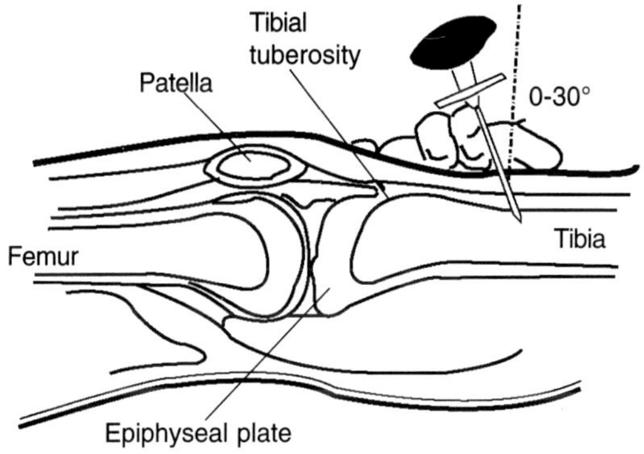

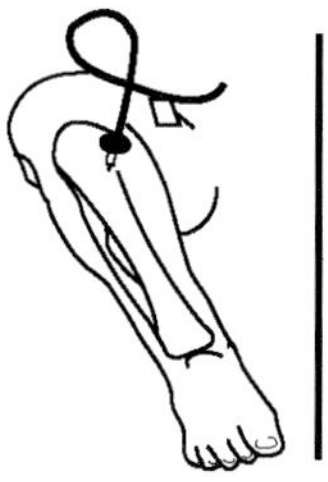

Fixation of intra-osseous line

Following features suggest entry into bone marrow:
- A distinctive pop with insertion, or a give or release of resistance is felt.
- Bone marrow is easily aspirated.
- The needle stands without support.
- The needle flushes without significant subcutaneous infiltration.

- Unscrew and remove the stylet.
- Flush the needle with 5-10 mL of normal saline.
- Attach IV tubing and commence the infusion of medications or fluids by pump.

Contraindications

Absolute
- Osteogenesis imperfecta.
- Osteopetrosis.

Relative
- Limb is traumatized.
- Fracture.
- Osteomyelitis.
- Local infection.

Complications

- Extravasation of fluid, drugs or air into skin or periosteum.
- Sub-periosteal infusion.
- Through and through puncture if the needle is advanced too far.
- Blockage of the needle.
- Infection—Cellulitis, abscess formation, skin necrosis and osteomyelitis.
- Fat and bone marrow microemboli.

REFERENCES

1. de Caen A: Venous access in the critically ill child: when the peripheral intravenous fails! Pediatr Emerg Care 2007;23:422-424.
2. Engle WA: Intraosseous access for administration of medications in neonates, Clin Perinatol 2006;33:161-168, ix.
3. LaRocco BG, Wang HE: Intraosseous infusion, Prehosp Emerg Care 2003;7:280-285.
4. Ellemunter H, Simma B, Trawöger R, Maurer H: Intraosseous lines in preterm and full term neonates, Arch Dis Child Fetal Neonatal Ed 1999;80:F74-75.
5. International Liaison Committee on Resuscitation. The International Liaison Committee on Resuscitation (ILCOR) consensus on science with treatment recommendations for pediatric and neonatal patients: Pediatric basic and advanced life support, Pediatrics 2006;117:e955-77.

6. Evans RJ, McCabe M, Thomas R: Intraosseous infusion, Br J Hosp Med 1994;51:161-164.

22. PROCEDURE FOR INVERTED NIPPLE

- Inverted or retracted nipples make attachment to the breast difficult.
- Treatment is started after birth of the baby. Nipple is manually stretched and rolled out several times a day.
- A plastic syringe is used to draw out the nipple and the baby is then put to the breast.

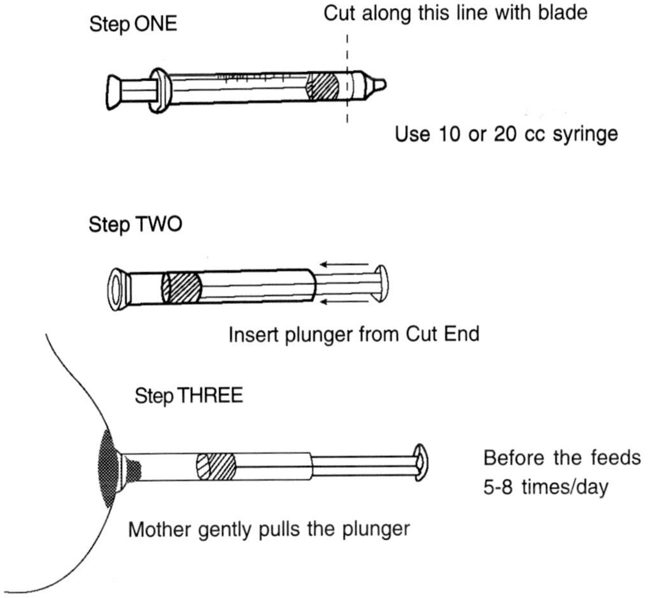

REFERENCE

1. Essential Newborn Nursing for Small Hospitals. In resource restricted countries, Learners Guide. Published by Division of Neonatology, Department of Pediatrics, AIIMS, New Delhi 2004.

23. KANGAROO CARE (KC)

Kangaroo care (also referred to as "skin to skin") is a special way of caring of LBW babies. It fosters their health and well being by promoting effective thermal control, breastfeeding, infection prevention and bonding. KC is initiated in the hospital and continued at home.

Indications

KC can be started as soon as the baby is stable.

1. Infants stable enough to tolerate traditional holding within 4 hours of birth.
2. A clinically stable ventilated infant, who does not require labile respiratory support.
3. A clinically stable infant requiring less than 0.5 FiO_2 via CPAP or nasal cannula.

Supplies

- Comfortable chair with arms.
- Pillows/footstool as required.
- Privacy screens/curtains.
- Baby hat/blanket.

Procedure

- Provide a hospital gown with facility to keep the front open.
- Providers of KC must have clean, dry skin, free of perfumes, oils, smoke, odor, with no rashes and/or lesions.
- Set up a comfortable environment
- Assess infant's vital signs prior to initiating KC.
- Prepare infant by placing him or her in a diaper and putting a hat on the infant.
- Transfer the infant onto the caregiver's chest; ensuring the attached lines, leads and tubings are carefully monitored for security. KC can last a varied length of time from 30 minutes to all day, depending on the caregiver and response/tolerance of the infant.
- Position the infant so that the caregiver and infant are chest to chest. The caregiver's hands support the infant's buttocks and back while the infant's legs are tucked into flexion. The infant's head and neck are positioned to protect the airway.
- Cover the infant with the caregiver's shirt or gown and a blanket as necessary.
- Assess vital signs for all infants 15 minutes after initiating KC. For infants <1000 g assess vitals every 30 minutes after initial assessment.
- Ensure that baby's neck is not too flexed or too extended, breathing is normal, and feet and hands are warm.
- Remain immediately available for support or assistance.
- Feedings may take place during KC.
- Assess vital signs and infant tolerance at the end of KC.

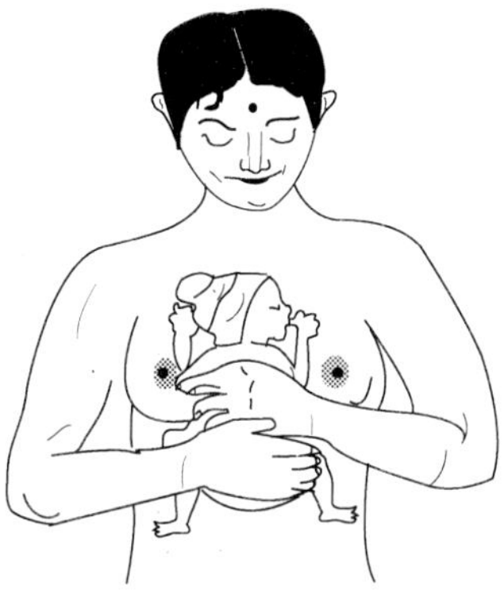

Monitoring

Nursing staff should make sure that baby's neck position is neither too flexed nor too extended, airway is clear, breathing is regular, color is pink and baby is maintaining temperature. Mother should be involved in observing the baby during KMC so that she herself can continue monitoring at home.

Document

1. Length of time of KC.
2. Infant's response/tolerance of the procedure.
3. Caregivers response to KC.
4. Patient education record.
5. All vital signs on flow sheet.
6. Any breast/enteral feeding on flow sheet.

Contraindications

1. Sick infants.
2. Unstable infants.
3. Infants with femoral or radial arterial lines or central line other than PICC.
4. Infants with chest drain.
5. Infants with abdominal defects or surgery.
6. Infants on high frequency ventilation.

Weaning off KC

When the mother and baby are comfortable, KC is continued for as long as possible, at the institution and then at home. Often this is desirable until the baby's gestation reaches term or the weight is around 2500 g. This is the time to wean the baby from KC.

REFERENCES

1. World Health Organization: Kangaroo mother care: A practical guide. Department of Reproductive Health and Research, WHO, Geneva 2003.
2. Charpak N, Ruiz-Pelaez JG, Charpak Y: Rey-Martinez Kangaroo Mother Program: An alternative way of caring for low birth weight infants? One-year mortality in a cohort study, Pediatrics 1994;94:804-810.
3. Conde-Agudelo, Diaz-Rosello JL, Belizan JM: Kangaroo mother care to reduce morbidity and mortality in low birth weight infants. Cochrane Database Syst Rev 2003; (2): CD002771.
4. Charpak N, Ruiz-Pelaez JG, Figueroa de C Z, Charpak Y: A randomized, controlled trial of kangaroo mother care: Results of follow-up at 1 year of corrected age, Pediatrics 2001;108:1072-1079.
5. Cattaneo A, Davanzo R, Bergman N, Charpak N: Kangaroo mother care in low-income countries. International Network in Kangaroo Mother Care, J Trop Pediatr 1998;44:279-282.
6. Sloan NL, Camacho LW, Rojas EP, Stern C: Kangaroo mother method: Randomised controlled trial of an alternative method of care for stabilised low-birthweight infants, Maternidad Isidro Ayora Study Team, Lancet 1994;344:782-785.
7. Ramanathan K, Paul VK, Deorari AK, Taneja U, George G: Kangaroo Mother Care in very low birth weight infants, Indian J Pediatr 2001;68:1019-1023.
8. Chwo MJ, Anderson GC, Good M, Dowling DA, Shiau SH, Chu DM: A randomized controlled trial of early kangaroo care for preterm infants: Effects on temperature, weight, behavior and acuity, J Nurs Res 2002;10:129-142.
9. Tessier R, Cristo M, Velez S, Giron M, de Calume ZF, Ruiz-Palaez JG, Charpak Y, Charpak N: Kangaroo mother care and the bonding hypothesis, Pediatrics 1998;102:e17.
10. Udani RH, Nanavati RN: Training manual on Kangaroo Mother Care. Published by the Department of Neonatology, KEM Hospital and Seth GS Medical College, Mumbai, September 2004.

24. LARYNGEAL MASK AIRWAY (LMA)

The laryngeal mask is a device for supporting and maintaining the airway without tracheal intubation. The LMA fills a niche between the face mask (FM) and tracheal tube (TT) in terms of both anatomical position and degree of invasiveness. It is manufactured from medical grade silicone rubber and is reusable.

Components of LMA

1. The **airway tube** is slightly curved to match the oropharyngeal anatomy, semirigid to facilitate atraumatic insertion and semitransparent, so that condensation and regurgitated material is visible. A black line runs longitudinally along its posterior curvature to aid in orientation. The distal

aperture of the airway tube opens into the lumen of an inflatable mask and is protected by two flexible vertical rubber bars, called mask aperture bars (MAB), to prevent the epiglottis from entering and obstructing the airway.

2. The **inflatable mask** is oval shaped with a broad, round proximal end and a narrower, more pointed distal end. It has an inflatable cuff and a semirigid, concave, shield like backplate. The cuff is attached to the outer rim of the backplate. The inner aspect of the mask is called the bowl, which is comprised the distal aperture, mask aperture bars, backplate and the inner aspect of the inflatable cuff.
3. The **mask inflation line,** which is attached to the most proximal portion of the cuff in the midline consists of four parts, the long narrow inflation line itself, the inflation indicator balloon (pilot balloon), a metallic valve and the syringe port.

Indications

1. Maintaining airway during difficult intubation.
2. Emergency management of airway in failed intubation.
3. Elective short surgical procedures under general anaesthesia excluding head and neck surgery.

Contraindication

1. Meconium stained liquor depressed infants.
2. Administration of drugs.
3. Preterm infants.

Supplies

- 5 cc syringe.
- Laryngeal mask airway – no 1.
- Water soluble lubricant.
- Adhesive tape.

Preparation

- Ensure laryngeal mask airway has been previously sterilized.
- Visually inspect the LMA cuff for tears or other abnormalities.
- Inspect the tube to ensure that it is free of blockage or loose particles.
- Deflate the cuff to ensure that it will maintain a vacuum.
- Inflate the cuff to ensure that it does not leak.

Procedure

- Choose the appropriate size LMA.
- Slowly deflate the cuff to form a smooth flat wedge shape, which will pass easily around the back of the tongue and behind the epiglottis.

- Use a water-soluble lubricant to lubricate the LMA. Only lubricate the LMA just prior to insertion. Lubricate the back of the mask thoroughly. Avoid excessive amounts of lubricant on the anterior surface of the cuff or in the bowl of the mask.
- Extend the head and flex the neck.
- Visualize the posterior oral airway.
- Grasp the LMA by the tube, holding it like a pen as near as possible to the mask end.
- Place the tip of the LMA against the inner surface of the patient's upper gum line
- Ensure that the LMA is not folding over in the oral cavity as it is inserted.
- Under direct vision: Press the mask tip upwards against the hard palate to flatten it out. Using the index finger, keep pressing upwards as you advance the mask into the pharynx to ensure the tip remains flattened and avoids the tongue.
- Keep the neck flexed and head extended: Press the mask into the posterior pharyngeal wall using the index finger.
- Continue pushing with your index finger. Guide the mask downward into position.
- Grasp the tube firmly with the other hand then withdraw your index finger from the pharynx. Press gently downward with your other hand to ensure the mask is fully inserted.
- A change of direction will be felt as the cuff tip follows the posterior pharyngeal wall downwards. The laryngeal mask is pushed as far as possible into the hypopharynx by the index finger. When the mask is fully advanced, resistance will be felt.
- If it is felt that the mask is not fully advanced into the hypopharynx, the laryngeal mask is pressed downwards by the non-dominant hand to complete placement.
- The cuff is inflated with an appropriate volume of air. The tube usually moves out of the mouth and the tissues overlying both the thyroid and cricoid cartilage bulge slightly when the cuff is inflated. The tube should not be held or connected to the breathing system during inflation. The tip of the mask is likely to be positioned too deeply if the tube is held during inflation.
- The laryngeal mask is connected to the breathing system and adequacy of ventilation is assessed.
- LMA can be secured utilizing the same techniques as those employed in the securing of an endotracheal tube.
- When adequate ventilation is not obtained, the mask is removed and placement reattempted. The cuff should be prepared between each attempt as initially described.
- When removal is planned, deflate the cuff and gradually withdraw the LMA.

Re-use

The laryngeal mask is autoclaved between uses. A maximum of 40 uses is recommended (i.e. 39 re-uses).

REFERENCES

1. International Liaison Committee on Resuscitation. The International Liaison Committee on Resuscitation (ILCOR) consensus on science with treatment recommendations for pediatric and neonatal patients: Pediatric basic and advanced life support, Pediatrics 2006;117:e955-77.
2. Takashi Asai: The laryngeal mask airway: Its features, effects and role, Can J Anaesth 1994;41:930-960.

25. LUMBAR PUNCTURE (LP)

Indications

1. Suspected CNS infection.
2. Suspected subarachnoid hemorrhage.
3. Therapeutic reduction of cerebrospinal fluid (CSF) pressure.
4. Positive blood culture.
5. Unexplained seizures.
6. To monitor efficacy of antibiotic therapy with repeat cell count and culture.

Contraindications

1. Local skin infections over proposed puncture site.
2. Uncontrolled bleeding diathesis.
3. Spinal column deformities.
4. Cardiorespiratory instability.

Supplies

- Alcohol, iodine, tincture benzoin cotton balls.
- Sterile gloves, Gauze pads, Towel, Fenestrated drape, Spot bandage.
- 1% lignocaine.
- 22 / 23 G needle.
- Sterile bulbs, 5 cc syringe.

Procedure

1. Obtain informed consent.
2. Provide necessary analgesia and/or sedation as required.
3. *Have the assistant restrain and position patient:* Lateral decubitus position with head and knees flexed and curling up. The head need not be flexed too far, as some infants develop increased respiratory difficulty with flexing of the head.

4. *Locate landmarks:* Palpate the spinous process that is even with the iliac crests. This is L4. Locate one interspace above (L3-L4) or one space below (L4-L5) as the site. Use this reference to locate the entry point. Aim the needle towards the navel.

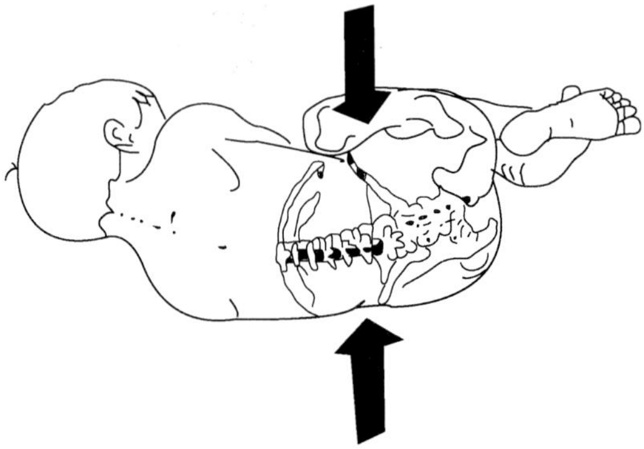

5. Prep and drape the area after identifying landmarks with iodine and alcohol from the proposed site of insertion to the periphery. Drape the area with proposed interspinous space open. Re-confirm the site of insertion. Use lidocaine (1%) 0.3 ml /kg, subcutaneously, 1-2 minutes prior to anesthetize the skin and the deeper tissues under the insertion site. However, the use of local anaesthetic is optional.
6. Assemble needle (23 or 24G). Hold the thumb of the left hand over L4 and with the right hand insert the needle with the bevel-up through the skin and advance through the deeper tissues. A slight pop or give is felt when the dura is punctured. Angle of insertion is on a slightly cephalad angle, between the vertebra. If you hit bone, partially withdraw the needle, reposition, and re-advance. You may need to rotate the needle slightly to increase or initiate the flow. If unsuccessful repeat attempt in next interspace up or down, but never go above the L2-L3 interspace.
7. When CSF flows, note the opening pressure and begin filling collection tubes with 1-2 ml of CSF each.

   Tube 1: Glucose, protein estimation.

   Tube 2: Gram's stain, bacterial and or viral cultures.

   Tube 3: Cell count and differential.

   Tube 4: Reserve tube for any special tests.
8. If CSF does not flow, or you hit bone, withdraw needle partially, recheck landmarks, and re-advance.
9. After tap, remove needle, and place a tincture benzoin bandage over the puncture site.

PRACTICE POINTERS

1. A traumatic "bloody tap" occurs when a spinal venous plexus is penetrated. Often the fluid will clear as succeeding tubes are filled. Spin down the first tube: if red blood cells have been in the spinal fluid for some time (for example, subarachnoid hemorrhage), xanthochromia will be present in the supernatant fluid. If the fluid is clear after it is spun down, the tap was only traumatic.
2. Supplemental O_2 is administered before and during LP to prevent hypoxia, in an infant who is receiving oxygen.
3. Make sure the specimen after collection reaches the lab promptly.
4. Early repeated CSF tapping cannot be recommended for neonates at risk of, or actually developing, post-hemorrhagic hydrocephalus.

Complications, Prevention and Management

Complication	*Prevention*	*Management*
Bleeding from puncture site post-tap	None	Local pressure
Bloody spinal fluid	None	Withdraw needle and perform tap at interspace either above or below
Infection	Do not perform tap through infected skin. Use sterile technique	Antibiotics
Hypoxia, bradycardia	Do not flex the head too much	Monitor vital parameters
Damage to spinal cord and nerves	Use interspace below L4	

Documentation

Document position of patient during the procedure, opening pressure and clarity/color of the CSF and clinical status pre and post procedure.

VENTRICULAR TAP

Indications

1. Drain cerebrospinal fluid in non-communicating hydrocephalus.
2. Diagnose ventriculitis.
3. Administer intraventricular drugs.

Prerequisite

1. Prior to a ventricular tap, an ultrasound should be performed to confirm ventriculomegaly and measurements taken to confirm the depth and direction of needle insertion.

2. Shave the scalp overlying the lateral angle of the anterior fontanelle.

Supplies

- Sterile drapes / Dressing pack.
- Lumbar puncture needle (size 22G or 23G).
- Specimen bottles.

Procedure

1. Clean a wide area of the shaved head with betadine and spirit using aseptic precautions.
2. Position the infant supine. Stand at the head end with the top of the infant's head facing towards you.
3. With a short beveled needle, preferably with a stylet, introduce along the lateral angle of the anterior fontanelle or into the coronal suture 2 cm lateral to the midline.
4. Advance perpendicularly the needle forwards, medially and superiorly aiming towards the nasion. Do not apply negative suction. The ventricle is generally reached at a depth of 2-4 cm. Allow the CSF to be drained. The needle should be inserted smoothly without change of direction to minimise trauma to the brain.
5. Seal with tincture benzoin.
6. Document the infant's tolerance of the procedure in the progress notes.

SUBDURAL TAP

Indication

1. Suspected subdural hematoma.
2. Suspected subdural effusion.

Prerequisite

1. USG skull or CT scan brain should be done.
2. Shave the scalp overlying the anterior fontanelle.

Supplies

- Sterile drapes / Dressing pack.
- Lumbar puncture needle (size 22G or 23G).
- Specimen bottles.

Procedure

1. Clean a wide area of the shaved head with betadine and spirit using aseptic precautions.
2. Position the infant supine. Stand at the head end with the top of the infant's head facing towards you.

3. With a short and wide bore needle enter just lateral to the lateral angle of the anterior fontanelle with the needle directed slightly laterally pointing to the tragus.
4. Withdraw the stylet and wait for a couple of minutes, as the subdural fluid is thick and viscid. If no fluid comes out advance further to a maximum depth of 1-1.5 cm. Do not apply negative suction.
5. If the tap is dry, attempt on the other side and more laterally in the coronal suture.
6. Seal with tincture benzoin.
7. Document the infant's tolerance of the procedure in the progress notes.

Complications

1. Injury to the cerebral cortex.
2. Intracranial hemorrhage.
3. Intraventricular hemorrhage.

REFERENCE

1. Manual of neonatal nursing, Ed. Lalitha Krishnan, Published by National Neonatology Forum, 1993.

26. MEASURING BLOOD GLUCOSE

Measure bedside blood glucose using paper reagent strips that are made for newborn babies.

Indications

- Screening for hypoglycemia in high-risk baby.
- Convulsing baby.
- Monitoring in sick newborn.

Supplies

1. An alcohol swab.
2. A sterile lancet.
3. A container for "sharps", i.e. for lancets.
4. Reagent strips such as Haemo-Glukotest.
5. Cotton wool swab to stop the bleeding.
6. A clock or watch.
7. Plastic squeeze bottle of water.
8. Paper towel and cotton wool.

Procedure

- Gather necessary equipment and supplies.

- Follow the instructions for the reagent strips.
- Wash hands.
- Clean the site with antiseptic. Allow it to air dry.
- Take a blood sample by piercing the heel of the baby with the lancet.

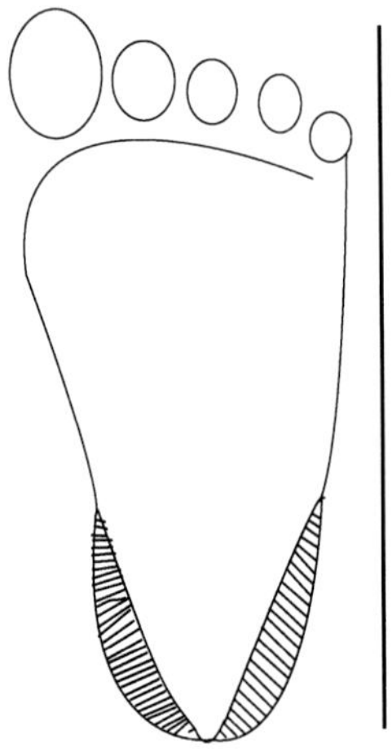

How to Use a Haemo-Glukotest Reagent Strip?

1. Place a large drop of blood onto the two reagent areas, which are found on the printed side of the plastic strip. Both reagent areas must be covered with blood.
2. Wait exactly 60 seconds then quickly wipe the blood off the reagent area with a piece of cotton wool. Do not touch the reagent area with your finger.
3. After a further 60 seconds compare the colour of the reagent areas by holding the strip against the colour chart on the container. A good light is essential.
4. The reagent area, closer to the end of the reagent strip that you hold, gives the more accurate measurement if the blood glucose concentration is in the normal or low range. The colour chart consists of 7 colour blocks ranging from yellow through grey-green to dark blue, which indicate blood glucose concentrations from 1 mmol/l (20 mg/dl) to 17 mmol/l (300 mg/dl) and above. The reagent area may match a colour block or fall between 2 adjacent colour blocks.

It is essential that the method described is strictly adhered to. Otherwise an incorrect reading may be obtained.

- Transfer the required volume of blood onto the reagent strip, usually in an area at the tip of the strip, taking care to cover all the required area with one or two drops of blood at the same time.

- Leave the blood on the strip for the required length of time — usually 30 to 60 seconds.
- Estimate the blood glucose by:
  a. Immediately compare the colour on the strip to a colour chart (usually on the container of the reagent strips) to estimate blood glucose.
  b. Reading displayed by the glucometer.
- If the blood glucose is less than 25 mg/dl (1.1 mmol/l), confirm by laboratory measurement.

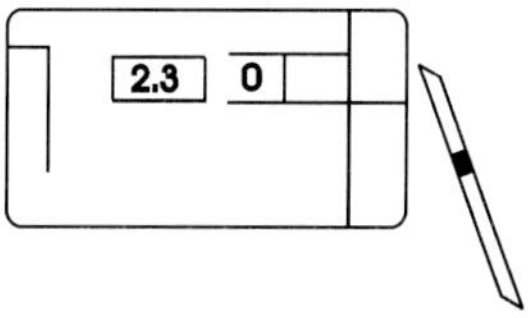

Glucometer with glucostix

PRACTICE POINTERS

Common Errors with Reagent Strips

1. The reagent strips must be fresh. Age, temperature, humidity or light may cause the reagents to deteriorate. This may result in a falsely low reading. The reagent strips must also be discarded if the expiry date on the bottle has been reached.
2. The whole reagent area must be covered with blood to prevent difficulty reading the colour change. A large drop of blood is, therefore, needed.
3. The blood must be wiped off after exactly 60 seconds. Waiting less than 60 seconds will give a falsely low reading while waiting too long will give a falsely high reading. It is advisable to use a watch or clock with a second hand to measure the 60 seconds accurately.
4. Do not attempt to wipe or wash off or rub off any pieces of adherent, dry blood, as excessive washing will give a falsely low reading.
5. A low packed cell volume (PCV) may give a falsely high reading while a high PCV may give a false low reading.
6. If possible, all readings below 2 mmol/l (40 mg/dl) should be confirmed with a blood glucose meter or by a laboratory measurement of the blood glucose concentration in venous or arterial blood.

   Reagent strips are subject to false positive and false negative results.

False Positive

- Low hematocrit values (<35%).
- Contamination with iso propyl alcohol.

False Negative

- High hematocrit values (>55%).

Appendix A

- Glucose values > 200 mg/dl.
- Hyperglycemic-hyperosmolar states with or without ketosis.
- Delay in lab analysis.

Do not perform blood glucose determination by reagent strip at temperature below 18 degree C or above 35 degree C.

REFERENCES

1. American Academy of Pediatrics, Committee on Fetus and Newborn, Routine Evaluation of Blood Pressure, Hematocrit and Glucose in Newborns (RE 9322), Pediatrics 1993;92:474-476.
2. Dextrostix [package insert], Mishawaka (IN)-Bayer Corporation.

27. MEASURING BLOOD PRESSURE (BP)

Arterial blood pressure remains the most frequently monitored indicator of neonatal circulatory status. Gold standard for blood pressure (BP) measurement is invasive BP monitoring. Non-invasive method (oscillometric method) is a rough guide to the actual BP. Although many sick newborns are treated for hypotension and hypertension, the normal physiologic blood pressure range ensuring appropriate organ perfusion is uncertain. For normal range of blood pressure follow postnatal age and gestational age related charts. A good rule of thumb is to aim for the baby's gestational age as the desired minimum mean blood pressure.

Techniques of blood pressure measurement

Direct method	*Indirect method*
• Intravascular	• Palpatory
	• Auscultatory
	• Flush method
	• Doppler
	• Oscillometric

Indications

1. For monitoring vital parameters.
2. For management of shock.
3. For management of hypertension.
4. Titrating drug therapy for dose and duration.

Supplies

- Cardio-respiratory monitor.
- Blood pressure cuffs.
- Noninvasive blood pressure monitor.

PROCEDURE FOR NON-INVASIVE BP MONITORING

- Properly fitting cuffs are essential for accurate measurements. Measure the infant's extremity and select cuff of correct size. Ensure that the 2/3rd of circumference of limb is covered with the cuff.
- Position cuff over artery.
- Upper arm or thigh measurements are recommended. Calf pressures have not been correlated with central arterial pressure readings. The difference in BP evaluation in lower or upper limb is miniscule till first year of life in normal infants.
- Optimal measurements are obtained when the infant is at rest. During measurement, keep extremity at heart level to maximize accuracy of readings. Support infant as needed; allow infant time to quiet before obtaining blood pressure.
- The infant is left undisturbed for at least 15 minutes or until the infant is sleeping or in a quiet awake state. Three successive BP recordings are taken at 2-minute intervals.
- Assess extremity for signs of circulatory impairment (discoloration, edema, poor perfusion, petechiae) especially when frequent measurements are being taken.
- Rotate BP cuff every 4 hourly.
- Disinfect probe/ cuff and extension tubes of BP apparatus in every shift.
- If the tubing to the BP cuff is loose do not use the cuff.

PROCEDURE FOR INVASIVE BP MONITORING

Supplies

- Cardiorespiratory monitor.
- Blood pressure transducer cable.
- Blood pressure transducer tubing set-up (prepackaged).
- 3-way stopcock.
  - Attach transducer tubing set-up to prepared IV fluid and tubing.
  - Flush through transducer tubing. Pinch clear plastic flush port while flushing tubing. Check carefully for bubbles in system. They will give false reading for blood pressure. Hold tubing to facilitate air bubbles to float up and out of the system.
  - Plug transducer wire into transducer cable.
  - Connect 3-way stopcock from the transducer pressure line to the umbilical artery catheter or T-connector on peripheral arterial line.
  - Place transducer at level of infant's right atrium with bed flat. Close the arterial line and open the transducer to air. Zero the transducer according to instructions in the individual Cardiorespiratory Monitor Operational Manual.

- A good wave pattern indicates that BP is being accurately monitored. If waveform is damped or questionable, a peripheral cuff pressure should be taken to check accuracy of transducer BP.
- If BP wave is continuously damped after troubleshooting efforts, notify the clinician and obtain cuff pressures according to relevant protocols. Under these circumstances, it is not necessary to document hourly blood pressures.
- Transducer set-up is changed every 24 hours with IV tubing change.
- Transducer should be zeroed every 8 hours.

Precautions

- The labelling of BP cuffs as preterm, very small preterm, term, infant and pediatric is misleading.
- Avoid applying the pulse ox probe and the BP cuff on the same limb.
- Palpatory, auscultatory and flush method have limitations hence are not used to diagnose and treat blood pressure problems.
- Rotate the BP cuff every 4-6 hourly for appropriate measurement.
- The relation between cuff size and limb circumference contributes substantially to the inaccuracy of the oscillometric blood pressure measurement. Appropriate size cuff is considered to be reasonably accurate for the clinical determination of systolic and mean blood pressure, provided that several consecutive measurements are performed and averaged in order to minimize the error of measurement in the absence of struggling, crying and movement of the newborn. Taking only one randomized measurement under these conditions would be enough and practical in daily newborn care practice instead of repeating and averaging many measurements.
- Assessment of blood pressure itself must be done in relation with gestational age and birth weight adapted norms.
- In low blood pressure there is a tendency to underestimate and in high blood pressure there is a tendency to overestimate by the oscillometric blood pressure measurement.
- Treatment decisions are based on statistically defined gestational and postnatal age-dependent normative blood-pressure values, combined with clinical intuition, rather than on data bearing physiologic reference, because of difficulties evaluating organ perfusion and adequacy of cerebral oxygen delivery.
- A systematic review was not able to define a threshold BP that was significantly predictive of a poor outcome, nor whether any interventions for hypotensive infants improved outcomes, nor which interventions were more likely to be beneficial.

REFERENCES

1. Kent AL, Kecskes Z, Shadbolt B, Falk MC: Normative blood pressure data in the early neonatal period, Pediatr Nephrol 2007;22:1335-1341.

2. Pejovic B, Peco-Antic A, Marinkovic-Eric J: Blood pressure in non-critically ill preterm and full-term neonates, Pediatr Nephrol 2007;22:249-257.
3. Hegyi T, Carbone MT, Anwar M, Ostfeld B, Blood pressure ranges in premature infants, I. The first hours of life, J Pediatr 1994;124:627-633.
4. Zubrow AB, Hulman S, Kushner H, Falkner B: Determinants of blood pressure in infants admitted to neonatal intensive care units: A prospective multicenter study, Philadelphia Neonatal Blood Pressure Study Group, J Perinatol 1995;15:470-479.
5. Nwankwo MU, Lorenz JM, Gardiner JC: A standard protocol for blood pressure measurement in the newborn, Pediatrics 1997;99:e10.
6. Pellegrini-Caliumi G, Agostino R, Nodari S *et al.*: Evaluation of an automatic oscillometric method and of various cuffs for the measurement of arterial pressure in the neonate, Acta Paediatr Scand 1982;71:791-797.
7. Pilossoff V, Schöber JG, Peters D, Bühlmeyer K: Non-invasive oscillometric measurement of systolic, mean and diastolic blood pressure in infants with congenital heart defects after operation: A comparison with direct blood pressure measurements, Eur J Pediatr 1985;144:324-330.
8. Dempsey EM, Barrington KJ: Treating hypotension in the preterm infant: When and with what: A critical and systematic review, J Perinatol 2007;27:469-478.

28. MEASURING TEMPERATURE

Indications

1. Pre-term/low birth weight or sick newborn on admission.
2. Admitted to hospital, regardless of the reason, periodically.
3. Suspected of being either hypothermic or hyperthermic.
4. Being re-warmed during management of hypothermia.
5. Being cooled down during management of hyperthermia.

Supplies

- Thermometer that measures temperatures as low as 35°C (axillary temperature).
- Thermometer that measures temperatures as low as 25°C (rectal temperature).
- Disinfectant solution.
- Water-based lubricant.

Site of Temperature Measurement

1. As a general rule, taking the axillary temperature is better than the rectal temperature because of safety, hygiene and ease.
2. Taking the axillary temperature involves no risk to the infant and if properly done gives a good approximation of body core temperature. Axillary

temperature tends to be about 1 degree lower (36°C) than the core temperature.

3. When hypothermia is suspected, the rectal temperature is more useful because it is a more accurate measure of the body core temperature. Rectal temperatures are slow to change in relation to changing core temperature, and they have been shown to stay elevated well after the patient's core temperature has begun to fall and vice versa. The depth of insertion affects rectal readings, conditions affecting local blood flow and the presence of stool. Rectal perforation is a rare but serious complication, which can be avoided if the procedure is undertaken correctly. Without proper sterilization techniques, rectal thermometry has the capacity to spread contaminants that are commonly found in stool.
4. Despite its low sensitivity and specificity in detecting fever, axillary temperature is recommended by the American Academy of Pediatrics as a screening test for neonates.

Procedure of Temperature Measurement

1. Gather necessary supplies.
2. Wash hands.
3. Roll the thermometer until you can see the thin ribbon of mercury. Ensure that the thermometer is clean.
4. Keep the baby as warm as possible during the procedure (e.g. warmly wrapped or on a warm surface).
5. Place the baby on her/his back or side.
6. Shake the thermometer until it is below 35°C if using glass thermometer.
7. Place the tip of the thermometer at axilla or rectum for at least 2 minutes.
8. Remove the thermometer and read the temperature.
9. If the temperature is too low to be recorded by this thermometer (less than 35°C), measure rectal temperature.
10. Wipe the thermometer with a disinfectant solution after use.

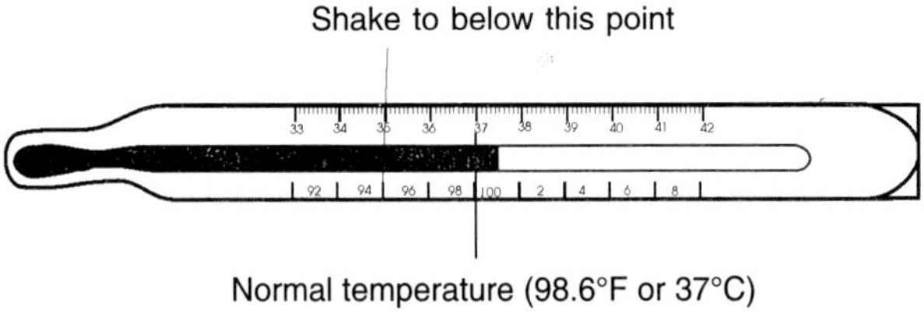

Taking Axillary Temperature

- Put the tip of the thermometer in an armpit. Make sure the armpit is dry.
- Close the armpit by holding the elbow against the chest. If you are using a glass thermometer, leave it in for 2 to 3 minutes. If you are using a digital

thermometer, take it out when you hear the signal (usually a series of beeps).

- Newborn has fever if the armpit temperature is over 99.0°F (37.2°C).
- If you have any doubt, take temperature by the rectum.

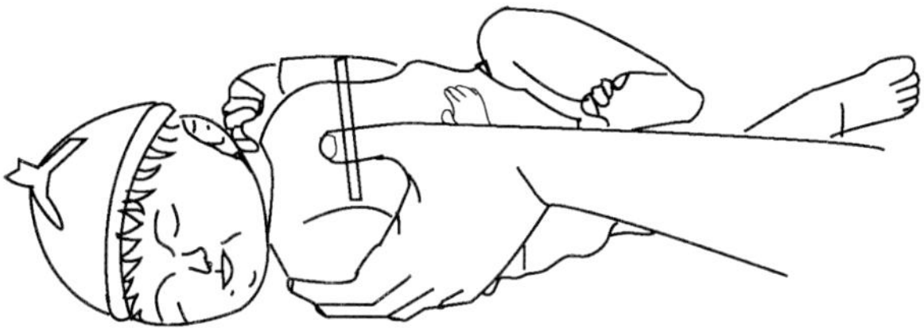

Taking Rectal Temperature

- Have the newborn lie stomach down on your lap.
- Put some petroleum jelly on the end of the thermometer and on the rectum.
- Put the thermometer gently into the rectum about 1 inch.
- Hold the baby still. If you are using a glass thermometer, leave it in for 2 minutes. If you are using a digital thermometer, take it out when you hear the signal (usually a series of beeps).
- The newborn has a fever if the rectal temperature is over 100.4°F (38°C).

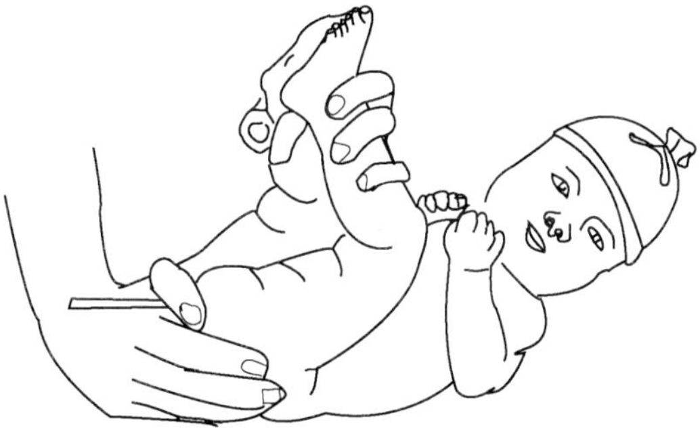

Choice of Thermometer

The thermometers available are glass thermometers and digital thermometers. The accuracy of both the devices is the same. The advantage of digital thermometer is ease of use, display of reading after set period of time and convenience. The disadvantage is availability and high cost.

Clinical Thermometer

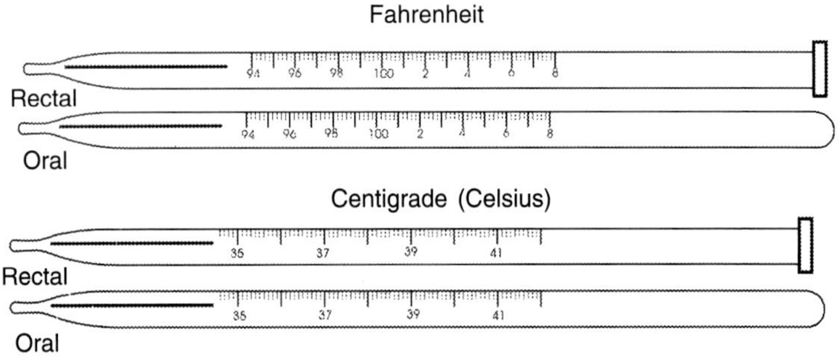

Digital Thermometer

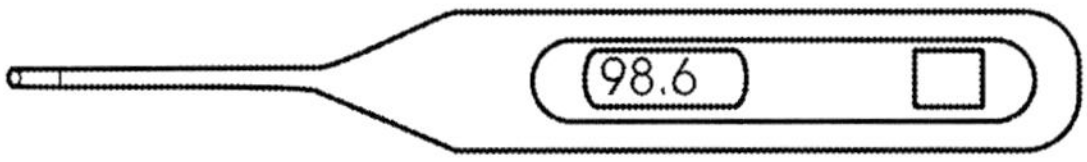

Body temperature in the newborn infant (°C)

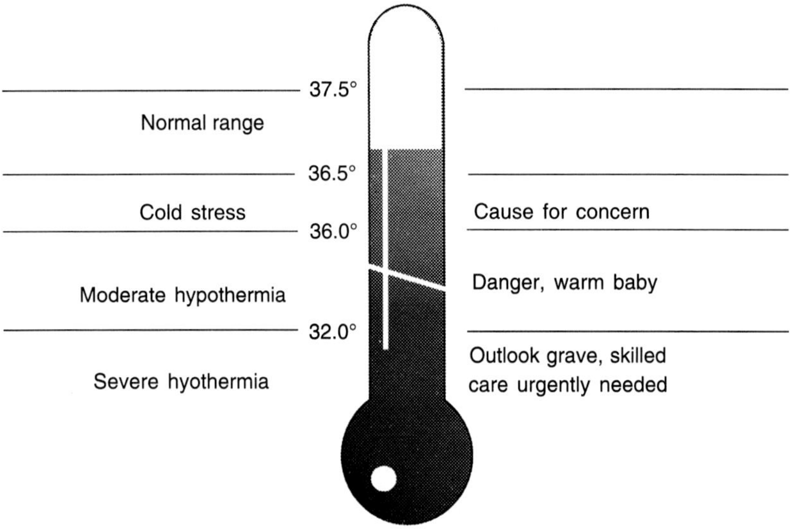

Frequency of temperature measurement:

< 2500 grams	< 1500 grams	Stable baby	Sick baby
6-12 hourly	4-6 hourly	Once a day	Every hour

Conversion of Fahrenheit to Celsius or vice versa

- To convert Fahrenheit to Celsius, subtract 32 and multiply by 5/9.
- To convert Celsius to Fahrenheit, multiply by 9/5 and add 32.

REFERENCES

1. Thermal protection of the newborn: A practical guide. Department of Reproductive Health and Research (RHR), World Health Organization, 1997.
2. Brown PJ, Christmas BF, Ford RP: Taking an infant's temperature: Axillary or rectal thermometer? N Z Med J 1992;105: 309-311.
3. Azzopardi D, Edwards AD: Hypothermia, Semin Fetal Neonatal Med 2007;12:303-310.

29. METABOLIC SCREENING TESTS

- Metabolic disorders are individually rare, but when considered together as a disease entity is relatively frequent, occurring in 1 in 1000 to 1 in 3000 infants. Some disorders can have devastating and irreversible outcomes if not diagnosed early and treated promptly.
- Newborn screening is more than a lab test. It is a coordinated and comprehensive system consisting of education, screening, follow-up, diagnosis, treatment, management and program evaluation.
- Newborn screening is a vital step in identifying infants with inborn metabolic disorders, hemoglobinopathies, infectious processes, and congenital endocrinopathies; the goal is early recognition and treatment. Inborn errors of metabolism often mirror other more common conditions and, as such, may be a diagnostic afterthought.
- Screening test results are insufficient information upon which to base diagnoses or long-term treatment.
- Milder disorder may be missed by newborn screening programs.

The common conditions screened for are:

1. Congenital hypothyroidism (CH).
2. Cystic fibrosis (CF).
3. Congenital adrenal hyperplasia (CAH).
4. Galactosaemia.
5. Phenylketonuria.
6. Fatty acid oxidation disorders including medium chain acyl CoA dehydrogenase deficiency (MCAD).
7. Some organic acidopathies (e.g. methymalonic acidaemia).
8. Some amino acidopathies (e.g. maple syrup urine disease, homocystinuria, and some urea cycle disorders).

Timing of Test

1. It is advisable that tests be taken within 72 hours of birth regardless of feeding regime and health status.
2. If a blood transfusion or antibiotic therapy is essential, obtain an initial screening sample prior to beginning therapy.
3. Samples should be taken as soon as possible after this time as some of the conditions—if untreated—can kill babies in the neonatal period.
4. Sensitivity of screening for some disorders is reduced if screening is delayed.
5. Repeat screening is recommended by the American Academy of Pediatrics for infants screened prior to 24 hours of life.
6. If an infant is transfused prior to collecting the newborn screen, repeat screening for hemoglobinopathies will need to be done 4 months after the last transfusion.

Obtaining Blood Sample

- Obtain *informed consent* from parent(s)/caregiver.
- Do not touch the specimen collection paper (circles).
- Check expiry date.
- Fill out all requested information on test card.
- Capillary blood is preferred over venous blood for convenience.
- No anticoagulant must be added as it interferes with laboratory analysis.
- The blood should completely saturate the filter paper and be applied to 1 side only.
- Filter-paper spots should not be handled, placed on wet surfaces, or contaminated by coffee, milk, or other substances.
- Warm the foot, if necessary.
- Sterilise the puncture site using a medi-swab.
- Wait for the area to dry.
- Make puncture with lancet with tip shorter than 2.0 mm. Wipe off first small drop.
- Gently apply collection paper to a large drop of blood. Allow blood to soak through completely.
- If blood does not fill the circle another drop may be applied immediately. Collect from one side of the paper only and check the circle is completely filled from both sides.
- Repeat step 8 to fill other 3 circles.
- Allow to dry.

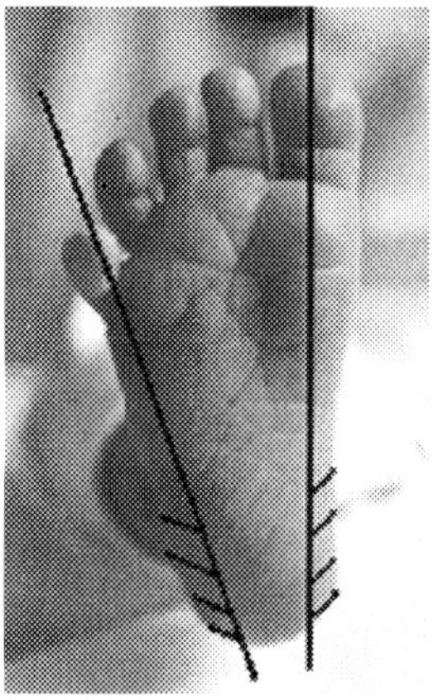

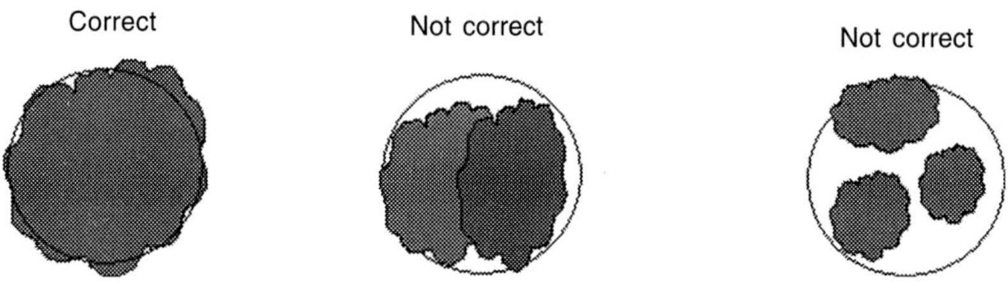

Filter paper collection

SOAK BLOOD FROM THE OTHER SIDE

Hospital name and ward				
USE BLOCK LETTERS OR HOSPITAL ID LABEL UR/Comments				
Doctor's name and initials				
Infant's full name				Twin 1 2
Date of birth	/ /	time		24:00 hr
Date of sample	/ /	time		24:00 hr
Gestation:	weeks	Current weight:		g
Breast Feed ☐	Formula type ☐	TPN ☐	Male ☐	Female ☐
Relevant Family History				
Collector's name				

Sample newborn screening card

Unsatisfactory Specimens

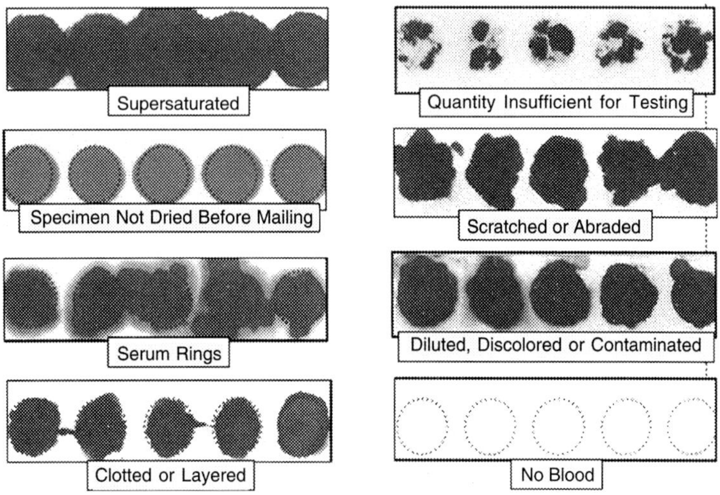

Tandem Mass Spectroscopy

- A tandem mass spectrometer is referred to as MS/MS because it is composed of 2 mass analyzers separated by a collision chamber.
- Over 20 different disorders can be identified from a single blood spot and can be reliably analyzed in about 2 minutes.
- It requires a few droplets of blood on filter paper. This technique can identify and quantify most amino acids and generate an acylcarnitine profile to screen for disorders of fatty acid oxidation and organic acidemias.
- Infants in the NICU may be at particularly high risk for false-positive results, which may be caused by prematurity, medium chain triglyceride (MCT) oil supplementation, carnitine supplementation, and hyperalimentation. To take advantage of the speed of this technology, specimens must get to the laboratory in a timely manner, ideally within 24 hours of collection.
- The MS/MS technology is quicker and has better sensitivity to detect inborn errors of metabolism than earlier techniques. It has improved both the sensitivity and specificity of detecting disorders.

Lab Tests for Inborn Error of Metabolism

Screening tests for inborn error of metabolism

Level I	*Level II*	*Level III*
B glucose	Arterial blood gas	Urine organic acids
S electrolytes	S ammonia	Plasma amino acids
B urea	S lactate	S carnitine

Contd.

Contd.

Urine analysis – non glucose / ketones	Urine metabolic screen	Blood or tissue DNA mutation analysis
CBC	S uric acid	Tissue biopsy for histology and biochemical analysis

REFERENCE

1. Essentials of Neonatal Screening: Pediatrics 2006;118;934-963.

30. NASOPHARYNGEAL AIRWAY (NPA)

The most effective way to relieve upper airway obstruction is by using a nasopharyngeal airway (NPA). Nasopharyngeal airways are inserted through one nostril to create an air passage between the nose and the nasopharynx.

Indication

1. Hypoplastic mandible.
2. Pierre-Robin sequence.

Contraindication

- Severe head or facial injuries.
- Evidence of basal skull fracture.

Procedure

- Use a nostril that is unobstructed.
- The length of the nasal airway can be estimated as the distance from the nares to the meatus of the ears.
- Lubricate the NPA with water-soluble lubricant prior to insertion.
- Insert through the nose and advance at an angle perpendicular to the face.
- If the airway meets an obstruction in one nostril, withdraw it and try to pass it up the other nostril.
- Once the airway has been passed a lateral neck x-ray must be performed as soon as possible.
- **If the airway becomes blocked or it falls out it must be immediately replaced.**
- Completely prepared spare airway of the correct size along with spare tapes must be kept at the bedside. An NPA, which is 0.5 mm smaller in diameter, must also be available.
- Oxygen, suction and resuscitation equipment must be kept by the bedside.

Care of the NPA

- Clean the nostrils regularly.
- Observe pressure areas for redness or breakdown.

- Use cushioned hypoallergenic adhesive dressing, to protect any potential pressure points especially around the cheeks. Cut this dressing into a small 'donut' shape to fit under the NPA where it meets the nostril.

Monitor

- Oxygen saturation.
- Respiratory rate.
- Heart rate.
- Vomiting, retching and coughing.

REFERENCE

1. International Liaison Committee on Resuscitation, The International Liaison Committee on Resuscitation (ILCOR) consensus on science with treatment recommendations for pediatric and neonatal patients: Pediatric basic and advanced life support, Pediatrics 2006;117:e955-977.

31. NEEDLE ASPIRATION FOR PNEUMOTHORAX

Drainage of a pneumothorax is often a matter of urgency especially when the air collection is under pressure.

Clinical signs include:

- Unequal or decreased air entry.
- Displaced apex beat.
- Transillumination. This sign is unreliable in:
  - Infants with increased thickness of the chest wall e.g. term infants and oedema.
  - Infants with pulmonary interstitial emphysema (who may show a 'false positive' result).

Equipment

- 21-gauge butterfly needle.
- 3 way stopcock.
- 10 ml syringe.
- 70% isopropyl alcohol swab.
- 1 pair sterile gloves.

Procedure

- Infant supine, prepare area with alcohol wipe.
- Insert needle into the pleural space (directly over the top of the rib in the 2nd or 3rd intercostal space in the mid-clavicular line) until air is aspirated into the syringe, and then expel air through the 3-way stopcock.
- Apply firm pressure following withdrawal of needle.

Ongoing Care

Following needle aspiration, insertion of an intercostal catheter is required for ongoing management.

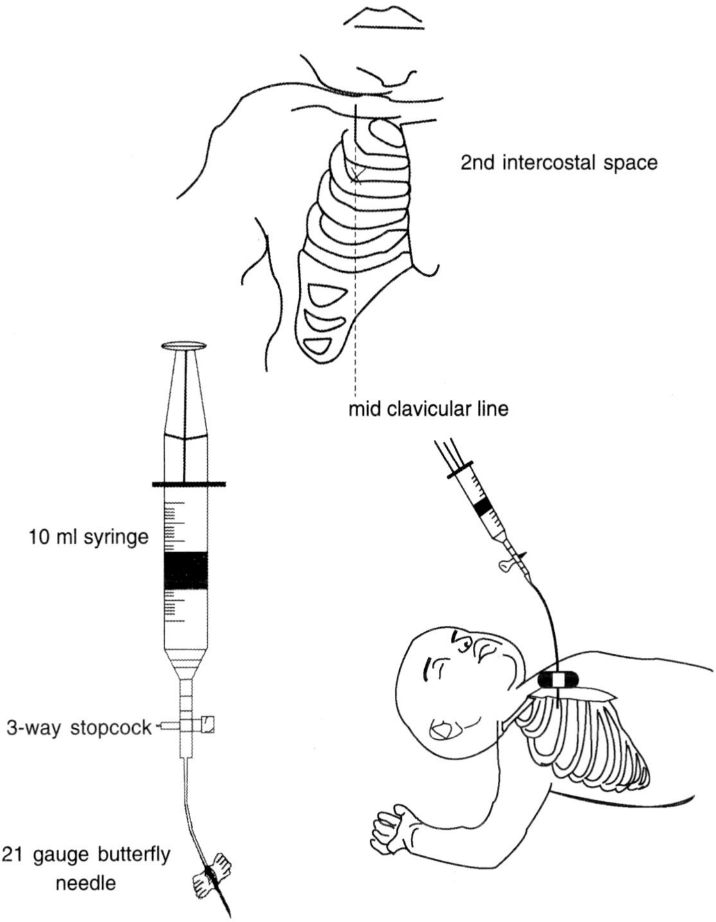

REFERENCE

1. Kirby C, Trotter C: Pneumothorax in the neonate: Assessment and diagnosis, Neonatal Netw 2005; 24:49-55.

32. NITROGEN WASHOUT TEST

Indication

To resolve a pneumothorax in term infants with radiological evidence of a non-tension pneumothorax.

Contraindication

Preterm and infants who are at risk for developing retinopathy of prematurity.

Procedure

- 100% oxygen is delivered to the infant to facilitate an increase in the oxygen level within the extrapleural space. As oxygen is absorbed more readily than nitrogen into surrounding tissues, the pneumothorax resolves more quickly.
- Regardless of the infant's oxygen saturation readings, the infant must continue to receive 100% oxygen for the required time.
- The outflow of gas from the headbox may need to be minimised to achieve an oxygen concentration of 100%.
- Confirm resolution of pneumothorax by X-ray.
- Watch for tension pneumothorax.

Ongoing Care

- Monitor respiratory rate, effort and distress.
- Oxygen saturation.
- Cry, colour and activity.
- Air entry.

Complication

Air leak syndrome.

REFERENCE

1. Carey B: Neonatal air leaks: Pneumothorax, pneumomediastinum, pulmonary interstitial emphysema, pneumopericardium, Neonatal Netw 1999;18:81-84.

33. OXYGEN THERAPY

Oxygen is a drug. As much as it can be life saving, it can be a very dangerous medicine with potentially significant side effects if not used properly. Avoiding hypoxia is important, but prolonged hyperoxia can be equally detrimental as it can lead to oxidative stress and injury. Care should be taken to include oxygen saturation (SpO_2) targets in daily practice to avoid fluctuating episodes or prolonged episodes of hypoxia/hyperoxia in infants receiving supplemental oxygen.

Supplies

- Hood / Nasal prongs / Nasal catheter / Nasopharyngeal catheter.
- Humidification device.
- Tubings.

- O_2 supply.
- Flow meter.
- Oxygen monitor.
- Pulse oximeter.

Indications for Oxygen Therapy

1. *Unintubated Infant Receiving Blow by Supplemental Oxygen*
   - Blow by 100% oxygen via tubing from the manual resuscitator attached to the flow meter set at 5 liters/minute.
   - Initially position tubing 4-6 inches from mouth and nares. If no improvement in saturation has occurred within 30 seconds move the tubing closer to the infant's mouth and nares.
2. *Unintubated Infant Receiving Positive Pressure Ventilation (PPV) via Manual Resuscitator*
   - Begin PPV with initial positive pressure breathes in room air (Keep oxygen flow meter off).
   - If no improvement in saturation has occurred within 30 seconds, adjust the oxygen flow meter to 5 liters.
3. *Nasal Cannula*
   - Begin resuscitator positive pressure breaths with using current oxygen concentration (flow set at 5 liters).
   - If no improvement in saturation has occurred within 30 seconds, gradually adjust FiO_2.
4. *Head Box Delivery*
   - Blended humidified oxygen flow meter adjusted to maintain infant within target range.
   - Adjust FiO_2 to maintain saturations in the target range.
5. *Intubated/NCPAP/NIPPV Infants Requiring PPV*
   - Manual resuscitator set at 5 liters oxygen via ventilator adjusted to maintain infant within target range.
   - Adjust FiO_2 via ventilator to avoid hyperoxia (>94 % saturation) and hypoxia (saturations between 80-84% for greater than thirty seconds or saturations <80% for any length of time).

Special Consideration

Use in delivery room / Emergency care

(Receiving blow by supplemental oxygen / positive pressure ventilation / nasal cannula)

"A nurse may administer blow by oxygen or bag and mask ventilation with oxygen when an emergency occurs, without a written order."

- During the first few minutes of life, saturations of 70 to 80% may be acceptable, as long as the heart rate is increasing, the baby is ventilating, and the SpO_2 is increasing.
- If the SpO_2 at 5 minutes of age remains less than 85% and is not increasing: Gradually increase the oxygen concentration being delivered from the blender.
- If the SpO_2 is greater than 94%: Gradually decrease the oxygen concentration to maintain an SpO_2 between 85 to 94%.

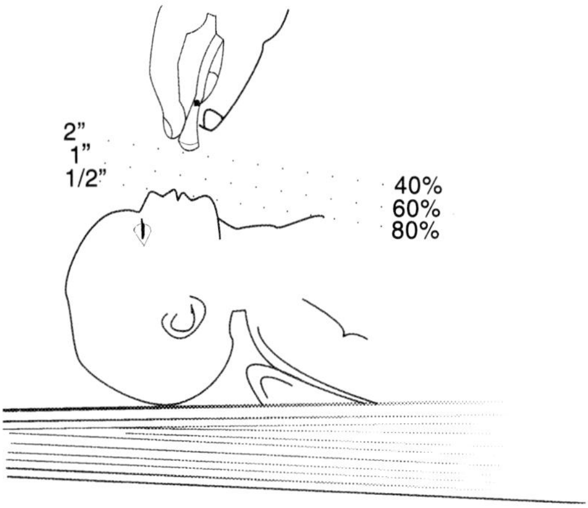

Monitoring of Supplemental Oxygen–Using Pulse Oximeter

1. All infants admitted to NICU should be monitored continuously with a cardiorespiratory monitor with SpO_2 capability.

Setting Alarms

1. Heart rate and respiratory rate alarms should be individualized based on gestational age and clinical condition.
2. Alarm settings should not change because the monitor alarms frequently.
3. Saturation alarms and orders for target ranges for infants receiving supplemental oxygen will be as follows unless specified:

	High	*Low*	*Desat*
Acceptable SpO_2 Target Range	93	85	80
Alarm Limits	94	84	80

4. Verify the High, Low and Desat alarms.
   - Saturations between 80-84% for short periods of time (< 30 seconds) with a stable heart rate and respiratory pattern may be well tolerated.

Appendix A

- A saturation < 80% or > 94% is considered clinically significant and requires assessment and immediate intervention.

Placing Pulse Ox Probes

1. Proper sequencing of probe placement is a must to minimize artifact. Attach the oximeter probe to the patient prior to attaching it to the cable. Once secured, attach the probe to the cable. Press the Power/Standby button on the pulse oximeter.
2. Suspected shunt pathology
   - Infants ≥ 35 weeks requiring supplemental oxygen with saturation consistently < 85%, consider placing a second pulse oximeter on the right hand.
   - Initial pulse oximeter probe will be placed on the infant's lower extremity. Post-ductal saturation tells you the "worst the infant can be".
   - The difference between the pre/post (pre > post) will identify if the infant is shunting right to left at the ductal level.
   - Infants at risk for maintaining ductal shunting should maintain pre/post ductal saturation monitoring until normal postnatal shunting is established.

TROUBLE SHOOTING FOR PULSE OXIMETER ALARMS

a. Saturation Alarms Below Target Range

- Respond to the baby first rather than the monitor.
- Check for heart rate and respiratory effort.
- If heart rate and respiratory efforts are good, consider motion artifacts.
- Saturations between 80-84% for short periods of time (< 30 seconds) with a stable heart rate and respiratory pattern may be well tolerated.
- Multiple episodes of intermittent saturations between 80-84% for short periods of time (<30 seconds) that increase the total % of time the infant is below target range require evaluation and possible intervention.
- Saturations < 80% (Desaturation Alarm) are considered clinically significant and require assessment, with immediate intervention.
- Intervene if saturations < 80% or between 80-84% for > 30 seconds.

In Non-Intubated Patient

- Use tactile stimulation first (if apneic). Do not spend time in stimulation in an apneic baby.
- Initiate bag-mask ventilation at the current FiO_2.
- If no response after 30 sec, increase FiO_2 to avoid hyperoxia (SpO_2 > 94%) and hypoxia (SpO_2 < 84%).
- If no response or FiO_2 must be significantly increased to maintain infant within target range, consider assisted ventilation.

In Intubated Patient

- Assess ventilation by chest expansion and air entry. Check for the ETT marking at the lip. Consider need for suctioning.
- If ventilation adequate and no need for suctioning and there is no response, provide 10-15 manual ventilator breaths at current FiO_2 for 30 seconds.
- If still no response, increase FiO_2 in increments of 5-10% and decrements of 2-5% are acceptable to avoid hyperoxia (SpO_2 > 94%) and hypoxia (SpO_2 < 84%).
- If still no response use manual resuscitator breathes with adjusted FiO_2.

b. Saturation Alarms Above Target Range

- FiO_2 should be weaned by decrements of 2% to 5% at a time to avoid periods of hyperoxia.
- Weaning may be done steadily until the infant comes within his target range as long as the SpO_2 is stable.
- When the infant and the oxygen saturation have remained stable (within target range) at a certain FiO_2 for at least an hour, that will be the FiO_2 charted on the infant's flowsheet, as the last stable FiO_2.
- Exercise caution to avoid an exaggerated decrease in FiO_2 that can produce hypoxia (and then a subsequent abrupt increase in FiO_2 with a risk for hyperoxia).

Special Circumstances—Increasing FiO_2

1. ETT Suctioning

- Suctioning should preferably be performed using an in-line suction port. In-line suctioning devices help to maintain functional residual capacity (FRC) and oxygen delivery during suctioning and minimizes the need for ventilator/FiO_2 adjustments.
- If in line suction is not available, increase FiO_2 by 10% prior to suctioning.
- After suctioning, observe the infant for at least 10 minutes, because adjustments of respiratory settings may be needed.
- Revert to preset FiO_2

2. Surfactant Administration

- Surfactant is administered through the in-line suction port.
- See *surfactant administration* section (# 37).

Documentation

1. During initial stabilization record saturation in SpO_2 Pre/Post column on flowsheet until saturation range and trending have been established.
2. When dual SpO_2 monitoring is required, record Pre/Post saturations along with % in ranges.

3. When the infant and the oxygen saturation have remained stable (within target range) at a certain FiO_2 for at least an hour, that will be the FiO_2 charted on the infant's flowsheet, as the last stable FiO_2.
4. *Notify if:*
   a. It is necessary to keep the FiO_2 >5% above the previous "stable" FiO_2 to maintain the infant's saturation within the pre-established saturation range.
   b. Saturations below the pre-established saturation range unresponsive to changes in FiO_2 or ventilator adjustments.

OXYGEN TOXICITY

The risk of oxygen damage is determined by the PaO_2 or SaO_2 and not by the FiO_2. A high FiO_2 is not dangerous if the PaO_2 or SaO_2 are normal (e.g. with severe respiratory distress). A high FiO_2 is most dangerous if there are no lung or heart problems, e.g., oxygen given to healthy preterm infants during transport. No FiO_2 above 0.21 can be regarded as safe unless the PaO_2 or SaO_2 are measured and found to be in the normal range. An increased FiO_2 is most dangerous in a preterm infant with recurrent apnea but no respiratory distress, as the PaO_2 can become very high.

Following are complications due to oxygen toxicity:

1. *Retinopathy of prematurity:* Immaturity is the most important risk factor but oxygen also plays a role. Other factors attributed are vitamin E deficiency; ambient light; clinical conditions including acidosis, shock, sepsis, apnea, anemia, and patent ductus arteriosus; and prolonged ventilatory support (especially when accompanied by episodes of hypoxia and hyperoxia) have been associated with ROP. ROP has occurred in premature infants who have never received supplemental oxygen and in infants with cyanotic congenital heart disease. Current evidence suggests that ROP is linked to the duration of oxygen rather than the concentration.
2. *Chronic lung disease:* With $FiO_2 \geq 0.5$, absorption atelectasis, oxygen toxicity, and or depression of ciliary and/or leukocytic function may occur.
3. With $PaO_2 \geq 60$ mmHg, ventilatory depression may occur in spontaneously breathing patients with elevated $PaCO_2$.
4. Increased PaO_2 can contribute to closure or constriction of the ductus arteriosus—a possible concern in infants with ductus-dependent heart lesions.
5. Fire hazard is increased in the presence of increased oxygen concentrations.
6. Bacterial contamination associated with certain nebulization and humidification systems is a possible hazard.

Ongoing Care

1. Analyze FiO_2 at hourly intervals to ensure that desired FiO_2 is maintained.
2. Report saturations that are consistently greater or lesser than ordered parameters.

3. Use adequate flow in system (at least 2L/minute) to prevent excessive CO_2 build-up (Exception: Nasal cannula).
4. Maintain neutral thermal environment with incubator temperature and by administering warm inspired gases.
5. Avoid stressful and unnecessary procedures, if possible, which may increase oxygen consumption. Use supportive measures to minimize discomfort and distress during procedures.
6. Humidify all oxygen that is administered.
7. Provide oral care at least every 8 hours.
8. Suction nose and mouth prn. A few drops of normal saline may be placed in the nares when infants are on nasal cannula to help maintain moistness and patency.
9. Maintain airway patency by positioning with head in extension.

Weaning Oxygen

Supplemental oxygen should be stopped when arterial oxygenation is adequate with the patient breathing room air. In patients without arterial hypoxaemia but at risk of tissue hypoxia, oxygen should be stopped when the acid-base state and clinical assessment of vital organ function are consistent with resolution of tissue hypoxia. Oxygen should be reduced in small steps of 0.10 (10%) at a time. A sudden, large drop in FiO_2 may cause severe hypoxia and collapse.

Oxygen Therapy in Low Resource Settings

Source of Oxygen

Oxygen supplies need to be available at all times. Oxygen source can be a cylinder, concentrator or central gas line depending upon resources. For reliable and uninterrupted oxygen delivery for a small nursery it is desirable to have central piped oxygen line.

Comparison of Oxygen Cylinders and Oxygen Concentrators

	Cylinders	*Concentrators*
Capital cost	Low	High
Running cost	High	Low
Reliability	Excellent	Good on selected models
Regular maintenance	Simple care only	Needed
Electricity	Not needed	Needed
Continuity of oxygen delivery	Liable to run out	Good, unless they break down or power fails
Supply system	Transport needed	Transport not needed

Selection of an Oxygen Delivery Device

A wide variety of oxygen delivery systems are available. The concentration of oxygen that patients inspire depends on the ventilatory minute volume (MV) and the flow rate of oxygen. The greater the ventilation, the lower the FiO_2 for a given flow rate of supplemental oxygen. The choice of device would depend upon the gestational age, wellness of infant, oxygen requirement and available resources.

Head Box Oxygen

Advantages	*Disadvantages*
Precise FiO_2 delivery.	Limitations on mobility.
No need for humidification.	Difficulty in feeding and suction procedures.
No risk of airway obstruction.	High flow oxygen required.
No gastric dilatation.	CO_2 buildup.

1. Place neonate in hood (use shoulder roll, if necessary).
2. Do not seal space between infant's neck and hood.
3. Initiate oxygen flow of at least 5 liters/min from flow meter.
4. Monitor baby for respiratory rate, distress and colour.
5. Remove hood in case of accidental disruption of O_2 supply.

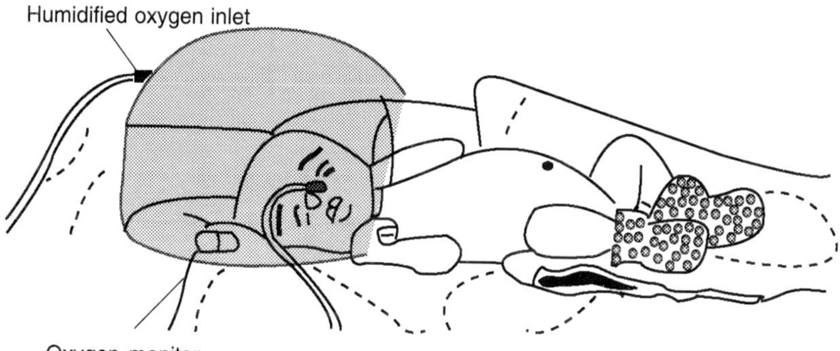

Oxygen therapy with oxygenhood

Facemask Oxygen

Advantages	*Disadvantages*
No risk of airway obstruction.	Variable FiO_2 delivery.
No gastric dilatation.	Difficulty in feeding and suction procedures.
	High flow oxygen required.
	CO_2 buildup

Nasal Cannula

Advantages	*Disadvantages*
Positive distending pressure.	Risk of airway obstruction.
No need for humidification.	Variables affecting are cannula flow rate, ratio of nasal prongs and nasal diameters, minute ventilation, ratio of inspiration to expiration, mouth breathing, use of sedatives.
No gastric dilatation.	

Variability in oxygen delivery is minimal when nasal cannula flow is reduced to the lowest possible flow by using undiluted (100%) oxygen; only then should the cannula oxygen concentration be reduced below 100%.

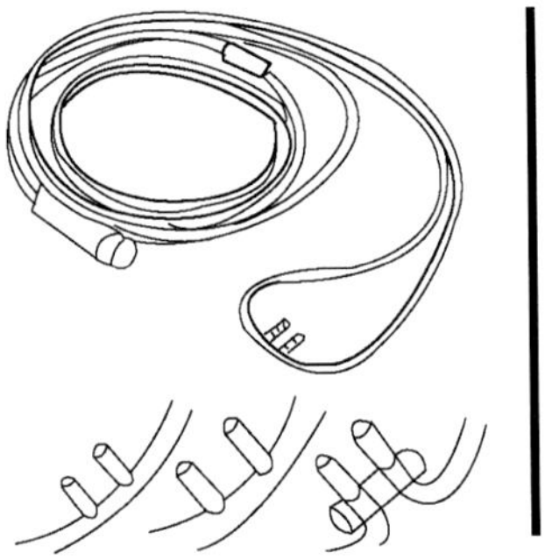

Oxygen Prongs and Tubings

Nasal Catheter

Advantages	*Disadvantages*
No need for humidification.	Require high oxygen flow.
No gastric dilatation.	
Unlikely to be dislodged.	

A catheter passed for a distance that is equal to the distance from the side of the nostril to the inner margin of the eyebrow usually reaches the posterior part of the nasal cavity.

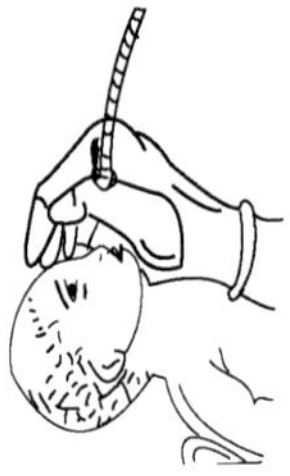

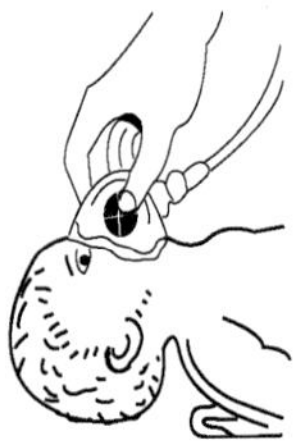

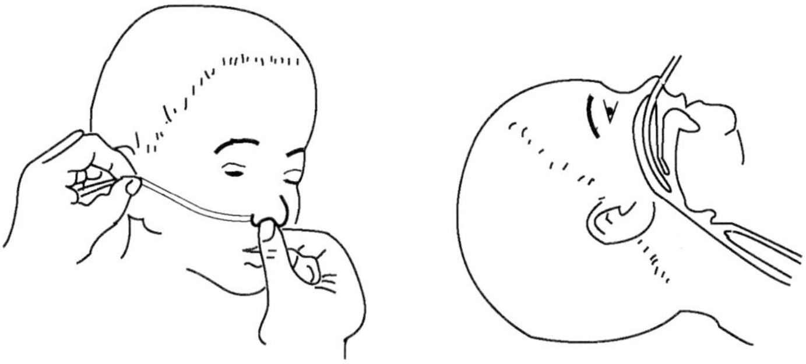

Nasopharyngeal Oxygen Catheter

Nasopharyngeal Catheter

Advantages	*Disadvantages*
No danger of hypercarbia if the oxygen is turned off or the tubing disconnects.	Risk of airway obstruction.
Continuous distending pressure.	Requires humidification.
	Risk of dislodgement into esophagus.
	Gastric dilatation.
	Removing and cleaning the catheter twice a day is required.

Catheters are inserted into the nose to a depth equal to the distance from the side of the nose to the front of the ear. 0.5 litres/min oxygen through an 8 F nasopharyngeal catheter in newborn infants with pneumonia, and 1 litre/min in infants upto 12 months.

Practical Considerations in Oxygen Delivery

All methods of oxygen administration need supervision by trained personnel to detect and manage complications appropriately.

Comparison of Different Modes of Oxygen Delivery

Criterion	*Nasal prongs*	*Nasal catheter*	*Nasopharyngeal catheter*	*Headbox*	*Face-mask*
Oxygen conc. (%)	30-35	35-40	45-60	> 90	> 90
Safety	High	High	Medium	Low	Low
Efficiency	Medium	Medium	High	Low	Low
Simplicity	High	Medium	Medium	Low	Medium
Tolerability	High	Medium	Medium	High	Low
Availability	Medium	High	High	Low	Low

Choosing Appropriate Oxygen Delivery Device

Nasal prong	Low level supplement of oxygen required.
Nasopharyngeal catheter	Feed the infant without interrupting oxygen delivery.
Oxygen masks	Provide supplemental O_2 in the moderate range (0.35-0.50, depending on size and minute ventilation) for short periods of time (e.g., during procedures, for transport, in emergency situations).
Partial rebreathing masks	Conserve the oxygen supply when higher concentrations ($FiO_2 > 0.4, < 0.6$) are warranted (e.g., during transport).
Non-rebreathing masks	Used to deliver concentrations ≥0.60 or specific concentrations (as from a blender).
Oxygen hood	1. Controlled FiO_2 in infant and small children. 2. Controlled FiO_2 and/or increased heated humidity to patients who cannot tolerate other devices. 3. Controlled FiO_2 when the chest, abdomen, and extremities must be accessible to caregivers. 4. The oxygen concentrations necessary for oxygen challenge (hyperoxia) tests in the spontaneously breathing neonate.

Role of Humidification

Because unhumidified gas is very dry and will irritate the linings of the nose, throat and airways it is recommended to humidify oxygen for administration when nasopharynx is bypassed or if the oxygen flow rate is more than 4 l/ m. Simple humidifier filled with sterile water can achieve this or temperature controlled electric humidifiers.

KEY POINTS

1. Oxygen is a *therapy*, i.e., an *intervention.*
2. In many acute situations, oxygen is the first drug to be given and is life saving. It should always be considered along with management of the airway, delivery system, the circulation, constant monitoring and reassessment of the treatment.
3. Maintenance of blood flow to the most hypoxia sensitive organs should be a primary therapeutic goal. Prevention, early identification, and correction of tissue hypoxia are essential skills.
4. Arterial oxygen saturation and PaO_2 remain the principal clinical measures of arterial hypoxaemia, but the values may be normal despite tissue hypoxia in low output cardiac states and anaemia.

5. All methods of oxygen administration need supervision by trained personnel to detect and manage complications appropriately. Oxygen therapy should be targeted to levels appropriate to the condition, gestational age and postnatal age of the infant.

REFERENCES

1. Win Tin: Oxygen Therapy: 50 Years of Uncertainty, Pediatrics, 2002;110:615-616.
2. DF Treacher, RM Leach: ABC of oxygen: Oxygen transport—Basic principles, British Medical Journal 1998;317:1302-1306.
3. Bateman NT and Leach RM: ABC of oxygen: Acute Oxygen Therapy, British Medical Journal 1998;317:798-801.
4. Dobson MB: Oxygen concentrators for the smaller hospital—A review, Tropical Doctor 1992;22:56-58.
5. World Health Organisation: Oxygen therapy for acute respiratory infections in young children in developing countries, Geneva: World Health Organisation 1993:WHO/ARI 93.28.
6. AARC Clinical Practice Guideline: Selection of an Oxygen Delivery Device for Neonatal and Pediatric Patients, Respir Care 1996;41:637-646.
7. B Frey, F Shann: Oxygen administration in infants: Archives of Disease in Childhood Fetal and Neonatal Edition 2003;88:F84.
8. Askie LM, Henderson-Smart DJ: Gradual versus abrupt discontinuation of oxygen in preterm or low birth weight infants, Cochrane Database Syst Rev 2000; (2): CD001075.
9. Askie LM: Early versus late discontinuation of oxygen in preterm or low birth weight infants, Cochrane Database Syst Rev 2000; (2): CD001076.

OXYGEN THERAPY ADJUVANTS

1. Using a Flow Meter with Humidifier

- It is important to measure the flow rate of gas given to an infant with a flow meter. The flow meter is usually plugged into an oxygen/air blender. However, the flow meter can also be plugged directly into an oxygen wall plug.
- The flow of gas is measured in litres per minute and can be adjusted by turning an adjusting wheel. A flow rate of 5 litres per minute is usually used into a head box. A high flow rate wastes gas and cools the infant while a low flow rate may allow carbon dioxide to accumulate in the head box.

2. Using a Humidifier

- Sterile or boiled water (which has been allowed to cool) is added to the humidifier so that the water level reaches the full mark. When the water level approaches the empty mark more water must be added.

- The water must be changed and the humidifier must be cleaned every day or when the humidifier is to be used for another infant. Dangerous bacteria such as *Pseudomonas* can grow well in water and, therefore, the humidifier should only be filled with water when it is being used.
- The humidifier should be cleaned with detergent or soap and water, and be allowed to drip dry. The switch on the humidifier must be kept on "bubbles" and not "jet". The humidifier must be dry during storage.
- Some humidifiers also warm the air. When infants are ventilated via an endotracheal tube (except during resuscitation) warmed, humidified gas should be used.

3. Using an Air-Oxygen Blender

- Except during an emergency resuscitation, 100% oxygen from a cylinder or piped source should not be used as pure oxygen is toxic to many tissues especially the retina of the eye. Therefore, oxygen should always be mixed (blended) with medical air using a blender or a venturi.
- *Gas Pipes:* The pipe for oxygen is usually white while the pipe for medical air is usually black. Each pipe ends in a steel connector that must be plugged into a wall gas fitting or a reduction valve on a cylinder. The shape of the 2 connectors differs to prevent the pipe being connected to the incorrect source. The oxygen connector is 6 sided while the medical air connector has 2 flat sides and 2 curved sides. The wall fitting for oxygen is white and the wall fitting for medical air is grey.
- *The Blender Unit:* This, with the gas pipes, is usually attached to a supporting rail on the wall. The blender also has emergency escape valves, which operate if the gas pressure gets too high. An alarm will sound if one of the pipes is not plugged in properly, or the pressure of oxygen or air is too low. The dial which controls the mixture of oxygen and air can be set at any combination from 21% oxygen (i.e. pure medical air) to 100% oxygen (pure oxygen).

4. Using an Oxygen Monitor

Whenever an infant is given oxygen into a head box, the FiO_2 must be measured with an oxygen monitor as too high or too low a concentration of oxygen may be dangerous for that infant if it results in too much or too little oxygen in the blood. The FiO_2 CANNOT be controlled accurately with a flow meter alone. If an oxygen monitor is not available then a blender or venturi should be used to determine the approximate FiO_2, provided a flow of 5 litres or more is used.

The Components of an Oxygen Monitor

1. *The Monitoring Unit:* This is usually attached to a rail or stands on a shelf. On the front of the unit is an on/off switch, a display of the FiO_2, high and low settings, a calibration knob and an alarm light. Batteries that have to be replaced at intervals power the monitor. Most models have a "low battery" display to warn that the battery is getting flat.

2. *The Oxygen Sensor:* This is attached to the monitoring unit by a thin cable. The sensor is placed in the head box (oxygen hood) next to the infant's head.

Calibrating the Oxygen Monitor

Place the sensor in room air and switch on the monitor. The display should read 21%. If not, adjust the calibration knob until the display reads 21%. The monitor should always be calibrated before it is used. It should also be calibrated at least daily while in use.

Using the Oxygen Monitor

Calibrate the monitor with room air as described above. Then place the sensor into the head box. The display should now give the FiO_2. Set the high and the low alarm limits to 5% above and 5% below the required FiO_2. If the display falls outside these limits, the red alarm light will come on and the alarm buzzer will sound. Silence the alarm by correcting the air/oxygen mixture. The display should be read and recorded on the observation chart at regular intervals while the infant is receiving extra oxygen. Remember that the monitor measures the FiO_2 but does not control the FiO_2. The FiO_2 cannot be changed by simply adjusting the oxygen monitor.

34. PERIPHERAL VASCULAR CATHETERS

Indication

- Administration of IV fluids.
- Deliver medications.
- Provide parenteral nutrition.

Supplies

- Gloves.
- Tourniquet or rubber band.
- 24 gauge IV catheter.
- Isopropyl alcohol swabs.
- Transparent dressing.
- 7 inch microbore extension tubing with needleless access cap.
- Neonatal limb board with slings.
- Cotton ball.
- Scissors.
- 1 ml syringes filled with normal saline.
- IV solution and administration set.
- Sterile gauze pieces.

Site of IV Insertion

- Peripheral veins on the back of the hand or top of the foot (the most common and preferred sites).

- Veins on the forearm, the front of the elbow, or around the ankle or knee (minimize use of the veins around the knee because there is a greater risk of the needle coming in contact with the bone).
- Scalp veins.

Procedure

- Prepare sucrose pacifier for elective IV insertions.
- Prepare IV solutions and place end of tubing within easy reach. Flush tubing and catheter with IV fluids. Air embolism can occur easily in babies. It is essential to ensure that all components of the IV infusion set are filled with fluid and that there are no air bubbles in the set before beginning the infusion.
- Cut transparent tape into appropriate lengths for securing IV catheter.
- Select vein. It is useful to select the "Y" region of the vein, where two veins join together. The IV device can be inserted in the crotch of the veins.
- Immobilize the extremity or have an assistant hold the extremity to reduce movement.
- Wash hands and put on gloves.
- Apply a tourniquet proximal to the puncture site.
- Clean the puncture site with povidone iodine followed by alcohol. Always prep in a circular pattern from center progressing outward, covering a 1-2 inch diameter. Allow the povidone iodine to dry before applying alcohol. Povidone iodine needs to be on the skin for at least 30 seconds as a skin disinfectant and then allowed to dry. Use of alcohol improves visualization of the IV site and reduces the possible adverse effects of povidone iodine.
- Use a "no touch" technique following the cleansing of skin.
- Pull skin taut to stabilize the vein.
- Place catheter between thumb and index finger so that the bevel of the needle is in an upward position. Puncture skin at a 15-45 degree angle just distal to planned site of vein puncture. Advance needle and catheter assembly slowly to puncture vein until blood enters the hub or "pop" is felt when entering the vein. Blood return will not always occur. By inserting the stylet back into the catheter and attempting to reposition the catheter, you run the risk of shearing the catheter. This may damage the catheter or create an embolus. A damaged catheter increases the irritation to the vein and the likelihood of phlebitis or infiltration.
- If resistance is met or the vein is not punctured, withdraw needle and catheter assembly slowly to just below the level of the skin, locate vein, and advance the needle again.
- Push the catheter off the needle into the vein until the hub of the catheter meets the skin. Attach the T-Connector and flush the IV. Sterile water or normal saline solution is used to flush the line.
- Secure catheter (without covering insertion site) to skin with strip or transparent dressing and flush with normal saline to confirm patency. Stabilize extremity on arm board as needed to prevent dislodgement of IV catheter.
- Attach tubing of in-line closed IV medication system to the distal end of the

T-Connector. Manually infuse the saline slowly while observing the IV site. At the end of the flush infusion, clamp the T-Connector while exerting positive pressure on the syringe. The positive pressure will help to keep the vein patent.

- Peripheral IVs not being used for continuous fluid administration should be flushed with normal saline solution every 8 hours.
- One individual should make no more than 2 attempts at cannulation. After 2 unsuccessful attempts, someone with more experience should make additional attempts.
- An IV site should be changed preferably after 3 or 4 days of use.
- Antibacterial ointments should not be used on IV dressings. They may increase the potential for fungal overgrowth.

Monitoring

Site check for infiltration, phlebitis, and signs of infection and equipment integrity should include:

- Skin temperature.
- General condition or appearance of site.
- Swelling or inflammation around device/site.
- Pain or tenderness around device/site.
- Unexplained fever.
- Presence and integrity of tape and transparent dressing.
- Presence and security of extension tubing.

Documentation

- *Document IV placement:* Date, time, location of insertion and gauge of catheter.
- *General condition of patient:* How insertion was tolerated, any manifestations of adverse reaction.
- Observation of patient and IV site hourly throughout infusion.

Securing and Fixation of IV Device

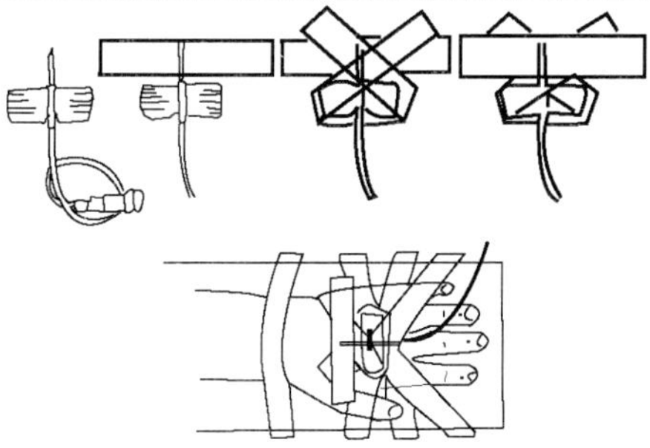

Securing at insertion site

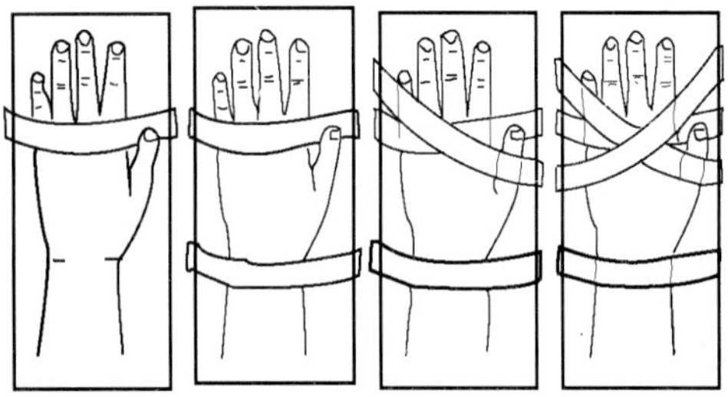

Immobilising hand

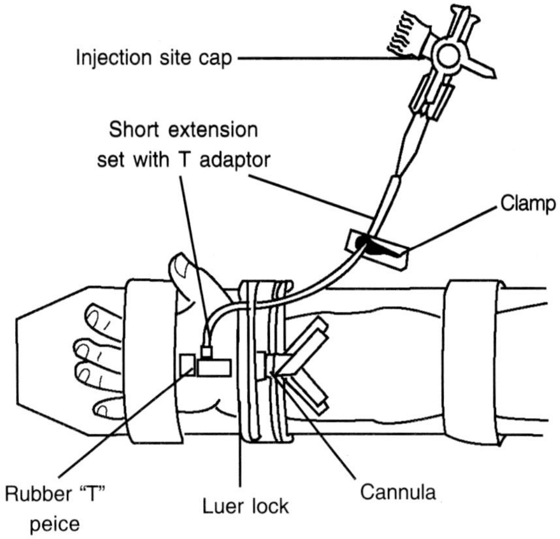

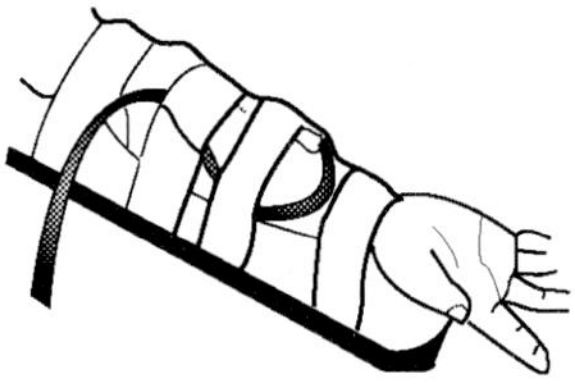

Spinting the extremity

Site Care and Dressing Change

Complete site care will be performed when an IV device dressing is not dry, clean or securely intact.

Supplies

- Cleansing agent (alcohol, or povidone iodine).

- Transparent dressing.
- Tape.
- Gloves.

Procedure

- Remove the old dressing carefully.
- Clean the insertion site and surrounding area with cleansing agent and allow to dry. Careful handling and securing of the catheter and extension set may be necessary in order to prevent catheter dislodgement.
- Secure catheter hub and extension tubing with tape.
- Cover site with a transparent dressing. Insertion site must be visible at all times. Do not cover the insertion site with gauze or other dressings.
- Label the dressing with date of dressing change, gauge of catheter and your initials.

REMOVAL OF IV DEVICE

Supplies

- Gloves.
- Gauze.
- Tape.
- Povidone-iodine or polysporin ointment.
- Transparent dressing.

Procedure

- Wash hands and put on gloves.
- Remove dressing from insertion site.
- Observe site condition. Note any signs/symptoms of complications.
- Pull catheter device straight out slowly. Observe catheter and catheter tip for integrity.
- Apply pressure to site with sterile gauze until bleeding has stopped.

DOCUMENTATION

Document on the Patient Care Record or unit specific flow sheet:

- Integrity of catheter.
- Insertion site condition.
- Date and time of removal.

PERIPHERAL IV INFILTRATE TREATMENT

Hyaluronidase is the primary treatment choice for IV infiltrates. Hyaluronidase is not indicated for blood infiltrates; blood is a natural substance that will be broken down and absorbed by the body. Phentolamine is the drug of choice when the infiltrate has been caused by a vasoconstrictive pressor.

Treatment should be done within the first few minutes to one hour after infiltration was noted for best results.

Supplies

- 26 gauge needle(s) and TB syringe(s).
- Medication (Hyaluroidase or Phentolamine).
- Normal saline (for dilution).
- Povidone-iodine swab.
- Rolls to elevate extremity.

Procedure

- Elevate the extremity whether treatment is required or not. Do not apply heat or compression to site.
- Reconstitute phentolamine with 1ml normal saline (5 mg/1cc). Phentolamine will need to be further diluted with 0.9% normal saline to 1mg/1cc (add 0.2 cc phentolamine to 0.8 cc normal saline) for injection.
- Hyaluronidase will need to be reconstituted and then diluted with 0.9% normal saline to 15 units/cc (add 0.1 cc Hyaluronidase to 0.9 cc normal saline) for injection.
- Standard dose: 0.5 cc = babies < 1500 grams 1.0 cc = babies > 1500 grams.
- Prepare infiltrate site with Betadine gently. Allow Betadine to dry on skin prior to injection.
- Subcutaneously inject the infiltrate with the medication using a new 26 gauge TB needle. Administer in four aliquots as ordered. Medication is NOT to be administered through infiltrated peripheral IV. Remove IV catheter prior to subcutaneous administration.

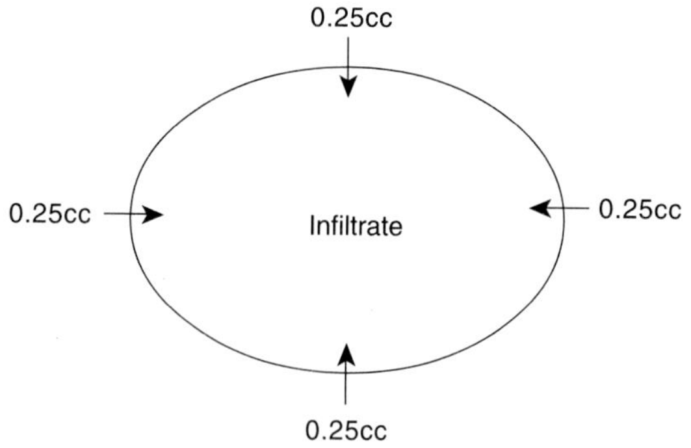

- Elevate the extremity for 2 hours to facilitate venous return and minimize dependent edema.

RADIAL ARTERY CANNULATION

Indications

- Peripheral exchange transfusion.
- ABG sampling.
- Continuous blood pressure monitoring.

Supplies

- Gloves.
- 24 gauge IV catheter.
- Isopropyl alcohol swabs.
- Transparent dressing.
- Three-way stopcock.
- Neonatal limb board with slings.
- Cotton ball.
- 1 ml syringes filled with normal saline.
- Sterile gauze pieces.

Procedure

- Perform Allen's test. If collateral circulation is not adequate, *DO NOT PERFORM* arterial puncture.
- Keep the extremity firm and fixed.
- Palpate artery with index and middle finger of the non-dominant hand.
- Cleanse area with antiseptic solution going in a circular motion moving from inward to outward. Allow to dry for at least 30 sec. prior to puncture.
- *Do not touch* prepped insertion site with fingers.
- Infiltrate the skin if local anesthetic is to be used or apply EMLA cream (1 hour prior). Insert 24 G intracath at a 5-15 degree angle with the bevel directed upward such that it only extends into the epidermis. The entire bevel should be covered and lay just under the skin.
- Gently and slowly insert intracath into artery using a 30°-45° angle. A pulsatile backflow of blood into the tubing of the butterfly or the hub of the syringe indicates the artery has been punctured. Withdraw the stylet.
- Attach the intracath to a 3-way valve and secure it with adhesive. Start heparin infusion using a syringe infusion pump 1U/ ml at 1 ml / hour.
- Label the line as "Arterial line – Do not inject".

Complications

- Hematoma.
- Occlusion of artery.
- Infection.

- Local necrosis.
- Embolisation.

Monitoring and Care

- Inspect site 6 hourly for signs of inflammation.
- Always flush the catheter with heparinised saline after withdrawal of blood samples.
- If catheter is suspected to be blocked, do not try forced flushing. Remove it.
- Check all tube connections and secure them tightly.

REFERENCES

1. Manual of neonatal nursing, Ed, Lalitha Krishnan, Published by National Neonatology Forum, 1993.
2. Stovroff M, Teague WG: Intravenous access in infants and children, Pediatr Clin North Am 1998;45:1373-1393.
3. Pettit J: Assessment of the infant with a peripheral intravenous device, Adv Neonatal Care 2003;3:230-240.
4. Gauderer MW: Vascular access techniques and devices in the pediatric patient, Surg Clin North Am 1992;72:1267-1284.
5. Möller JC, Reiss I, Schaible T: Vascular access in neonates and infants—Indications, routes, techniques and devices, complications, Intensive Care World 1995;12:48-53.
6. Thigpen JL: Peripheral intravenous extravasation: Nursing procedure for initial treatment, Neonatal Netw 2007;26:379-384.
7. Salzman MB, Rubin LG: Intravenous catheter-related infections, Adv Pediatr Infect Dis 1995;10:337-368.

35. PERICARDIAL TAP

Indications

1. Cardiac tamponade due to pericardial effusion.
2. Pneumopericardium.

Supplies

- Sterile gloves, towel.
- 10 cc syringe, 3-way stopcock, 22 G needle.
- Spirit and betadine cotton balls.

Procedure

- Place a cardioscope monitor on the infant.
- Clean the xiphoid area.
- Insert a 22 G needle attached to a 10 ml syringe via a 3-way tap at an angle of 30 degrees directed towards left shoulder upto a depth of 1 cm.

- Elevation of ST segment or appearance of ectopic beats indicates that the needle has touched the epicardium. In that case, withdraw the needle slightly.
- Aspirate pus or air.
- Remove the needle and seal with tincture benzoin.

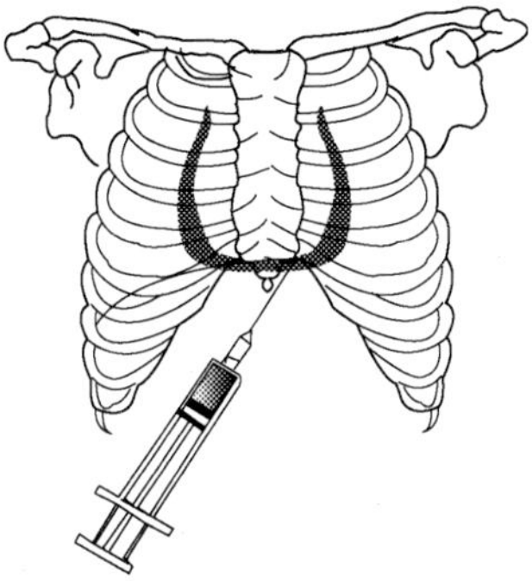

Complications

- Arrhythmia.
- Collapse.
- Infection.
- Injury to the myocardium.

REFERENCE

1. Carey B: Neonatal air leaks: Pneumothorax, pneumomediastinum, pulmonary interstitial emphysema, pneumopericardium, Neonatal Netw 1999;18:81-84.

36. STOOL HEME OCCULT TEST

Guaiac-based slide tests (e.g., Hemoccult) are used most commonly to screen for occult blood in stool. In full-term neonates, the initial meconium is devoid of occult blood.

The site of bleeding in gastrointestinal tract varies from proximal to distal gastrointestinal tract (GIT) which, in turn, results in different blood derived compounds being found in the stool. However, there are multiple extraintestinal sources of blood in stool, including swallowed maternal blood (ingested during delivery or from cracked nipples) and neonatal blood from catheter-induced trauma to the upper airway or gastric mucosa.

Blood Products in the Stools

Haemoglobin undergoes degradation in the gut (and stool) proportional to the time it spends in contact with digestive processes and gut microorganisms. Hence distal bleeds and large proximal bleeds result in intact haemoglobin in stool; small proximal bleeds are significantly degraded to heme and ultimately porphyrins.

TESTS

Guaiac Tests

- Detects both haem and intact haemoglobin by their peroxidase activity.
- These tests are thus able to detect proximal and distal GIT bleeds. Blood is present in the sample of stool; the mixing of the solution with blood causes the guaiac to turn visibly blue. The blue color is caused by the interaction (promoted by the oxidizing agent) of the heme portion of the hemoglobin molecule, the oxygen-carrying molecule in red blood cells and the guaiac.
- The test is cheap and easy to perform.

Heme-Porphyrin Test

- Quantifies porphyrins from haemoglobin
- Measures amount of stool blood present.
- Expensive and requires increased lab staff time.
- High false positive rate.

37. SURFACTANT ADMINISTRATION

Surfactant is indicated for prevention and treatment ("rescue") of respiratory distress syndrome (RDS). The incidence of RDS is related more to lung immaturity than to gestational age. Risk for developing RDS increases with decreasing gestational age. Surfactant administration may take place in:

a. Delivery room.

b. NICU.

Definite Indications

1. Newborn infants with clinical signs of RDS.
2. Newborns at high risk of RDS.

Relative Indications

1. Intubated infants with meconium aspiration syndrome requiring more than 50% oxygen.
2. Sick newborn infants with pneumonia and an oxygenation index greater than 15.
3. Intubated newborn infants with pulmonary hemorrhage, which leads to clinical deterioration.

Supplies

- Syringe and 18-gauge needle.

- Surfactant warmed to room temperature (8 cc or 4 cc vial).
- Endotracheal tube (ETT) with side port.
- Extra prepared ETT at bedside.

Prerequisite

- Any infant being given surfactant must be on a cardiorespiratory monitor and pulse oximeter.
- ETT placement will be evaluated by clinical assessment. Chest X-ray is not necessary.
- A trained personnel equipped with airway emergency management should be present at bedside during dosing so that ventilator changes be made in a timely manner. They should be available until the tidal volume stabilizes.
- Warm the surfactant preparation to room temperature by leaving at room temperature for 20 minutes and gently turn the vial upside down to achieve a uniform suspension. Do not shake or agitate. Do not put in incubator or under radiant warmer to warm.
- Calculate the dose based on weight. Any remaining surfactant left in the vial should be returned to the refrigerator, with the date and time of opening written on it. Discard Curosurf 12 hours after opening and discard Survanta 24 hours after opening.
- If vial is warmed to room temperature for less than 24 hours and not used it may be returned to the medication refrigerator and reused.

Procedure

- Double check dose.
- Obtain an assistant to help administer dose. Identify who will give the dose and who will position the infant.
- Prepare sterile field and drop onto the field the sterile syringe, contents of the suture removal set, and the 5 Fr feeding tube. Cut the feeding tube to the desired length – the length of the cut ETT plus 3 cm for the adaptor.
- Measure from the hub of the feeding tube, taking care not to contaminate the feeding tube with the tape measure. A second person should hold the tape measure to assist with this step.
- Holding syringe upright and have assistant place the needle on the syringe. The assistant will then remove the needle cap. Draw up the surfactant dose while the assistant holds the vial in an inverted position.
- Remove the needle from the syringe, and prime the catheter (approximately 0.4 cc). The dose to be given should equal the amount in the syringe.
- To determine the proper catheter advancement position, add 5.0 cm to cut length of ETT.
- Disconnect the ETT adaptor from the ventilator circuit or the resuscitation bag.
- Instill the surfactant-filled feeding tube into the ETT. Instill the desired aliquot volume of surfactant then withdraw the catheter, holding securely with the gloved hand so it is not contaminated.

- Surfactant is administered in 2 to 4 equal aliquots as per manufacturer's instruction with the bed flat and the infant in a neutral position with head and body in alignment. There is no evidence to support the practice of placing the infant in multiple different positions during the administration of surfactant.
- Position the infant in accordance with recommendations specific to the surfactant preparation and gently instill the first aliquot over 2-3 seconds.
- Following every aliquot administration allow 30-60 seconds to stabilize by connecting to the ventilator. Administer the ordered dosage of medication and retract the catheter from the ETT.
- Reattach ventilator circuit or resuscitation bag and assess for adverse effects of dosing. Marked improvements in oxygenation may occur within minutes of administration.
- Use of a ventilator is preferred for improved consistency of breath rate and pressure and to avoid volutrauma. If hand bagging, use a rate of 60 breaths per minute, FiO_2 sufficient to prevent cyanosis, and sufficient positive pressure to provide adequate air exchange and chest wall excursion.
- If the infant has adverse effects such as bradycardia and decreasing oxygen saturations, stop the procedure, provide supportive measures to stabilize infant, and then resume dosing when infant is stable.
- After the final aliquot is given and the infant is stabilized, slowly wean ventilator settings and FiO_2 back to pretreatment settings as tolerated.
- The clinician should remain at the bedside to make needed ventilator changes.
- Do not suction for one hour after the dose of surfactant is administered unless patient's condition warrants (i.e., airway obstruction, increased work of breathing, decreased breath sounds).
- Rales and moist breath sounds can occur transiently after administration.
- Overdosage might result in acute airway obstruction.
- Do an ABG, 30 minutes after dosing with surfactant.

CLINICAL ASSESSMENT AND CARE

1. Continually assess the infant during the administration of surfactant for signs of intolerance of the procedure such as:
   a. Bradycardia.
   b. Agitation.
   c. Tachycardia.
   d. Regurgitation of drug into ETT/adapter.
   e. Decreased oxygen saturations.
2. After administration of surfactant assess respiratory status every 30 minutes times four and then every hour times two, including:
   a. Respiratory rate (may be unobtainable for infants receiving oscillatory ventilation).
   b. Work of breathing.

c. Chest wall compliance.
d. Breath sounds (will not be able to assess for infants receiving oscillatory ventilation).

Suctioning is done if clinically indicated but this is not routine practice.

Monitoring for surfactant administration

During therapy	*After therapy*
• Heart rate, respirations	• Heart rate, respirations
• Chest expansion	• Chest expansion
• Skin color and vigor	• Skin color and vigor
• Chest-wall movement	• Breath sounds
• Oxygen saturation	• Blood pressure
• Proper placement and position of delivery device	• Chest radiograph
• FiO_2 and ventilator settings	• Ventilator settings (PIP, PEEP, Paw) and FiO_2
• Reflux of surfactant into ETT	• ABG
• Position of patient (i.e., head direction)	

Repeat Dose of Surfactant

1. Dose no sooner than 6 hours (for Survanta) and 12 hours (for Curosurf) after the preceding dose if the infant remains intubated and requires at least 30% inspired oxygen to maintain a PaO_2 less that or equal to 80 torr.
2. Radiographic confirmation of RDS should be obtained before administering additional doses to those who received a prevention dose.
3. Manual handbag ventilation should not be used to administer repeat doses.

Causes of Non-response to Surfactant

a. Lung injury prior to birth.
b. Lung injury after birth and prior to treatment.
c. Pulmonary hypoplasia.
d. Cardiovascular disease.

Surfactant Preparations

- There are many surfactants currently available; no two are alike. Use of animal-derived surfactants leads to reductions in mortality, a lower occurrence of pneumothorax, and faster weaning compared with synthetic surfactants.
- The advantages of these animal-derived surfactants over Exosurf are primarily faster weaning and a reduced risk of pneumothorax when used

for treatment of RDS. Presence of surfactant protein-B (SP-B) in animal-derived surfactants primarily affords advantages in short-term outcomes over synthetic surfactants that contain only phospholipids.

- Comparisons of the animal-derived surfactants Survanta and Infasurf, which essentially differ mainly in their SP-B content, have not shown any advantages in mortality or bronchopulmonary dysplasia.
- There may be a survival advantage of using a high initial dose of Curosurf, which provides more phospholipids and SP-B, compared with Survanta, but no differences in other important outcomes have been observed.
- Caution must be exercised when interpreting these data, however, because they are derived from studies of lesser quality and with a lower number of infants than other surfactant comparisons.

	Survanta	*Curosurf*	*Infasurf*
Prophylaxis for RDS	Yes	No	Yes
Treatment of RDS	Yes	Yes	Yes
Initial dose	4 cc/kg	2.5 cc/kg	3 cc/kg
Aliquots	4	2	2-4
Maximum repeat doses	3	2	3
Criterion for repeat dose	FiO_2 greater than 0.3.	Still intubated 12 hours after the last dose.	FiO_2 >0.3, but no sooner than six hours after the last dose OR Post 12 hours, if still intubated.

Complications of Surfactant Administration

Procedural	*Physiologic*
• Plugging of endotracheal tube. • Hemoglobin desaturation • Bradycardia • Tachycardia • Pharyngeal deposition • Administration to only one lung • Suboptimal dose delivery secondary to miscalculation or error in reconstitution	• Apnea • Pulmonary hemorrhage • Mucus plugs • Increased necessity for treatment for patent ductus arteriosus (PDA) • Barotrauma

KEY POINTS

1. Natural surfactants should be used in preference to any of the synthetic surfactants.

2. Infants who are at a significant risk of RDS should receive prophylactic natural surfactant therapy as soon as they are stable within a few minutes after intubation.
3. There is no evidence to support the practice of placing the infant in multiple different positions during the administration of surfactant.
4. Lower total dose is required in infants treated prophylactically compared with rescue therapy. Thus, it appears that improvements in outcomes are seen upto a dose of about 120 mg phospholipids/kg body weight for the first dose, larger initial doses do not lead to further improvements in outcomes.
5. Infants with RDS who have persistent or recurrent oxygen and ventilatory requirements within the first 72 hours of life should have repeat doses of surfactant. Administering more than three doses has not been shown to have a benefit.
6. Intubated infants with RDS should receive exogenous surfactant therapy before transport.
7. No adverse side effects have been reported in the short or the long-term in use of surfactant therapy.
8. Individualising the surfactant regime to match the infant's disease severity offers perhaps the best and most readily available method to reducing costs but at the same time improving outcomes in those infants with more severe disease.
9. The clinician administering the drug must be experienced in neonatal intensive care, including endotracheal intubation, mechanical ventilation and cardiorespiratory and oxygen monitoring.

REFERENCES

1. Sinha SK, Gupta S, Donn SM: Immediate respiratory management of the preterm infant, Semin Fetal Neonatal Med 2008;13:24-29.
2. Sweet D, Bevilacqua G, Carnielli V, Greisen G, Plavka R, Didrik Saugstad O, Simeoni U, Speer CP, Valls-I-Soler A, Halliday H, Working Group on Prematurity of the World Association of Perinatal Medicine, European Association of Perinatal Medicine, European consensus guidelines on the management of neonatal respiratory distress syndrome, J Perinat Med 2007;35:175-186.
3. Spragg R: Surfactant for acute lung injury, Am J Respir Cell Mol Biol 2007;37:377-378.
4. El Shahed AI, Dargaville P, Ohlsson A, Soll RF: Surfactant for meconium aspiration syndrome in full term/near term infants, Cochrane Database Syst Rev 2007;(3):CD002054.
5. Halliday HL: Recent clinical trials of surfactant treatment for neonates, Biol Neonate 2006;89:323-329.

38. TRANSILLUMINATION

Transillumination is the transmission of light through tissues of the body. It is mainly used to shine light in specific areas in infants and observe the amount of scattered light. Since their skeleton is not fully calcified, light can easily penetrate tissues. Areas filled with air or fluid that is not supposed to be in that location have increased light transmission and transilluminate when they should not. Transillumination is a useful initial screening test for infants with abnormal findings in the office or in hospital settings where CT or MRI scanning may not be immediately available. Transillumination is a safe, nonionizing, and noninvasive diagnostic technique. In addition, its portability, minimal expense, and facility make it a useful and necessary tool for the neonatal intensive care unit.

Indications

1. Suspected pneumothorax.
2. Suspected hydrocephalus, hydranencephaly, subdural effusion, subdural hematoma and porencephaly.
3. Cannulation of peripheral vein.
4. Cannulation of peripheral artery.
5. Suspected hydrocele.
6. Suspected cystic lesion over the body.
7. Suspected pneumo-peritoneum.

Supplies

Fibreoptic cold light source.

Procedure

- Connect the transilluminator to a power source and switch it on.
- Apply the fibreoptic cold light source over the site of interest.
- Dim the lights of the nursery.
- Look for the glow along the margins of the cold light source.
- Barotrauma–compare the glow on opposite side.
- Transillumination of more than 1 cm around the edge of the beam or asymmetry of the transillumination suggests underlying pathology. However, this parameter will vary significantly depending on prematurity, age, light source and operator technique.
- False positive transillumination of thorax is seen in pulmonary interstitial emphysema and subcutaneous edema.
- False negative transillumination of thorax is seen in small pneumothorax.

Complications

1. Erythematous to purpuric papules and vesicles.

REFERENCES

1. Sanklecha MU: Transillumination–A lost clinical skill, Indian J Pediatr 1993;60:835-836.

2. Donn SM, Faix RG: Transillumination in neonatal diagnosis, Clin Perinatol 1985;12:3-20.
3. Mattson D, O'Connor M: Transilluminator assistance in neonatal venepuncture, Neonatal Netw 1986;5:42-45.
4. Demaret P, Detaille T: Torch on a baby's tummy, Lancet 2007 Oct 13;370:1346.
5. Perman MJ, Kauls LS: Transilluminator burns in the neonatal intensive care unit: A mimicker of more serious disease, Pediatr Dermatol 2007;24:168-171.

39. UMBILICAL VESSEL CANNULATION

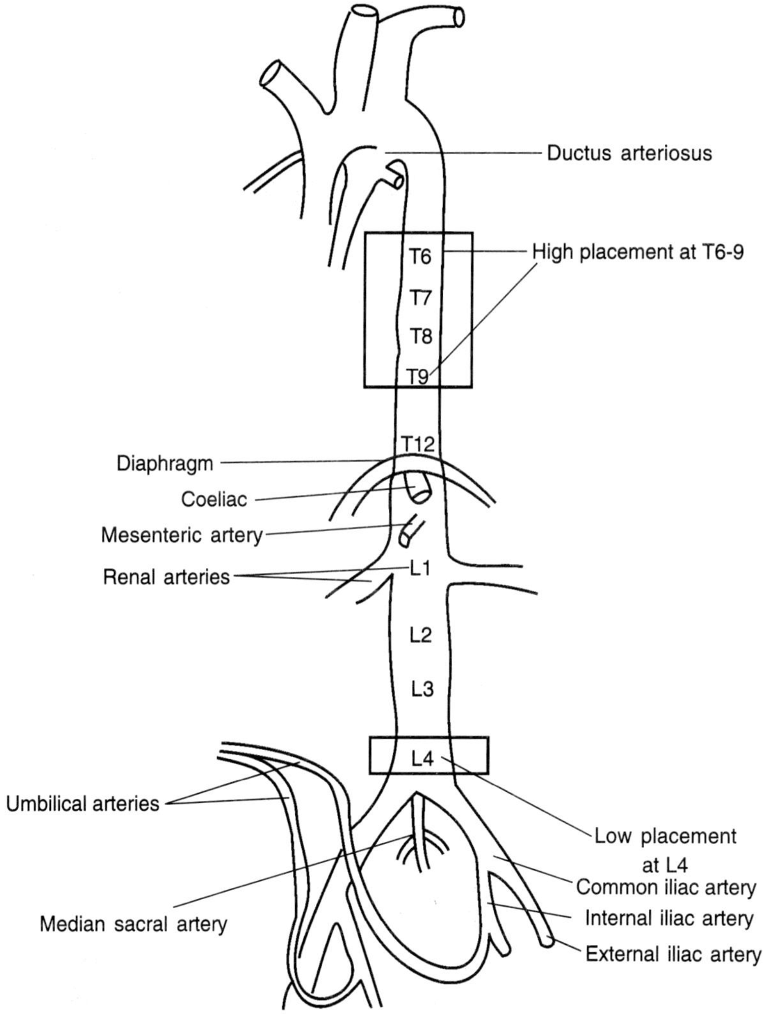

UMBILICAL VEIN (UV) CATHETERIZATION

Anatomy

- The umbilical vein is 2-3 cm long and 4-5 mm in diameter.
- From the umbilicus, it passes cephalad and a little to the right. It joins the left branch of the portal vein after giving off several large intrahepatic branches.
- The ductus venosus arises from the point where the UV joins the left portal vein.

Position

- It can be difficult to pass the catheter through the ductus venosus. There are some manoeuvres that can assist in placement. These include:
  i. Pulling the catheter back to about 4-5 cm, then advancing the catheter whilst rotating the catheter clockwise.
  ii. Passing another catheter down beside the already malplaced catheter. The path of the second catheter may be through the ductus venosus.
- Do not force a catheter in if there is resistance.
- In an emergency, an UV catheter (UVC) that remains in the portal circulation may be withdrawn until it lies in the umbilical vein. Solutions, which are not isotonic, can be infused through this for a short period of time until more suitable access is obtained.

Catheter Size

< 1500 g	3.5 F
> 1500 – 3500 g	5 F

Catheter Choice

- For infants who are term or near-term and sick enough to require central access (for example, sepsis, meconium aspiration syndrome or persistent pulmonary hypertension of the newborn), a 5F double-lumen UVC should be inserted.
- For infants <1000 g, a 3.5F double-lumen catheter should be considered if the infant is likely to need inotropes or multiple infusions. This will be decided on an individual basis.

Insertion Distance

- If the shoulder-to-umbilicus distance is measured, the catheter can be inserted the appropriate distance according to the graph below.
- Remember to measure from the skin at the base of the stump where it connects to the anterior abdominal wall.
- Remember to add the length of the umbilical stump to the distance inserted.
- Another method is to calculate the distance according to the weight of the baby. See the graph below to evaluate UVC position.

- An approximation of this is to use the calculation of: UVC length (cm) = (1.5 × birthweight (kg)) + 5.5 or half the umbilical artery catheter (UAC) length (calculated below) + 1 cm.

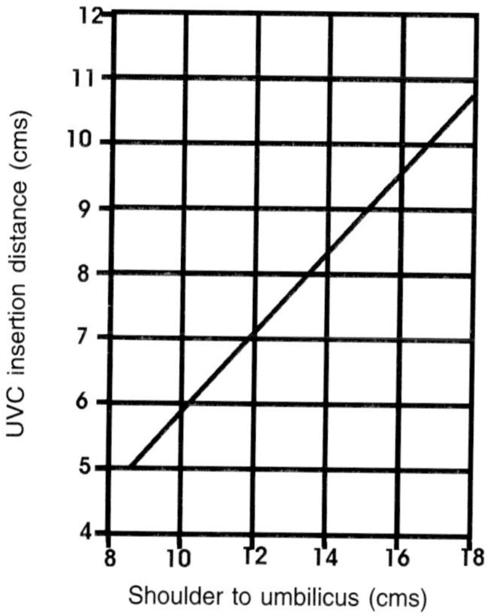

Indications

- Urgent vascular access at birth or in emergency.
- Infusion of hypertonic solutions (greater than 10%).
- Administration of vaso-active drugs.
- Initial delivery of parenteral nutrition until percutaneous central venous access is established.
- Delivery of blood and blood products—platelets should not be administered via this route.
- Measurement of central venous pressure.
- Exchange transfusion.

Supplies

- UVCs single lumen size 3.5 Fg for all infants.
- Consider 5 Fg for infants needing:
  - Exchange transfusion, or
  - Large volume replacement.
- Gown and gloves.
- Sterile green drapes.
- Dressing pack.
- Umbilical drip insertion set (scalpel blade/sutures included).

- Sterile linen cord tie.
- Additional gauze swabs.
- Assorted needles/syringes.
- 3 way taps × 2.
- Tape measure.
- Heparinised saline.

Contraindications

- Omphalitis.
- Omphalocele.
- Necrotizing enterocolitis.
- Peritonitis.

Procedure

- Wash hands.
- Open sterile towels and aseptically place on the clean surface to create a sterile field. Open central line kit and other contents of onto the sterile field.
- Set up sterile field; open packages of antiseptic swabs and organize supplies in the order of use. Traffic around the sterile field needs to be minimized. Every effort should be made to avoid distracting the person who is performing the procedure.
- Open the sterile pack and fill the sterile syringe with normal saline. Attach the catheter to the syringe and fill the catheter with saline to displace any air.
- The infant should be placed naked on its back in a warm environment. A good light is essential.
- While the assistant lifts up the umbilical cord stump with an artery forcep, clean the cord and periumbilical skin.
- Cleanse the catheter site with 3 alcohol swabs. Cleanse from the catheter outward to a distance of about 2.5 cm using a circular motion. Change the swab with each pass. Allow the alcohol to air dry.
- Cleanse the catheter site with 3 povidone iodine swabs. Cleanse from the catheter outward to a distance of about 2.5 cm using a circular motion. Change the swab with each pass. Allow the povidone to air dry.
- Assess the catheter site for erythema, induration, drainage or odor. Assess the integrity of the catheter.
- Place a sterile towel around the umbilicus.
- Loosely tie a sterile tape around the base of the umbilical cord. This is done so that the tape can be quickly tied if the cut umbilical vessels start to bleed.
- Grasp the base of the cord between the thumb and index finger of one hand. Do not release the pressure on the base of the cord until the catheter has been inserted and the tape around the base of the cord has been firmly tied. This is very important to prevent bleeding from the cord vessels.

- While squeezing the base of the cord, ask the assistant to hold up the cord away from the infant's abdominal wall. Now cut the cord off about 2 cm from the skin. Immediately after cutting the umbilical cord, the scalpel blade must be dropped into a special container for "sharps".
- On the cut end of the cord you will now see the one umbilical vein and two umbilical arteries. The umbilical vein is thin walled and situated towards the infant's head (at 12 O'clock) while the umbilical arteries have thick walls and are situated towards the infant's feet (at 4 and 8 O'clock).
- Measure the shoulder to umbilicus distance. Using the graph to determine how far to insert catheter so it is placed safely in the inferior vena cava above the level of the diaphragm. Position of catheter tip to be confirmed by X-ray or ultrasound and should be sited between T6-T10. The nurse may only commence infusions of 10% dextrose and morphine prior to confirmation of catheter tip placement.
- Preparation of the skin at the insertion site is regarded as one of the most important measures for preventing catheter related infection. Apply chlorhexidine 0.5% in alcohol solution to stump and surround, allow to dry for 2 minutes. **Do not allow solution to pool under the infant as it may burn the skin of the very low birth weight infant.** Change any damp or wet linen under the infant immediately following the procedure.
- Insert the tip of the saline filled catheter into the umbilical vein. Only gentle pressure is needed to introduce the catheter. Feed about 10 cm of the catheter into the vein, when you should be able to aspirate blood.
- Tighten the knot of the tape around the umbilical cord to prevent bleeding from the arteries. Only now should you release your grip on the base of the umbilical cord.
- The UVC should be sutured to the umbilical stump (not skin) using a 3/0 silk suture. The stump is nerve free and therefore there will be no discomfort for the infant. A separate suture should be used for the UVC and UAC lines. Do not suture catheter to the surrounding skin area as this is painful and increases the risk of infection. Secure to prevent catheter movement without occlusion.

  Note: UVC will become less secure as cord sloughs and separates.
- If the position of the UVC requires adjustment *the catheter may be withdrawn the desired length.* Under no circumstances should the catheter be advanced– a new catheter is to be inserted under sterile conditions. Remove all lines curving into lobe of the liver.
- The type of UVC inserted, size, markings at skin/stump, radiological findings and manipulations to be documented by registrar/fellow.
- Apply "Comfeel" to protect the skin and make "goal posts" using leucoplast tape. Circle catheters separately between tapes and document markings at skin/stump in the progress notes (see figure).
- To leave the catheter tip 1cm above the diaphragm. Measure the perpendicular distance from an imaginary line drawn between the two shoulders to the level of the umbilicus. Plot on the chart and read off the insertion distance from the skin level.

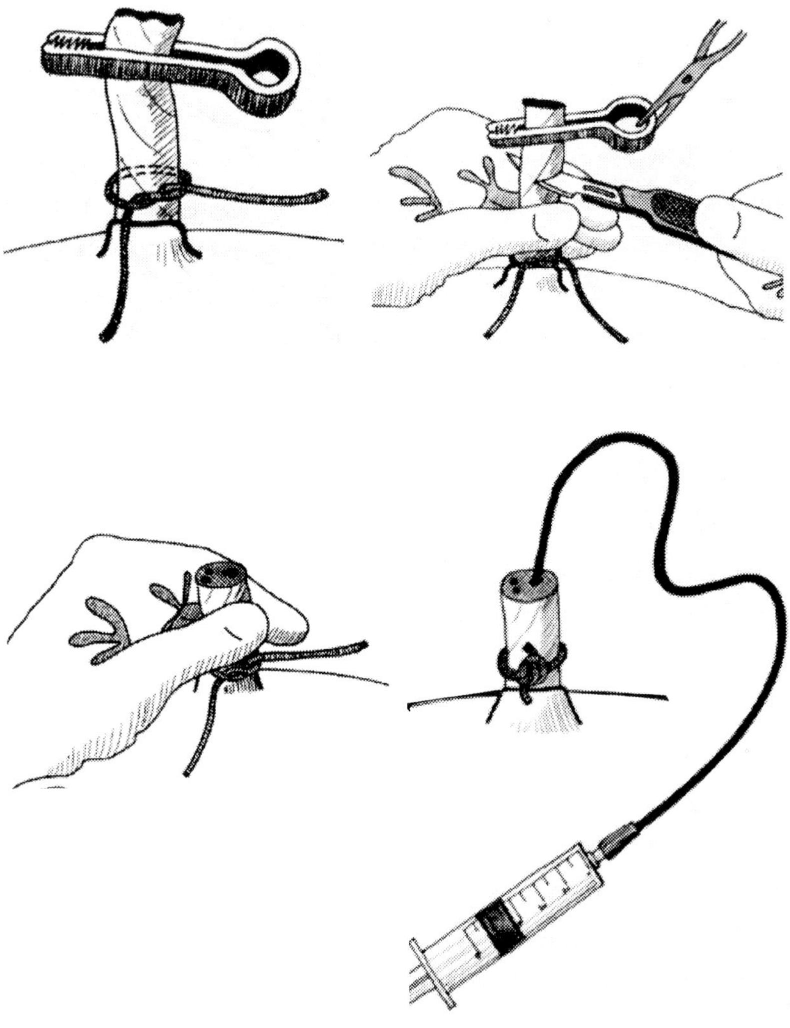

Securing of Umbilical Catheters in Babies under 1500 g

- To secure catheter wrap one suture thread around the catheter × 2 firmly and close to the base. Double knot and repeat.
- Take a 5 cm length of elastoplast. Attach to the catheter close to the base. Position the threads along the length of the catheter and wrap half the tape around and around.
- Fold back the thread lengths and continue wrapping the tape around catheter, catching the threads again.
- At the end, turn under the last bit of tape to make a tag.

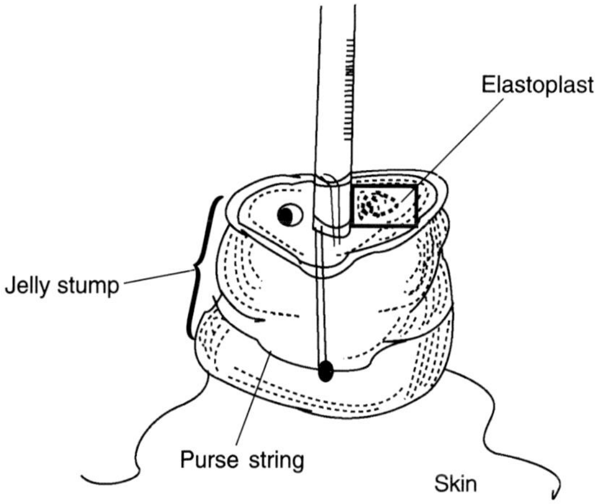

Securing of the UVC using "H tapes"

1. Cut 2 pieces of "comfeel" and leucoplast tape.

   The two pieces of "comfeel" should be cut and positioned to fit under the leucoplast. The "comfeel" is used to protect the skin and provides a barrier against epidermal stripping should the tape be removed in the first days following birth.

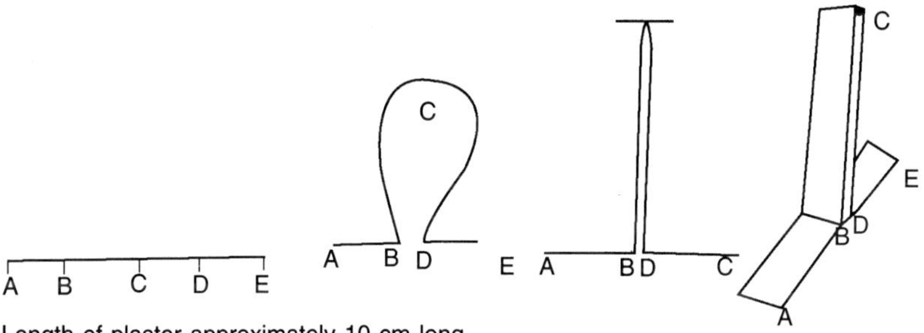

Length of plaster approximately 10 cm long.

2. Fix tapes as illustrated below:

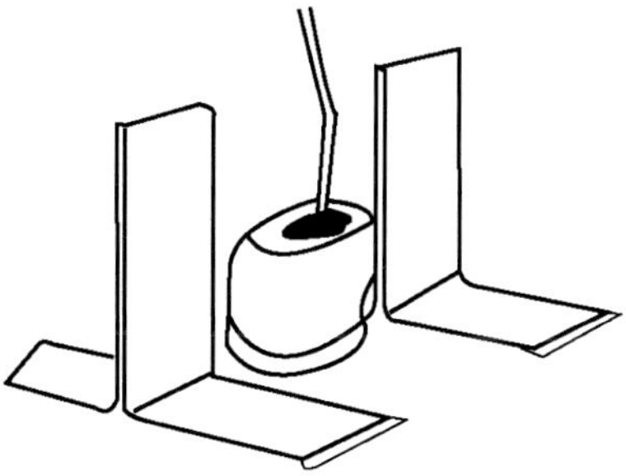

3. Cut strapping, loop UVC and UAC separately and fix as demonstrated below:

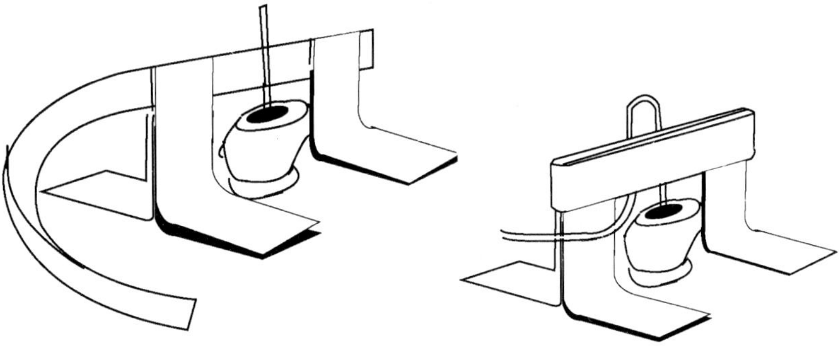

Ensure tape is secure and catheter is looped so that accidental tension to line will not displace catheter.

Complications

1. Infection.
2. Thromboembolism.
3. Catheter malposition:
   - Pericardial effusion/tamponade – more commonly seen when the UVC is sited in the right atrium or superior vena caval/right atrial junction.
   - Arrhythmia – withdraw line.
   - Hydrothorax (catheter lodged in or perforated in pulmonary vein).
   - Hepatic necrosis.
   - Extravasation in the liver may lead to ascites and cyst formation.
   - Portal vein thrombosis.
4. Sepsis.

Removal of UVC

- Remove UVC as soon as its use is no longer clinically indicated.
- The UVC may remain in situ for 7-14 days without complications. The registrar/fellow should plan to site a percutaneous central venous catheter (PCVC) for infants who require ongoing central venous access prior to removing the UVC.
- Universal precautions include the wearing of protective goggles when UVCs are removed on an open care cot.
- The UVC may be removed by trained nursing staff when the registrar/fellow is in unit.
- Cease infusion.

- Cut suture/remove tape.

  Note: In some instances UVC is removed with UAC remaining in situ. Care must be taken not to dislodge UAC. Ensure H-tapes remain firmly secured to the skin.
- Remove catheter slowly using a sterile technique.
- Ensure catheter is complete and note tip of catheter is complete.
- UVCs are not routinely sent for culture.
- Control bleeding by applying gentle pressure superior to stump site for 5 minutes using sterile gauze.
- The infant should remain supine for 6 hours to observe stump for excessive ooze or haemorrhage.
- Document procedure.

UMBILICAL ARTERY (UA) CATHETERISATION

Anatomy

The umbilical arteries are the direct continuation of the internal iliac arteries. A catheter passed into an umbilical artery will usually (but not always) enter the aorta via the internal iliac artery. Occasionally it will pass into the femoral artery via the external iliac artery or into the gluteal arteries. The femoral artery or gluteal artery is unsuitable sites for sampling, infusion, or blood pressure monitoring.

Position

- There are two potential positions for the UAC. These are described as "high" or "low".
- The high position is at the level of thoracic vertebral bodies T6-T9. This position is above the coeliac axis (T12), the superior mesenteric artery (T12-L1), and the renal arteries (L1). This position is essentially "above the diaphragm".
- The low position is at the level of lumbar vertebral bodies L3-L4. This position is below the structures as above, and is above the aortic bifurcation (L4-L5). The inferior mesenteric artery arises from L3-L4. This position is essentially "above the bifurcation".
- There is debate over whether one position is better. The Cochrane Systematic Review suggests that a high position is preferred as it is associated with fewer obvious vascular complications, a probable reduction in the incidence of aortic thrombus, and longer catheter life.

Catheter Size

< 1200 g	3.5 F
> 1200 g	5 F

Insertion Distance

- If you know the length of the infant, you can refer to the graph below which

Appendix A

relates UAC distance to total body length. This will result in placement at approximately T8. Note that of all the birth measurements, length is the least reliable.

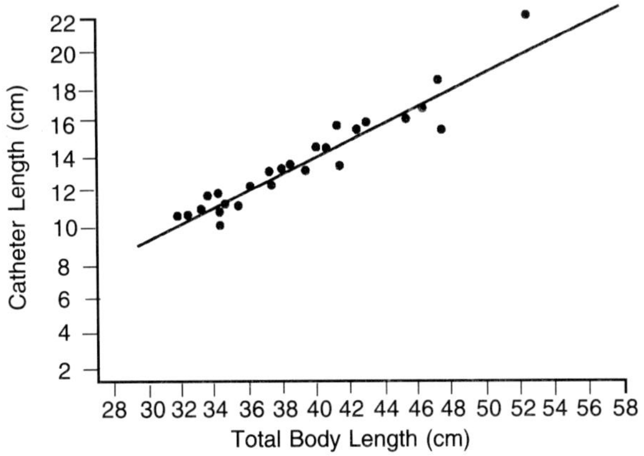

- Another option—and one which is particularly good if you forget to measure the shoulder-to-umbilicus length—is to calculate the insertion distance using the birthweight and referring to the graph below, or using the formula: UAC distance (cm) = (birthweight (kg) × 3) + 9.
- The top lines on the graph below are for UAC position. The bottom lines on the graph below are for UVC position. The curved lines above and below the straight lines are the 95% confidence intervals.

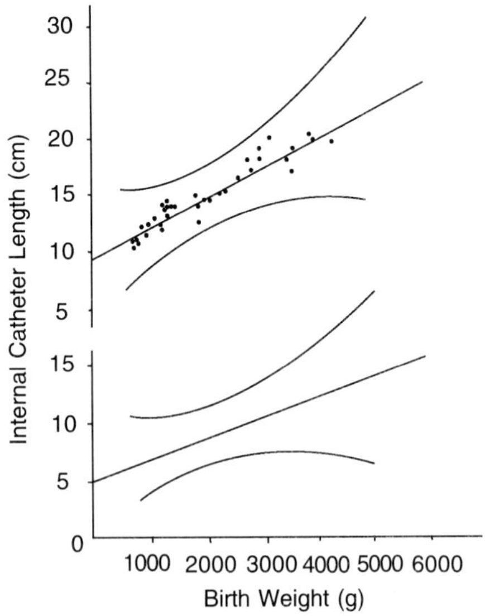

- It does no harm to insert the line a centimetre further than calculated, as the line can be pulled back slightly if needed. However, you should avoid inserting the UAC so far that it needs to be removed from the carotid or subclavian arteries.

Indications

- Blood gas monitoring.
- Continuous monitoring of arterial blood pressure.

Contraindications

- Local sepsis.
- Omphalocele.
- Necrotising enterocolitis.
- Peritonitis.

Supplies

- Arterial tray – 1 scalpel blade holder, 1 Probe, 4 Mosquito artery forceps – 2 curved and 2 straight, 2 pair dissecting forceps–toothed and non toothed, 1 Iris forceps, 1 pair of scissors, 1 needle holder, cotton wool swabs, sterile gauze pads.
- Sterile drape, gowns, gloves.
- 1 Scalpel blade.
- Umbilical artery catheter.
- 3 way tap.
- 3/0 black silk sutures.
- 10 ml syringe.
- Povidone iodine, alcohol swabs.
- Strapping bridge.
- Infusion pump with normal saline with 1 U/1 ml heparin.

Procedure

- Infants with a birth weight of less than 1.5 kg will usually require a 3.5-Fr catheter for arterial catheterization. 5-Fr catheters are used for arterial placement in larger infants regardless of infant size. Catheters (4 and 5-Fr) with PaO_2 monitoring capability (Neocath) are also available for umbilical artery catheterization. This device allows continuous monitoring of PaO_2.
- Measure shoulder umbilical length from lateral end of clavicle to a horizontal line drawn from the umbilicus to determine desired length of catheter to be inserted.
- Decide whether low (between L3 and L4) or high placement (T8 and T10) is to be done. Mark the length of catheter to be inserted.

- Assemble and check all the equipment.
- Restrain the baby.
- Follow universal precautions.
- The infant's abdomen and cord are cleaned with alcohol. The alcohol should be sparingly applied to prevent pooling under the infant's back and buttocks. The area is then draped so that only the cord is exposed.
- Tie a piece of umbilical tape around the base of the umbilical cord tightly enough to minimize blood loss but loosely enough so that the catheter can be passed easily through the vessel.
- Using a surgical blade, the cord is cut cleanly 1.0 to 2.0 cm from the skin.
- The cord is stabilized with a forceps or hemostat, and the vessels identified. The single, large, thin walled oval vein can readily be distinguished from the two smaller, thick-walled round arteries.
- The arteries are usually constricted, so that the lumens appear pinpoint in size. Gently inserting the closed tips of the curved iris forceps into the lumen of the artery until the cut end of the artery is at the bend in the forceps, and then allowing the spring of the forceps to gently spread the tips, can dilate the artery.

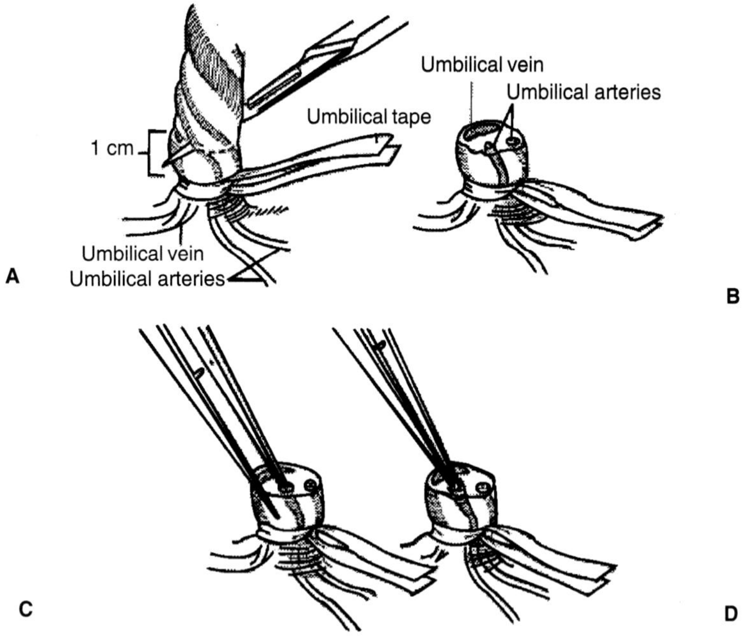

A: The umbilical cord should be amputated, leaving a1-cm stump. B: Identification of the umbilical vessels. C and D: A forceps is used to gently dilate the umbilical artery

Appendix A

- Grasping the catheter between the thumb and forefinger or with a forceps, the catheter can be inserted into the lumen of the dilated artery. Supporting the stump is usually necessary. Once the catheter has been inserted, it may encounter resistance at the level of the anterior abdominal wall or at the bladder. This resistance can usually be overcome by application of gentle steady pressure. Repeated probing movements or excessive pressure must be avoided. If unsuccessful, wait 2-3 minutes until the vasospasm ceases, or attempt the other umbilical artery.
- After the catheter is advanced the appropriate distance, the position of the catheter should be confirmed by X-ray. If, after sterile technique has been broken, the catheter is found to be in the wrong position, it can only be pulled back—IT MUST NEVER BE ADVANCED.
- Observe both legs for evidence of blanching, cyanosis or mottling. If a "blue leg" develops (presumably from vasospasm), the catheter should be removed or carefully observed for a short period of time to allow for resolution of the impaired circulation.
- After placement of the catheter, a purse-string suture is placed around the umbilicus taking care not to puncture the catheter.

Complications

- Thromboembolism involving various branches of abdominal artery leading to:
  a. Renal–Hematuria, hypertension, acute renal failure.
  b. Mesentric–Gut ischaemia, bowel infarct, necrotizing enterocolitis.
  c. Illiac vessels–Blanching, cyanosis of back, buttocks and or lower extremity.
    - Infection.
    - Disseminated intravascular coagulation (DIC).
    - Hemorrhage.
    - Vasospasm.

Monitor

- Observe colour of skin of back, buttocks and legs.
- Bowel sounds.
- Urine for RBC.
- Blood pressure.
- Platelet count.

Catheter Removal

The catheter is removed slowly over a period of 60 seconds allowing the umbilical artery to go into spasm at its proximal end while the catheter is still occluding its distal end.

REFERENCES

1. Sehgal S (1995): CSMC NICU Teaching Files: Umbilical vein catheterisation. Cedars—Sinai Medical Center LA. http://www.cs.nsw.gov.au/rpa/neonatal/html/newprot/uvc.html.
2. Nash P: Umbilical catheters, placement and complication management, J Infus Nurs 2006;29:346-52.
3. Hermansen MC, Hermansen MG: Intravascular catheter complications in the neonatal intensive care unit, Clin Perinatol 2005;32:141-156, vii.
4. Bradshaw WT, Furdon SA: A nurse's guide to early detection of umbilical venous catheter complications in infants, Adv Neonatal Care 2006;6:127-138.
5. Kabra NS, Kumar M, Shah SS: Multiple versus single lumen umbilical venous catheters for newborn infants, Cochrane Database Syst Rev 2005;(3):CD004498.
6. Moclair A and Bates I: The efficacy of heparin in maintaining peripheral infusions in neonates, Eur J Pediatr 1995;154:567-570.

40. URINE SPECIMEN COLLECTION

Indications

1. Monitoring urine output.
2. For culture and sensitivity study.

A. INDWELLING URINARY CATHETER

Supplies

- Uricath tray.
- Sterile glove.
- ½ inch paper tape.
- Small transparent dressing.

Procedure

- Set up sterile field.
- Choose appropriate size catheter. 2.5 umbilical vessel catheters should also be available for use with extremely low birth weight babies.
- While maintaining sterility, lubricate catheter tip.
- Locate urethral meatus.
- Prep meatus with Betadine.
- For the female patient, separate the labia; identify the urinary meatus and use the wipe in a downward motion (front to back) to cleanse the insides of the labia and the meatus, using new wipe for each part. For the male patient, retract the foreskin (if uncircumcised), use the wipe to clean urinary meatus in a circular fashion.
- Use a second person to provide support, immobilization, and to minimize pain and distress during procedure.

- Insert lubricated catheter until urine is obtained. Do not force catheter if resistance is met.
- Attach catheter to drainage system.
- Secure catheter to thigh or abdomen (boys) with transparent dressing. Securing catheter to abdomen in males is associated with decreased likelihood of urethral strictures.
- Wash off Betadine with soap and water.
- Wash the perineum with soap and water as part of the daily bath and as needed, when feces or drainage contaminates perineum.

Monitoring

- Report urine leakage around catheter.
- Report significant increase or decrease in volume.
- Report change in color especially if urine is bloody.
- Perform catheter care every 8 hours: Cleanse gently around meatus and tubing with soap and water.
- Palpate abdomen to assess for bladder distention if catheter is not draining.

B. NON-INVASIVE URINE COLLECTION

- Use the **diapers** and weigh them every 6 hourly. Urine passed is absorbed in the diaper. The weight of the diapers in grams is equivalent to the amount of urine passed in ml. This gives a rough estimate of the amount of urine output.
- Use a simple **test tube** of about 10 cm in length or a 20 cc **plastic syringe** with the flange removed and allows the penis to be dipped in it. Secure the test tube or the syringe to the perineum with tape. Place a feeding tube with the distal end attached to the 10 ml syringe. The amount of urine passed is checked frequently by aspirating the syringe.
- **Urine collection bags** are available and can be stuck to the perineum. The amount of urine passed is checked periodically. Apply collecting bag firmly around groin area adjacent to labia majora/scrotum so that the opening is exposed to receive urine.

REFERENCE

1. Manual of neonatal nursing: Ed Lalitha Krishnan, Published by National Neonatology Forum, 1993.

41. GASTRIC ASPIRATE SHAKE TEST

A sample of gastric aspirate collected from a newborn infant within 30 minutes after delivery consists mainly of swallowed lung fluid and amniotic fluid. Therefore, gastric aspirate can be used to assess whether surfactant is present in the infant's lungs at birth. If the gastric aspirate shake test indicates that surfactant is present, then the infant's lungs are mature and hyaline membrane disease is very unlikely. The gastric aspirate shake test should be done on all infants who develop respiratory distress within the first 30 minutes after delivery and in all infants who weigh less than 1500 g at birth.

Supplies

1. A F5 or F6 nasogastric tube.
2. Three 1 ml plastic syringes.
3. A clean glass test tube.
4. An ampoule of normal saline.
5. A bottle of 95% alcohol with a tight fitting top.
6. A rubber stopper or piece of Parafilm.

Collection of the Gastric Aspirate

A nasogastric tube is passed after delivery within 30 minutes of birth. The stomach contents are aspirated into a plastic syringe.

Procedure

- Inject 0.5 ml of gastric aspirate from the syringe into a clean glass test tube.
- Aspirate 0.5 ml of saline into a second clean syringe and inject the saline into the test tube containing the gastric aspirate.
- Close the end of the test tube with a rubber stopper or piece of Parafilm and shake the 1 ml mixture of gastric aspirate and saline well for 15 seconds. Remove the stopper or Parafilm.
- Aspirate 1 ml of 95% alcohol into the third clean syringe and inject the alcohol into the test tube containing the gastric aspirate-saline mixture.
- Again close the test tube with the stopper or Parafilm and shake the 2 ml mixture of gastric aspirate, saline and alcohol well for a further 15 seconds.
- Let the test tube stand upright for 15 minutes and then examine the surface of the fluid to decide the result of the shake test.

Interpreting Shake Test

The result of the shake test is determined by observing the number of bubbles present on the surface of the mixture after it has been allowed to stand for 15 minutes:

1. If no bubbles are present then the test is NEGATIVE. This result indicates that the infant's lungs are probably immature and that very little surfactant is present. As a result, the infant is at high risk of developing RDS.
2. If bubbles are seen around the top of the fluid but not enough bubbles are present to completely cover the surface, then the test is INTERMEDIATE. This result indicates that only some surfactant is present in the lungs and the infant may still develop mild RDS.
3. If bubbles are present right across the surface of the fluid, then the test is POSITIVE. This indicates that the lungs are mature and are producing

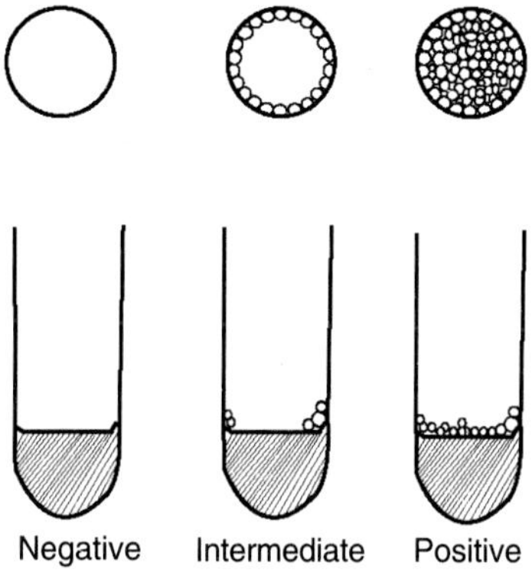

The method of evaluating the shake test

adequate amounts of surfactant. Any respiratory distress that the infant might develop is very unlikely to be due to RDS.

Practical Issues

- If collected later than 30 minutes after birth the shake test may give an incorrect result.
- The exact amount of gastric aspirate, saline and alcohol must be measured correctly.
- The test tube must be clean.

  The test tube must be closed with a rubber stopper or piece of Parafilm before shaking. Covering the opening with your finger may give a false positive result, which means that no surfactant is present even though the test is positive.
- The alcohol must be 95%. Always close the top of the alcohol bottle immediately after use as this keeps the alcohol concentration constant. If the top is left off, the alcohol absorbs moisture from the air. As a result, the concentration of the alcohol will fall.
- You must always mix the gastric aspirate with saline first before adding the alcohol or you will get an incorrect result.
- You must wait for 15 minutes before reading the result. Examining the number of bubbles earlier may give a false positive result. Reading the result too early is the most common mistake made when doing the shake test.
- If the gastric aspirate is blood or meconium stained you should not do the shake test as the result may be falsely positive.

REFERENCES

1. Chaudhari R, Deodhar J, Kadam S, Bavdekar A, Pandit A: Gastric aspirate shake test for diagnosis of surfactant deficiency in neonates with respiratory distress, Ann Trop Paediatr 2005;25:205-209.
2. Smith ML, Curnock D, Forshaw F: Value of the gastric aspirate shake test, Arch Dis Child 1981;56:230-231.

APPENDIX B

COMMON MEDICATIONS

Shaik Ashfaq Hussain
and Srinivas Murki

ANTIBIOTICS

Ampicillin (Semi-synthetic Broad Spectrum Bactericidal Aminopenicillin)

- Indication: Listeria, Gr B streptococci, pneumococci, hemophilus, enterococci, coliform infections.
- Dose: 25 to 50 mg/kg/dose, 100 mg/kg/dose for meningitis.

PMA (weeks)	*Postnatal days*	*Interval (hours)*
≤ 29	0-28	12
	>28	8
30-36	0-14	12
	>14	8
37-44	0-7	12
	>7	8
> 45	All	6

- Route
  - Slow IV push.
  - Intramuscular.
- Supply and administration
  - 125 mg, 250 mg, 500 mg, 1g and 2g vials.
  - Mix with sterile water and use within 1 hour for best potency.
  - Final concentration is 100 mg/ml concentration for IV and 250 mg/ml for IM.
- Side effects
  - Hypersensitivity reactions (rash, urticaria, fever).
  - Lower seizure threshold with high doses.

Cefotaxime (3rd Generation Cephalosporin, Bactericidal)

- Indication Gram negative (E. coli, H. Influenzae, Klebsiella, Pseudomonas) bacterial infections/meningitis, Gonococcal Infections.
- Dose 50 mg/kg/dose.

PMA (weeks)	*Postnatal days*	*Interval (hours)*
≤ 29	0-28	12
	>28	8
30-36	0-14	12
	>14	8
37-44	0-7	12
	>7	8
>45	All	6

- Route
  - Intravenous infusion over 30 minutes.
  - Intramuscular.
- Supply and administration
  - 250 mg, 500 mg, 1g and 2g vials.
  - Mix with sterile water.
  - Final concentration is 100 mg/ml concentration for IV.
- Side effects
  - Rash, phlebitis, diarrhea, leucopenia, granulocytopenia, eosinophilia.

Ceftriaxone (3rd Generation Cephalosporin, Bactericidal)

- Indication
  - Gram negative (E.coli, H.influenzae, Klebsiella, Pseudomonas).
  - Bacterial infections/meningitis, Gonococcal infections.
- Dose
  - 50 mg/kg/dose/24 hours, single dose.
  - Meningitis: 100 mg/kg as loading and then 80 mg/kg/day Q 24 hours.
- Route
  - Intravenous infusion over 30 minutes.
  - Intramuscular (to reduce pain reconstitute with 1% lignocaine).
- Supply and administration
  - 250 mg, 500 mg, 1g and 2g vials.
  - Mix with sterile water.
  - Final concentration is 40 mg/ml concentration for IV.
- Side effects
  - Not recommended for babies with jaundice.
  - Eosinophilia, thrombocytosis, leucopenia, increase in bleeding time.

- Biliary sludge, diarrhea, increase in BUN, creatinine, transaminases.

Ceftazidime (3rd Generation Cephalosporin, Bactericidal)

- Indication
  - Gram negative (E.coli, H.influenzae, Neisseria, Klebsiella and Proteus sp), especially Pseudomonas.
  - Bacterial infections/meningitis.
- Dose 30 mg/kg/dose.

PMA (weeks)	*Postnatal days*	*Interval (hours)*
≤ 29	0-28	12
	>28	8
30-36	0-14	12
	>14	8
37-44	0-7	12
	>7	8
>45	All	8

- Route
  - Intravenous infusion over 30 minutes.
  - Intramuscular (reduce pain by reconstituting with 1% lignocaine).
- Supply and administration
  - 500 mg, 1g and 2g vials.
  - Mix with sterile water.
  - Final concentration is 50 mg/ml concentration for IV.
- Side effects
  - Rash, phlebitis, diarrhea, eosinophilia, elevated transaminases, positive Coombs test.

Pipericillin (Semi-synthetic Penicillin)

- Indication
  - Gram negative (E.coli, Serratia, Klebsiella, Enterobacter, Citrobacter and proteus sp), especially Pseudomonas.
  - Group B streptococcal infections.
- Dose 50-100 mg/kg/dose.

PMA (weeks)	*Postnatal days*	*Interval (hours)*
≤ 29	0-28	12
	>28	8
30-36	0-14	12
	>14	8
37-44	0-7	12
	>7	8
>45	All	6

- Route
  - Intravenous infusion over 30 minutes.
  - Intramuscular .
- Supply and administration
  - 2g, 3g, 4g vials.
  - Mix with sterile water.
  - Final concentration is 100 mg/ml concentration for IV.
- Side effects
  - Eosinophilia, hyperbilirubinemia, elevated transaminases, azotemia.

Aztreonam (Synthetic B-lactum Antibiotic)

- Indication
  - Gram negative (E.coli, Serratia, Klebsiella, Enterobacter, Pseudomonas).
  - Used in combination with aminoglycoside.
- Dose 30 mg/kg/dose.

PMA (weeks)	*Postnatal days*	*Interval (hours)*
≤ 29	0-28	12
	>28	8
30-36	0-14	12
	>14	8
37-44	0-7	12
	>7	8
>45	All	6

- Route
  - Intravenous infusion over 10 minutes.
- Supply and administration
  - Powder for injection 500 mg, 1g and 2g vials.
  - Mix with sterile water for a concentration of 50 mg/ml. Shake immediately and vigorously.
- Side effects
  - Eosinophilia, hypoglycemia, elevated transaminases, phlebitis.

Imipenem/Cilastin (Broad Spectrum Carbapenem Combined with Cilastin 1:1 Ratio)

- Indication
  - Reserve antibiotic used for gram negative ***Non-CNS infections*** especially Entero-bacteriaceae and anaerobes, resistant to other antibiotics.
- Dose 20-25 mg/kg/dose Q12 hours.
- Route

- Intravenous infusion over 30 minutes.
- Supply and administration
  - 250 mg, 500 mg vials.
  - Mix with ***Normal saline*** to obtain concentrations of 5 mg/ml. Use reconstituted solution in 10 hours at room temperature and if refrigerated, within 48 hours.
- Side effects
  - Seizures in neonates with CNS infections or CNS pathology.
  - Phlebitis and thrombocytosis.
  - Eosinophilia, elevated transaminases, diarrhea.

Meropenem (Broad Spectrum Carbapenem with CSF Penetration)

- Indication
  - Pneumococcal meningitis, gram negative infections resistant to other antibiotics, ESBL producing Klebsiella.
  - Meningitis and infections by Pseudomonas.
- Dose
  - 20 mg/kg/dose Q12 hours.
  - 40 mg/kg/dose Q 8 hours for meningitis.
- Route
  - Intravenous infusion over 30 minutes
- Supply and administration
  - 250 mg, 500 mg, 1g vials.
  - Mix with ***Normal saline*** to obtain concentrations of 50 mg/ml. Use reconstituted solution in 2 hours at room temperature and if refrigerated, within 12 hours.
- Side effects
  - Diarrhea, nausea, vomiting, rash, phlebitis.
  - Development of cephalosporin resistance in enterobacter, pseudomonas, serratia, proteus, citrobacter and acinetobacter species.
  - Pseudo-membranous colitis and fungal infections.

Netilmycin (Aminoglycoside)

- Indication
  - Gram negative bacilli (E.coli, Klebsiella, Pseudomonas).
  - Usually used in combination with penicillins/cephalosporins.
- Dose

PMA (weeks)	*Postnatal days*	*Dose (mg/kg)*	*Interval (hours)*
≤ 29	0-7	5	48
	8-28	4	36

Contd.

Contd.

	> 28	4	24
30-34	0-7	4.5	36
	>7	4	24
>34	All	4	24

- Route
  - Intravenous infusion over 30 minutes. Separate from penicllins.
- Supply and administration
  - 100 mg/ml in 1.5 ml.
  - Mix with sterile water/D5W/NS.
- Side effects
  - Renal tubular dysfunction with loss of sodium, calcium and magnesium.
  - Ototoxicity and nephrotoxicity, especially when combined with other toxic drugs.
  - Neuromuscular blockade with pancuronium.

Amikacin (Aminoglycoside)

- Indication
  - Gram negative bacilli (E.coli, Klebsiella, Pseudomonas) resistant to other amino-glycosides.
  - Usually used in combination with B-lactams.
- Dose

PMA (weeks)	*Postnatal days*	*Dose (mg/kg)*	*Interval (hours)*
≤ 29*	0-7	18	48
	8-28	15	36
	> 28	15	24
30-34	0-7	18	36
	>7	15	24
>34	All	15	24

* In case of PDA/Indomethacin treatment/asphyxia follow the dosage schedule as that of ≤ 29 weeks.

- Route
  - Intravenous infusion over 30 minutes. Separate from penicllins.
- Supply and administration
  - 50 mg/ml or 250 mg/ml.
  - Mix with sterile water/D5W/NS.
- Side effects
  - Renal tubular dysfunction with loss of sodium, calcium and magnesium.
  - Ototoxicity and nephrotoxicity, especially when combined with other toxic drugs.
  - Neuromuscular blockade with pancuronium.

Gentamicin (Aminoglycoside)

- Indication
  - Gram negative bacilli (E.coli, Klebsiella, Pseudomonas).
  - Usually used in combination with penicillins/cephalosporins.
- Dose

PMA (weeks)	*Postnatal days*	*Dose (mg/kg)*	*Interval (hours)*
≤ 29*	0-7	18	48
	8-28	15	36
	> 28	15	24
30-34	0-7	18	36
	>7	15	24
>34	All	15	24

* In case of PDA/Indomethacin treatment/asphyxia follow the dosage schedule as that of ≤ 29 weeks.

- Route
  - Intravenous infusion over 30 minutes. Separate from penicllins.
- Supply and administration
  - 10 mg/ml.
  - Mix with sterile water/D5W/NS.
- Side effects
  - Renal tubular dysfunction with loss of sodium, calcium and magnesium.
  - Ototoxicity and nephrotoxicity, especially when combined with other toxic drugs.
  - Neuromuscular blockade with pancuronium.

Tobramycin (Aminoglycoside)

- Indication
  - Aerobic gram negative bacilli (E.coli, Klebsiella, Pseudomonas).
  - Usually used in combination with penicillins/cephalosporins.
- Dose

PMA (weeks)	*Postnatal days*	*Dose (mg/kg)*	*Interval (hours)*
≤ 29	0-7	5	48
	8-28	4	36
	> 28	4	24
30-34	0-7	4.5	36
	>7	4	24
>34	All	4	24

* In case of PDA/Indomethacin treatment/asphyxia follow the dosage schedule as that of ≤ 29 weeks.

- Route
  - Intravenous infusion over 30 minutes. Separate from penicillins.
- Supply and administration
  - 10 mg/ml.
  - Mix with sterile water/D5W/NS.
- Side effects
  - Renal tubular dysfunction with loss of sodium, calcium and magnesium.
  - Ototoxicity and nephrotoxicity, especially when combined with other toxic drugs.
  - Neuromuscular blockade with pancuronium.

Oxacillin (Cloxacillin) (Anti-staphylococcal Penicillin)

- Indication Penicillinase producing staphylococci.
- Dose
  - 25 mg/kg/dose over 10 minutes.
  - Meningitis 50 mg/kg/dose.

PMA (weeks)	*Postnatal days*	*Interval (hours)*
≤ 29	0-28	12
	>28	8
30-36	0-14	12
	>14	8
37-44	0-7	12
	>7	8
>45	All	6

- Route
  - Intravenous infusion over 10 minutes.
- Supply and administration
  - 250 mg, 500 mg, 1 g and 2 g powder vials.
  - Mix with sterile water.
  - Final concentration is 40 mg/ml concentration for IV.
- Side effects
  - Interstitial nephritis, bone marrow depression, phlebitis, elevated transaminases.

Vancomycin (Methicillin Resistant Anti-Staphylococcal and Anti-Pneumococcal)

- Indication
  - Methicillin resistant staphylococcal infections.
  - Methicillin resistant pneumococcal infections.

- Dose
  - Usual dose 10 mg/kg/dose.
  - Meningitis 15 mg/kg/dose.

PMA (weeks)	*Postnatal days*	*Interval (hours)*
≤ 29	0-28	12
	>28	8
30-36	0-14	12
	>14	8
37-44	0-7	12
	>7	8
>45	All	6

- Route
  - Intravenous infusion over 60 minutes.
- Supply and administration
  - 500 mg, 1 g vials.
  - Mix with sterile water.
  - Final concentration is 50 mg/ml concentration for IV.
- Side effects
  - Nephrotoxicity and ototoxicity increased by combined aminoglycosides.
  - Rash and hypotension (Red Man syndrome).
  - Neutropenia and phlebitis.

Clindamycin (Bacteriostatic for Anaerobic Infections)

- Indication
  - Bacteremia and deep seated infections by anaerobes and gram positive cocci.
  - Do not use for meningitis.
- Dose
  - 5-7.5 mg/kg/dose.

PMA (weeks)	*Postnatal days*	*Interval (hours)*
≤ 29	0-28	12
	>28	8
30-36	0-14	12
	>14	8
37-44	0-7	12
	>7	8
>45	All	6

- Route
  - Intravenous infusion over 30 minutes.
- Supply and administration
  - 150 mg/ml in 2 ml, 4 ml and 6 ml vials.

- Dilute with NS/D5W for a final concentration of 6 mg/ml concentration for IV.
- Side effects
  - Pseudo membranous colitis (bloody diarrhea, pain abdomen and fever).

Metronidazole (Bactericidal for Anaerobic Infections)

- Indication
  - Meningitis, ventriculitis and endocarditis caused by bacteroides fragilis and other anerobes resistant to penicillins.
  - Treatment of trichomonas vaginalis and C. difficile colitis.
- Dose
  - 15 mg/kg/dose as loading and maintenance of 7.5 mg/kg/dose.

PMA (weeks)	*Postnatal days*	*Interval (hours)*
≤ 29	0-28	48
	>28	24
30-36	0-14	24
	>14	12
37-44	0-7	24
	>7	12
>45	All	8

- Route
  - Intravenous infusion over 60 minutes.
- Supply and administration
  - 5 mg/ml in 100 ml ready to use solutions.
  - Tablets 250 mg and 500 mg.
- Side effects
  - Seizures and sensory polyneuropathy.

Rifampin (Semi-synthetic, Bacterial DNA Transcription Inhibitor)

- Indication
  - Persistent staphylococcal infections in combination with vancomycin.
  - Prophylaxis for N. meningitis and H. influenza type B.
- Dose
  - Oral dose: 10 to 20 mg/kg/dose Q 24 hours.
  - Intravenous: 5 to 10 mg/kg/dose Q12 hours.
- Route
  - Oral.
  - Intravenous infusion over 30 minutes.
- Supply and administration
  - 150 mg and 300 mg capsules.

- Powder for injection 600 mg.

- Side effects
  - Orange or red discoloration of secretions.
  - Phlebitis.

Penicillin G (Crystalline Penicillin)

- Indication
  - Group B streptococcal infections, congenital syphilis and gonococcal infections.
- Dose
  - Bacteremia : 25,000 to 50,000 units/kg/dose.
  - Meiningitis : 75,000 to 1,00,000 unit/kg/dose.

PMA (weeks)	*Postnatal days*	*Interval (hours)*
≤ 29	0-28	12
	>28	8
30-36	0-14	12
	>14	8
37-44	0-7	12
	>7	8
>45	All	6

- Route
  - Intravenous infusion over 30 minutes.
- Supply and administration
  - Powder for injection.
  - Diluted with sterile water for a final concentration of 1,00,000 unit/ml.
- Side effects
  - Cardiac arrest on rapid infusion.
  - CNS toxicity with high doses.
  - Granulocytopenia, hepatitis.
  - No hypersensitivity in neonates.

ANTIVIRAL DRUGS

Acyclovir (Antiviral Drug)

- Indication
  - Herpes simplex infection and varicella zoster infection with CNS and pulmonary involvement.
  - Herpes simplex encephalitis.
- Dose
  - 20 mg/kg per dose Q 8 hours intravenous ***infusion*** over 1 hour.

- Prolong the dosing interval in
  - Premature infants <34 weeks.
  - In neonates with renal impairment or hepatic failure.
  - Treat localized Herpes simplex infection for 14 days and disseminated or CNS infection for 21 days.

- Route
  - Intravenous.
- Supply and administration
  - 500 mg and 1 gm vials.
  - Dissolve contents of 500 mg vial in 10 ml of sterile water for injection.
  - 1 ml of this 50 mg/ml solution is further diluted with 9 ml of NS to get 5 mg/ml of concentration. Such reconstituted solution is stable at room temp for 12 hours. Do not refrigerate.
- Side effects
  - Neutropenia (20%), phlebitis, transient renal dysfunction and crystalluria.
  - Minimize side effects by slow infusion rates and adequate patient hydration.

Ganciclovir (Acyclic Nucleoside Analog of Guanine)

- Indication
  - Prevention of progressive hearing loss for symptomatic congenital CMV.
  - Treatment of congenital CMV infection.
- Dose
  - 6 mg /kg per dose Q 12 hours intravenous ***infusion*** over 1 hour.
  - Duration for atleast 6 weeks.
  - Reduce dose by half for significant neutropenia <500 cells /mm^3.
  - Chronic oral suppression; 30-40 mg/kg per dose Q 8 hours oral.
- Route
  - Intravenous or Oral.
- Supply and administration
  - 500 mg per vials.
  - Reconstituted with 10 ml sterile water to get concentration of 50 mg/ml.
  - Dilute 1 ml of 50 mg/ml solution with 9 ml of NS/D5W to get 5 mg/ml concentration.
- Side effects
  - Significant neutropenia in majority. Discontinue treatment if neutropenia does not resolve after reducing dose by half.
  - Anemia and thrombocytopenia.

Zidovudine (Thymidine Analog Antiretroviral Drug)

- Indication
  - Prophylaxis of neonates born to HIV infected mothers.
- Dose
  - Intravenous: 1.5 mg /kg per dose via ***infusion*** pump over 1hour.
  - Oral: 2 mg /kg per dose.
  - Term babies: 2 mg/kg by mouth or 1.5 mg /kg IV once every 6 hours for 6 weeks starting in 8-12 hours after birth.
  - Preterm babies: 2 mg/kg/dose. 12 hourly if gestation < 34 weeks. Change to 8 hourly after 2 weeks if gestation >30 weeks and after 4 weeks if gestation <30 weeks.
- Route
  - Intravenous or Oral.
- Supply and administration
  - 10 mg /ml in 20 ml single use vial.
  - Dilute to a concentration not exceeding 4 mg /ml before infusion.
  - Oral suspension has 50 mg/5 ml.
- Side effects
  - Anemia, Neutropenia if serum concentration is greater than 3 micromol /l.
  - Lactic academia if exposure to in-utero antiretroviral therapy.

Nevirapine (Non-nucleoside Antiretroviral Drug)

- Indication
  - Prophylaxis of neonates born to HIV infected mothers along with zidovudine.
- Dose
  - Oral: 2 mg /kg single dose at 48-72 hours.
  - If the mother received nevirapine less than one hour before delivery, give one dose at birth and again at 48 to 72 hours.
- Route
  - Oral.
- Supply and administration
  - 10 mg/ml Oral suspension.
- Side effects
  - None reported.

ANTIFUNGAL DRUGS

Fluconazole (Triazole Antifungal Agent)

- Indication

- Treatment of systemic infections, meningitis and severe superficial infections caused by candida species.
- Prophylaxis in ELBW infants with high fungal infection rates.

• Dose
- 12 mg/kg loading dose followed by 6 mg/kg.

PMA (weeks)	*Postnatal days*	*Interval (hours)*
≤ 29	0-14	72
	>14	48
30-36	0-14	48
	>14	24
37-44	0-7	48
	>7	24
>45	All	24

• 3 mg/kg/dose infusion twice weekly.

• Route
- Oral.
- Intravenous by infusion in 30 minutes.

• Supply and administration
- 2 mg/ml concentration in 100 ml and 200 ml vials.
- 50 mg, 100 mg tablets.

• Side effects
- Elevations in transaminases, contraindicated with cisapride.

Amphotericin B (Fungicidal or Fungistatic, Ergosterol Affinity)

• Indication
- Systemic fungal infections and severe superficial mycosis.

• Dose
- 0.5-1 mg/kg Q 24 hours.
- Stop therapy for 2 to 5 days if serum creatinine increases by 0.4 mg/dl.

• Route
- Intravenous infusion over 2 to 6 hours.

• Supply and administration
- 50 mg powder for injection in a vial.
- Mix with D5W to get a concentration of 0.1 mg/ml.
- Do not mix with normal saline.
- Protect from light.

• Side effects
- Renal tubular dysfunction with loss of potassium, magnesium and sodium.
- Renal tubular acidosis and decreased GFR.

  - Anemia, thrombocytopenia, hypokalemia, nauseas/vomiting and fever.
  - Toxic doses may cause cardiac arrest.

Amphotericin B Lipid Complex (Complexed with Phospholipids)

- Indication
  - Systemic fungal infections and severe superficial mycosis resistant to conventional amphotericin and in neonates with hepatic and renal dysfunction.
- Dose
  - 5 mg/kg Q 24 hours.
- Route
  - Intravenous infusion over 2 hours.
- Supply and administration
  - 5 mg/ml in 10 ml and 20 ml ready to use suspension.
  - Mix with D5W to get a concentration of 1-2 mg/ml.
  - Do not mix with normal saline.
  - Protect from light.
- Side effects
  - Anemia, thrombocytopenia, hypokalemia, nauseas/vomiting and fever.

Amphotericin B Liposome (Intercalated in Bilayer Liposomal Drug Delivery System)

- Indication
  - Systemic fungal infections and severe superficial mycosis resistant to conventional amphotericin and in neonates with hepatic and renal dysfunction.
- Dose
  - 5 to 7 mg/kg Q 24 hours.
- Route
  - Intravenous infusion over 2 hours.
- Supply and administration
  - 50 mg powder vials.
  - Initially dilute with sterile water for injection to get a concentration of 4 mg/l.
  - Further dilute with D5W to get a concentration of 1-2 mg/ml.
  - Do not mix with normal saline.
  - Protect from light.
- Side effects
  - Anemia, thrombocytopenia, hypokalemia, nauseas/vomiting and fever.

Nystatin (Polyene Antifungal)

- Indication
  - Mucocutaneous candidal infections.
- Dose
  - Apply ointment or cream to affected site Q 6 hours till the subsidence of symptoms and another 3 days after that.
  - For oral thrush, apply 1 ml (preterm) or 2 ml (term) of 1,00,000 units/ml suspension to each side of mouth with a cotton swab.
- Supply and administration
  - Ointment/cream 1,00,000 units/gram in 15 and 30 gm tubes.
  - Suspension 1,00,000 units/ml in 5 ml and 60 ml bottles. Do not mix with milk.
- Side effects
  - Rash.

Gentian Violet (Triphenyl Methane Antiseptic Dye)

- Indication
  - Candida infection of the skin and active against gram positive organisms including staphylococci.
  - Twice daily for 3-4 days.
- Route
  - Topical (avoid mucosal contact), deep penetration.
- Supply
  - 0.5% aqueous solution.
- Side effects
  - Stains everything it touches including skin.

CARDIOVASCULAR DRUGS

Alprostadil (Prostaglandin E1): Pulmonary Vasodilator

- Indication Dilatation of ductus arteriosus in duct dependent congenital heart diseases.
- Dose
  - Initial 0.05 -0.1 mcg/kg/minute by infusion.
  - Maintenance As low as 0.01 mcg/kg/min. Titrate with infants response (Oxygenation versus adverse effects).
- Route
  - Only intravenous (avoid extravasations).
- Supply and administration
  - 500 mcg in 1ml vial.

- Dilute with D5W or NS.
- Mix one ampoule (1 ml) in 49 ml of D5W (concentration obtained is 10 mcg/ml) and run at rate 0.6 ml/kg/hour to get 0.1 mcg/kg/min.

• Side effects
- Apnea, fever, leucocytosis, cutaneous flushing, bradycardia.
- Uncommon: Seizures, edema, hypotension.
- Prolonged therapy results in edema, widened fontanels, cortical hyperostosis.

Adenosine (Anti-arrhythmia Agent for PSVT)

• Indication PSVT.

• Dose
- Initial dose 50 mcg/kg.
- Subsequent doses in increments of 50 mcg/kg to a maximum of 250 mcg/kg.

• Route
- Rapid intravenous push (1 to 2 seconds).

• Supply and administration
- 2 ml vial contains 6000 mcg. Do not refrigerate.
- Dilute 1 ml of adenosine with 9 ml of NS (1 ml/300 mcg).
- Connect a 3 way to the IV canula. Push adenosine through one port and immediately flush with NS through the other port.
- Watch for reversal of arrhythmia.

• Side effects
- Flushing, dyspnea, irritability. Recurrence of PSVT in 30% of treated neonates.

Indomethacin (Prostaglandin Inhibitor)

• Indication Closure of ductus arteriosus. Prevention of IVH.

• Dose
- <48 hours: 0.2 mg/kg, 0.1 mg/kg and 0.1 mg/kg at 12 hourly intervals.
- 2-7 days: 0.2 mg/kg, 0.2 mg/kg and 0.2 mg/kg at 12 hourly intervals.
- >7 days: 0.2 mg/kg, 0.25 mg/kg and 0.25 mg/kg at 12 hourly intervals.
- Prolonged course 0.2 mg/kg/day for 5 to 7 days.

• Route
- IV infusion over 30 minutes.
- Oral.

• Supply and administration
- 1 mg vials, 25 mg tablet.
- Dilute with NS or sterile water.

- Side effects
  - Oliguria, feed intolerance, hypoglycemia, platelet dysfunction.
  - Decreased blood flow to brain, GI and kidneys.
  - Monitor for platelets, urine output, urea, creatinine and bleeds before and during treatment.

Ibuprofen Lysine (Prostaglandin Inhibitor)

- Indication Closure of ductus arteriosus.
- Dose
  - 1st dose 10 mg/kg.
  - 2nd and 3rd dose 5 mg/kg/dose every 24 hours.
- Route
  - IV infusion over 15 minutes.
  - Oral.
- Supply and administration
  - 2 ml vial with 10 mg/ml. May dilute with NS, D5W.
  - Syrup 20 mg/ml.
  - Protect from light.
- Side effects
  - Oliguria, platelet dysfunction, increased oxygen dependency.

Milrinone (Selective Phosphodiesterase Inhibitor)

- Indication Short term (<72 hours) treatment of acute low cardiac output after cardiac surgery or due to septic shock.
- Dose
  - Loading dose 0. 75 mcg/kg IV infused over 60 min.
  - Maintenance Infusion of 0.5 to 0.75 mcg/kg/min.
  - **Premature babies <30 weeks GA.**
  - Loading dose: 0.75 mcg/kg per min for 3 hours immediately followed by.
  - Maintenance: Infusion of 0.2 mcg/kg per min.
- Supply
  - 1 mg/ml solution for injection in 10, 20, 50 ml single dose vials.
  - Dilution with DW or NS.
- Side effects
  - BP will likely to fall 5 to 9% after the loading dose but should return to baseline by 24 hours (Continuous monitoring of heart rate, rhythm and BP is necessary).
  - Thrombocytopenia occurs rarely.

Dopamine (Catecholamine)

- Indication Treatment of neonatal hypotension.
- Dose
  - 2-20 mcg /kg per min continuous IV infusion. Begin with low dose and titrate by monitoring effects.
- Supply and administration
  - Available as 40 mg/ml, 80 mg/ml, 160 mg/ml vials for injection.
  - Add weight * 5 mg of dopamine to 50 ml of D5W or NS and run at 1ml/hour for 1 mcg/kg/min.
- Side effects
  - Tachycardia, arrhythmias, increase in pulmonary artery pressure, reversible suppression of prolactin, thyrotropin.
  - Monitor heart rate, intra-arterial pressure, urine output and peripheral perfusion frequently to avoid side effects.

Dobutamine (Synthetic Catecholamine with Primarily Beta Adrenergic Activity)

- Indication Treatment of hypoperfusion, especially if myocardial dysfunction.
- Dose 2-25 mcg/kg per min continuous IV infusion.
- Route
  - Intravenous infusion only.
- Supply and administration
  - 250 mg per 20 ml vial(12.5 mg/ml).
  - Add weight * 5 mg of dobutamine to 50 ml of D5W or NS and run at 1ml/hour for 1 mcg/kg/min.
  - Reconstituted solution stable for 6 hours at room temp and 48 hours if refrigerated.
- Side effects
  - Hypotension if patient is hypovolemic, tachycardia at high dosages, arrhythmias, cutaneous vasodilation and increased myocardial oxygen consumption.

Epinephrine (Sympathomimetic, Agonist on Alpha and Beta Adrenoreceptors)

- Indication Acute cardiovascular collapse, short term use for cardiac failure that is resistant to other drugs.
- Dose
  - Severe bradycardia and hypotension: 0.1-0.3 ml/kg 1 in 10,000 conc. equal to 0.01- 0.03 mg/kg.

- 0.1 mcg/kg/min to 1 mcg/kg/min.
- Correct acidosis to improve efficacy of epinephrine.

- Route
  - Can be given by ET tube immediately followed by 1ml NS.
  - Intravenous infusion.
- Supply and administration
  - 1 ml ampoule contains 1 mg epinephrine (1 in 1000).
  - Dilute with D5W or NS to prepare 1 in 10,000 concentration.
- Side effects
  - Cardiac arrhythmias, renal vascular ischaemia, severe hypertension with intracranial hemorrhage, increase myocardial oxygen consumption and hypokalemia.

Noradrenaline (Directly Acting Sympathomimetic Agent)

- Indication Potent vasoconstrictor used to treat refractory hypotension.
- Dose
  - Start with 0.1 mcg/kg/min and increase to a max of 1.5 mcg /kg per min.
- Route
  - Intravenous infusion.
- Supply and administration
  - 2 ml, 4 ml ampoules contain 2 mg/ml of nor-adrenaline.
  - Dilute with D10/DW.
- Side effects
  - Tachycardia, severe hypertension leading to cerebral hemorrhage and rarely ventricular arrhythmias.

Digoxin (Digitalis Glycoside with Positive Inotropic and Negative Chronotropic Effect)

- Indication
  - Heart failure caused by diminished myocardial contractility.
  - Supra ventricular tachycardia , atrial flutter and atrial fibrillation.
- Dose

Weight	*Loading dose*	*Maintenance dose*
<1.5 kg	20 mcg/kg IV or 25 mcg/kg Oral	5 mcg/kg
1.5-2.5 kg	30 mcg/kg IV or 35 mcg/kg Oral	7.5 mcg/kg
> 2.5 kg	35 mcg/kg IV or 45 mcg/kg Oral	10 mcg/kg

- Route
  - Intravenous.
  - Oral elixir.
- Supply and administration
  - 1 ml ampoule contains 100 mcg.
  - Oral digoxin elixir 1 ml=500 mcg.
  - Give half of the total loading dose immediately and quarter of total dose after 8 hours and 16 hours, check each dose carefully as overdose can cause arrhythmias.
- Side effects
  - Toxic cardiac side effects: PR interval prolongation, sinus bradycardia, ventricular arrhythmias, ectopic beats.
  - Nontoxic cardiac side effects: Heart slowing, QTc shortening, ST segment sagging.
  - Other side effects: Vomiting, feeding intolerance, diarrhea, lethargy.

Lignocaine (Type 1 b Anti-arrhythmic Agent)

- Indication
  - Short-term control of ventricular arrhythmias/ventricular tachycardia.
  - Premature ventricular contractions.
  - Arrhythmias resulting from digitalis intoxication.
- Dose
  - Initial bolus dose – 0.5 to 1 mg/kg IV push over 5 min repeat Q10 min.
  - Max total bolus should not exceed 5 mg/kg.
  - Maintenance IV infusion of 10-50 mcg /kg/min.
- Route
  - Intravenous.
- Supply and administration
  - Multiple concentrations ranging from 1% to 20%. To make a dilution for bolus dosing dilute 10 mg lidocaine (0.5 ml of 2% solution) in 9.5 ml NS.
- Side effects
  - CNS toxicity: Early signs of drowsiness, agitation, vomiting and muscle twitching. Late signs include seizures, loss of consciousness, respiratory depression and apnea.
  - Cardiac toxicity with excessive doses: Bradycardia, hypotension, heart block, cardiovascular collapse.

Captopril (Angiotensin Converting Enzyme Inhibitor)

- Indication
  - After load reduction in congestive cardiac failure.

  - Hypertension.
- Dose
  - 0.01-0.05 mg/kg per dose Q 8 to12th hours.
- Route
  - Oral.
- Supply and administration
  - 25 mg tablets.
  - Dissolve in 25 ml of water to 1mg/ml solution. Stable for 24 hours.
  - Further dilution may be done with sodium ascorbate to decrease oxidation.
- Side effects
  - Decrease in cerebral and renal blood flow in premature infants with chronic hypertension at higher doses.
  - Acute renal failure in bilateral renal vascular disease, renal artery stenosis in a solitary kidney.
  - Hyperkalemia.
  - Chronic therapy causes seizures, apnea, lethargy, oliguria.

Enalapril Maleate (Potent ACE Inhibitor)

- Indication
  - Moderate to severe hypertension.
  - After load reduction in congestive cardiac failure.
- Dose
  - Intravenous: 0.01 mg/kg/dose over 5 minutes.
  - Oral: 40 mcg/kg/dose Q 24 hours. Maximum dose 150 mcg/kg/dose Q 6 hours.
- Route
  - Oral.
- Supply and administration
  - 2.5 mg, 5 mg, 10 mg, 20 mg tablets.
  - Oral suspension is prepared by dissolving 2.5 mg tablet in 25 ml of isotonic citrate buffer to get 0.1 mg/ml concentration. Solution is stable for 30 days on refrigeration.
- Side effects
  - Hypotension, oliguria, rise in serum creatinine, hyperkalemia, cough.

Hydralazine (Direct Relaxant of Arteriolar Smooth Muscle)

- Indication
  - Mild to moderate hypertension.
  - Afterload reduction in congestive cardiac failure.
- Dose
  - Intravenous: 0.1-0.5 mg/kg/dose Q 6-8 hours. Maximum 2 mg/kg/dose Q6 hours.

- Oral: 0.25 mg to 1mg /kg per dose Q 6 -8 hours.

- Route
  - Oral.
  - Intravenous.
- Supply and administration
  - 20 mg/ml in 1 ml vial. Dilute 0.5 ml of intravenous injection with 9.5 ml of NS to obtain 1mg /ml dilution. Solution stable for 24 hours.
  - Tablet of 10 mg, 25 mg, 50 mg and 100 mg.
  - Crush 50 mg tablet in 4 ml of 5% mannitol. Add 46 ml of sterile water to make final concentration of 1 mg/ml. Solution is stable for 7 days on refrigeration.
- Side effects
  - Diarrhea, vomiting, tachycardia, hypotension, headache, drug fever, rash, bone marrow suppression, temporary agranulocytosis.

CENTRAL NERVOUS SYSTEM DRUGS

Acetaminophen (Anti-pyretic, Analgesic)

- Indication Fever and Pain.
- Dose
  - 15 mg/kg/dose.
  - Term Q 6 hours.
  - Preterm Q 8 hours if gestation > 32 weeks and Q 12 hours if gestation ≤32 weeks.
- Route
  - Oral.
  - Rectal.
- Supply and administration
  - Drops 100 mg/ml.
  - Syrup 125/5 ml, 250/5 ml.
  - Suppositories: 80 mg, 120 mg, 325 mg.
- Side effects
  - Liver toxicity with excessive doses.
  - Rash, fever, thrombocytopenia, leukopenia, neutropenia.

Chloral Hydrate (Oral Sedative)

- Indication
  - Sedative/hypnotic for short term use only.
  - No analgesic properties, may cause excitement in some with pain.
- Dose
  - 25 to 75 mg/kg/dose.

- Supply and administration
  - 50 mg/ml and 100 mg/ml.
  - Dilute and give after feeds.
- Side effects
  - Gastric irritation, bradycardia.
  - CNS, respiratory, myocardial depression on prolonged usage.

Morphine (Opioid Analgesic)

- Indication
  - Analgesia and sedation.
  - Narcotic withdrawal and abstinence syndrome.
- Dose
  - Bolus 0.05-0.2 mg/kg over 5 minutes Q 4 hours.
  - Infusion 10-20 mcg/kg/hour after a loading dose of 100 mcg/kg.
- Route
  - Intravenous.
  - Intramuscular.
  - Subcutaneous.
- Supply and administration
  - 0.5 mg/ml to 50 mg/ml vials.
  - Dilute with D5W, NS or sterile water.
- Side effects
  - Respiratory depression (Naloxone is an antidote).
  - Hypotension and bradycardia.
  - Urinary retention, delayed gastric emptying, ileus.
  - Tolerance on prolonged usage.

Midazolam (Short-acting Benzodiazepine)

- Indication Neonatal seizures, Sedation, Hypnotic, Anesthesia.
- Dose
  - Bolus 0.05-0.15 mg/kg over 5 minutes.
  - Infusion 0.01-0.06 mg/kg/hour.
- Route
  - Intravenous.
  - Intramuscular.
  - Intranasal and sublingual.
- Supply and administration
  - 5 mg/ml, 1 mg/ml in 1 ml, 2 ml, 5 ml and 10 ml vials.
  - Dilute with D5W, NS or sterile water.

- Side effects
  - Respiratory depression.
  - Hypotension.
  - Seizure like myoclonus in premature infants on infusion.

Fentanyl (Synthetic Opioid Analgesic)

- Indication Analgesia, Sedation and Anesthesia.
- Dose
  - Sedation and analgesia (Bolus: 1-4 mcg/kg slow IV push, 1-5 mcg/kg/hour by infusion).
  - Anesthesia (5-50 mcg/kg/dose).
- Route
  - Intravenous
- Supply and administration
  - 50 mcg/ml in 2 ml, 5 ml and 10 ml vials.
  - Dilute with D5W, NS or sterile water.
- Side effects
  - Respiratory depression.
  - Chest wall rigidity, sometimes with laryngospasm (antidote is Naloxone).
  - Withdrawal symptoms, if used for 5 or more days.

Pancuronium (Skeletal Muscle Relaxant)

- Indication
  - Skeletal muscle relaxation or paralysis in infants fighting mechanical ventilation and to improve oxygenation / ventilation / reduce barotrauma and fluctuations in cerebral blood flow.
- Dose
  - 0.1 mg /kg (0.04- 0.15 mg /kg). Intravenous push with dosing intervals of 1-2 hours.
- Route
  - Intravenous.
- Supply and administration
  - 2 ml ampoules with concentration of 2 mg/ml.
  - Dilute 0.5 ml from the ampoule with 0.5 ml of NS in 1 ml syringe to obtain preparation containing 0.1mg in 0.1ml.
- Side effects
  - Hypoxemia, tachycardia, hypotension and hypertension, increased salivation, bronchospasm.

Vecuronium (Shortacting Skeletal Muscle Relaxant)

- Indication Skeletal muscle relaxation or paralysis in infants requiring mechanical ventilation to improve oxygenation/ventilation/reduce barotrauma and fluctuations in cerebral blood flow.

- Dose
  - Bolus: 0.1 mg/kg (0.03-0.15 mg/kg) every 1-2 hourly.
- Route
  - Intravenous.
- Supply and administration
  - 10 mg vials.
  - Dissolve the powder in 5 ml of sterile water to give solution of 2 mg / ml.
  - Further dilute 1 ml of this solution with 1ml of NS or D5W to obtain 100 mcg (0.1 mg) in 0.1 ml for neonatal administration.
  - After reconstitution, can be stored for 24 hours.
- Side effects
  - Hypoxemia, hypotension, delayed ventilation.
  - Cardiac side effects are minimal.

Methadone (Longacting Synthetic Opioid Analgesic)

- Indication
  - Opioid withdrawal symptoms/signs.
- Dose
  - 0.05-0.2 mg/kg/dose once or twice daily.
- Route
  - Oral or Intramuscular.
- Supply and administration
  - Oral mixture contains 1 mg /ml of methadone.
  - I/M preparation contains 10 mg/ml.
- Side effects
  - Respiratory depression, ileus, delayed gastric emptying.

Nalaxone (Potent Opioid Antagonist)

- Indication
  - Narcotic antagonist, reversal of narcotic induced respiratory depression.
- Dose
  - Bolus dose 0.1 mg /kg (max 2 mg/dose) repeat every 2-3 minutes until desirable response achieved, max dose 10 mg.
- Route
  - Intravenous.
- Supply and administration
  - 1 ml contains 400 mcg (0.4 mg). Also available in 1 mg/ml.

- Do not mix in an alkaline solution.

- Side effects
  - Vomiting, sweating, tachycardia , tremulousness, seizures.

ANTICONVULSANT DRUGS

Phenobarbital (Increases Inhibitory Neurotransmission)

- Indication
  - Control of seizures.
  - Cholestasis. Before Tc^{99} IDA scan.
  - Criggler Najjar Type II.
- Dose
  - Loading 20 mg/kg intravenous infusion over 15 minutes. Additional doses of 10 mg/kg upto a maximum of 40 mg/kg.
  - Maintenance dose of 3 to 4 mg/kg Q 24 hours.
- Route
  - Intravenous infusion.
  - Oral.
- Supply and administration
  - 30 mg/ml and 60 mg/ml injections.
  - Oral elixirs of 20 mg/5 ml.
- Side effects
  - Sedation, respiratory depression at high doses, irritant to veins.

Phenytoin

- Indication
  - Control of seizures.
- Dose
  - Loading 20 mg/kg intravenous infusion over 30 minutes. Additional dose of 10 mg/kg upto a maximum of 30 mg/kg.
  - Maintenance dose of 4 to 8 mg/kg Q 24 hours.
- Route
  - Intravenous infusion (maximum rate of infusion is 0.5 mg/kg/minute).
  - Oral (absorption is erratic).
- Supply and administration
  - 50 mg/ml injections.
  - Oral suspensions 30 mg/5 ml.
- Side effects
  - Phlebitis, seizures at high doses, hypersensitivity.

- Long-term therapy causes cardiac arrhythmias, hypotension, gingivitis, nystagmus, rickets, hyperglycemia and hypoinsulinemia.

Lorazepam (Benzodiazepine Anticonvulsant)

- Indication
  - Control of seizures refractory to conventional treatment.
- Dose
  - 0.05 to 0.1 mg/dose slow IV push.
- Route
  - Slow intravenous push.
- Supply and administration
  - 2 mg/ml and 4 mg/ml vials.
  - Dilute with sterile water to obtain a concentration of 0.4 mg/ml.
- Side effects
  - Respiratory depression.
  - Rhythmic myoclonic jerks in premature infants.

Fosphenytoin (Pro-drug of Phenytoin)

- Indication
  - Control of seizures.
- Dose
  - Loading 15-20 mg/kg intravenous infusion over 10 minutes.
  - Maintenance dose of 4 to 8 mg/kg Q 24 hours. Dosing interval of Q 8 hours after 7 days in term infants.
- Route
  - Intravenous infusion (maximum rate of infusion is 1.5 mg/kg/minute).
  - Intramuscular.
- Supply and administration
  - 50 mg/ml injections in 2 ml and 10 ml vials.
- Side effects
  - Caution in neonates with jaundice. Risk of phenytoin overdosing.
  - Drowsiness.

Lidocaine (Newer Anticonvulsant)

- Indication
  - Control of refractory neonatal seizures.
- Dose
  - Loading 2 mg/kg intravenous infusion over 10 minutes followed immediately with maintenance infusion of 6 mg/kg/hour till 12 to 24 hours.

- Route
  - Intravenous infusion.
- Supply and administration
  - 1% to 20% injections.
  - Dilute with D5W or saline to obtain concentration of 1 mg/ml for intravenous bolus.
- Side effects
  - Arrhythmia and bradycardia.

DIURETICS

Furosemide (Diuretic at Ascending Loop of Henle)

- Indication
  - Diuretic for congestive cardiac failure, PDA, BPD and fluid overload.
- Dose
  - 1 mg/kg slow IV push. Maximum of 2 mg/kg/dose for IV and 6 mg/kg/dose for oral.
- Route
  - Intravenous bolus.
  - Oral.
- Supply and administration
  - 10 mg/ml injections.
  - Dilute with normal saline or sterile water for injection.
  - Do not use dextrose solutions.
- Side effects
  - Hyponatremia, hypokalemia, hypochloremic alkalosis.
  - Hyperacalciuria and ototoxicity on chronic use.

Hydrochlorthiazide (Diuretic Acting on Distal Nephron)

- Indication
  - Diuretic for congestive cardiac failure, PDA, BPD and fluid overload.
  - Mild and moderate hypertension.
  - Used in combination with spironolactone.
- Dose
  - 1 mg-2 mg/kg Q 12 hours.
- Route
  - Oral.
- Supply and administration
  - 50 mg/5 ml solution.
- Side effects
  - Hypokalemia, hyperglycemia and hyperuricemia.

Spironolactone (Mineralocorticoid Antagonist)

- Indication
  - Diuretic for congestive cardiac failure, PDA, BPD and fluid overload.
  - Used in combination with hydrochlorothiazide.
- Dose
  - 1 mg-3 mg/kg Q 24 hours.
- Route
  - Oral.
- Supply and administration
  - 25 mg, 50 mg and 100 mg tablets.
- Side effects
  - Rash, vomiting, diarrhea, paresthesias.
  - Gynaecomastia in male neonates.

GASTROINTESTINAL DRUGS

Ranitidine (Histamine, H2-receptor Antagonist)

- Indication
  - Symptomatic oesophagitis, gastritis, peptic ulceration.
  - Prevention and treatment of stress ulcers and GI hemorrhage aggravated by gastric acid secretion.
- Dose
  - Oral 2 mg/kg per dose Q 8 hourly.
  - Intravenous: Term babies–1.5 mg/kg per dose Q 8 hours slow push and Preterm-0.5 mg/kg per dose Q12 hours slow push.
  - Continuous intravenous infusion–0.0625 mg/kg per hour.
- Supply and administration
  - 2 ml and 6 ml vial with 25 mg /ml concentration.
  - Oral tablets 150 mg and 300 mg.
- Side effects
  - Rarely, thrombocytopenia.

Omeprazole (Proton Pump Inhibitor)

- Indication
  - Short term (less than 8 weeks) treatment of documented reflux esophagitis or duodenal ulcer refractory to conventional therapy.
- Dose 0.5 mg-1.5 mg/kg per dose oral once a day.
- Route
  - Oral.

- Supply and administration
  - Delayed release capsules with 10 mg , 20 mg , 40 mg omeprazole as enteric coated granules.
  - Prepare a 2 mg/ml concentration by mixing five 20 mg capsule granules with 50 ml sodium bicarbonate. Reconstituted solution stable for 30 days if refrigerated.
- Side effects
  - Hypergastrinemia and elevation in transaminases after prolonged use.

Domperidone (Dopamine D2 Receptor Antagonist)

- Indication
  - Nausea, vomiting, gastroesophageal reflux disease.
- Dose
  - 300 mcg/kg per dose Q 4 to 8 hours.
- Route
  - Oral.
- Supply and administration
  - 1 mg/ml sugar free suspension.
- Side effects
  - Very rarely extra pyramidal side effects, flatulence.

Metaclopramide (Derivative of Procainamide, Dopamine Receptor Antagonist and Peripheral Cholinergic Agent)

- Indication
  - Nausea, vomiting and gastroesophageal reflux disease.
- Dose
  - 30 mcg to 100 mcg/kg Q 6 to 8 hours orally.
- Route
  - Intravenous.
  - Oral.
  - Intramuscular.
- Supply
  - 10 mg tablets.
  - 1 mg/ml suspension.
  - 5 mg/ml in 2 ml ampoules.
- Side effects
  - Dystonic reactions and extra pyramidal symptoms at higher doses.

Erythromycin (Macrolide Antibiotic, Motilin Receptor Agonist)

- Indication

- Neonatal gut dysmotility.
- Conjunctivitis and pneumonia due to chlamydia.

- Dose
  - Gut Dysmotility: 10 mg/kg per dose Q 6 hours for 2 days followed by 4 mg/kg Q 6 hours for 5 days.
  - Infections: 12.5 mg/kg per dose Q 6 hours for 14 days.
- Route
  - Oral.
  - Intravenous.
- Supply and administration
  - 200 mg and 500 mg per 5 ml.
  - Mix with EBM or formula and administer to decrease GI upset.
  - 500 mg and 1g powder for injection vials. Dilute with sterile.
- Side effects
  - Diarrhea, abdominal discomfort, eosinophilia, arrhythmias, thrombophlebitis.

Ursodiol (Ursodeoxycholic Acid—A Choleretic Agent)

- Indication Cholestasis and to dissolve gallstones.
- Dose
  - 10 to 15 mg/kg/dose every 12 hourly.
- Route
  - Oral.
- Supply and administration
  - 150 and 300 mg tablets.
  - The powder from capsules to be mixed with glycerin, Ora Plus and Orange syrup and obtain a solution with a final concentration of 25 mg/ml. Mixture can be stored at room temperature for 60 days.
- Side effects
  - Nausea/vomiting, pain abdomen, constipation and flatulence.

HEMATOLOGICAL DRUGS

Erythropoietin (Synthetic Glycoprotein with Erythropoeitic Activity)

- Indication
  - Stimulate erythropoiesis and decrease RBC transfusions in high risk preterm infants.
- Dose
  - 200 to 400 units/kg/dose 3 to 5 times per week for 2 to 6 weeks.

- Route
  - Intravenous infusion over 4 hours.
  - Subcutaneous.
- Supply and administration
  - 1 ml vial with contents of either 2000, 3000, 4000 and 10,000 units.
  - Always administer iron therapy along with erythropoietin.
- Side effects
  - Neutropenia.

Enoxaparin (Low Molecular Weight Heparin)

- Indication
  - Anticoagulation. Preferred over heparin.
- Dose
  - Treatment of thrombosis: 1.5 mg/kg/dose Q 12 hours. Adjust dosage to maintain antifactor Xa levels between 0.5 to 1units/ml.
  - Preterm require higher doses 2 mg/kg/dose Q 12 hours.
  - Prophylaxis of thrombosis. 0.75 mg/kg/dose Q12 hours. Adjust dosage to maintain antifactor Xa levels between 0.1 to 0.4 units/ml.
- Route
  - Subcutaneous.
- Supply and administration
  - 100 mg/ml prefilled syringes or ampoules.
  - Administer subcutaneous.
- Side effects
  - Serious and minor bleeding.

Heparin (Anti-thrombin III Activator)

- Indication
  - Anticoagulation. Bilateral renal vein thrombosis or extension into IVC.
  - Patentcy of central venous lines.
- Dose
  - Central lines: 0.5 to 1 unit/ml of IV fluid.
  - Thrombosis: 75 units/kg bolus, 28 units/kg/hour. Adjust dose for a anti-factor Xa level of 0.3 to 0.7 (aPTT of 60 to 85 seconds).
- Route
  - Intravenous infusion or bolus.
- Supply and administration
  - 10 units/ml, 1000 units/ml and 10,000 units/ml.
  - For central lines, mix 36 ml of NS with 4 ml of 10 units/ml heparin and run at 0.5 to 1 ml/hour.

- Side effects
  - Thrombocytopenia.
- Osteoporosis on long-term use
  - Acute bleeding on overdose. Antidote is protamine sulphate 1mg for 100 units of heparin given in last 4 hours.

Alteplase (Tissue Plasminogen Activator t-PA)

- Indication
  - Dissolution of intravascular thrombi of acute onset (arterial or life threatening).
  - Adjuvant for infective endocarditis.
- Dose
  - 200 mcg/kg/hour for 6 to 48 hours. Discontinue heparin hours before t-PA.
- Route
  - Intravenous infusion.
- Supply and administration
  - Lyophilized powder in 2 mg (2000 mcg) vials.
  - Reconstitute with sterile water/NS.
- Side effects
  - Intracranial hemorrhage. Bleeding from venipuncture sites.

Immunoglobulin (Immunoprotective)

- Indication Rh isoimmunisation, Alloimmune thrombocytopenia.
- Dose
  - 500 to 750 mg/kg/dose. Infuse over 2 to 6 hours.
- Route
  - Intravenous.
- Supply and administration
  - Available as 1, 2.5, 5 and 10 g vials. Reconstitute with supplied diluents.
  - Also available as 10, 50, 100 and 200 ml vials (50 mg/ml).
  - Compatible with D5W, Dextrose/Amino acids.
- Side effects
  - Hypoglycemia, tachycardia and hypotension (stop the infusion).

RESPIRATORY SYSTEM DRUGS

Aminophylline (Respiratory Stimulant)

- Indication Apneas, post-extubation and post anesthesia, bronchodilator
- Dose

- Loading 8 mg/kg over 30 minutes.
- Maintenance 1.5 to 3 mg/kg per dose 8 hourly or 12 hourly.
- Therapeutic concentration 7 to 12 mcg/ml for apnea management.

- Route
  - Intravenous or Oral (increase the dose by 20% when changing to oral).
- Supply and administration
  - 25 mg/ml in 10 or 20 ml vials.
  - Dilute 1 ml with 4 ml of D5W or NS.
  - Stable for 4 days when refrigerated.
- Side effects
  - Tachycardia, vomiting, jitteriness, hyperreflexia, lower seizure threshold and hyperglycemia.
  - Antidote for toxicity is activated charcoal 1 g/kg 2 hourly or 4 hourly.

Caffeine Citrate (Respiratory Stimulant)

- Indication Apneas, post extubation and post anesthesia.
- Dose
  - Loading 20 to 40 mg/kg of caffeine citrate over 30 minutes.
  - Maintenance 5 to 8 mg/kg/dose once every 24 hours.
- Route
  - Intravenous or Oral.
- Supply and administration
  - 20 mg/ml in 3 ml vial (20 mg of caffeine citrate is equivalent to 10 mg of caffeine base).
- Side effects
  - Restlessness, vomiting, decreased cerebral and intestinal blood flow.

Surfactant (Surface Tension Reducing Agent)

- Indication
  - Rescue treatment of infants with moderate to severe RDS.
  - Prophylaxis of infants at high risk of RDS (<29 weeks gestation).
  - Severe MAS.
- Dose
  - 100 to 200 mg/kg/dose of phospholipids.
  - Survanta 4 ml/kg/dose in four aliquots.
  - Curosurf 2.5 ml/kg/dose for initial doses and 1.25 ml/kg for later doses.
  - Infasurf 3 ml/kg/dose.
  - Exosurf 5 ml/kg/dose.
- Route
  - Intratracheal.

- Supply and administration
  - Survanta 4 ml and 8 ml vials. Curosurf 1.5 ml and 3 ml vials. Infasurf 3 ml and 6 ml vials. Exosurf to be reconstituted with supplied diluent.
  - Allow the vial to reach room temperature by gently swirling. Do not use artificial warming. Do not shake.
  - Administer in aliquots of 1 to 2 ml. Do not allow desaturations during administration.
  - No need to shift position for administration of aliquots.
- Side effects
  - Transient desaturations, bradycardia, leakage/reflux of surfactant.
  - Pulmonary hemorrhage may occur in 2 to 4% of treated infants, primarily in extreme premature with untreated PDA.

VITAMINS AND MINERALS

Pyridoxine (Vitamin B_6)

- Indication
  - Diagnosis and treatment of pyridoxine dependent seizures. Pyridoxine dependent seizures are due to defective binding of pyridoxine in the formation of GABA. Administration of pharmacological doses of pyridoxine will correct this GABA deficiency.
- Dose
  - Initial diagnostic dose 50-100 mg Intravenous push or Intramuscular.
  - Maintenance dose 50-100 mg PO Q 24 hours.
- Route
  - Intravenous.
  - Intramuscular.
  - Oral.
- Supply and administration
  - 100 mg/ml in 1ml vials.
  - Injectable form can be used orally, mix in simple syrup if desired.
- Side effects
  - Risk of profound sedation and ventilatory support may be necessary.

Hydroxocobalamin (Vitamin B_{12})

- Indication
  - Breast fed babies of vitamin B_{12} deficient vegetarian mothers, and in deficient older children due to malabsorbtion.
  - Transcobalamin 2 deficiency.
- Dose
  - Dietary deficiency: Single intramuscular injection between 250 mcg and

1 mg and ensure later that the diet is adequate (1 mcg/kg per day is sufficient).
  - Absorptive defect: 1mg intramuscular at monthly intervals.
  - In transcobalamin 2 deficiency: 1mg intramuscular three times a week is given during first year of life later reducing to 1mg once a week with haematological monitoring.
  - Metabolic disease: Initial maintenance dose is 1mg daily irrespective of the weight, also it can be reduced to 1-3 injections a week.
- Route
  - Intramuscular.
- Supply and administration
  - 1 ml ampoules with 1 mg hydroxocobalamin.

Vitamin E (Alpha Tocopherol, the Most Active Antioxidant)

- Indication
  - To prevent hemolytic anemia in vitamin E deficient babies.
  - Malabsorbtion due to cholestasis.
  - Abetalipoproteinaemia.
- Dose
  - Neonatal prophylaxis: Single 20 mg/kg intramuscular injection to babies less than 1 kg or 1.5 kg at birth.
  - Nutritional deficiency: 10 mg/kg by mouth once a day.
  - Malabsorbtion: 50 mg supplement once a day by mouth.
  - Biliary artesia: 10 mg/kg twice a month intramuscular.
  - Abetalipoproteinaemia: 100 mg/kg once a day by mouth.
- Route
  - Intramuscular.
  - Oral.
- Supply and administration
  - 2 ml vials containing 50 mg/ml.
  - Oral suspension containing 100 mg/ml.
- Side effects
  - Feeding intolerance, due to hyperosmolarity of the preparation.
  - Pharmacological doses associated with increased rates of sepsis and NEC (osmolarity of oral formulation).

Vitamin D

- Indications and doses
  - Irrespective of weight all babies need 5 mcg (200 units) once a month.
  - Maternal prophylaxis: 5 mg Intramuscular in the third trimester to women likely to have limited stores.

  - In malabsorbtion (complete Biliary obstruction): 750 mcg once a month.
  - Renal disease; 20 nanogms of oral or intravenous once a day.
- Route
  - Oral.
  - Intramuscular.
  - Intravenous.
- Supply and administration
  - Ergocalciferol (D2): 1ml ampoules for intramuscular use.
  - 10 mcg tablets containing redundant calcium.
  - 3000 unit /ml oral liquid.
  - Alfacalcidol-10 ml bottles of sugar free oral liquid (100 nanogms/drop).
  - 1 mcg 0.5 ml ampoules for intravenous use.

Folic Acid /Folinic Acid

- Indication
  - Prevent megaloblastic anemia.
  - Supplementation prior to conception can decrease the risk of the fetus developing various defects such as anencephaly or spina bifida.
  - Refractory neonatal seizures.
- Dose
  - Megaloblastic anemia in infancy (not due to B_{12}) 1mg folic acid.
  - Preterm babies fed heat treated human milk may benefit from 500 mcg supplement once a week if suitable milk fortifier is not used.
- Route
  - Oral.
- Supply and administration
  - A sugar free oral suspension containing 500 mcg/ml.

Ferrous Sulphate

- Indication
  - Iron supplementation for prevention and treatment of anemia.
- Dose
  - 2 mg/kg per day of elemental iron for growing premature infants (max 15 mg /day). Begin therapy after 2 weeks of age.
  - ELBW infants may need 4 mg/kg per day.
  - 6 mg/kg per day of elemental iron for patients receiving erythropoietin. Administer oral in 1 or 2 divided doses.
- Route
  - Oral.

- Supply and administration
  - Drops: 25 mg in 1ml.
  - Elixir: 44 mg elemental iron per 5 ml.
- Side effects
  - In growing premature infants iron supplementation should not be started until adequate vitamin E is supplied in the diet, otherwise iron may increase hemolysis, nausea, constipation, black stools, lethargy, hypotension and erosion of gastric mucosa.

Zinc

- Indication
  - Acrodermatitis enteropathica (perioral, and perianal dermatitis pustular lesions on the hands and feet, alopecia, irritability).
  - Diarrhea.
  - Preterm infants.
- Dose
  - 1 mg/kg of zinc per day will rapidly cure any symptoms due to simple dietary deficiency.
  - A regular daily 5 mg/kg oral supplement for acrodermatitis enteropathica.
- Route
  - Oral.
- Supply and administration
  - 125 mg effervescent tablets of zinc sulphate monohydrate with 45 mg of zinc.
  - One tablet is dissolved in 4.5 ml of water to give a 10 mg/ml solution.
- Side effects
  - No serious or reported side effects.

Vitamin K1 (Phytonadione)

- Indication
  - Prophylaxis and therapy of hemorrhagic disease of newborn.
  - Treatment of hypoprothrombinemia secondary to factors limiting absorbtion or synthesis of vitamin K (cholestasis, liver disease, malabsorption etc.).
- Dose
  - Prophylaxis: 0.5 to 1 mg Intramuscular at birth.
  - Preterm infants: <32 weeks gestation and BW>1000 gms: 0.5 mg intramuscular: BW <1000 gms: 0.3 mg/kg.
  - Oral dose: Healthy term, exclusively breast fed infants: 2mg with first feed, 1 week, 4 weeks and 8 weeks of age.
  - Severe hemorrhagic disease: 1 to 10 mg slow intravenous push.

- Route
  - Intramuscular.
  - Intravenous.
  - Oral.
- Supply and administration
  - 2 mg/ml aqueous dispersion in 0.5 ml ampoules and 10 mg/ml acqueous dispersion in 1 ml ampoules and 2 ml, 5 ml vials.
- Side effects
  - Pain and swelling.
  - Rarely shock and cardiac and respiratory arrest reported in adults.

Calcium Gluconate

- Indication
  - Hypocalcaemia.
  - Hyperkalemia to protect the heart from arrhythmias.
- Dose
  - Acute treatment: 100-200 mg/kg per dose or 1-2 ml/kg per dose intravenous infusion slowly under cardiac monitoring.
  - Maintenance treatment: 200-800 mg/kg per day or 2-8 ml/kg per day by infusion for 3 to 5 days. Same dose can be given orally.
- Route
  - Intravenous.
  - Oral.
- Supply
  - 10% calcium gluconate injections with 9.3 mg/ml elemental calcium.
  - 10% calcium chloride for intravenous injections.
  - Oral calcium in combination with gluconate, chloride or phosphates.

Phosphate

- Indication
  - Supplemental phosphate (as oral sodium phosphate) to prevent neonatal rickets in very low birth weight babies.
- Route
  - Oral.
  - Intravenous.
- Dose
  - Oral administration: VLBW infants developing a plasma phosphate level < 1.5 mmol/l in the first few weeks of life should be offered 250 micro mol of extra phosphate twice a day by mouth.
- Supply
  - 10 ml ampoules containing 2.16 g of anhydrous sodium glycerophosphate suitable for continuous intravenous infusion.

Arginine (Essential Nutritional Supplements for Neonates with Urea Cycle Disorder)

- Indication
  - Inborn error of metabolism affecting urea cycle such citrullinaemia (CL), arginosuccinic aciduria (AC), ornithine transcarbamoylase (OTC) and carbamoyl phosphate synthetase (CPS) deficiency.
- Dose
  - For OCT and CPS: 25-35 mg/kg Q 6 hours and 200 mg/kg/day intravenous in case of acute hyperammonemia.
  - CL and AC: 175 mg/kg Q 6 hours and 600 mg/kg of loading dose followed by 25 mg/kg/hour intravenous infusion in case of acute hyperammonemia.
- Route
  - Oral.
  - Intravenous.
- Supply and administration
  - 10 g/100 ml vial for intravenous infusion.
  - *Sugar free medicine in 20 ml bottles, add 185 ml of purified water to the contents of the bottle to obtain 200 ml of 100 mg/ml liquid. Solution is stable for 2 months.*
- Side effects
  - Vomiting, hypotension, hyperchloremia.

MISCELLANEOUS DRUGS

Insulin (Hypoglycemic Agent)

- Indication Hyperglycemia with BS >250 mg/dl or for hyperkalemia.
- Dose
  - Infusion 0.01 to 0.1 unit/kg per hour. For hyperkalemia add 1U of Insulin for every 5 grams of glucose infused.
  - Intermittent 0.1 to 0.2 unit/kg every 6 or 12 hourly.
- Route
  - Intravenous (recommended).
  - Subcutaneous.
- Supply and administration
  - 100 Unit/ml in 10 ml vials.
  - Dilute with sterile water. First dilute 1 ml of insulin with 9 ml of sterile water to get 10 U/ml of insulin. Dilute further in 2 more steps to get 0.1 U/ml.
  - Always use insulin syringe for administration.
  - Extreme care is required during dilution.

- Side effects
  - Hypoglycemia.
  - Insulin resistance on prolonged usage.

Levothyroxine (T4)

- Indication Hypothyroidism.
- Dose
  - Initial oral dose 10 to 14 mcg/kg once a day.
  - Initial IV dose 5 to 8 mcg/kg.
- Route
  - Oral.
  - Intravenous.
- Supply and administration
  - 25 mg, 50 mg or 100 mg tablets.
  - Crush the tablet and dissolve in 2 ml of sterile water/breast milk/ non soya formula.
  - Use the same brand and try to avoid switching brands.
  - Monitor at 2 weeks, bimonthly T4/ TSH after starting therapy. Keep T4 between 10-16 mcg/dl and TSH <15 mU/L.
- Side effects
  - Thyrotoxicosis: Hyperactivity, tachycardia, perspiration, fever, exophthalmos and goiter.
  - Prolonged over treatment causes craniosynostosis and accelerated bone age.

Cyclopentolate (Mydriatic)

- Indication
  - Mydriasis and cycloplegia for ophthalmic procedures such as ROP screening and laser therapy.
- Dose
  - 1 or 2 drops in the eye 15 to 30 minutes before the procedure.
- Supply and administration
  - 0.5%, 1% and 2% in 2 ml to 15 ml bottles.
  - Use 0.5% or less for neonates.
  - Use in combination with 1 drop of 2.5% phenylephrine.
  - Apply pressure on lachrymal sac for 2 minutes after application to reduce systemic side effects.
- Side effects
  - Fever, tachycardia, vasodilatation, dry mouth, restlessness, delay in gastric emptying, urinary retention.

Phenylephrine (Mydriatic)

- Indication
  - Mydriasis and cycloplegia for ophthalmic procedures such as ROP screening and laser therapy.
- Dose
  - 1 drop in the eye 10 minutes before the procedure.
- Supply and administration
  - 0.12%, 2.5% and 10% in 2 ml to 15 ml bottles.
  - Use 2.5 % for neonates.
  - Use in combination with 1 drop of 0.5% cyclopentolate and 0.5% tropicamide.
  - Apply pressure on lachrymal sac for 2 minutes after application to reduce systemic side effects.
- Side effects
  - Decreased pulmonary compliance.
  - Do not use in neonates on propranolol (β blockers).
  - Hypertension or tachycardia.

Tropicamide (Mydriatic)

- Indication
  - Mydriasis and cycloplegia for ophthalmic procedures such as ROP screening and laser therapy.
- Dose
  - 1 drop in the eye 10 minutes before the procedure.
- Supply and administration
  - 0.5% and 1% in 2 ml to 15 ml bottles.
  - Use 0.5% for neonates.
  - Use in combination with 1 drop of 0.5% cyclopentolate and 2.5% phenylephrine.
  - Apply pressure on lachrymal sac for 2 minutes after application to reduce systemic side effects.
- Side effects
  - Fever, tachycardia, vasodilatation, dry mouth, restlessness, delay in gastric emptying, urinary retention.

Hyaluronidase (Mucolytic Enzyme)

- Indication
  - IV extravasations of medications such as calcium, aminophylline, cloxacillin, phenytoin, KCl, $NaHCO_3$, Vancomycin, TPN etc.
  - Do not use for extravasation of vasoconstrictors.

- Dose
  - 1 ml (150 units) for extravasation.
- Route
  - Subcutaneous.
- Supply and administration
  - 150 units/ml in 2 ml vials.
  - Inject subcutaneous 1 ml (150 units) as 5 separate 0.2 ml injections around the periphery of extravasations.
- Side effects
  - Nil if injected subcutaneous.

EMLA (Eutectic Mixture of Local Anesthetics)

- Indication
  - Topical analgesia for venipuncture, circumcision but not for heel prick.
- Dose
  - Apply 1 to 2 gm to distal half of penis for circumcision or over the venipuncture site 30 minutes to 60 minutes before procedure.
- Route
  - Topical application.
- Supply and administration
  - 5 gm and 30 gm tubes.
- Side effects
  - Blanching, redness, methemoglobinemia.

INDEX

D

E

I

J

K

L

Index

Index

U

V

W

X